Digital Resources for Learning

New!
Global Health Watch

CENGAGE LEARNING'S
GLOBAL HEALTH WATCH
— GLOBAL HEALTH RESOURCE CENTER —

One-stop access to the most current information about health from Cengage Learning!

Easy to use and endlessly resourceful, *Global Health Watch* provides thousands of trusted health sources, is updated daily, and is searchable by topic or key word, making it easy for you to find the most current news related to health.

This dynamic resource provides:

▶ Convenient access to thousands of trusted sources, including academic journals, newspapers, magazines, videos, podcasts, and more.

▶ New articles and resources—updated daily—to help students remain current in this ever-changing field.

▶ A powerful search engine to quickly locate the most current information on hot topics.

▶ One-stop access to the most current information about health.

View a demo of *Global Health Watch*!

www.cengage.com/rc/globalhealthwatch/demo

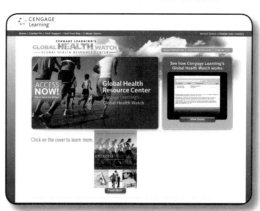

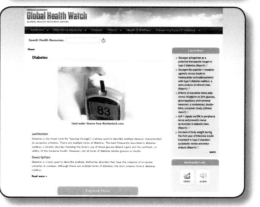

Health CourseMate

Set your sights on success in health with this interactive online learning tool

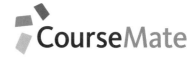

Cengage Learning's **Health CourseMate** brings course concepts to life with interactive learning, study, and exam preparation tools that support this text. With **Health CourseMate** as one of your tools, you can better prepare for class, review for tests, and study at your own pace.

CourseMate gives you access to:

Flashcards • Animations • Quizzes • Interactive eBook • Glossary • Crossword puzzles • and much more!

For more information about these products go to

www.cengage.com/health

Exercise Physiology

An Integrated Approach

Peter B. Raven, Ph.D., F.A.C.S.M.
Professor of Integrative Physiology
University of North Texas Health Science Center
Fort Worth, Texas

David H. Wasserman, Ph.D., F.A.C.S.M
Professor of Molecular Physiology and Biophysics
Annie Mary Lyle Chair of Biomedical Sciences
Director, Mouse Metabolic Phenotyping Center
Vanderbilt University Medical Center
Nashville, Tennessee

William G. Squires, Jr., Ph.D., F.A.C.S.M.
Professor of Biology and Kinesiology
Dr. Frederick C. Elliot Chair in Health, Fitness and Nutrition
Texas Lutheran University
Seguin, Texas

Tinker D. Murray, Ph.D., F.A.C.S.M.
Professor of Health and Human Performance
Texas State University
San Marcos, Texas

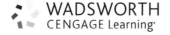
WADSWORTH
CENGAGE Learning

Australia • Brazil • Canada • Mexico • Singapore • Spain • United Kingdom • United States

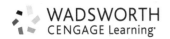

WADSWORTH
CENGAGE Learning

Exercise Physiology: An Integrated Approach
Peter B. Raven, David H. Wasserman, William G. Squires, Jr.,
Tinker D. Murray

Sr. Acquisitions Editor: Aileen Berg

Developmental Editor: Samantha Arvin

Assistant Editor: Shannon Elderon

Media Editor: Katie Walton

Marketing Manager: Tom Ziolkowski

Marketing Assistant: Jing Hu

Marketing Communications Manager: Darlene Macanan

Sr. Content Project Manager: Tanya Nigh

Design Director: Rob Hugel

Art Director: John Walker

Print Buyer: Becky Cross

Rights Acquisitions Specialist: Dean Dauphinais

Production Service: Megan Greiner, Graphic World Inc.

Text Designer: RHDG | Riezebos Holzbaur

Photo Researcher: Bill Smith Group

Text Researcher: Karyn Morrison

Copy Editor: Graphic World Inc.

Cover Designer: Riezebos Holzbaur/Brie Hattey

Cover Images: Top: Phase4Photography; Bottom Left: Aleksandr
Markin; Bottom Center: © Erik Isakson/Tetra Images/Corbis;
Bottom Right: Photographer: DIBYANGSHU SARKAR/Stringer;
Credit: AFP/Getty Images

Compositor: Graphic World Inc.

For product information and technology assistance, contact us at
Cengage Learning Customer & Sales Support, 1-800-354-9706
For permission to use material from this text or product, submit all
requests online at **www.cengage.com/permissions**
Further permissions questions can be e-mailed to
permissionrequest@cengage.com

Library of Congress Control Number: 2011934851

ISBN-13: 978-0-495-11024-8

ISBN-10: 0-495-11024-8

Wadsworth
20 Davis Drive
Belmont, CA 94002-3098
USA

Cengage Learning is a leading provider of customized learning solutions with
office locations around the globe, including Singapore, the United Kingdom,
Australia, Mexico, Brazil, and Japan. Locate your local office at
www.cengage.com/global

Cengage Learning products are represented in Canada by Nelson Education, Ltd.

To learn more about Wadsworth, visit **www.cengage.com/wadsworth**
Purchase any of our products at your local college store or at our preferred
online store **www.CengageBrain.com**

Printed in the United States of America
1 2 3 4 5 6 7 15 14 13 12 11

brief contents

Chapter

contents

preface

In the April 19, 2005, edition of *Circulation* (the primary journal of the American Heart Association), in the article "Obesity, risk factors, and predicting cardiovascular events," Michael Criqui, M.D., reported that a large body of scientific evidence associated with increases in obesity also "predicts large increases in insulin resistance/diabetes, hypertension, hypertriglyceridemia, and HDL cholesterol, as well as unfavorable changes in endothelial function and a host of inflammatory, thrombotic, and fibrinolytic factors." These factors (as well as others currently being studied) contribute to the two major causes of death: cardiovascular disease and cancer.

More recently, exercise physiology–related research has supported the importance of participating in regular physical activity and exercise to control the host of factors associated with the metabolic syndrome and to prevent the development of chronic diseases associated with sedentary behavior (Physical Activity Guidelines Advisory Committee, *Physical activity guidelines advisory committee report, 2008*. Washington, D.C.: U.S. Department of Health and Human Services). Examples from the exercise physiology literature now show that: (a) exercise genes help determine how active one is (Hagberg, J. M. 2010. Exercise genes? And no, not Levi's 501s! *J. Appl. Physiol.* 109:619–620; and Lightfoot, J. T., L. Leamy, D. Pomp, et al. 2010. Strain screen and haplotype association mapping of wheel running in inbred mouse strains. *J. Appl. Physiol.* 109:623–634); (b) exercise interventions can help reverse metabolic syndrome and control obesity (Touati, S., F. Meziri, S. Devaux, et al. 2011. Exercise reverses metabolic syndrome in high-fat diet-induced obese rats. *Med. Sci. Sports Exerc.* 43:398–407); and (c) lifestyle factors such as exercise are keys to the prevention and management of many chronic diseases (American College of Sports Medicine; American Diabetes Association. 2010. Exercise and type 2 diabetes: American College of Sports Medicine and the American Diabetes Association: Joint position statement. Exercise and type 2 diabetes. *Med. Sci. Sports Exerc.* 42:2282–2303; and Defronzo, R. A. 2009. Banting Lecture. From the triumvirate to the ominous octet: A new paradigm for the treatment of type 2 diabetes mellitus. *Diabetes* 58:773–795). This text is designed to teach students about the traditional and emerging concepts of exercise physiology so that they can, in turn, develop and deliver interventions to help curb the daunting global societal challenge that Criqui described.

This text focuses on the field of exercise physiology and the subfields that include the scientific basis for developing practical exercise training and physical activity for health, disease prevention/control, athletic performance, and clinical rehabilitation. Examples in this text promote the avoidance of physical inactivity, the achievement of long-term functional health, and strategies to optimize human performance.

The field of exercise physiology for entry-level professionals has expanded rapidly as career paths (categories) have changed, even as we write this preface. Currently, a diverse array of professional job opportunities exists for those trained in exercise physiology and the exercise sciences. For example, a graduate majoring in exercise science, kinesiology, nursing, pre-physical therapy, pre-athletic training, and/or pre-medicine (with only a one-course experience in exercise physiology) can now find opportunities for employment in a variety of fields, including personal training, athletic coaching, fire–police–military trainers, rehabilitation specialists, nursing, pre-medicine, pre-athletic training, pre-physical therapy, wellness instructors, athletic trainers, physical education teaching, physical activity specialist, among others. The philosophy of this text is to promote the translation of exercise physiology to help young professionals develop effective strategies to meet the metabolic and physiologic challenges and implications of physical inactivity and caloric imbalance that have developed worldwide since the late 1990s.

We also designed this text to help instructors develop strategies to help students answer relevant questions with regard to exercise physiology and biochemistry and to help correct the most **common misconceptions** (Morton, J. P., D. A. Doran, and D. P. Maclaren. 2008. Common student misconceptions in exercise physiology and biochemistry. *Adv. Physiol. Educ.* 32:142–146) such as:

1. Lactate is only produced when muscle contracts under anaerobic conditions.

2. Lactate causes fatigue.

3. Fat is used as an energy source only during exercise when carbohydrate sources run out.

4. To maximize fat loss during exercise, exercise intensity should be high.

5. The process of muscle contraction consists solely of peripheral processes.

6. When a muscle shortens in length during contraction, the A-band also shortens.

7. Maximal oxygen uptake ($\dot{V}O_2$ max) is the most important determinant of endurance performance.

8. Oxidation reactions involve only oxygen molecules.

9. Blood pressure is higher during prolonged exercise in hot conditions compared with normal conditions.

This text contains 14 chapters (plus 2 additional specific "call out" sections on the exercise biology of metabolic syndrome and diabetes). In addition, some laboratories (labs) have been identified to serve as a guide to undergraduates to help them integrate the concepts of biology, chemistry, biochemistry, exercise training, and kinesiology for future professional success. The book contents were designed so that the material could be taught completely in a typical one-semester course, lasting 16 weeks.

This text provides scientific evidence across a spectrum of disciplines from genetic and molecular biologic influences to the epidemiology of exercise and health. As you work through the various chapters and practical experiences in the book, you will be able to develop strategies to integrate the fundamental physiologic concepts pertinent to physical activity to help guide you through the problem-solving process and apply exercise interventions for your specific areas of interest (for example, health/fitness, clinical, rehabilitation). The emphasis throughout the book is on teaching you how to work with clients to avoid physical inactivity and understand how to improve human performance while preventing/controlling chronic disease and improving quality of life and longevity (Booth, F. W., M. V. Chakravarthy, S. E. Gordon, and E. E. Spangenburg. 2002. Waging war on physical inactivity: Using modern molecular ammunition against an ancient enemy. *J Appl. Physiol.* 93:3–30; and Baldwin, K. M., and F. Haddad. 2010. Research in the exercise sciences: Where we are and where do we go from here—Part II. *Exerc. Sport Sci. Rev.* 38:42–50).

Details about this First Edition

The contents of all chapters in this first edition of *Exercise Physiology: An Integrated Approach* have been developed and arranged according to the combination of specific and applied scientific principles related to exercise. This text begins by providing an overview of the public health challenges related to exercise and the basics of exercise training and then moves into the specifics of scientific principles that influence exercise interventions. Innovative features in this text include:

1. *Warm-Up*—pre-test questions to help you determine what you already know about topics in each chapter and your level of need for review

2. *Quick Start*—practical questions to help you think about how you can use information in the chapter with clients

3. *Hot Links*—several notations per chapter that refer you to other readily available sources for more information about topics discussed in the text

4. *Parenthetical Questions*—questions throughout each chapter that challenge you to read or reread pertinent portions of this text, enabling you to interpret this text and answer the question

5. *In Retrospect*—an example of classical exercise physiology experiments that were used to investigate the topics covered in each chapter

6. *In the Spotlight*—a biography of an expert in each chapter topic area that is covered

7. *Concepts, Challenges, & Controversies*—a feature that provides more in-depth information about exercise physiology topics that seem to be "ever changing"

8. *In Practice*—brief examples that provide perspectives related to health/fitness, medicine, athletic performance, and rehabilitation

9. *Chapter Summary*—a bulleted review of the chapter to help you study the information provided

10. *Exercise Physiology Reality*—interactive labs available through CengageNOW™ help reinforce concepts presented in each chapter

11. *Exercise Physiology Web Links*—numerous worldwide web links related to the material covered in each chapter

12. *Terms to Know*—key terms covered in each chapter, together with page references

13. *Study Questions*—10 general questions that represent all the material covered in each chapter

14. *Selected References*—select references provide additional information for further study

Chapter Highlights

- **Chapter 1** introduces you to the public health challenges of sedentary living and how the application of exercise physiology concepts can help your clients obtain functional health and optimize their performance goals. The concept of applying the scientific method in exercise physiology is covered, and examples of exercise dose–response actions for specific health and performance goals are provided. The *2008 Physical Activity Guidelines for Americans*, the *Physical Activity Guidelines Advisory Committee Report, 2008*, and *Healthy People 2020* are all included in this chapter.

- **Chapter 2** discusses the basics of exercise screening and exercise prescription. The components of exercise that contribute to specific dose–response relationships are introduced and described to give you practical perspectives that you can apply for designing exercise interventions with regard to physiologic challenges presented in later chapters. The spectrum of energy demands is introduced and reviewed as a prerequisite for understanding material in later chapters. Specific Hot Links provide you with a variety of web resources that make designing exercise programs more accessible. The *ACSM Guidelines for Exercise Testing and Prescription*, the U.S. National Physical Activity Plan, and the Toronto Charter for Physical Activity are all included in this chapter.

- **Chapter 3** discusses neuromuscular integration. The basics of bone, nerve, and muscle activity are reviewed initially; then the specifics of the physiology of muscular contraction during exercise are presented. Muscle fiber type, fiber recruitment, and muscle fiber adaptations to training are then discussed, together with specific training program responses (strength, power, and muscular endurance). Factors associated with muscular fatigue and muscular soreness are highlighted. The chapter Spotlight features Kenneth M. Baldwin, Ph.D. (2011 ACSM Honor Award recipient), an internationally recognized muscle physiologist who advises both the National Aeronautics and Space Administration and the National Institutes of Health.

- **Chapter 4** covers the basics of exercise metabolism. The chemical reactions and metabolic pathways by which the primary fuels used during exercise, glucose and fatty acids, are discussed. The chapter includes a section on turning chemical energy extracted from glucose and free fatty acids into adenosine triphosphate (ATP) and a featured topic about the formation of reactive oxygen species.

- **Chapter 5** covers fuel utilization and includes a discussion of substrate metabolism that focuses on three physiologic objectives: (a) maintaining glucose homeostasis, (b) metabolizing the most efficient substrate, and (c) sparing muscle glycogen. Included is a specific section that highlights the coordinated mobilization and utilization of the signals that control fuel metabolism.

- **Chapter 6** initially covers hormonal regulation of metabolism during exercise and describes how endocrine and neural metabolic regulators respond to exercise.

Subsequently, the chapter discusses the regulation of muscle glucose uptake and glycogen breakdown and the means by which lipids are mobilized from adipose tissues. The final sections of the chapter highlight the control of lipid metabolism by the liver and the regulation of fat uptake and metabolism by the working muscles.

- **Chapters 6A and 6B** are special "call out" sections that focus on the lifestyle intervention of exercise as an essential part of management plans for the prevention and control of metabolic syndrome (Chapter 6A) and diabetes (Chapter 6B). These chapters provide details about the metabolic factors associated with the metabolic syndrome and diabetes that are essential for helping clients achieve and maintain functional health. Chapter 6A explores the relationship between genes and environment with regard to the metabolic syndrome and exercise. The case is made for how behavioral and metabolic challenges shape gene action. Chapter 6B discusses how individuals with type 1 and type 2 diabetes respond to exercise; it also highlights the rationale for why individuals with diabetes should exercise and lead active lifestyles, together with taking precautions for participation in exercise programming.

- **Chapter 7** covers the cardiovascular system's response to exercise. The basics of the cardiovascular system are initially reviewed; then the specifics of cardiovascular functions during dynamic and resistance exercise are discussed. Descriptions of how cardiac output and oxygen consumption change to meet the metabolic demands of the skeletal muscles and the brain during exercise are provided. In addition, explanations of how the neural control of the circulation integrates the distribution of blood flow to the working muscles while maintaining regulation of arterial blood pressure during exercise are detailed.

- **Chapter 8** discusses the cardiovascular adaptations to endurance and resistance exercise training programs. The chapter includes material that explains how participation in regular dynamic exercise increases $\dot{V}O_2$ max via changes in cardiac output (remodeling of the heart) and to the peripheral vasculature. The chapter also includes a section about the cardiovascular adaptations to resistance training and the negative effects of deconditioning (bed rest and exposure to microgravity of spaceflight) on the cardiovascular system.

- **Chapter 9** discusses the response of the respiratory system to exercise. The basics of the respiratory system initially are reviewed; then the specifics of the mechanics of lung function ventilation, gas exchange, and transport to and from the lungs and tissues during endurance exercise are discussed. Specific note is made of the following:

(a) how the lungs function in acid–base regulation during exercise, (b) exercise-induced arterial hypoxemia, and (c) Hi-Lo altitude training.

- **Chapter 10** provides the underlying physiology of many protocols used in measuring common anaerobic and aerobic capacities. The current concepts about how to choose and interpret the specific exercise tests of anaerobic and cardiorespiratory functions are highlighted with numerous in-text examples of specific tests with links that provide web resources and options for test selection.

- **Chapter 11** covers the basics of nutrition and exercise. The concepts of basal metabolic rate are explained together with the importance of understanding caloric balance and how it can be markedly influenced by high-intensity, prolonged exercise. Specific strategies are discussed about how to coordinate and implement a basic nutrition plan for the beginning exerciser, as well as those interested in optimizing exercise performance.

- **Chapter 12** discusses selected strategies with regard to basic physiologic concepts that can enhance exercise performance. The importance of maintaining carbohydrate stores and methods to optimize recovery from high-intensity exercise are discussed. A section on the "female athletic triad" syndrome is included, and legal and illegal means of performance enhancement are discussed to conclude the chapter.

- **Chapter 13** introduces the basics of body composition and weight control management. Laboratory and field methods to determine and interpret body composition are discussed. This chapter builds on the metabolic issues discussed in Chapters 4, 5, 6, 6A, and 6B by teaching you about the physiologic, environmental, and behavioral factors that influence weight control and how to apply effective strategies that you can use with clients for weight management and good health, as well as for achieving peak performance.

- **Chapter 14** is the final chapter in this text, and it focuses on exercise adaptations related to the environmental extremes of heat, cold, altitude, and air pollution. Explanations of how each environmental challenge can affect physiologic performance are provided, and discussions about how specific physiologic adaptations to environmental challenges occur and/or are limited are included.

Authors' Notes

It is usual for the appendix to contain a number of conversion tables; for example:

1. Yards to meters for distances
2. Feet to meters for altitude
3. Fahrenheit to Centigrade (or Celsius) for temperature
4. International units of pressure

In addition, it is usual to include specific descriptions of exercise test protocols common to the exercise laboratory and field testing; however, because these conversion tables and testing protocols are readily available on computer search engines, we decided to provide practical examples of exercise programs for training competitive and recreational athletes and preventative and rehabilitative medical exercise programs.

ancillaries

CourseMate with eBook When you adopt *Exercise Physiology: An Integrated Approach,* you and your students will have access to a rich array of teaching and learning resources that you won't find anywhere else. The CourseMate brings course concepts to life with interactive learning, study, and exam preparation tools that support the printed textbook. The CourseMate includes an interactive eBook and interactive teaching and learning tools, including quizzes, flashcards, videos, and more. It also contains the Engagement Tracker, a first-of-its-kind tool that monitors student engagement in the course.

- 1-Semester Instant Access Code:
  ISBN-13: 978-1-111-68001-5
- 1-Semester Printed Access Code:
  ISBN-13: 978-1-111-68002-2

WebTutor with eBook on Blackboard WebTutor enables you to quickly and easily jump-start your course with customizable, rich text-specific content within Blackboard. Using WebTutor allows you to assign online labs, provide access to a robust eBook, and deliver online text-specific quizzes and tests to your students. Give your students all their course materials through Blackboard with WebTutor from Cengage Learning.

- 1-Semester Instant Access Code:
  ISBN-13: 978-0-8400-5552-1
- 1-Semester Printed Access Code:
  ISBN-13: 978-0-8400-5553-8

WebTutor with eBook on WebCT WebTutor enables you to quickly and easily jump-start your course with customizable, rich, text-specific content within your Course Management System. Using WebTutor allows you to assign online labs, provide access to a robust eBook, and deliver online text-specific quizzes and tests to your students. Give your students all their course materials through your Course Management System with WebTutor from Cengage Learning.

- 1-Semester Instant Access Code:
  ISBN-13: 978-0-8400-5550-7
- 1-Semester Printed Access Code:
  ISBN-13: 978-0-8400-5551-4

CengageNOW™ with eBook and InfoTrac® College Edition Get instant access to CengageNOW™. This exciting online resource is a powerful learning companion that helps students gauge their unique study needs and provides them with a personalized learning plan that enhances their problem-solving skills and conceptual understanding. A click of the mouse allows students to access online assessments, an interactive eBook, videos, and other interactive learning tools whenever they choose, with no instructor setup necessary. CengageNOW also includes the Behavior Change Planner, which guides students through a behavior change process tailored specifically to their needs and personal motivation. An excellent tool to give as a project, this plan is easy to assign, track, and grade, even for large sections.

- 1-Semester Instant Access Code:
  ISBN-13: 978-0-495-39284-2
- 1-Semester Printed Access Code:
  ISBN-13: 978-0-495-39283-5

Online Instructor's Manual with Test Bank. ISBN-13: 978-0-495-11026-2. The Instructor's Manual provides discussion questions, suggested class activities, and additional resources. The Test Bank provides matching, true/false, multiple-choice, and short answer questions.

PowerLecture DVD with ExamView® Computerized Testing. ISBN-13: 978-0-495-11029-3. Designed to make lecture preparation easier, this DVD includes more than 500 customizable PowerPoint® presentation slides with images from the text, new BBC video clips, and electronic versions of the Instructor's Manual and Test Bank. Also included is the ExamView Computerized Test Bank, which allows you to create, deliver, and customize tests (both print and online) in minutes with this easy-to-use assessment and tutorial system.

Global Health Watch Updated with today's current headlines, Global Health Watch is your one-stop resource for classroom discussion and research projects. This resource center provides access to thousands of trusted health sources, including academic journals, magazines, newspapers, videos, podcasts, and more. It is updated daily to offer the most current news about topics related to your health course.

- Instant Access Code: ISBN-13: 978-1-111-37733-5
- Printed Access Card: ISBN-13: 978-1-111-37731-1

Diet Analysis Plus, 10th Edition Take control. Reach your goals. Experience Diet Analysis Plus. Diet Analysis Plus allows students to track their diet and physical activity, as well as analyze the nutritional value of the food they eat so they can adjust their diets to reach personal health goals—all while gaining a better understanding of how nutrition relates to and impacts their lives. Diet Analysis Plus includes a 20,000+ food database; customizable reports; new assignable labs; custom food and recipe features; the latest Dietary Reference Intakes; and goals and actual percentages of essential nutrients, vitamins, and minerals. New features include enhanced search functionality with filter option, an easy-to-use instructor page, and a resources tab with helpful information.

- 2-Semester Instant Access Code:
  ISBN-13: 978-0-538-49509-7
- 2-Semester Printed Access Code:
  ISBN-13: 978-0-538-49508-0

Careers in Health, Physical Education, and Sports, 2e. ISBN-13: 978-0-495-38839-5. This unique booklet takes students through the complicated process of picking the type of career they want to pursue; explains how to prepare for the transition into the working world; and provides insight into different career paths, education requirements, and reasonable salary expectations. A designated chapter discusses some of the legal issues that surround the workplace, including discrimination and harassment. This supplement is complete with personal-development activities designed to encourage students to focus on and develop better insight into their future.

Walk4Life® Pedometer. ISBN-13: 978-0-495-01315-0. Provided through an alliance with Walk4Life, the Walk4Life Elite Model pedometer tracks steps, elapsed time, and distance. A calorie counter and a clock are included in this excellent class activity and tool to encourage students to track their steps and walk toward better fitness awareness.

This book is dedicated to Shirley and to my mentors in the UK; Nigel Tucker and Bryan Woods, my colleagues and friends in the USA; Jere Mitchell, Ken Baldwin, Charles Tipton, John Johnson, Mike Joyner, Marc Kaufmann, Bill Morgan, and Barbara Drinkwater, along with colleagues and friends in Denmark; Niels Secher and Bengt Saltin, all of whom have influenced my career. In addition, I dedicate this book to all my past graduate students and post-doctoral fellows and especially my close colleague Shigehiko Ogoh, to whom I owe a great deal.

PBR

To my wife, Doris.
To my children, Micah Joe and Mira.
To my parents, Gail and Karl.
To my teachers and colleagues.
To my students and fellows.
To the battle against the diseases of physical inactivity.

DHW

This is dedicated to my mom and dad, Bill and Alverda; my three sons, Bill, Joshua, and David; and my daughter, Cara, an exercise physiologist.

WGS

I dedicate the book to my parents, Bob and Louise, who have always encouraged my scholarly efforts. I want to also thank Karen Mitchell for her love and support. Lastly, thanks to all my students who keep teaching me new things.

TDM

author biographies

Peter B. Raven

University of North Texas Heath Science Center

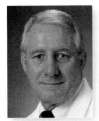

Peter B. Raven was born and raised in London, England, and was certified as a physical education teacher from St. Luke's College, University of Exeter in 1965. In 1959, at the age of 19, he was selected to play for the first team of the London Saracens, a first-class Rugby Union club side. However, after graduating from St. Luke's as an honor student in 1965, he emigrated to the United States and entered the University of Oregon in Eugene, Oregon, to pursue the study of the Scientific Basis of Physical Education. He received his Ph.D. in 1969 and was awarded an NIH Post-Doctoral Training Fellowship in Exercise Physiology under the Mentorship of Steven M. Horvath, Ph.D., at the Institute of Environmental Stress at the University of California at Santa Barbara (UCSB). Between 1969 and 1975, Dr. Raven was promoted through the academic ranks to associate professor. In his tenure at UCSB, he received some $1 million in research funding and published 30 peer-reviewed articles as first author and coauthor on environmental effects of heat, cold, and air pollution on exercise performance.

From 1975 to 1977, Dr. Raven moved to Dallas to work with Michael Pollock at the Institute of Aerobic Research and develop a program of environmental physiology. Subsequently, he joined the fledgling medical school, the Texas College of Osteopathic Medicine (TCOM)/1993-UNTHSC as an associate professor of physiology. He was promoted to professor in 1986 and served as the chair of the Department of Integrative Physiology from 1993 to 2001. Currently, he is professor of integrative physiology and orthopedics. From 1965 through 1995, he continued to play and coach rugby for the University of Oregon, UCSB, and the Dallas and Fort Worth rugby football clubs. Since 1977, Dr. Raven has worked with and mentored 18 M.S., 17 Ph.D. graduate students, and 10 post-doctoral fellows and was continuously funded by the NIH from 1983 to 2007 and again in 2011, as well as being periodically funded by NASA, AHA, and DoD. He has served as a "Viva Voce" examiner for the faculty of medicine at Kuwait University, an external examiner

of three Ph.D. degrees, two in Australia and one in Canada, and an external examiner of the awarding of three D.Sc. degrees in the United Kingdom. During his career, he has served as a visiting professor/consultant to the Division of Cardiology's Space Physiology Laboratory at UT Southwestern, the Institute of Exercise and Environmental Medicine at Presbyterian Hospital/UT Southwestern, and the Veteran's Administration Hospital in Dallas. He has a visiting professorship at the University of Copenhagen's Danish Academy of Science and the Copenhagen Muscle Research Center. His professional collaborations extend across the United States and internationally between Canada, Australia, Japan, the United Kingdom, Denmark, Italy, and the Netherlands.

In 1971, Dr. Raven joined the American Physiological Society and the American College of Sports Medicine as his two major professional societies. In addition to these, he is currently a member of the American Heart Association, the American Autonomic Society, and the Physiological Society. In 1987, he was elected to be president of the American College of Sports Medicine (ACSM), and from 1989 to 2001 served as the editor-in-chief of ACSM's official *Journal Medicine and Science in Sports and Exercise*. Currently, he serves on the editorial boards of the *Journal of Applied Physiology and Experimental Physiology* and has served on the board of the *American Journal of Physiology-Heart, Circulation,* and *Physiology*. Dr. Raven has served on study section reviews of NIH and DoD grant applications and currently reviews annual applications for ACSM's Steven M. Horvath Travel award and the University of Oregon Foundation's Eugene Evonuk Memorial Graduate Fellowship awards.

In 1989, Dr. Raven was the ACSM representative to the President's Council on Physical Fitness Exchange visit to Moscow and Leningrad (St. Petersburg) to the then-named USSR. He was awarded the ACSM Citation Award in 1995, the Korr Award for Basic Science Research in the American Osteopathic Association (AOA) in 2001, and the Benjamin L. Cohen Outstanding Research Award of the AOA in 2006. In 2011, he was awarded the American Physiological Society's Exercise and Environmental Section's Honor Award.

David H. Wasserman
Vanderbilt University Medical Center

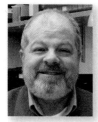

David H. Wasserman was born in New Orleans, Louisiana, and raised in California. He received a B.Sc. and an M.Sc. from UCLA in kinesiology in 1979 and 1981. He obtained his Ph.D. in physiology in 1985 at the University of Toronto under the guidance of Mladen Vranic, M.D., D.Sc. He continued his training in the Department of Molecular Physiology and Biophysics at Vanderbilt University School of Medicine, where he received fellowships from the NIH and the Juvenile Diabetes Research Foundation. He joined the faculty at Vanderbilt in 1987 and was appointed to full professor in 1997. In 2001, he became the founding director of the Vanderbilt-NIH Mouse Metabolic Phenotyping Center. In that capacity, he and his colleagues have developed and applied physiological tools to study diabetes, obesity, and metabolism in genetically modified mice. In 2007, he was named the Ron Santo Chair in Diabetes Research, and in 2010, he was named the Annie Mary Lyle Professor of Molecular Physiology and Diabetes. Dr. Wasserman has received continuous funding from the NIH since 1987. Dr. Wasserman has dedicated his research career to defining the endocrine regulation of glucose metabolism with a special emphasis on exercise and diabetes. He has published more than 160 papers and more than 25 book chapters. He has trained 10 graduate students and 10 postdoctoral fellows and served on the mentor committee or as examiner of 30 graduate students from seven different academic institutes.

Dr. Wasserman is a long-standing and active member of the American Diabetes Association, American Physiological Society, and American College of Sports Medicine. He served as chair of the Council on Exercise of the American Diabetes Association from 1999 to 2001 and chair of the Steering Committee of the Endocrinology and Metabolism Section of The American Physiology Society from 1997 to 2001. He coauthored technical papers on exercise and type 1 diabetes in 1994 and on exercise and type 2 diabetes in 2004 for the American Diabetes Association. He coauthored the most recent position paper of the American Diabetes Association on diabetes and exercise. Dr. Wasserman has served on NIH Study Sections and Research Review Panels for the American Diabetes Association and the Juvenile Diabetes Research Foundation. He has served on the editorial boards for several notable journals. Honors Dr. Wasserman has received include the Henry Pickering Bowditch Award (1997) and Solomon A. Berson Award from the American Physiology Society (2008), the C.R. Park Award for Excellence in Research from Vanderbilt University (2010), and an NIH M.E.R.I.T. Award (2008).

William G. Squires, Jr.
Texas Lutheran University

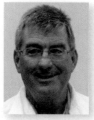

William G. Squires, Jr., has his bachelor's and master's from Texas State University and his Ph.D. in exercise physiology from Texas A&M University and Baylor College of Medicine in cardiac rehabilitation, where he was certified both as an ACSM exercise specialist and as a program director. Dr. Squires's next stop was at the Johnson Space Center working in the cardiopulmonary lab, performing crew pre-flight testing for STS 1. Dr. Squires then accepted a position at Texas Lutheran University, dual-appointed in biology and kinesiology, where he holds the Dr. Fredrick C. Elliot Chair in Health Fitness and Nutrition. He holds adjunct positions at Baylor College of Medicine and at the University of North Texas Health Science Center. Dr. Squires returned to NASA in 1989 to work in the biomechanics lab, where he served on the Exercise Countermeasures Task, which made recommendations to NASA for in-flight exercise programs for the shuttle program. Two-time president of the Texas chapter of the American College of Sports Medicine, Dr. Squires received the chapter's Honor Award in 2010. In 2008, Dr. Squires was awarded a sabbatical, during which he studied pediatric obesity at the University of Texas School of Public Health in Austin, Texas. He now puts his scientific effort into working with disadvantaged at-risk kids in the Seguin community.

Tinker D. Murray
Texas State University

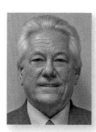

Tinker D. Murray is a professor in the Department of Health and Human Performance at Texas State University in San Marcos, Texas. He earned his Bachelor's of Science in physical education at the University of Texas–Austin in 1973. He earned a Master's of Education degree in physical education from Southwest Texas State University in 1976 and completed his Ph.D. in physical education from Texas A&M University in 1984. Dr. Murray served as director of cardiac rehabilitation at Brooke Army Medical Center from 1982 to 1984 and was twice recognized for his exceptional performance. He has been at Southwest Texas and Texas State University since 1984 and served as the director of Employee Wellness from 1984 to 1988 and director of the Exercise Performance Laboratory from 1984 to 2000. He was a voluntary assistant cross-country and track coach at Southwest Texas from 1985 to 1988 and helped win three Gulf Star Conference titles.

From 1985 to 1988, Dr. Murray was a sub-committee member for the Governor's Commission on Physical Fitness that developed the Fit Youth Today Program. Dr. Murray has been a lecturer and examiner for the USA Track and Field Level II Coaching Certification Program (1988 to 2008). He served as the vice chair (for Governor Ann Richards) of the Governor's Commission for Physical Fitness in Texas from 1993 to 1994.

Dr. Murray is a fellow of the American College of Sports Medicine (ACSM) and certified as an ACSM program director. He is a former two-time president of the Texas regional chapter of ACSM (1987 and 1994). He served on the national ACSM Board of Trustees from 1998 to 2001. In the fall of 2003, he was a guest researcher at the Centers for Disease Control and Prevention (CDC), Division of Nutrition and Physical Activity. In the fall of 2011, he participated in a developmental leave at the UT School of Public Health–Austin Regional campus.

Dr. Murray served on a five-year study intervention (HEALTHY) as a Co-I (Roberto Trevino, M.D., PI) funded by the National Institutes of Health (NIH) to prevent type 2 diabetes in middle school minority students in San Antonio, Texas, and nationwide. The HEALTHY Study group has recently (2010) reported the key findings of the intervention in *The New England Journal of Medicine*.

Dr. Murray has worked with the Professional Development Cooperative (PDC) in coordination with the Texas High School Coaches Association (THSCA) and D.W. Rutledge (executive director) since 2003 to promote continuing education experiences for coaches. He has chaired numerous master's thesis and served on more than 20 thesis and dissertation committees since 1984. He has authored or coauthored several books and book chapters, refereed journal articles, edited articles, and published abstracts. He has also been professionally involved in annual professional meeting presentations and invited talks.

Acknowledgments

The completion of the first edition of *Exercise Physiology: An Integrated Approach* was made possible through the contributions of many individuals. Thanks to Samantha Arvin, Aileen Berg, and all the folks at Cengage Learning for their hard work on making this book a reality. To Nedah Rose, thanks for giving us the initial opportunity to write the book.

We would also like to express our gratitude to the reviewers of this text; their valuable comments and suggestions are most sincerely appreciated. Finally, special thanks and appreciation to Anthony J. Clapp, Ph.D. from Augsburg College, and David J. Szymanski, Ph.D., CSCS*D, RSCC*D, FNSCA from Louisiana Tech University, who provided their expertise in helping complete the ancillary teaching package for the text.

reviewers

Nicholas Boer
University of Tennessee, Chattanooga

Melinda Bolgar
Jacksonville State University

Philip Buckenmeyer
SUNY, Cortland

Craig Cisar
San Jose State University

David Criswell
University of Florida

Phyllis Croisant
Eastern Illinois University

Deborah Dailey
Louisiana State University

Elizabeth Dowling
Old Dominion University

J. Andrew Doyle
Georgia State University

John D. Emmett
Eastern Illinois University

Hermann-J. Engels
Wayne State University

Paul Fadel
University of Missouri

William Farquhar
University of Delaware

Judith Flohr
James Madison University

Julie Franks Gill
Louisiana State University, Alexandria

Allan Goldfarb
North Carolina University, Greensboro

Felicia Greer
California State University, Fresno

Chris Harman
California University of Pennsylvania

Craig Harms
Kansas State University

Michael Harris-Love
George Washington University

Deborah Johnston
Baylor University

Michael Kalinski
Kent State University

Tom Kernozeck
University of Wisconsin, LaCrosse

Kristen Lagelly
Illinois State University

Greg Martel
Coastal Carolina College

Tim Michael
Western Michigan University

Robert J. Moffat
Florida State University

Burch Oglesby
University of Tennessee, Chattanooga

Brian Parr
University of South Carolina, Aiken

David Pavlat
Central College

Brian L. Pritschet
Eastern Illinois University

Kelly Quick
University of Sioux Falls

Roberto Quintana
California State University, Sacramento

Jacalyn Robert-McComb
Texas Tech University

Marc Rogers
University of Maryland

Donald Rudd
University of Evansville

William Ryan
Slippery Rock University of Pennsylvania

Timothy Scheet
College of Charleston

Richard J. Schmidt
University of Nebraska, Lincoln

Molly Smith
Weber State University

Ann Snyder
University of Wisconsin, Milwaukee

Curt Spanis
University of Montana

Wayland Tseh
University of North Carolina, Wilmington

Mary Visser
Minnesota State University

Michael Webster
University of Southern Mississippi

Leslie White
University of Georgia

David Wittenberg
University of Texas, Brownsville

Frank Wyatt
Midwestern State University

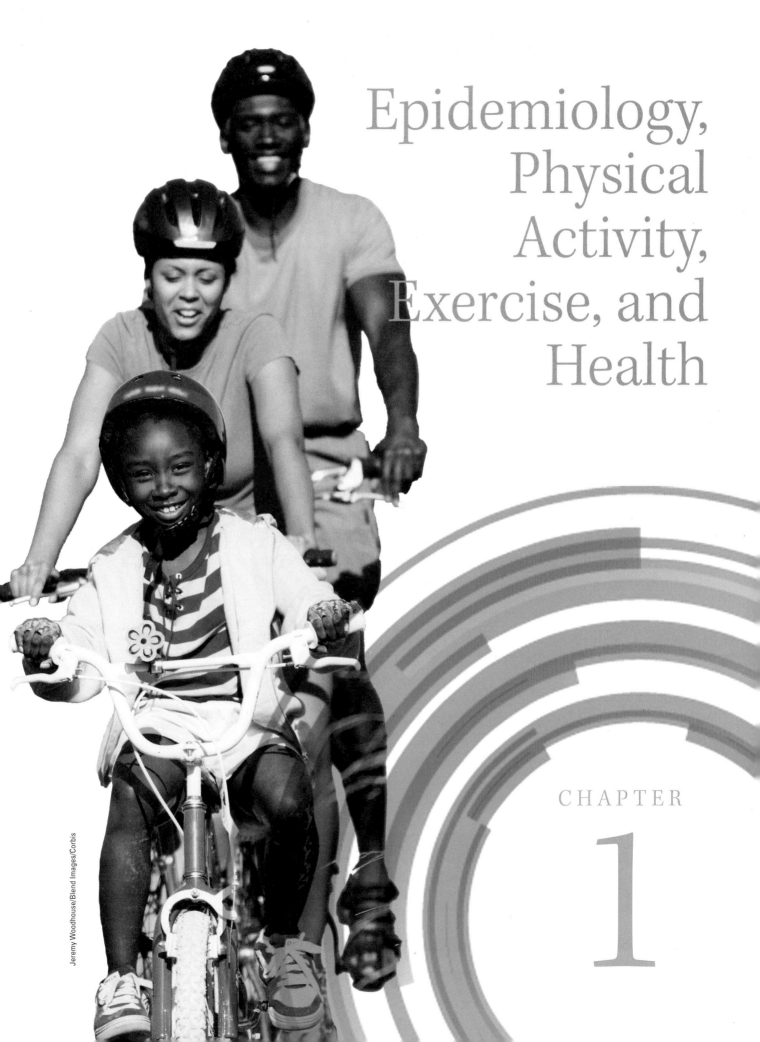

Epidemiology, Physical Activity, Exercise, and Health

CHAPTER

1

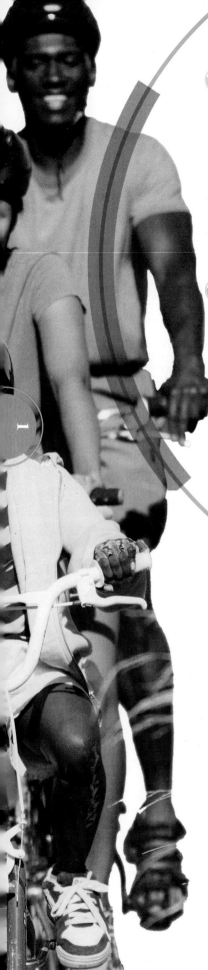

⊙ Warm-Up

CENGAGE **brain**.com

What do you already know about epidemiology, physical activity, exercise, and health?

- Use the following Pre-Test or the online evaluation tools for Chapter 1 to determine how much you already know. To access the course materials and companion resources for this text, please visit www.cengagebrain.com. See the preface on page xiii for details.

- Need more review? Let the online assessments, animations, and tutorials for Chapter 1 help prepare you for class.

⊙ Pre-Test

1. What are the bodily movements produced by skeletal muscle contractions collectively called?

2. Most people in the United States get a(n) _____ level of physical activity to maintain good health.

3. From 2000 to the present, the amount of obesity in the United States has _____.

4. What is the first stage of behavioral change related to physical activity?

5. Research on the effects of fitness on mortality indicates that the largest drop in premature mortality is seen between the _____ fit and _____ fit groups.

6. Name a component of health-related fitness.

7. Homeostasis refers to the controlled internal environment at _____.

8. The leading cause of death in the United States is _____.

9. During the past decade, health care costs in the United States have _____.

10. What is the greatest health benefit of being physically active 150 minutes per week?

1. physical activity; 2. insufficient; 3. increased; 4. pre-contemplation 5. least, moderately; 6. cardiorespiratory endurance, body composition, agility, muscular strength, endurance, or muscular flexibility; 7. rest; 8. cardiovascular disease; 9. increased; 10. maintenance of functional health

What You Will Learn in This Chapter

- How to apply the scientific method to the field of exercise physiology to improve your critical thinking and decision-making skills

- What the field of epidemiology has to do with promoting health and exercise messaging for the United States and international communities

- Basic terminology related to epidemiology, physical activity, exercise, and health

- The measurement of exercise and surveillance in epidemiology

- How to promote positive behaviors associated with recommended programs of exercise related to Health/Fitness, Medicine, Athletic Performance, and Rehabilitation

QUICKSTART!

Have you thought about how healthy you will be when you are 40, 50, 60, or 70+? How many of the health changes you will experience will be influenced by your genetics versus your personal behaviors? Do you think that engaging in regular exercise, eating healthy foods, and avoiding risky behaviors can improve your long-term health? If so, how?

Introduction to Epidemiology, Physical Activity, Exercise, and Health

Welcome to the course that explores the discipline of exercise physiology. This is a key course in your academic preparation for a future career in the exercise sciences. Exercise sciences, as you are learning, include disciplines such as exercise physiology, biomechanics, sports and behavioral psychology, nutrition, motor learning, and motor control.

Throughout this book, you will be asked to explain, demonstrate, and experience the concepts presented to you by participating in and practicing exercise physiology concepts. By completing these activities, you will become better at planning, developing, and implementing exercise physiology concepts into your professional career.

According to Lauralee Sherwood, Ph.D., author of *Human Physiology*, and a consensus of other physiology professionals, **exercise physiology** is the study of both the functional changes that occur in response to a single session of exercise and the adaptations that occur as a result of regular, repeated exercise sessions. Exercise physiology also studies the integration and coordination among most body systems, including the muscular-skeletal, nervous, circulatory, respiratory, immune, endocrine (hormone-producing), digestive, renal, integumentary (skin), and reproductive systems (see Figure 1.1). Indeed, exercise physiology is the sine qua non (the essential ingredient) of "human integrative physiology."

Health/Fitness, Medicine, Athletic Performance, and Rehabilitation

As noted earlier, exercise physiology is a key course in your academic preparation for a future career in the exercise sciences. Your future work or career options in the exercise sciences will most likely fall within one of the four areas that will be focused on throughout the text: Health/Fitness, Medicine, Ath-letic Performance, and Rehabilitation. Some examples of exercise physiology-related careers that you may find yourself pursuing and that are related to the four focus areas just listed include those in Table 1.1.

> What future career are you preparing for, and how do you think you will use exercise physiology as part of your work?

Basic Definitions

Exercise physiology, like every other science, has its own vocabulary. Some examples of basic terms that you need to quickly become familiar with in the course include *physical activity, kilocalories* (kcal), *physical fitness, health-related* and *skill-related fitness, moderate-to-vigorous physical activity* (MVPA), and *functional health.*

Physical activity and **exercise** are terms that are often used synonymously by exercise science practitioners, but in reality, they mean different things. Physical activity is any movement that works larger muscles of the body, such as the arm, leg, and back muscles. Engaging in physical activity causes you to expend energy or **kilocalories** (kcal; see other related scientific definitions in Chapters 4 and 11) versus remaining **sedentary** (or inactive), and the *2008 Physical Activity Guidelines for Americans* (**http://www.health.gov/paguidelines**) highlights the health benefits of physical activity for all age groups. Exercise is physical activity that is planned, structured, and repetitive and that results in an outcome, such as an improvement in **physical fitness**. In the remainder of this text, the term *exercise* will also include physical activities that promote an improvement or the maintenance of good

exercise physiology The study of both the functional changes that occur in response to a single session of exercise and the adaptations that occur as a result of regular, repeated exercise sessions.

physical activity Any movement that works larger muscles of the body, such as the arm, leg, and back muscles.

exercise Physical activity that is planned, structured, and repetitive and that results in a desired outcome.

kilocalories (kcal) The amount of energy required to raise the temperature of 1 kilogram of water 1 degree centigrade. The term *kilocalorie*, or *Calorie*, is also used to describe the energy value of food or for energy expenditure during exercise.

sedentary Inactive lifestyle with regard to participating regularly in physical activity or exercise. Expending few calories above resting levels and associated with lots of sitting.

physical fitness The outcome of participating in physical activity exercise that improves the body's ability to carry out daily tasks and still have enough reserve energy to respond to unexpected demands.

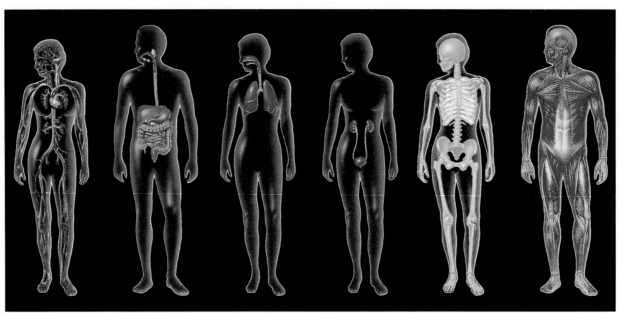

Circulatory system
heart, blood vessels, blood

Digestive system
mouth, pharynx, esophagus, stomach, small intestine, large intestine, salivary glands, exocrine pancreas, liver, gallbladder

Respiratory system
nose, pharynx, larynx, trachea, bronchi, lungs

Urinary system
kidneys, ureters, urinary bladder, urethra

Skeletal system
bones, cartilage, joints

Muscular system
skeletal muscles

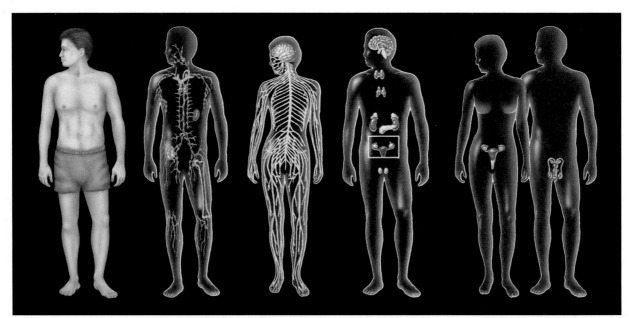

Integumentary system
skin, hair, nails

Immune system
lymph nodes, thymus, bone marrow, tonsils, adenoids, spleen, appendix, and, not shown, white blood cells, gut-associated lymphoid tissue, and skin-associated lymphoid tissue

Nervous system
brain, spinal cord, peripheral nerves, and, not shown, special sense organs

Endocrine system
all hormone-secreting tissues, including hypothalamus, pituitary, thyroid, adrenals, endocrine pancreas, gonads, kidneys, pineal, thymus, and, not shown, parathyroids, intestine, heart, skin, and adipose tissue

Reproductive system
Male: testes, penis, prostate gland, seminal vesicles, bulbourethral glands, and associated ducts

Female: ovaries, oviducts, uterus, vagina, breasts

◉ FIGURE 1.1 Components of the body systems. (From Sherwood, L. 2010. Figure 1.4 in *Human physiology.* 7th ed. Belmont, CA: Brooks/Cole-Cengage Learning.)

Health/Fitness	Medicine	Athletic Performance	Rehabilitation
Physical education teacher	Physician	Coach	Physical therapist
Physical activity specialist	Nurse	Sporting goods representative	Athletic trainer
Firefighter	Researcher	Biomechanist	Rehabilitation specialist
Police/Military	Nutritionist	Facility owner	Occupational therapist
Personal trainer	Wellness coach	Consultant	
	Clinical exercise physiologist		Diabetes/Obesity prevention physiologist

Look for "In Practice" sections on the four career areas highlighted in this table throughout each chapter of the text; they will provide you with real-life examples of how your understanding and application of exercise physiology principles will enhance your work in your future career areas.

health/fitness, medical management, athletic performance, and rehabilitation. Physical fitness is an outcome of participating in physical activity or exercise, or both, that improves the body's ability to carry out daily tasks and still have enough reserve energy to respond to unexpected demands (see Figure 1.2).

Physical fitness includes several components, and these are often subdivided into the categories of health- and skill-related fitness (see Figure 1.3).

Functional health and longevity

● **F I G U R E 1.2** Model of the relationships between physical activity, exercise, physical fitness, functional health, and longevity. (© Cengage Learning 2013)

Health-related fitness refers to your ability to stay healthy and fit and includes obtainable optimal levels of cardiovascular fitness, body composition, muscular strength, muscular endurance, and flexibility.

Skill-related fitness (sometimes called *motor-skill*, *athletic*, or *performance fitness*) refers to your ability to perform successfully in various games and sports. The components of skill-related fitness include the ability to demonstrate high levels of agility, balance, speed, power, coordination, and reaction time. An effective way to achieve these themes is by engaging regularly in **moderate-to-vigorous physical activity (MVPA)** or exercise. Numerous exercise physiologists are beginning to apply the concept of promoting programs of exercise training to improve an individual's capacity to perform physical activity and exercise, assist in disease prevention, improve one's physical fitness or athletic ability, and recover from injury or disease.

As a future exercise physiologist, you should begin to promote some common outcomes of regular participation in exercise that can include the attainment or maintenance of functional health and personal fitness. **Functional health** is the ability to maintain high levels of health and wellness by reducing or controlling your health risks for development of health problems and maintaining your physical movement independence to perform **functional abilities** (for example, physical movement for transportation—walking, preventing avoidable falls, and so on) and **activities of daily living (ADL)**.

health-related fitness The ability to stay healthy and fit; includes obtainable optimal levels of cardiovascular fitness, body composition, muscular strength, muscular endurance, and flexibility.

skill-related fitness (Sometimes called motor-skill, athletic, or performance fitness.) The ability to perform successfully in various games and sports. The components of skill-related fitness include the ability to demonstrate high levels of agility, balance, speed, power, coordination, and reaction time.

moderate-to-vigorous physical activity (MVPA) Threshold for physical activity or exercise where intensities between 3 to 5.9 METs are considered moderate intensity and those above 6 METs are considered to be vigorous intensity.

functional health The ability to maintain high levels of health and wellness by reducing or controlling your health risks for developing health problems and maintaining your physical movement independence.

functional abilities Activities such as physical movement used for transportation (walking, preventing avoidable falls, etc.).

activities of daily living (ADL) Physical activities one must perform daily for self-care.

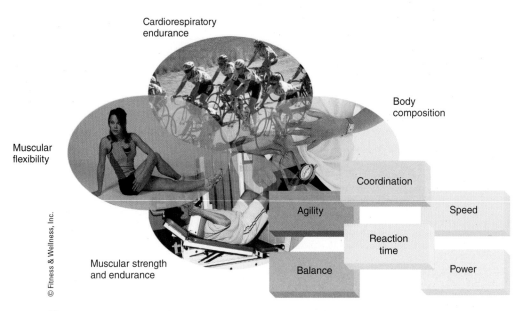

Cardiorespiratory
endurance

Body
composition

Muscular
flexibility

Coordination

Agility

Speed

Reaction
time

Muscular strength
and endurance

Balance

Power

© Fitness & Wellness, Inc.

FIGURE 1.3 Components of health-related and motor-skill–related fitness. (From Hoeger, W. W. K., and S. A. Hoeger. 2010. Figures 1.11 and 1.12 in *Lifetime physical fitness & wellness*, 11th ed. Belmont, CA: Brooks/Cole-Cengage Learning.)

personal fitness Individual attainment and maintenance of both functional health and physical fitness.

regular exercise Working most days of the week at the MVPA threshold for several minutes (30 minutes total, per session, or accumulated in multiple sessions each day).

Personal fitness incorporates individual attainment and maintenance of both functional health and physical fitness. You should help your clients achieve personal fitness by engaging in **regular exercise**, following a healthy eating plan, and avoiding harmful substances. Figure 1.4 shows the dose relationship between the level of physical activity and the risk for functional/mobility limitations. The development and maintenance of functional health and physical fitness is beneficial at any age, but is particularly important in the later decades of life. You will learn more about functional health and personal fitness later in this chapter.

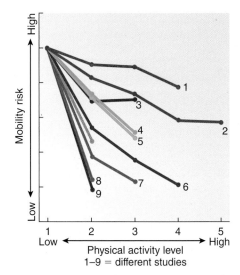

FIGURE 1.4 Physical activity levels and mobility risk. (From Physical Activity Guidelines Advisory Committee. 2008. *Physical activity guidelines advisory committee report*, 2008. Washington, DC: U.S. Department of Health and Human Services. Retrieved from http://www.health.gov/PAGuidelines/)

The Scientific Method and Exercise Physiology

scientific method A systematic process for testing hypotheses.

Scientists conduct research in an ordered way, using the **scientific method,** which is a systematic process for testing hypotheses.

By reviewing and applying the basics of the scientific method, you can become a better and more effective exercise physiologist, as well as a more analytical problem solver. You have probably used the scientific method without even thinking about it to "problem solve" and provide friends or relatives with quality feedback that helped improve their performance or understanding of exercise science concepts through "critical thinking." For example, what if a collegiate male long jumper who consistently jumped 26 feet told you that in recent practices he could jump only 24 feet? You would probably want to observe him. Most likely you would make a video of several jumps to observe his takeoff speed, steps, technique, and landing. If he jumped poorly, and you noticed that he took off a foot behind the takeoff board and had a slow approach, you could help him correct those factors and regain his 26-foot form. In making this analysis, you have applied the scientific method.

Table 1.2 provides a simplified model of the scientific method, which you should begin to apply as you problem solve both in and outside of the exercise physiology class.

You do not have to be a research scientist to use the scientific method. You can use it in the locker room, on the playing field, or in the classroom just by thinking more critically and seeking out resources that can help you make better decisions. You can practice the steps of the scientific method in many situations, and the tips that follow can help you apply them effectively. In each chapter, you will find examples of how scientists have used the scientific method to address their questions. By collecting and translating scientific evidence related to exercise, new knowledge is acquired and the entire field of exercise science advances.

Suggestions for Effectively Applying the Scientific Method

The first step is to think about the way a question is asked. For example, consider the question: "What is the best replacement fluid to drink during exercise?" The first answer that comes to mind might be "water." And although water is an excellent replacement fluid in sporting activities that last 30 minutes or less, for events that last several hours (such as a cycling race) or those that have elimination rounds (such as an all-day soccer competition), better choices are available (see Chapters 11, 12, and 14 for more examples). It would probably be much better to recommend that an athlete drink a nutrient replacement drink because these drinks contain a variety of substances such as protein, carbohydrates (sugar), and electrolytes like sodium and magnesium that are associated with enhanced performance. They are also needed to help athletes balance what they have lost (by expending calories and sweating) during longer periods of exercise. So, to receive a good answer to commonly asked exercise science questions, you will probably have to ask more specific questions to determine how exactly to answer your client's question.

Once you have a good question or set of questions, the next step is deciding how to gather the best scientific evidence to help you determine the answer. You will use the following three levels of scientific evidence to make more informed decisions:

1. Strong scientific evidence from many published research reports in credible scientific journals (*Note:* Although Wikipedia has many

● **T A B L E** **1.2** **Steps of the Simple Scientific Model**

1. Make sure you have a good exercise physiology question to solve—one that can be answered.

2. Observe the situation related to the question, if possible.

3. Describe what you observe.

4. Explain your observation(s) and description(s).

5. Predict future outcomes related to the question more precisely than by guessing.

documented scientific facts, many reported facts are scientifically questionable. Therefore, Wikipedia is not an acceptable reference source.)

2. The best scientific evidence that we can find based on fewer reports than found at level one in the published literature

3. Expert opinion

The best evidence to answer the question is found at level one, but it may not be possible to access recent research reports, particularly if only a few studies have been conducted in an area. When using expert opinion, it is important to look carefully at the expert whose opinion you are using, especially if you rely on opinions expressed on television or in popular publications. The "experts" may really only want to sell product(s) and may have little regard for scientific evidence.

Even if your only goal in taking this course and reading this book is to be an exercise practitioner, you should understand that all scientific disciplines require you to read and understand the research that provides the basis of knowledge in that discipline. In the case of exercise physiology, you need to understand that physical educators, athletic coaches, exercise leaders, personal trainers, and physical therapists are all professions based on the history of scientific discovery in the medical sciences. Reading and referring to peer-reviewed published research in scientific journals, together with research presentations at open forums, is considered critical to promoting the discipline of exercise physiology. Peer-reviewed journals have editorial boards and expert reviewers in the field who help exercise physiologists edit and interpret their research findings with the ultimate goal of achieving agreement on scientific issues. The peer-review process helps ensure that more questions are raised about scientific issues, and this enables exercise physiologists to accept or refute hypotheses over time. Read the article "What Is Science," by two of your textbook authors (Raven and Squires 1989) for more about research in the field of exercise physiology.

> When was the last time you tried to answer a question about exercise posed by one of your friends or relatives? What components of the scientific method (if any) did you use to help solve the problem or issue?

Linkages of Epidemiology and Exercise Physiology to Health

epidemiology The study of how a disease or health outcome is distributed in populations and what risk factors influence or determine this distribution. Epidemiologists study infectious or communicable diseases such as influenza or tuberculosis, as well as chronic diseases such as heart disease and cancer. They also study behaviors that may positively impact those chronic diseases.

According to Dr. Leon Gordis, a professor at John Hopkins University, **epidemiology** is the study of how a disease or health outcome is distributed in populations and what risk factors influence or determine this distribution. Epidemiologists study infectious or communicable diseases such as influenza or tuberculosis, as well as chronic diseases such as heart disease and cancer. They also study behaviors that may positively impact those chronic diseases. Since 1900, with better hygiene and pharmaceuticals, the health burden of infectious diseases has diminished in the United States, and now the most frequent causes of death among adults is chronic diseases. Because many of these diseases can be prevented with better lifestyle habits, epidemiologists now study ways of promoting better lifestyle habits.

The science of epidemiology and the promotion of physical activity and exercise provide all individuals interested in exercise physiology, and the exercise sciences in general, with a unifying goal: the understanding of, and the promotion to the general public, the health benefits of regular participation in physical activity and exercise. Research outcomes about the health benefits associated with regular participation in physical activities (see Table 1.3) provided the basis for the development of the *2008 Physical Activity Guidelines for Americans.*

In the United States, the average life expectancy is approximately 80 years for women and 75 years for men. However, many individuals lose their functional health (primarily because of adopting a sedentary lifestyle) long before they die and as a result often reduce their quality of life.

The epidemiological scientific evidence provided by researchers of the stature of Drs. Ralph Paffenbarger (deceased) and Jeremy Morris (deceased), together with Steven N. Blair (University of South Carolina), William Haskell (Stanford University), Arthur Leon (University of Minnesota), and others suggests that fit, physically active persons have a lower risk for dying prematurely than physically inactive or unfit persons. More recently, Jackson and col-

TABLE 1.3 Health Benefits Associated with Regular Physical Activity

Children and Adolescents

Strong evidence
- Improved cardiorespiratory and muscular fitness
- Improved bone health
- Improved cardiovascular and metabolic health biomarkers
- Favorable body composition

Moderate evidence
- Reduced symptoms of depression

Adults and Older Adults

Strong evidence
- Lower risk for early death
- Lower risk for coronary heart disease
- Lower risk for stroke
- Lower risk for high blood pressure
- Lower risk for adverse blood lipid profile
- Lower risk for type 2 diabetes
- Lower risk for metabolic syndrome
- Lower risk for colon cancer
- Lower risk for breast cancer
- Prevention of weight gain
- Weight loss, particularly when combined with reduced calorie intake
- Improved cardiorespiratory and muscular fitness
- Prevention of falls
- Reduced depression
- Better cognitive function (for older adults)

Moderate to strong evidence
- Better functional health (for older adults)
- Reduced abdominal obesity

Moderate evidence
- Lower risk for hip fracture
- Lower risk for lung cancer
- Lower risk for endometrial cancer
- Weight maintenance after weight loss
- Increased bone density
- Improved sleep quality

Note: The Advisory Committee to *2008 Physical Activity Guidelines for Americans* rated the evidence of health benefits of physical activity as strong, moderate, or weak. To do so, the committee considered the type, number, and quality of studies available, as well as consistency of findings across studies that addressed each outcome. The committee also considered evidence for causality and dose response in assigning the strength-of-evidence rating.
Source: *2008 physical activity guidelines for Americans.* 2008. Washington, DC: U.S. Department of Health and Human Services. Retrieved from http://www.health.gov/PAGuidelines/

leagues (2009) reported that individuals who remain physically active, maintain their weight, and abstain from smoking as they age maintain their functional fitness levels (in this case, as measured by cardiorespiratory fitness) longer than those who do not (see Figure 1.5).

Indeed, the research findings reported by these investigators and the many exercise epidemiologists who continue their work were instrumental in persuading the Surgeon General of the United States in classifying Physical Inactivity as an "independent risk factor" for Heart Disease (1996 U.S. Surgeon General's report on *Physical Activity and Health*). This became the first additional behavioral risk factor

identified since the initial five major risk factors were established by the historical Framingham Heart Study.

HOTLINK *See* **http://www.framingham-heartstudy.org/** *for more about the Framingham Heart Study that began in 1948.*

) Can you name the five major risk factors for heart disease? (

More recently, epidemiologists from the Centers for Disease Control and Prevention (CDC) and the academically based national and international epidemiologists have identified obesity as an established disease in the adult population and one

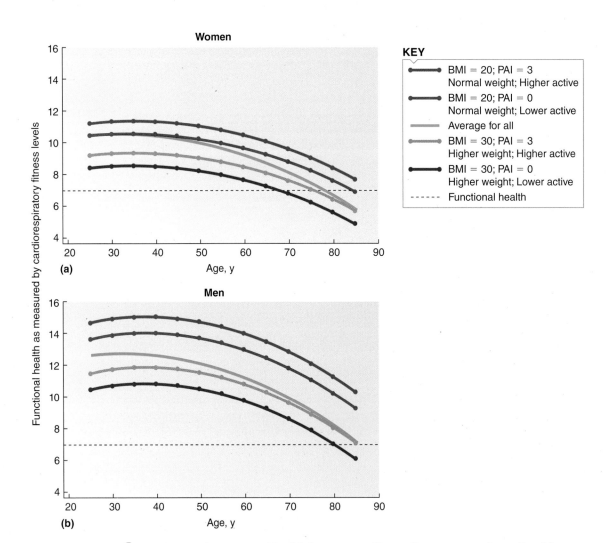

FIGURE 1.5 Functional health (as measured by cardiorespiratory fitness levels) levels in relationship to aging and changes in weight and physical activity levels. (From Jackson, A. S., X. Sui, J. R. Hébert, T. S. Church, and S. N. Blair. 2009. Role of lifestyle and aging on the longitudinal change in cardiorespiratory fitness. *Arch. Int. Med.* 169(19):1781–1787.)

that is becoming more readily identified in children as young as 2 to 5 years of age. As you will learn in Chapters 6, 6A, and B, lack of exercise, obesity, and metabolic dysfunctions are major contributors to diagnosed and undiagnosed diabetes, which has become a major accelerating health and economic challenge for more than 23 million Americans (or 7.8 percent of the population in 2007, according to the CDC). In 2010, the CDC estimated that 1 in 3 U.S. adults will experience development of diabetes in their lifetime (up from 1 in 5 just a few years ago).

Exercise Prescription

Because of its importance in maintaining health, exercise can be prescribed in a similar manner as a physician prescribes medicine to combat a disease, according to John O. Holloszy, M.D., of the Washington University School of Medicine (Holloszy 2004). Just as with a medication, a **dose–response relationship** exists between the amount of exercise you prescribe for a client and the health outcomes for that client. In other words, the epidemiological scientific research supports the concept of prescribing a program of exercise, because exercise has some of the same effects as medications prescribed by a physician. Indeed, an international movement entitled "Exercise Is Medicine" is sponsored by the American College of Sports Medicine, and was formally established in 2009.

The dose of exercise that you prescribe should be determined by the type of activity selected. It should be based on the intensity of effort, the duration, and the frequency of participation. (You will learn more about these concepts in Chapter 2). The dose effects of exercise provide varying acute and long-term physiological benefits that can influence a client's health and physical fitness, as shown in Figure 1.6.

The 1996 U.S. Surgeon General's report on Physical Activity and Health states that, in general, the harder you work, the greater the benefits to your health and fitness. Figure 1.6 further illustrates that even moderate activity results in health benefits, whereas higher intensities (moderate to high) of exercise are required to achieve higher fitness goals (like jogging a 10-kilometer run without stopping). Finally, it also indicates that engaging in too much exercise may potentially be detrimental to an individual's health and fitness, as with overtraining (you will learn more about this concept in Chapter 2).

Figure 1.7 illustrates the dose relationships between regular participation in exercise (minutes per week) and a variety of health benefits for Health/Fitness-, Medicine-, Athletic Performance-, and Rehabilitation-

dose–response relationship The amount of exercise needed to get the desired health or performance outcomes for a client.

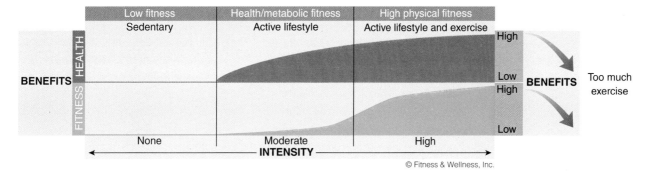

© Fitness & Wellness, Inc.

FIGURE 1.6 Health benefits based on the type of lifestyle and exercise program. (From Hoeger, W. W. K., and S. A. Hoeger. 2010. Figure 1.15 in *Lifetime physical fitness & wellness,* 11th ed. Belmont, CA: Brooks/Cole-Cengage Learning.)

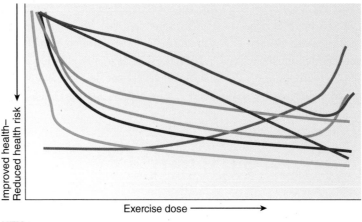

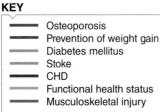

KEY

━━━ Osteoporosis
━━━ Prevention of weight gain
━━━ Diabetes mellitus
━━━ Stoke
━━━ CHD
━━━ Functional health status
━━━ Musculoskeletal injury

● **FIGURE 1.7** **With an increased dose of exercise, some health factors improve (functional health), whereas risks for musculoskeletal injury increase, and risks like stroke decrease and then increase at higher doses.** (From Kohl, H. W., and T. D. Murray. 2012. *Foundations of physical activity and public health.* Champaign, IL: Human Kinetics.)

exercise physiology integration
The understanding and the development of exercise physiology strategies to promote exercise to achieve functional fitness and higher levels of human performance.

relapse Discontinuing a regular program of exercise.

related situations. Notice that the concepts illustrated in Figure 1.7 show that for each variable (or goal) listed, there is variability (just as for prescription medications) in how much exercise is required. For example, Figure 1.7 shows the dose (that is, amount of exercise) needed to produce a change, the amount of change that can be expected per dose (that is, the rate of change), and the maximal effect that can be expected based on the dose of exercise (the lower the dose, the fewer benefits to be expected). Finally, you should remember that individual differences exist among clients for acquiring health/fitness benefits when they participate in regular exercise via their inherent trainability (adaptations; you will learn more about trainability in Chapter 2) and how they tolerate negative side effects (like injury or overtraining).

Moderate-to-strong epidemiological evidence exists for many of the relationships illustrated, but some are estimated based on sports-specific and rehabilitation-specific predictions. Some estimates are required because the concept of exercise promotion in exercise physiology for health

has emerged as a new paradigm in the 2000s that emphasizes exercise for health maintenance and promotion across a performance spectrum (**exercise physiology integration**). Exercise physiology integration involves understanding and developing strategies to promote exercise on a spectrum from achieving and maintaining basic functional fitness and continuing all the way to acquire peak performance (athletic-like). You will need to be able to prescribe exercise for your clients while adjusting for their ever-changing health status and lifestyle behaviors. **Relapses** in exercise behaviors (becoming more sedentary) and/or lifestyle changes of clients because of genetic factors, unhealthy eating, and/or risky behaviors can result in lower levels of functional health or compound challenges to mobility, medical management issues, and rehabilitation success. Figure 1.8 illustrates how basic functional health should be a primary goal for all your clients, from which further participation in physical activity and exercise can lead to higher levels of performance goals similar to those of athletes. You need to understand basic

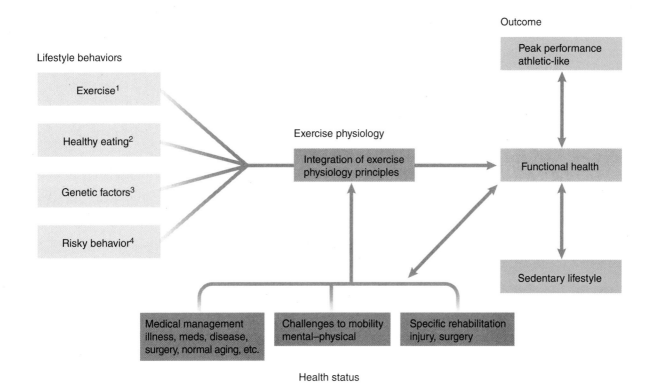

Lifestyle behaviors

Exercise[1]

Healthy eating[2]

Genetic factors[3]

Risky behavior[4]

Exercise physiology

Integration of exercise physiology principles

Outcome

Peak performance athletic-like

Functional health

Sedentary lifestyle

Medical management illness, meds, disease, surgery, normal aging, etc.

Challenges to mobility mental–physical

Specific rehabilitation injury, surgery

Health status

Relapse in exercise behaviors (becoming more sedentary) and/or lifestyle changes due to genetic factors, healthy eating, and/or risky health behaviors can result in lower levels of functional helath or compound challenges to mobility, medical management outcomes, and rehabilitation success. Prolonged sedentary periods are associated with increased risks for chronic disease and loss of functional health.

1. Exercise–see www.health.gov/pageuidelines for more
2. Healthy eating–see http://www.cnpp.usda.gov/DGAs2010-DGACReport.htm for more
3. Genetics factors–see http://healthfinder.gov/ for more
4. Risky behaviors–see http://healthfinder.gov/ for more

FIGURE 1.8 Primary factors that influence the acquisition and maintenance of functional health. (From Kohl, H. W., and T. D. Murray. 2012. *Foundations of physical activity and public health.* Champaign, IL: Human Kinetics.)

principles of exercise physiology so that you can help individuals acquire and maintain functional fitness even when facing the challenges to health such as medical management issues and exercise rehabilitation. Your clients will need to maintain or regain their functional health to optimize medical management in disease processes and/or reverse the disease process (for example, type 2 diabetes; see Chapter 6B) or during rehabilitation (after athletic injury—relapse). Once functional fitness is obtained, they can once again strive to optimize performance if that is their goal. A primary message to share with your clients is that "research clearly demonstrates the importance of avoiding inactivity," with regard to developing and maintaining functional health and optimizing performance

(*2008 Physical Activity Guidelines for Americans*).

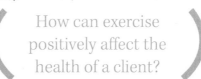

How can exercise positively affect the health of a client?

As shown in Figure 1.9, the risk for dying prematurely declines as people become more physically active. The *2008 Physical Activity Guidelines for Americans* recommends that individuals acquire 150 minutes of physical activity per week for most health benefits. However, to achieve higher performance goals like preventing weight regain after significant weight loss (10–20 pounds), most clients will need to exercise more (≥200–300 minutes/week) and sometimes at higher intensities to be successful.

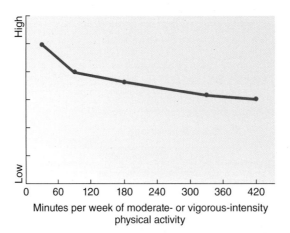

High

Low

0   60   120   180   240   300   360   420

Minutes per week of moderate- or vigorous-intensity
physical activity

FIGURE 1.9 The risk for dying prematurely declines as people become physically active. (From Physical Activity Guidelines Advisory Committee. 2008. Physical activity guidelines advisory committee report, 2008. Washington, DC: U.S. Department of Health and Human Services. Retrieved from http://www.health.gov/PAGuidelines/)

Defining Levels of Exercise Activity

To better understand how to apply concepts across the disciplines of exercise physiology and epidemiology, you need to become aware of how regular exercise has been generally defined from epidemiologic research and health promotion. It includes the descriptors listed in Table 1.4.

Table 1.5 lists moderate-to-vigorous activities for children and adults as described in the *2008 Physical Activity Guidelines for Americans.*

How Much Exercise Is Enough for Health?

As you learned in the dose–response section earlier in the chapter, the number of minutes of exercise that exercise physiologists and epidemiologists often recommend for specific health/fitness/performance benefits vary greatly depending on the goals that clients are trying to accomplish. The *Physical Activity Guidelines Advisory Committee Report* (PAGACR) from 2008 provides a detailed review of what is known, and not known, about the health benefits of

TABLE 1.4 Definitions

Regular Exercise
- Most days of the week, preferably daily
- 5 or more days of the week if moderate intensity activities are chosen
- 3 or more days per week if vigorous intensity activities are chosen
- The accumulation (multiple short bouts of exercise such as 3 times for 10 minutes) of moderate exercise activities daily can also result in health/fitness benefits, if done regularly

Moderate-Intensity Physical Activity or Exercise
- A perceived exertion of 11–14 on a rating of Perceived Exertion Scale; a numerical scale (Borg Scale) used to have individuals rate how they perceive the effort they are using to exercise (see Chapter 2 for a more detailed explanation for perceived exertion and METs)
- Working at 3–5.9 METs per minute (1 MET is the equivalent of energy you expend sitting at rest); exercising at this intensity will make you feel warm and slightly out of breath
- Examples of moderate activities and exercise for adults include walking briskly (3 miles/hour or faster), general gardening, bicycling at ≤10 miles/hour, and carrying groceries

Vigorous-Intensity Physical Activity or Exercise
- A perceived exertion rating of ≥15
- Working at >6 METs; when exercising at this intensity you will be sweating and breathing hard
- Examples of activities and exercise include jogging, chopping wood, high-impact aerobic dance, swimming continuous laps, lifting 3–5 sets of 6–10 repetitions for 10–12 major muscle areas, or cycling uphill (see Chapter 2 for more on weight lifting details)

Modified from *Promoting physical activity: A guide for community action* (p. 17). Champaign, IL: Human Kinetics, 1999; and the 2008 *Physical Activity Guidelines for Americans.*

T A B L E 1.5 Examples of Moderate- and Vigorous-Intensity Aerobic Physical Activities and Muscle- and Bone-Strengthening Activities for Children and Adolescents

Type of Physical Activity	Children	Adolescents
Moderate-intensity aerobic	• Active recreation, such as hiking, skateboarding, rollerblading • Bicycle riding • Brisk walking	• Active recreation, such as canoeing, hiking, skateboarding, rollerblading • Brisk walking • Bicycle riding (stationary or road bike) • Housework and yard work, such as sweeping or pushing a lawn mower • Games that require catching and throwing, such as baseball and softball
Vigorous-intensity aerobic	• Active games involving running and chasing, such as tag • Bicycle riding • Jumping rope • Martial arts, such as karate • Running • Sports such as soccer, ice or field hockey, basketball, swimming, tennis • Cross-country skiing	• Active games involving running and chasing, such as flag football • Bicycle riding • Jumping rope • Martial arts, such as karate • Running • Sports such as soccer, ice or field hockey, basketball, swimming, tennis • Vigorous dancing • Cross-country skiing
Muscle strengthening	• Games such as tug-of-war • Modified push-ups (with knees on the floor) • Resistance exercises using body weight or resistance bands • Rope or tree climbing • Sit-ups (curl-ups or crunches) • Swinging on playground equipment/bars	• Games such as tug-of-war • Push-ups and pull-ups • Resistance exercises with exercise bands, weight matches, handheld weights • Climbing wall • Sit-ups (curl-ups or crunches)
Bone strengthening	• Games such as hopscotch • Hopping, skipping, jumping • Jumping rope • Running • Sports such as gymnastics, basketball, volleyball, tennis	• Hopping, skipping, jumping • Jumping rope • Running • Sports such as gymnastics, basketball, volleyball, tennis

Note: Some activities, such as bicycling, can be moderate or vigorous intensity, depending on level of effort.
Source: *2008 physical activity guidelines for Americans.* 2008, p. 18. Washington, DC: U.S. Department of Health and Human Services. Retrieved from http://www.health.gov/PAGuidelines/

exercise. The scientific evidence summarized in the PAGACR indicates that participation in regular physical activity and exercise are associated with positive health outcomes. The report contains major findings related to the following categories:

• Mortality

• Cardiorespiratory health

• Metabolic health

• Energy balance

• Musculoskeletal health

• Functional health

• Cancer

• Mental health

• Youth

• Adverse events or risks of participating in various physical activities

HOTLINK *See part E of the* Physical Activity Guidelines Advisory Committee Report *2008 for specific health comes related to the categories summarized by the PAGACR at* http://www.health.gov/paguidelines/.

In this section, recommendations about how much exercise is necessary are provided for youth, adults (ages 18–65), and older adults (>65 years). The recommendations in Tables 1.6 through 1.8 are based on the best available scientific evidence from the *2008 Physical Activity Guidelines for Americans.* It is important for you to understand and learn to use these guidelines to provide simple health messages about exercise to your clients. Past guidelines for physical activity and exercise provided by professional organizations, governmental agencies, corporate groups, and others have varied so greatly that they created confusion about effective messaging for the general public and exercise profession-als alike. It has been proposed to the U.S. Department of Health and Human Services that the physical activity guidelines will be reviewed and updated every 5 years or so, much like the *Dietary Guidelines for Americans* have been since 1980.

School-age youths should participate daily in 60 minutes or more of MVPA that is developmentally appropriate, enjoyable, and involves a variety of activities. Regular bouts of physical activity lasting 60 minutes or longer can be helpful in the following ways (compiled from Strong and Malina 2005):

1. Helping youth control their body weight (reduce the incidence of obesity)
2. Helping achieve better lipid (cholesterol and triglyceride) profiles
3. Reducing blood pressure and the risks for hypertension
4. Increasing cardiovascular fitness on an average of about 10 percent
5. Becoming part of a management plan to control asthma
6. Reducing anxiety and depression
7. Improving academic performance
8. Improving bone health

(Do you meet the key exercise guidelines for your age group? Why or why not?)

TABLE 1.6 Key Guidelines for Children (>6 years) and Adolescents

- Children and adolescents should do 60 minutes (1 hour) or more of physical activity daily.
  - *Aerobic:* Most of the 60 or more minutes a day should be either moderate- or vigorous-intensity aerobic physical activity, and should include vigorous-intensity physical activity at least 3 days a week.
  - *Muscle-strengthening:* As part of their 60 or more minutes of daily physical activity, children and adolescents should include muscle-strengthening physical activity on at least 3 days of the week.
  - *Bone-strengthening:* As part of their 60 or more minutes of daily physical activity, children and adolescents should include bone-strengthening physical activity on at least 3 days of the week.
- It is important to encourage young people to participate in physical activities *that are appropriate for their age, that are enjoyable, and that offer variety.*

Source: *2008 Physical activity guidelines for Americans.* 2008, p. 16. Washington, DC: U.S. Department of Health and Human Services. Retrieved from http://www.health.gov/PAGuidelines

TABLE 1.7 Key Guidelines for Adults

- All adults should avoid inactivity. Some physical activity is better than none, and adults who participate in any amount of physical activity gain some health benefits.
- For substantial health benefits, adults should do at least 150 minutes (2 hours and 30 minutes) a week of moderate-intensity or 75 minutes (1 hour and 15 minutes) a week of vigorous-intensity aerobic physical activity, or an equivalent combination of moderate- and vigorous-intensity aerobic activity. Aerobic activity should be performed in episodes of at least 10 minutes, and preferably, it should be spread throughout the week.
- For additional and more extensive health benefits, adults should increase their aerobic physical activity to 300 minutes (5 hours) a week of moderate-intensity or 150 minutes a week of vigorous-intensity aerobic physical activity, or an equivalent combination of moderate- and vigorous-intensity activity. Additional health benefits are gained by engaging in physical activity beyond this amount.
- Adults should also do muscle-strengthening activities that are moderate or high intensity and involve all major muscle groups on 2 or more days a week, because these activities provide additional health benefits.

Source: *2008 Physical activity guidelines for Americans.* 2008, p. 22. Washington, DC: U.S. Department of Health and Human Services. Retrieved from http://www.health.gov/PAGuidelines

TABLE 1.8 Key Guidelines for Older Adults (same as for adults plus the following)

- When older adults cannot do 150 minutes of moderate-intensity aerobic activity a week because of chronic conditions, they should be as physically active as their abilities and conditions allow.
- Older adults should do exercises that maintain or improve balance if they are at risk for falling.
- Older adults should determine their level of effort for physical activity relative to their level of fitness.
- Older adults with chronic conditions should understand whether and how their conditions affect their ability to do regular physical activity safely.

Source: *2008 Physical activity guidelines for Americans.* 2008, p. 30. Washington, DC: U.S. Department of Health and Human Services. Retrieved from http://www.health.gov/PAGuidelines

Relationships between Risk Factors, Epidemiology, and Exercise

Risk factors are conditions and behaviors that represent a potential threat to an individual's well-being. Figure 1.10 illustrates several common chronic disease processes and their contributing risk factors that have been identified by epidemiologists.

Once epidemiologists have identified specific risk factors for chronic diseases, they can also identify human behaviors (both changeable and unchangeable or less modifiable) that are linked to each risk.

Individuals can modify or influence many risk factors, at least in part, if they practice positive health behaviors like participating in regular exercise, eating healthy foods, and avoiding risky behaviors. In fact, research has shown that the health behaviors that are established as a young adult will most likely continue into later adult life. Put another way, the health behaviors you adopt now may either benefit or injure your health in the future.

Less modifiable risk factors may not be able to be changed as much with an intervention (like physical activity and exercise) as compared with modifiable risk factors.

However, the overall risk (like heredity/genetic risk) may become down-regulated or inhibited versus becoming up-regulated, which may accelerate a disease process. Lightfoot et al. (2010) have reported further evidence (first suggested in the 1975 biological literature by J. K. Choo) that exercise behaviors are moderately to highly inherited and that the study of how physical activity and exercise influence functional health and risk factors for disease are complex, yet exciting, areas for future investigations in exercise physiology.

Depending on a gene or cluster of genes impacted by adopting a health behavior-like exercise, a down-regulation or an up-regulation may be considered positive, depending on the overall change in risk. For example, if a person is at greater risk for being obese (because both parents are obese), the person may participate in regular physical activity and exercise and control body weight, and therefore reduce, down-regulate, or inhibit (but may not eliminate) the risk for metabolic dysfunction (associated with increased risk for type 2 diabetes and cardiovascular disease)

risk factors Conditions and behaviors that represent a potential threat to an individual's well-being.

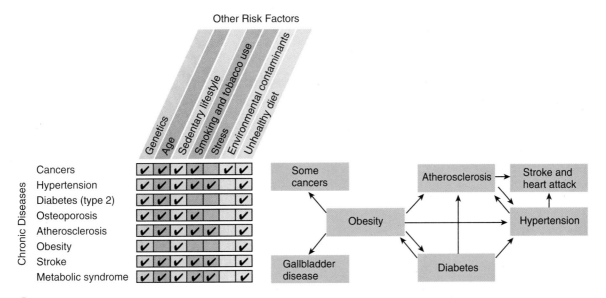

● FIGURE 1.10 Exercise, risk factors, and chronic disease. (From Whitney, E. N., and S. R. Rolfes. 2004. Figure 18.3 in *Understanding nutrition*, 10th ed. Belmont, CA: Wadsworth.)

versus being inactive and increasing type 2 diabetes and cardiovascular disease risk. Thus, it is important to recognize the risk factors that we currently have and those we can prevent. Strategies can then be developed and practiced in a plan to reduce or eliminate these risk factors for ourselves, as well as for others, if possible.

HOTLINK *See the Centers for Disease Control and Prevention website at* **http://www.cdc.gov** *for more information on risk factors.*

Risk Factors That You Can Modify

A person who is inactive throughout life is at an increased risk for health problems (or chronic disease) such as:

- Cardiorespiratory (lung and blood vessels) disease
- Cardiovascular heart disease (CHD)
- Hypertension
- Low back pain
- Osteoporosis
- Obesity
- Diabetes
- Negative emotional stress
- Colon cancer
- High blood cholesterol and triglyceride concentrations

Epidemiological research has shown that adults who are sedentary or unfit die of chronic diseases at much higher rates than do more active or fit individuals. Figure 1.11 shows that if you have numerous risk factors (>1–2), you are at a much greater risk for development of chronic disease—in this case, risk for heart attack (cardiovascular disease).

Smoking

Chronic smokers (people who have smoked consistently for 10, 20, or even 30 years) have an increased risk for heart and lung disease compared with nonsmokers. For example, smokers are two times as likely as nonsmokers to have a heart attack (damage to the heart). Smokers tend to be less active than nonsmokers, which increases their risk for premature chronic disease.

Smokers who stop smoking and choose an active lifestyle can reduce their heart attack risk to that of nonsmokers in 2 to 3 years. Although it is very difficult to stop smoking, it is never too late to quit smoking and begin a more active lifestyle.

Hypertension

A person with high blood pressure, or hypertension, is at an increased risk for stroke (damage to the brain), heart attack, kidney disease, and other serious health problems. Hypertension has few symptoms, which is one reason why it can be so dangerous. Hypertension is associated with genetic makeup, aging, a high salt or

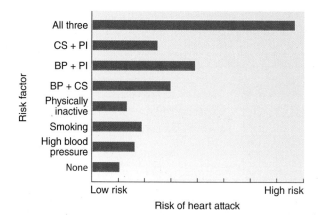

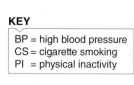

KEY

BP = high blood pressure
CS = cigarette smoking
PI = physical inactivity

FIGURE 1.11 Relationship between risk factors and heart attack risk. (Based on data from Paffenbarger, R. S., W. E. Hale, R. J. Brand, et al. Physical Activity as an Index of heart Attack Risk in College Alumni. *American Journal of Epidemiology,* 108:161–175, 1978.)

sodium intake, obesity, and excessive alcohol consumption.

When physicians diagnose people as having hypertension, they may recommend weight loss, lower sodium diets, and more physical activity. Appetite-suppressive drugs, prescribed by a physician, are oftentimes helpful if lifestyle changes do not help. Self-medication and abuse of appetite-suppressive drugs can be an indication of low self-esteem.

HOTLINK *To learn more about how high blood pressure can influence your personal fitness, see the website for the National Heart, Lung, and Blood Institute (NHLBI) at* **http://www.nhlbi.nih.gov**.

High Levels of Cholesterol and Triglycerides

A person with an increased concentration of **cholesterol** in the blood is at an increased risk for the development of **atherosclerosis**. The total amount of cholesterol in the blood is determined by the combination of the fats we eat and the fats produced by our bodies.

Cholesterol is often classified as either "good cholesterol" or "bad cholesterol." It is carried in the blood by lipoproteins (complexes or compounds of lipids and protein that transport lipids in blood). **High-density lipoprotein (HDL)** is "good cholesterol," and higher amounts of HDL are associated with a lower risk for heart disease (>60 mg/dl). **Low-density lipoprotein (LDL)** (>100–130 mg/dl) and **very low-density lipoprotein (VLDL)** are types of "bad cholesterol," and higher amounts of LDL and VLDL are associated with higher heart disease risk.

Triglycerides are another type of blood fat. High concentrations of triglycerides in the blood are associated with a greater heart disease risk (>150 units mg/dl). Therefore, it is important to limit fat intake in the diet and take lipid medications as prescribed by a physician. In that way, individuals can manage their blood cholesterol and triglyceride concentrations. Regular participation in exercise can also help to manage blood cholesterol and triglyceride concentrations independent of the exercise

weight loss effect by metabolic up-regulation (see Chapters 4–6, 6A, 6B, and 11 for more information).

Diabetes

Diabetes is a disease in which concentrations of glucose (sugar) in the blood cannot be regulated at a normal healthy value of 80 to 100 mg/dl. Diabetes can be either a type 1 or 2 variety. **Type 1 diabetes** was initially thought to be a genetic disease. However, type 1 diabetes has been diagnosed in people of all ages, and causes an individual's immune system to attack and destroy the insulin-producing beta cells of the islets of Langerhans in the pancreas (treatable with insulin). Pregnancy also appears to increase the risk for type 1 diabetes after birth and is known as gestational diabetes, particularly for women who become pregnant after age 35.

Type 2 diabetes, or adult-onset diabetes, was initially linked to excessive weight gain and causes insulin resistance at the tissues, thereby slowing down or inhibiting the glucose uptake (more specific mechanisms and their metabolic consequences are presented in Chapters 6A and 6B). Type 2 diabetes used to been seen only in adults older than 40 years. However, in recent years, as many as 50 percent of new type 2 diabetic cases are seen in childhood and adolescence (for more information, see Chapters 6A, 6B, and 11). Type 2 diabetes is linked to lack of physical activity, being overweight (increased waist circumference), and genetic factors predisposing the individual to obesity. It is important to control diabetes risks because this disease can lead to premature health problems such as diabetic ulcers, limb gangrene, limb amputation, blindness, renal nephropathy, and kidney failure, which requires renal dialysis and transplantation. Figure 1.12 illustrates the increases in diabetes from 1994 to 2008 in the United States.

Body Composition

The amount of water, bone, muscle, and fat in the body helps determine **body composition** (you will learn more about these concepts in Chapter 13). A person who carries

cholesterol A fat-like substance that is manufactured in the body and found in animal foods.

atherosclerosis Narrowing and hardening of the arteries.

high-density lipoprotein (HDL) A fat transporter called *good cholesterol* because it has a higher proportion of protein and lower proportion of triglyceride and cholesterol.

low-density lipoprotein (LDL) A fat transporter called *bad cholesterol* because it has a moderate proportion of protein, a low proportion of triglyceride, and a high proportion of cholesterol.

very low-density lipoprotein (VLDL) A fat transporter also called *bad cholesterol* because it has a higher proportion of triglyceride and serves as a precursor to the formation of low-density lipoproteins.

triglyceride A fat made up of three fatty acids attached to a glycerol molecule; major storage form of fat in humans.

type 1 diabetes This was initially thought to be a genetic disease. However, type 1 diabetes has been diagnosed in people of all ages and causes an individual's immune system to attack and destroy the insulin-producing beta cells of the islets of Langerhans in the pancreas (treatable with insulin).

type 2 diabetes Also known as adult onset diabetes, type 2 diabetes was initially linked to excessive weight gain and causes insulin resistance at the tissues, thereby slowing down or inhibiting the glucose uptake. Type 2 diabetes is linked to lack of physical activity, being overweight (increased waist circumference), and genetic factors predisposing the individual to obesity.

body composition Components such as the amount of water, bone, muscle, and fat in the body.

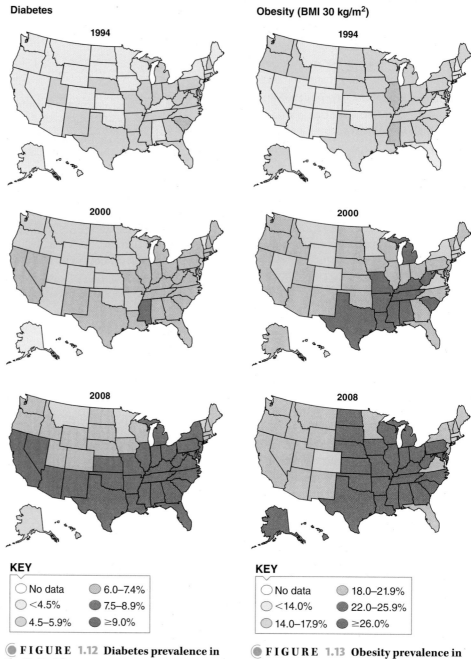

Diabetes

1994

2000

2008

Obesity (BMI 30 kg/m²)

1994

2000

2008

KEY

○ No data	◐ 6.0–7.4%
◯ <4.5%	◕ 7.5–8.9%
◔ 4.5–5.9%	● ≥9.0%

◉ FIGURE 1.12 Diabetes prevalence in the United States. (Centers for Disease Control and Prevention's Division of Diabetes Translation, http://www.cdc.gov/diabetes/statistics/slides/maps_diabetesobesity94.pdf)

KEY

○ No data	◐ 18.0–21.9%
◯ <14.0%	◕ 22.0–25.9%
◔ 14.0–17.9%	● ≥26.0%

◉ FIGURE 1.13 Obesity prevalence in the United States. (Centers for Disease Control and Prevention's Division of Diabetes Translation, http://www.cdc.gov/diabetes/statistics/slides/maps_diabetesobesity94.pdf)

too much body fat is at an increased risk for problems such as hypertension, heart disease, and type 2 diabetes. Increased body weight (measured by a body mass index [BMI] > 25; see Chapter 13 for a more detailed discussion) and obesity (BMI > 30) often begin in childhood and usually persist into adulthood, unless a person alters his or her diet and adopts an active lifestyle. A person with too little body fat (excessive leanness), in contrast, appears to be at risk for problems such as osteoporosis and certain forms of cancer. Excessive leanness is often also associated with abnormal eating and psychological or addictive behaviors that require professional attention. Figure 1.13 illustrates the often-reported U.S. increases in adults who are overweight and obese. This trend has become a global challenge. As the economies in developing countries enable a greater supply of more processed foods and technology reduces the physical ADL, the sedentary lifestyle results in obesity.

HOTLINK *You can learn more about BMI in Chapter 13.*

Stress

Stress is defined as the physical and psychological responses of your body as you try to adapt to stressors. A **stressor** is anything that requires you to adapt and cope with either positive or negative situations. **Distress** is excess negative stress, caused by fear, anger, confusion, or other similar mood states in one's life. Distress can increase the risk for chronic disease (such as heart attack) or can make a disease process worse. Distress can produce negative physical responses (increases in heart rate, increases in stress hormone concentrations, headaches, and so on). It can also have negative emotional effects such as anxiety, sleeplessness, and depression, among others.

Eustress is positive stress and is healthy. It is an enjoyable type of stress, such as what you might feel prior to becoming elected class president, scoring well on an exam, or obtaining your driver's license.

A few ways to cope positively with stress and distress include changing one's diet (for example, by eating breakfast regularly and reducing caffeine intake), meditation (it can be as simple as reflecting about a pleasant event in one's life), or engaging regularly in exercise (such as brisk walking, weight lifting, climbing stairs). Dealing with stress and distress in a positive way is something that will challenge you daily for the rest of your life.

Less Modifiable Risk Factors

Three health risk factors related to death or disability caused by chronic disease are age, sex (male or female), and heredity (genetics).

Age

An older person tends to be at increased risk for diseases such as high blood pressure, heart disease, and cancer as compared with younger individuals. However, a chronic disease process can exist without evidence of symptoms in childhood or early adulthood and not manifest itself until later in life (ages 70, 80, 90, and beyond). You cannot change your age. However, you can optimize your functional health as you age and live a higher quality lifestyle by being physically active and by eating a healthy diet throughout your life. In fact, you may know someone much older than you who has better functional health than you because that person has been active throughout his or her life. This fact provides you, the exercise practitioner, with a strong argument to promote a healthy lifestyle to people of all ages.

Sex

Some health risk factors are influenced by the individual's sex. For example, men between the ages of 40 and 50 have a greater risk for heart disease than do women of the same age range. The risk for heart disease for women increases dramatically after the onset of menopause (usually age 50–55 years) and then matches that of men. Women have a greater risk than men for osteoporosis beginning at ages 45 to 50 years, and the risks are exacerbated by menopause. The risk for osteoporosis for men increases dramatically after age 65 to 75, a period known as the "climacteric," and is similar to the menopause of women because it is a period of loss of the sex steroid testosterone.

It is important to recognize the health risk factors associated with sex. Even if you have an increased health risk because of your sex, certain behaviors can help you modify and minimize that risk. For example, to reduce the risk for osteoporosis, many women take calcium supplements and exercise regularly to modify and reduce that risk. The exercise regimen for both women and men should include weight training to help maintain bone health. In fact, the biggest medical problem that will confront astronauts on future long-term space flights is the loss of bone mass caused by weightlessness. Heavy resistance training has been recommended to slow down this loss of bone mass during space flight.

stress The physical and psychological responses of your body as you try to adapt to a new situation that can be threatening, frightening, or exciting.

stressor Anything that requires one to adapt and cope with either positive or negative situations.

distress Excess negative stress, caused by fear, anger, confusion, or other similar mood states in one's life.

eustress Positive stress that is healthy.

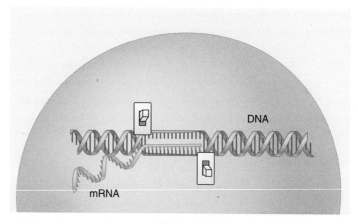

FIGURE 1.14 **Environmental and behavioral factors (for example, exercise) can modify the epigenetic markers or switches and help control gene expression associated with negative health risk and disease processes.** (Adapted from Whitney E. N., and S. R. Rolfes. 2011. Figure 6-7 in *Understanding nutrition*, 12 ed. Belmont, CA: Wadsworth.)

Heredity (Genetics) Markers

genetic predisposition Increased health risk for various disease processes.

A person may be born with a **genetic predisposition** (genetic link; see Chapters 4–6B for more information) to increased health risk for various disease processes. For example, some individuals are born with extremely high blood cholesterol concentrations. They experience development of atherosclerosis at an early age (in their 20s or 30s), which can cause them to have heart attacks and die prematurely. Often the genetic map that we are born with can be positively or negatively influenced by the dietary and physical activity behaviors we choose throughout life.

epigenetic markers These sit on top of the genes and help regulate gene function (or gene expression), at least in part, by up-regulating or down-regulating their cellular actions.

Since 2005, exercise scientists have identified and studied the epigenome or **epigenetic markers**. These epigenetic markers sit on top of the genes and help regulate gene function (or gene expression), at least in part, by up-regulating or down-regulating their cellular actions (see Figure 1.14). It has been reported that epigenetic markers are significantly negatively influenced by lifestyle factors, such as being physically inactive and consuming a high-calorie, high-fat diet. Participating in regular physical activity and exercise, in contrast, is associated with positive epigenetic effects. Adapting to or changing one's environment can also positively influence epigenetic markers, health, and longevity (see Figure 1.15).

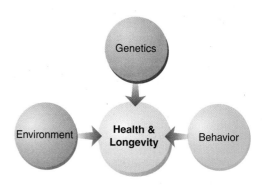

FIGURE 1.15 **Factors that determine health and longevity.** (From Hoeger, W. W. K., and S. A. Hoeger. 2010. Figure 1.2 in *Lifetime physical fitness & wellness*, 11th ed. Belmont, CA: Brooks/Cole-Cengage Learning.)

Fortunately, even if your family has a history of a disease, you can often modify your behaviors or lifestyle to reduce or optimize your own risks. For example, if your father or grandfather had a heart attack before age 60, you have most likely inherited some heart disease risk. However, according to the American Heart Association, by controlling health risk factors such as smoking, cholesterol intake, obesity, physical inactivity, and so on, you can significantly reduce your overall risk for a heart attack.

HOTLINK *To learn more about how genetics can influence your risk for sudden death during exercise, see the website for the Pennington Biomedical Research Center (PBRC; Louisiana State University, Baton Rouge, LA) at* **http://www.pbrc.edu**. *The director of the PBRC is Dr. Claude Bouchard, one of the world authorities on genetic linkages to obesity and physical activity.*

Now that you have learned about many of the risk factors associated with common chronic diseases and health problems, you will begin to explore why epidemiologists have studied the potential positive linkages between regular participation in physical activity programs and its modification of risk factors.

> Which risk factors
> do you have that you
> think you can modify
> with lifestyle changes?

Homeostasis and Steady-State Exercise

As you have learned in your previous anatomy/physiology courses, **homeostasis** refers to the maintenance of a relatively stable internal environment at rest, as shown in Figure 1.16. Homeostasis is essential for the survival of each cell, and each cell, through its specialized activities, contributes to the maintenance of the body's internal environment shared by all cells. In the body, homeostasis is primarily maintained by negative feedback mechanisms (see Figure 1.17) that respond to changes in normal resting values (for example, body temperature) by sensing the change, adapting to the change, and bringing about bodily actions to return the body back to homeostasis.

Steady state exercise refers to the body's ability to maintain homeostatic-like conditions during movement. Figure 1.18 shows the oxygen uptake response of an individual who attempts to jog at 50 percent of his or her maximal ability (or submaximal exercise; see Chapters 2, 7, 8, and 10 for further discussions) and achieves a steady state, whereas the demand for oxygen and energy is equal to that supplied (level line = steady state or demand for oxygen = supply of oxygen).

steady state exercise The body's ability to maintain homeostatic-like conditions during movement.

homeostasis The maintenance of a relatively stable internal environment at rest.

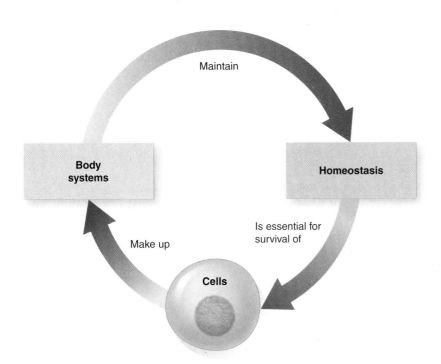

● **FIGURE 1.16 Interdependent relationship of cells, body systems, and homeostasis.**
Homeostasis is essential for the survival of cells, body systems maintain homeostasis, and cells make up body systems. This relationship serves as the foundation for modern-day physiology. (From Sherwood, L. 2010. Figure 1.6 in *Human physiology*, 7th ed. Belmont, CA: Brooks/Cole-Cengage Learning.)

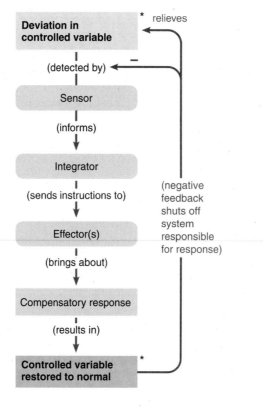

(a) Components of a negative-feedback control system

(b) Negative-feedback control of body temperature

KEY

Flow diagrams throughout the text
- **+** = Stimulates or activates
- **−** = Inhibits or shuts off
- ⬭ = Physical entity, such as body structure or a chemical
- ▭ = Actions
- ❘ = Compensatory pathway
- ❙ = Turning off of compensatory pathway (negative feedback)
- * Note that lighter and darker shades of the same color are used to denote, respectively, a decrease or an increase in a controlled variable.

FIGURE 1.17 Negative feedback and homeostasis. (From Sherwood, L. 2010. Figure 1.8 in *Human physiology*, 7th ed. Belmont, CA: Brooks/Cole-Cengage Learning.)

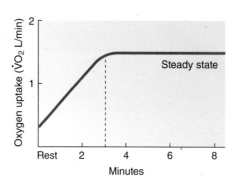

FIGURE 1.18 Exercise steady state.
(© Cengage Learning 2013)

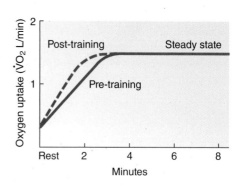

FIGURE 1.19 Exercise training effects (pre- and post-training) on achieving steady state. (© Cengage Learning 2013)

As you will learn in following chapters, the homeostatic challenges of exercise include factors such as increased heart rate, increased ventilation, redistribution of blood flow, maintenance of body temperature, energy production, and recovery from activity back to baseline levels. The ability to obtain a steady state during exercise cannot be achieved at high intensities of exercise (>90 percent of maximum effort for most). However, a normal response to exercise training is the obtainment of steady state sooner (see Figure 1.19). The adaptations acquired by engaging in regular steady state exercise promote improvements in functional health and enhance homeostatic control during exercise and in recovery.

HOTLINK *Visit the course materials for Chapter 1 for an animation that illustrates a detailed example of a negative feedback loop.*

Epidemiological Research and Its Relationship to Exercise

Physical activity or exercise epidemiology involves the application of epidemiologic principles to an examination of the benefits and risks of participation in exercise-related activities. The primary goals of physical activity and exercise epidemiologists are as follows:

- Determine the causes and risk factors associated with various preventable diseases that can be positively influenced by participation in a regular program of exercise.

- Determine the extent of preventable disease processes in the community and how they can be positively influenced by participation in a regular program of exercise.

- Monitor different intensities of physical activity and physical inactivity in populations to determine trends of effect, both positive and negative, on disease and health processes.

- Determine the history and progression of preventable disease processes and how they can be positively influenced by participation in a regular program of exercise.

- Determine proper treatment and therapy strategies to prevent disease processes, and improve health and human performance via participation in a regular program of exercise.

- Determine public policy messages to be promoted nationally and internationally to encourage individuals to participate in a regular program of exercise to prevent disease processes and enjoy improved health and performance.

Physical activity and exercise epidemiologists have used three common methods for the past half-century to measure or assess physical activity and/or exercise in relation to health and disease outcomes:

1. Self-reported intensities of exercise
2. A measure or estimate of cardiorespiratory fitness, such as $\dot{V}O_2$ max (maximal oxygen uptake) assessment performed on a treadmill or bicycle ergometer in a laboratory setting, which is associated with increased intensities of exercise
3. A review of occupational data relating the intensities of different occupations to exercise intensities

Regardless of the method or instrument of exercise used to study population behaviors, the accuracy of the information gathered depends on the following key criteria:

- **Validity**: degree to which an instrument measures what it is supposed to measure
- **Reliability**: ability to obtain repeatable results during different testing sessions

validity The degree to which an instrument measures what it is supposed to measure.

reliability The ability to obtain repeatable results during different testing sessions.

Wellness Lifestyle Questionnaire

Name: _____ Date: _____

Course: _____ Section: _____ Gender: _____ Age: _____

The purpose of this questionnaire is to analyze current lifestyle habits and help determine changes necessary for future health and wellness. Check the appropriate answer to each question and obtain a final score according to the guidelines provided at the end of the questionnaire.

	Always	Nearly always	Often	Seldom	Never
1. I participate in vigorous-intensity aerobic activity for 20 minutes on 3 or more days per week, and I accumulate at least 30 minutes of moderate-intensity physical activity on a minimum of 2 additional days per week.	5	4	3	2	1
2. I participate in strength-training exercises, using a minimum of eight different exercises, 2 or more days per week.	5	4	3	2	1
3. I perform flexibility exercises a minimum of 2 days per week.	5	4	3	2	1
4. I maintain recommended body weight (includes avoidance of excessive body fat, excessive thinness, or frequent fluctuations in body weight).	5	4	3	2	1
5. Every day, I eat three regular meals that include a wide variety of foods.	5	4	3	2	1
6. I limit the amount of saturated fat and trans fats in my diet on most days of the week.	5	4	3	2	1
7. I eat a minimum of five servings of fruits and vegetables and six servings from grain products daily.	5	4	3	2	1
8. I regularly avoid snacks, especially those that are high in calories and fat and low in nutrients and fiber.	5	4	3	2	1
9. I avoid cigarettes or tobacco in any other form.	5	4	3	2	1
10. I avoid alcoholic beverages. If I drink, I do so in moderation (one daily drink for women and two for men), and I do not combine alcohol with other drugs.	5	4	3	2	1
11. I avoid addictive drugs and needles that have been used by others.	5	4	3	2	1
12. I use prescription drugs and over-the-counter drugs sparingly (only when needed), and I follow all directions for their proper use.	5	4	3	2	1
13. I readily recognize and act on it when I am under excessive tension and stress (distress).	5	4	3	2	1
14. I am able to perform effective stress-management techniques.	5	4	3	2	1
15. I have close friends and relatives with whom I can discuss personal problems and approach for help when needed, and with whom I can express my feelings freely.	5	4	3	2	1
16. I spend most of my daily leisure time in wholesome recreational activities.	5	4	3	2	1
17. I sleep 7 to 8 hours each night.	5	4	3	2	1
18. I floss my teeth every day and brush them at least twice daily.	5	4	3	2	1
19. I avoid overexposure to the sun, and I use sunscreen and appropriate clothing when I am out in the sun for an extended time.	5	4	3	2	1
20. I avoid using products that have not been shown by science to be safe and effective. (This includes anabolic steroids and unproven nutrient and weight loss supplements.)	5	4	3	2	1
21. I stay current with the warning signs for heart attack, stroke, and cancer.	5	4	3	2	1
22. I practice monthly breast/testicle self-exams, get recommended screening tests (blood lipids, blood pressure, Pap tests), and seek a medical evaluation when I am not well or disease symptoms arise.	5	4	3	2	1
23. I have a dental checkup at least once a year, and I get regular medical exams according to age recommendations.	5	4	3	2	1
24. I am not sexually active. / I practice safe sex.	5	4	3	2	1
25. I can deal effectively with disappointments and temporary feelings of sadness, loneliness, and depression. If I am unable to deal with these feelings, I seek professional help.	5	4	3	2	1
26. I can work out emotional problems without turning to alcohol, other drugs, or violent behavior.	5	4	3	2	1

Parvomedics

GLUE STOCK/Shutterstock.com

A partial example of a self-report questionnaire and a metabolic assessment of physical activity and exercise levels. (From Dunford, M., and J. A. Doyle. 2007. Figure 2.15 in *Nutrition for sport and exercise.* Belmont, CA: Wadsworth; Hoeger, W. W. K., and S. A. Hoeger. 2010. Wellness Lifestyle Questionnaire in *Lifetime physical fitness & wellness* (p. 27). 11th ed. Belmont, CA: Brooks/Cole-Cengage Learning.)

- **Sensitivity**: ability of the method or assessment tool to measure and detect change in exercise patterns

Once each of the three measures of exercise is determined, they can be compared with the rates of disease or negative health conditions in a population. For example, Jeremy N. Morris, D.Sc., D.P.H., was the first to study the relationship between vocational and leisure-time physical activity and the impact on the incidence of CHD in London bus drivers and conductors of the double-decker bus in the early 1950s. Dr. Morris and his coworkers were the first epidemiologists to find that the conductors (ticket takers), who walked up and down the stairs of the transport bus all day to take tickets, were much less likely to experience development of CHD (and when they did it was less severe) than their inactive driver counterparts, who also had the added stress of driving a large bus in the traffic-congested narrow streets of London.

Epidemiologists also determine measures of **mortality** (death) and **morbidity**, or new cases, in terms of the number (**incidence**) and total in the population at a specific point in time (**prevalence**). Collection of these types of data allows physical activity and exercise epidemiologists to determine the **biological plausibility** (or theory) that there is a causal link between preventable diseases or health outcomes and exercise. Of course, epidemiologists must control their studies involving exercise measures to allow for **confounders** (or variables, such as age, body composition, or baseline health status) that might influence interpretation of the data—for example, the independent effect that age has on the incidence of CHD regardless of the exercise history, that is, the older one gets the greater the risk for having CHD.

Epidemiologists have used two main approaches to investigate the relationships between exercise and disease or specific health conditions. These include **observational** and **experimental** study designs. Observational studies, such as the one mentioned previously by Morris and colleagues, evaluate self-selected intensities of exercise by study subjects and often do not control for confounders that might influence the conclusions made by the researcher. Prospective experimental studies are more powerful and conclusive than observational studies because individuals can be **randomly** assigned to groups of exercise or control (inactivity) and various confounders can be statistically controlled. However, valuable data regarding the relationships between exercise participation and health and performance outcomes have been obtained from both observational and experimental epidemiological studies.

Table 1.9 outlines the different types of epidemiological study designs and describes how each of them provides a different level of understanding about how exercise can help prevent disease processes, improve health, and optimize human performance.

Common Assessments or Measures of Exercise and Considerations for Their Use

The assessment of participation in regular exercise by epidemiologists is an ongoing fundamental challenge for researchers who want to determine the behaviors associated with increased intensities of exercise and the dosages of exercise needed to positively affect areas related to Health/Fitness, Medicine, Athletic Performance, and Rehabilitation. Exercise physiologists and epidemiologists use both subjective and objective measures to evaluate the associations between different intensities of regular participation in a program of exercise and various outcome measures of interest.

Some common subjective instruments used to measure exercise intensity in epidemiological research include **exercise questionnaires and surveys** (an example of which is shown on the previous page). Numerous exercise questionnaires and surveys have been developed during the past 50+ years of scientific investigation, but all vary according to their complexity (simple or detailed?), time frame of recall (days, weeks, months, year, lifetime?), and the type of activities assessed (leisure, occupational, household/self-care, and transportation?).

sensitivity The ability of the method or assessment tool to measure and detect change in exercise patterns.

mortality Death.

morbidity The rate of incidence of a disease.

incidence Rate or range of occurrence.

prevalence The total number of cases of a disease in a given population at a specific point in time.

biological plausibility The theory that there is a causal link between preventable diseases or health outcomes and exercise.

confounders Variables, such as age, body composition, or baseline health status, which might influence interpretation of the data.

observational A study that evaluates self-selected intensities of exercise by study subjects and often does not control for confounders that might influence the conclusions made by the researcher.

experimental A study where the researcher can assign individuals to groups of exercise or control (inactivity) and various confounders can be statistically controlled.

randomly Individuals or groups are assigned by chance.

exercise questionnaires and surveys Tools that can be simple or detailed that use a time frame of recall (e.g. days, weeks, months, years, or a lifetime), and types of activities assessed (e.g. leisure, occupational, household/self-care, and/or transportation) to provide the researcher with exercise data.

cross-sectional This type of study uses individuals with and without a disease or health problem and compares subjects at one point in time to determine if participation in regular exercise has any relationship to the disease or health problem.

case-control This type of study uses individuals with and without a disease or health problem and compares past participation in regular exercise to determine if there was any relationship to the disease or health problem.

prospective This type of study uses individuals who are free of the disease or health problem of interest and monitors baseline exercise. Subjects are evaluated over time for the development of disease or the outcome with regards to their exercise.

clinical trial This type of study uses individuals free of disease or a health problem of interest who are randomly assigned to receive an exercise intervention or no exercise intervention. The groups are followed over time to determine if they differ in terms of the percentage of people who develop the disease or health problem.

direct observation A common measure of epidemiological and physical activity research; an example is charting minutes of participation during a middle-school physical education class.

indirect calorimetry Measuring oxygen consumption and energy expenditure in an exercise laboratory.

doubly labeled water A biochemical marker that estimates energy expenditure through the use of isotopes of water ingested by study subjects.

global positional systems (GPS) Geographical location devices that use satellite technology to document participation in exercise.

heart rate monitor Heart rate transmitters worn by study participants used to estimate energy expenditure.

accelerometers Usually worn on the hip at waist level, these assess the intensity, frequency, and duration of acceleration of movement associated with participation in exercise.

pedometers Monitors worn on the hip that use stride length and steps taken throughout the day to estimate exercise and energy expenditure. Pedometers can help measure distances but do not measure intensity, an important component in assessing exercise.

TABLE 1.9 Epidemiological Study Designs

Observational
- **Cross-sectional**: This type of study uses individuals with and without a disease or health problem and compares subjects at one point in time to determine whether participation in regular exercise has any relationship to the disease or health problem.
- **Case–Control**: This type of study uses individuals with and without a disease or health problem and compares past participation in regular exercise to determine whether there was any relationship to the disease or health problem.
- **Prospective**: This type of study includes individuals who are free of the disease or health problem of interest and monitors baseline exercise. Subjects are evaluated over time for the development of disease or the outcome with regard to their exercise.

Experimental
- **Clinical trial**: This type of study includes individuals free of disease or a health problem of interest who are randomly assigned to receive an exercise intervention or no exercise intervention (for example, health education only). The groups are followed over time to determine whether they differ in terms of the percentage of people who experience development of the disease or health problem.

Objective methods of measuring exercise participation include the following:

Direct observation: for example, charting minutes of participation during a middle-school physical education class

Indirect calorimetry: measuring oxygen consumption and energy expenditure in an exercise laboratory

Doubly labeled water: a biochemical marker that estimates energy expenditure through the use of isotopes of water ingested by study subjects

Global positional systems (GPS): geographical location devices that use satellite technology to document participation in exercise

Heart rate monitor: heart rate transmitters worn by study participants that are used to estimate energy expenditure

Accelerometers: monitors, usually worn on the hip at waist level, that assess the intensity, frequency, and duration of acceleration of movement associated with participation in exercise

Pedometers: monitors worn on the hip that use stride length and steps taken throughout the day to estimate exercise and energy expenditure; pedometers can help measure distances, but do not measure intensity, an important component in assessing exercise

Physical fitness assessments: the most commonly used are various health-related measures of cardiovascular

fitness, muscular fitness (strength and endurance), body composition, and/or flexibility to indicate changes in the intensities of the exercise associated with conditioning

All the techniques of the assessment of participation in regular exercise used by epidemiologists and exercise physiologists have "pros and cons" related to their ability to effectively measure exercise intensity and how behavioral interventions might impact changes in exercise behavior. For example, some of the techniques discussed earlier are costly and complex to implement, whereas others are simple and inexpensive. Typically the more complex and technical the exercise assessment tool, the more accurate it is; the more simplistic and easy it is to use, the less accurate the tool.

Some of the exercise assessment tools identified earlier have also been used by policy makers and practitioners to help promote increased amounts of physical activity and exercise in large populations (see Figure 1.20). For example, one can use "pedometer challenges" where participants receive free pedometers. Pedometer challenges have been used to successfully motivate subjects to increase their daily amount of exercise.

(How can you effectively evaluate regular participation in exercise?)

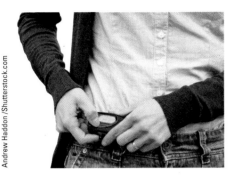 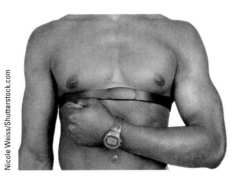

physical fitness assessments The most commonly used assessments are various health-related measures of cardiovascular fitness, muscular fitness (strength and endurance), body composition, and/or flexibility to indicate changes in the intensities of the exercise associated with conditioning.

Pedometers and heart rate monitors are used to assess exercise levels.

Healthy People 2020 goals and objectives for physical activity

PA–1: Reduce the proportion of adults who engage in no leisure-time physical activity.

PA–2: Increase the proportion of adults who meet current Federal physical activity guidelines for aerobic physical activity and for muscle-strengthening activity.

PA–3: Increase the proportion of adolescents who meet current Federal physical activity guidelines for aerobic physical activity and for muscle-strengthening activity.

PA–4: Increase the proportion of the Nation's public and private schools that require daily physical education for all students.

PA–5: Increase the proportion of adolescents who participate in daily school physical education.

PA–6: Increase regularly scheduled elementary school recess in the United States.

PA–7: Increase the proportion of school districts that require or recommend elementary school recess for an appropriate period of time.

PA–8: Increase the proportion of children and adolescents who do not exceed recommended limits for screen time.

PA–9: Increase the number of States with licensing regulations for physical activity provided in child care.

PA–10: Increase the proportion of the Nation's public and private schools that provide access to their physical activity spaces and facilities for all persons outside of normal school hours (that is, before and after the school day, on weekends, and during summer and other vacations).

PA–11: Increase the proportion of physician office visits that include counseling or education related to physical activity.

PA–12: (Developmental) Increase the proportion of employed adults who have access to and participate in employer-based exercise facilities and exercise programs.

   Potential data source: National Health Interview Survey (NHIS), CDC, NCHS.

PA–13: (Developmental) Increase the proportion of trips made by walking.

PA–14: (Developmental) Increase the proportion of trips made by bicycling.

PA–15: (Developmental) Increase legislative policies for the built environment that enhance access to and availability of physical activity opportunities.

F I G U R E 1.20 *Healthy People 2020* goals and objectives for physical activity. (From *Healthy People 2020*, U.S. Department of Health and Human Services, Centers for Disease Control and Prevention, http://www.healthypeople.gov/2020/topicsobjectives2020/objectiveslist.aspx?topicId=33)

іnRETROSPECT

Pioneers of Physical Activity and Public Health: Jeremy Morris, Ph.D., and Ralph Paffenbarger, Jr., Ph.D.

Drs. Jeremy Morris and Ralph Paffenbarger, Jr., were initial leaders in the field of study of exercise epidemiology. Their careers and key highlights from 1965 to the present related to significant accomplishments in exercise, health, and fitness are summarized.

Jeremy N. Morris: The first epidemiologist to study the relationship between vocational and leisure-time physical activity (self-reported) related to the development of CHD in London double-decker bus drivers and conductors (all men). Dr. Morris and his coworkers also found that postmen delivering mail on foot had lower rates of CHD than sedentary supervisors and telephonists. Working from the 1970s to the 1990s, Dr. Morris and coworkers extended their work and reported that civil servants (men) who engaged in regular vigorous exercise (>7.5 kcal/min) had half the risk for a first heart attack (and if they had a heart attack, they were half as likely to die) compared with their less active counterparts.

Ralph S. Paffenbarger, Jr.: Epidemiologist who studied two groups of several thousand men over several decades, including San Francisco Longshoremen and College Alumni of Harvard College and University of Pennsylvania. He found that those who engaged in the lowest intensity physical activity programs (for example, <150 kcal/week) had much greater rates of CHD and all causes of mortality than those who were more active (for example, >1,500 kcal/week) (see Figure 1.21).

1965—Adult Physical Fitness: A Program for Men and Women, President's Council on Physical Fitness

The first national recommendation by an organization or agency to urge Americans to improve their physical fitness (today the equivalent would be increasing physical activity and exercise).

1989—Surgeon General's Report on Nutrition and Health

The first national public health message issued by the U.S. Department of Health and Human Services (equivalent of the CDC today) that promoted the concept that Americans should control their weight.

1995—The American College of Sports Medicine (ACSM) and the Centers for Disease Control and Prevention (CDC) Physical Activity Recommendation

The authors of this report recommended that "every U.S. adult should accumulate 30 minutes or more of moderate-intensity physical activity on most, preferably all, days of the week" (Pate et al. 1995).

1996—Surgeon General's Report on *Physical Activity and Health*

Landmark report that concluded that "being physically inactive is bad for one's health" (U.S. Department of Health and Human Services 1996). The 278-page report provided extensive reviews of the scientific epidemiological and exercise physiological research that linked regular participation in MVPA to positive health outcomes. The report also

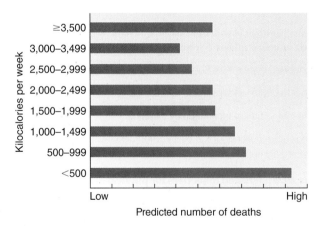

FIGURE 1.21 Relationship between expending kilocalories each week and predicted number of deaths in men. (Based on data from Paffenbarger, R.S., et al. Physical activity, all-cause mortality, and longevity of college alumni. *New England Journal of Medicine,* 314:605–613, 1986.)

identified that **physical inactivity** was an independent risk factor for coronary heart disease.

2008—The *2008 Physical Activity Guidelines for Americans and the Physical Activity Guidelines* Advisory Report 2008

Most comprehensive scientific review and recommendations for physical activity and health to date that provide the basis of a new approach to promoting exercise physiology concepts across the exercise spectrum described earlier in the chapter.

2010—*Healthy People 2010/2020* Objectives

Reports from the U.S. Department of Health and Human Services and the CDC representing various national organizations, agencies, and individuals that set public health (including physical activity and nutrition) objectives for the nation to achieve (see Figure 1.20 again for more).

HOTLINK *Search the internet to find out more about other significant contributors (including Drs. Steven Blair, Art Leon, Henry Blackburn, I. M. Lee, William Kannel, Ancel Keys, William Haskell, Daniel Levy, and Phillip Wolf) to the field of epidemiology and MVPA.*

physical inactivity An independent risk factor for coronary heart disease.

in*Practice*

Examples of the Relationship between Epidemiology and the Promotion of Exercise

We will now look at how epidemiologists have promoted participation in regular programs of exercise and some practical examples of how you will be using exercise promotional messages related to your area of interest (review the future career list in Table 1.1). The following questions/recommendations for exercise are based on the most current understanding of the link between the science of epidemiology and exercise promotion, which is continuing to evolve as you read this section.

Health/Fitness: How much exercise is enough to help adults lose weight and prevent weight regain? The American College of Sports Medicine Positions Stand of 2001 and *2008 Physical Activity Guidelines for Americans* recommends 225 to 300 minutes per week of exercise to meet this goal.

Medicine: How much exercise does one need to achieve to control type 2 diabetes? The American Diabetes Association recommends a minimum of 150 minutes of MVPA minutes per week to control and reduce one's risk for development of type 2 diabetes.

Athletic Performance: How much exercise does one need to accumulate to be a world-class marathoner like Meb Keflezighi, the 2004 U.S. Olympic Marathon Silver Medalist and 2009 New York City Marathon winner, who typically trains 100+ miles per week? Based on Meb's intensity ability (2:09.56 personal best or approximately 4:58/mile pace for 26.2 miles), one might estimate that you would need to accumulate 600 to 720 minutes of exercise per week to even think about competing with Meb.

Rehabilitation: How much exercise does one need to accumulate in a Phase 2 (outpatient 6–8 weeks post-heart attack or post-coronary bypass surgery) cardiac rehabilitation program?

Depending on the clinical status of the patient and the physician's recommendations, according to American College of Sports Medicine guidelines, a cardiac patient should accumulate 100 to 150 minutes of MVPA per week in Phase 2 of the patient's rehabilitation.

Behavioral Theories, Exercise, and Epidemiology

Physical activity or exercise epidemiologists often use various behavioral theories to help determine how regular participation in exercise can improve health or performance. There are literally dozens of behavioral models that exercise scientists might use to study exercise, and the associations between research interventions and positive behavioral change. However, the **transtheoretical model** of behavioral change (or Stages of Change Model) is one of the

transtheoretical model The transtheoretical model of behavioral change (or Stages of Change Model) is one of most popular models currently used by researchers and includes levels labeled pre-contemplation, contemplation, preparation, action, maintenance, and relapse.

most popular models currently used by researchers to help individuals achieve their personal fitness goals.

You will most likely use the Stages of Change Model in your career field to help your clients make a commitment to developing and adhering to behavioral changes. Figure 1.22 illustrates the Stages of Change Model and the steps related to how individuals think about changing behavior, adopting new behaviors, maintaining desired behaviors, perhaps suffering relapse, or ending desired behaviors. Stages include pre-contemplation, contemplation, preparation, action, maintenance, and relapse.

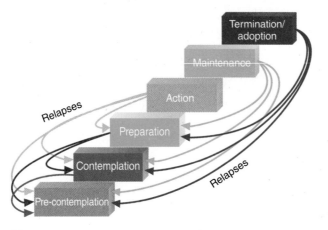

FIGURE 1.22 Stages of behavioral change. (From Hoeger, W. W. K., and S. A. Hoeger. 2010. Figure 2.4 in *Lifetime physical fitness & wellness*, 11th ed. Belmont, CA: Brooks/Cole-Cengage Learning.)

in*Practice*

Using the Stages of Change Model

Mary is a 45-year-old healthy but sedentary woman who 9 months ago had surgery to repair her anterior cruciate ligament (ACL) following an injury she sustained when she fell while shopping at a mall. Mary's physician has released her from physical therapy rehabilitation but has encouraged her to begin a regular walking and resistance-training program to control her weight and to help in the management of her knee rehabilitation. Mary is planning on beginning the program recommended by her physician but has not started as of yet.

At what stage of change is Mary currently? How would you help her move to the next stage?

CONCEPTS, *challenges,* **contro**versies

Metabolic Syndrome

In the April 19, 2005, edition of *Circulation* (the primary journal of the American Heart Association), Dr. Michael Criqui reported that a large body of scientific evidence associated with the increases in obesity also "predicts large increases in insulin resistance/diabetes, hypertension, hypertriglyceridemia, and low HDL cholesterol, as well as unfavorable changes in endothelial function and a host of inflammatory, thrombotic, and fibrinolytic factors" (J. P. Despres 2005, pp. 453–455). Collectively, these obesity-related factors are called "metabolic syndrome" today, but were known in the past as "syndrome x," the "deadly quartet," and cardiovascular dysmetabolic disease. These factors (as well as others currently being studied) contribute to the two major causes of death, cardiovascular disease and cancer. Metabolic syndrome is a topic of current interest and controversy, as indicated by a PubMed (http://www.ncbi.nlm.nih.gov/pubmed) search in 2005 that revealed more than 10,000 references to the term.

Many researchers have started recommending that low cardiorespiratory fitness is an important risk marker for metabolic syndrome. Therefore, many exercise physiologists and other exercise-related scientists have begun recommending that individuals with low cardiorespiratory fitness should improve their fitness to reduce their risk for development of metabolic syndrome. However, some exercise scientists have suggested that although the recommendations make logical sense, more scientific evidence is needed to truly understand the link between biological mediators of disease (fitness) and therapeutic targets.

For example, many questions about metabolic syndrome remain to be answered, such as: Does weight loss with caloric reduction alone reduce one's risk for development of metabolic syndrome? How much does genetics influence our ability to control metabolic syndrome? What physical activity or exercise intensities, durations, and frequencies optimize the reduction of risk for development of metabolic syndrome? In any case, it is likely that you will hear a lot more about the topic of metabolic syndrome in the future.

Andrii Muzyka/Shutterstock.com

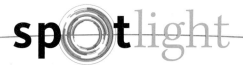

The Making of an Epidemiologist and the Link to Public Health Policies: Harold W. Kohl III, Ph.D.

Harold W. "Bill" Kohl III was born in St. Louis, Missouri, on April 11, 1960. He attended the University of San Diego in San Diego, California, where he earned his Bachelor's of Arts in Biology with a minor in Chemistry in 1982. Although his initial academic interest was in biology (not surprising because his father and grandfather were physicians), Kohl became interested in public health issues and statistics (the basics for the study of epidemiology). In 1984, Kohl earned his Master's of Science in Public Health from the University of South Carolina at Columbia, South Carolina, specializing in epidemiology and statistics. In 1993, he completed his Doctor of Philosophy in Community Health Studies (major in epidemiology, minors in biometrics and health promotion) from the University of Texas Health Science Center (UTHSC) in Houston, Texas.

During his graduate studies in epidemiology, statistics, and physical activity, he worked with mentors and notable epidemiologists Drs. Steven N. Blair and Ralph S. Paffenbarger. Kohl became the director of research at the Baylor Sports Medicine Institute in 1995 and expanded his epidemiological research interests to the area of orthopedic rehabilitation. In 1999, Kohl became an executive director of the Center for Health Promotion at the International Life Sciences Institute (ILSI) in Atlanta, Georgia. At ILSI, Kohl developed and helped market a variety of epidemiological-based products that help promote physical activity and healthy nutrition. In 2002, Kohl was selected to become a lead epidemiologist for the CDC (Physical Activity and Health Branch) in Atlanta, Georgia.

He is currently a professor in the departments of epidemiology and kinesiology at University of Texas Health Science Center (School of Public Health, Austin Regional Campus) and the Michael and Susan Dell Center for Healthy Living in Austin, Texas. He is a founder and the president of the International Society for Physical Activity and Public Health (http://www.ispah.org) and a co-editor of the *Journal of Physical Activity and Health.* He has also been involved professionally by serving in numerous organizations, scientific journal advisory boards, and by authoring and publishing more than 120 significant physical activity epidemiological scientific articles.

Chapter Summary

Exercise physiology is the study of both the functional changes that occur in response to a single session of exercise and the adaptations that occur as a result of regular, repeated exercise sessions. Exercise physiology, like most sciences, has its own vocabulary.

- All scientific disciplines investigate problems using a set of principles that we identify as the "scientific method."

- In this chapter, you learned how the disciplines of exercise physiology and epidemiology overlap and are involved in the promotion of exercise and public health.

- Epidemiology is the study of how a disease or health outcome is distributed in populations and what risk factors influence or determine this distribution.

- Moderate-to-vigorous physical activity (exercise) can be prescribed like medicine because there is a dose–response relationship. In other words, one can prescribe the proper dose of exercise to obtain the outcome, goal, or desired response.

- The number of minutes of regular exercise (or how much is enough) recommended by epidemiologists varies greatly, depending on one's goals and health status.

- Risk factors are conditions and behaviors that represent a potential threat to an individual's well-being. Some risk factors are more modifiable than others.

- Epidemiologists study risk factors associated with participation in exercise and make recommendations to promote positive health messages.

- Epidemiologists use a variety of observational and experimental research designs to study exercise.

- There are a variety of ways that epidemiologists and exercise physiologists can measure exercise participation.

Exercise Physiology Reality

CENGAGE brain.com   To reinforce the exercise physiology concepts presented above, complete the laboratory exercises for Chapter 1. To access labs and other course materials for this text, please visit www.cengagebrain.com. See the pref-ace on page xiii for details. Once you complete the exercises, evaluate your results based on the scales provided and develop a personal plan for successfully completing your exercise physiology course.

Exercise Physiology Web Links

Access the following websites for further study of topics covered in this chapter:

- Find updates and quick links to these and other epidemiology and exercise physiology–related sites at our website. To access the course materials and companion resources for this text, please visit www.cengagebrain.com. See the preface on page xiii for details.

- Search for further information about epidemiology, physical activity, and exercise at the Centers for Disease Control and Prevention (CDC) website: http://www.cdc.gov

- Search for information about physical activity, health, and the International Society of Physical Activity and Public Health at: http://www.ispah.org

- Search for information about epidemiology and the American College of Sports Medicine at: http://www.acsm.org

- Search for more information about epidemiology, physical fitness, and risk factors at: http://www.fitness.gov

- Search for more information about type 2 diabetes at the U.S. Government health information site: http://www.healthierUS.gov

- Search for more information about physical activity and the built physical environment at: http://www.activelivingbydesign.org

Study Questions

Review the Warm-Up Pre-Test questions you were asked to answer prior to reading Chapter 1. Test yourself once more to determine what you know now that you have completed the chapter.

The questions that follow will help you review this chapter. You will find the answers in the discussions on the pages provided.

1. Define the term *exercise physiology* and how this discipline relates to the field of epidemiology. *p. 3*

2. How does the discipline of epidemiology relate to the field of exercise physiology? *pp. 8–11*

3. Why can exercise be prescribed like medicine? *pp. 11–12*

4. Define the following terms: regular exercise risk factors, predisposition, functional health, and functional fitness. *pp. 5, 6, 17, 22*

5. How much exercise is enough for health? *pp. 14–16*

6. What is the relationship of validity, reliability, and sensitivity to epidemiology research? *pp. 25–26*

7. Provide one example of how your understanding of epidemiology and research findings from this area of exercise science will help prepare you for a career in the areas of Health/Fitness, Medicine, Athletic Performance, or Rehabilitation. *pp. 3, 5*

8. List two ways in which research study designs differ in epidemiological research. *p. 28*

9. Which two methods of exercise would you use to gather epidemiological data about the physical activity behaviors of a study population? Why? *p. 28*

10. Describe how you should use the "scientific method" to improve your critical thinking with regard to being a better exercise physiologist. *pp. 6–8*

Selected References

American College of Sports Medicine. 2010. *ACSM's guidelines for exercise testing and prescription*, 8th ed. Philadelphia: Lippincott Williams & Wilkins.

Choo, J. K. 1975. Genetic studies on walking behavior in *Drosophila melanogaster*. I. Selection and hybridization analysis. *Can. J. Genet. Cytol.* 17:535–542.

Després, J. P. 2005. Our passive lifestyle, our toxic diet, and the atherogenic/diabetogenic metabolic syndrome: Can we afford to be sedentary and unfit? *Circulation* 112:453–455.

Holloszy, J. O. 2004. Adaptations of skeletal muscle mitochondria to endurance exercise: A personal perspective. *Exerc. Sport Sci. Rev.* 32(2):41–43.

Jackson, A. S., X. Sui, J. R. Hébert, T. S. Church, and S. N. Blair. 2009. Role of lifestyle and aging on the longitudinal change in cardiorespiratory fitness. *Arch. Int. Med.* 169(19):1781–1787.

Lightfoot, J. T., L. Leamy, D. Pomp, et al. 2010. Strain screen haplotype association mapping of wheel running in inbred mouse strains. *Jour. Appl. Physiol.*, 109:623–634.

Pate, R. R., M. Pratt, S. N. Blair, et al. 1995. Physical activity and public health. A recommendation from the Centers for Disease Control and Prevention and the American College of Sports Medicine. *JAMA* 273:402–407.

2008 physical activity guidelines for Americans. 2008. Washington, DC: U.S. Department of Health and Human Services. Retrieved from http://www.health.gov/PAGuidelines/

Physical Activity Guidelines Advisory Committee. 2008. *Physical activity guidelines advisory committee report, 2008.* Washington, DC: U.S. Department of Health and Human Services. Retrieved from http://www.health.gov/PAGuidelines/

Raven, P. B., and W. G. Squires. 1989. What is science? *Med. Sci. Sports Exerc.* 21(4):351–352.

Sherwood, L. 2010. *Human physiology,* 7th ed. Belmont, CA: Brooks/Cole-Cengage Learning.

Strong, W. B., R. M. Malina, C. J., Blimkie, et al. 2005. Evidence based physical activity for school-age youth. *J. Pediatr.* 146:732–737.

U.S. Department of Health and Human Services. 1988. *Nutrition and health: A report of the Surgeon General* (DHHS publication [PHS] no. 88-50210). Atlanta, GA: U.S. Department of Health and Human Services, Public Health Service.

U.S. Department of Health and Human Services. 1996. *Physical activity and health: A report of the Surgeon General.* Atlanta, GA: U.S. Department of Health and Human Services, Centers for Disease Control and Prevention, National Center for Chronic Disease Prevention and Health Promotion.

U.S. Department of Health and Human Services, Public Health Service, Centers for Disease Control and Prevention, National Center for Chronic Disease Prevention and Health Promotion, Division of Nutrition and Physical Activity. 1999. *Promoting physical activity: A guide for community action.* Champaign, IL: Human Kinetics.

U.S. Department of Health and Human Services, Public Health Service, Centers for Disease Control and Prevention, National Center for Chronic Disease Prevention and Health Promotion, Division of Nutrition and Physical Activity; Brown, D. R., Heath, G. W., Martin, S. L. 2010. *Promoting physical activity: A guide for community action,* 2nd ed. Campaign, IL: Human Kinetics.

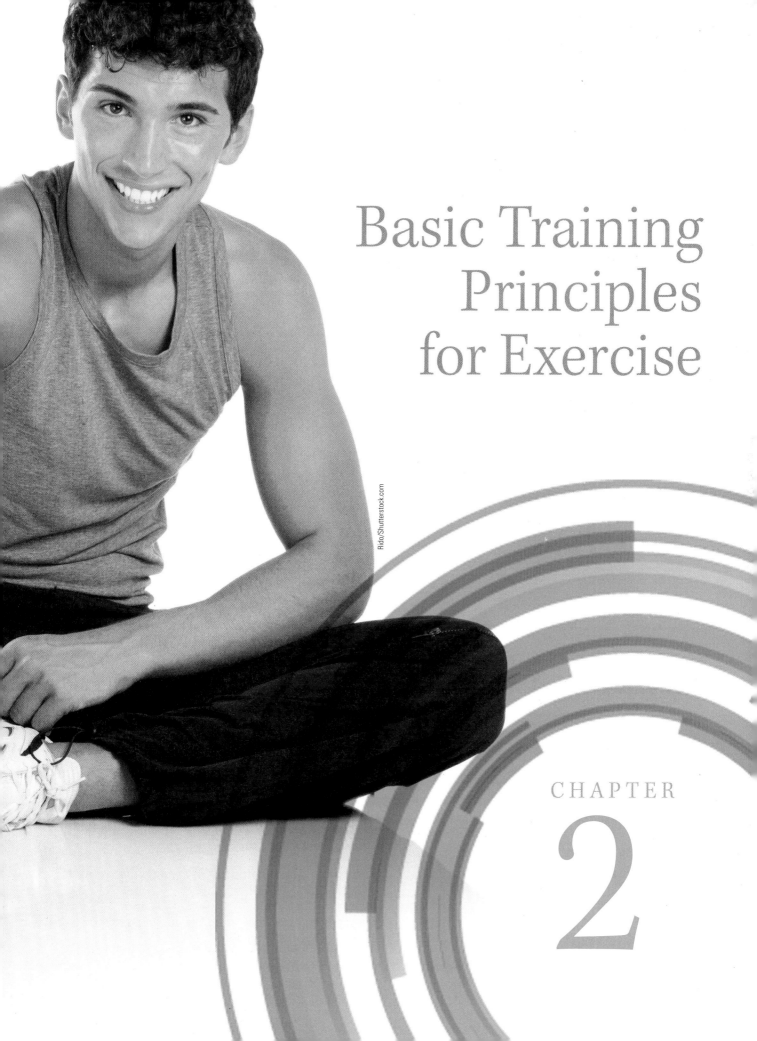

Basic Training
Principles
for Exercise

CHAPTER

2

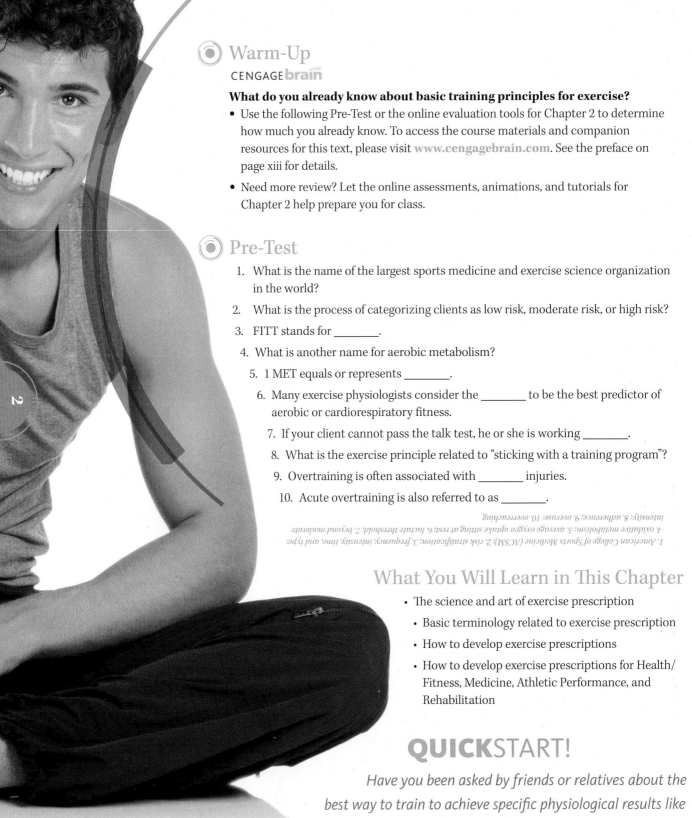

Warm-Up

CENGAGE brain

What do you already know about basic training principles for exercise?

- Use the following Pre-Test or the online evaluation tools for Chapter 2 to determine how much you already know. To access the course materials and companion resources for this text, please visit www.cengagebrain.com. See the preface on page xiii for details.

- Need more review? Let the online assessments, animations, and tutorials for Chapter 2 help prepare you for class.

Pre-Test

1. What is the name of the largest sports medicine and exercise science organization in the world?

2. What is the process of categorizing clients as low risk, moderate risk, or high risk?

3. FITT stands for _____.

4. What is another name for aerobic metabolism?

5. 1 MET equals or represents _____.

6. Many exercise physiologists consider the _____ to be the best predictor of aerobic or cardiorespiratory fitness.

7. If your client cannot pass the talk test, he or she is working _____.

8. What is the exercise principle related to "sticking with a training program"?

9. Overtraining is often associated with _____ injuries.

10. Acute overtraining is also referred to as _____.

1. American College of Sports Medicine (ACSM); 2. risk stratification; 3. frequency, intensity, time, and type; 4. oxidative metabolism; 5. average oxygen uptake sitting at rest; 6. lactate threshold; 7. beyond moderate intensity; 8. adherence; 9. overuse; 10. overreaching

What You Will Learn in This Chapter

- The science and art of exercise prescription
- Basic terminology related to exercise prescription
- How to develop exercise prescriptions
- How to develop exercise prescriptions for Health/Fitness, Medicine, Athletic Performance, and Rehabilitation

QUICKSTART!

Have you been asked by friends or relatives about the best way to train to achieve specific physiological results like weight loss, increasing speed, improving muscular strength, among others? If so, did you feel comfortable about your abilities to provide sound scientific advice, or did you just pass along information that you have heard from others?

Introduction to Basic Training Principles for Exercise

Chapter 1 described the relationship between the field of exercise physiology and exercise epidemiology, and provided insight about research questions related to scientific investigations that seek to clarify the impact of physical activity on health. Indeed, the *1996 Surgeon General's Report,* edited by Dr. Steven Blair, identified "Physical Inactivity" as an independent risk factor for cardiovascular disease, cancer, and non–insulin-dependent diabetes. Furthermore, it has been the combined efforts of exercise epidemiologists and exercise scientists studying the health benefits of exercise that have helped produce the recent *2008 Physical Activity Guideline for Americans* (see Chapter 1). You may be aware of national or international plans such as the U.S. National Physical Activity Plan (see **http://www .physicalactivityplan.org** for more information) and the Toronto Charter for Physical Activity (see **http://www.globalpa .org.uk** for more information) that propose policies for the promotion of healthy active lifestyles for all citizens and are part of exercise promotion advocacy.

In this chapter, you will learn how you can use the scientific principles from exercise physiology to develop prescriptions and recommendations for exercise in the areas of Health/Fitness, Medicine, Athletic Performance, and Rehabilitation. It is important to understand the basics of writing and developing individual **exercise prescriptions** so that you can learn how to apply the physiological principles presented in the remaining chapters to your specific areas of interest. You can also learn more about the specifics of exercise plans for communities by searching online for a sample state plan such as that developed in Texas by using the keywords "Active Texas 2020."

Coaches, therapists, physicians, personal trainers, and others have provided personal exercise prescriptions for individuals and athletes for centuries. The principles of exercise training for designing a program of exercise have been developed based on volumes of scientific research combined with empirical experience reported by researchers and clinicians. Organizations such as the American College of Sports Medicine (ACSM; the largest sports medicine organization in the world) have developed extensive guidelines. For example, the *ACSM Guidelines for Exercise Testing and Prescription* (8th edition, 2011) is used by health/fitness professionals when prescribing exercise.

Although several national agencies and organizations (for example, American Heart Association; American Alliance for Health, Physical Education, Recreation and Dance; ACSM; American Academy of Pediatrics) have made recommendations for appropriate amounts of physical activity and exercise for school-aged youth and adults, it has only been recently that exercise scientists have found more consensus as to how much is needed to promote good health, as well as specific health and performance goals. For example, Fulton et al.'s (2004) review of physical activity and physical fitness recommendations for youths notes that certain national agencies and organizations provided conflicting exercise guidelines and information. The authors also report that, although these organizations have, in general, promoted increased intensities of exercise, the lack of consensus about a consistent level of intensity has created a mixed message, causing confusion among professionals and the general public.

In this chapter, you will learn more about how exercise can be prescribed like medicine based on desired dose–response and its consequent physiological outcome. In addition, you will learn how to apply the

exercise prescriptions Individual or group exercise guides that provide the type, intensity, frequency, and duration of physical activities to achieve personal fitness goals.

principles of designing a program of exercise and how to develop specific training recommendations to achieve specific goals. It will become clear to you that the general principles of exercise prescription can be applied to all populations and individuals (from developing basic functional health across the spectrum of achieving peak performance; see Figure 1.8 in Chapter 1).

HOTLINK *For more information about "Make the Move," the 2010–2011 National Implementation of the U.S. Physical Activity Plan, visit* **http://www.nxtbook.com/nxtbooks/ncppa/make_the_move/index.php.**

(Why do you think it is important to know about basic physiological training principles for optimizing the effects of an exercise program?)

Health Screening before Developing Exercise Prescriptions

Before developing an exercise program, you will often need to make sure that your clients have been evaluated for health risks before they begin a program of exer-

cise that is beyond the level of intensity to which they are accustomed. By initially learning more about the health risks of your clients, you can better promote safe exercise testing and exercise programming, and more effectively control your personal liability as an exercise professional.

However, the *Physical Activity Guidelines Advisory Committee Report 2008* notes, "The protective value of a medical consultation for persons with or without chronic diseases who are interested in increasing their physical activity level is not established." For example, if an adult is planning to start a program of moderate-intensity exercise (like walking briskly at 4 miles/hour, gardening, yard work, dancing, swimming, or golf) by starting slowly (2–3 days/week for 15 minutes) and gradually working up to 150 min/week (the recommended number of min/week for adults to achieve health benefits), they will be at much lower risk for adverse cardiac events or musculoskeletal injuries than someone engaging in high-intensity exercise. Overall, the benefits of exercise outweigh the negative health effects of remaining sedentary.

The ACSM recommends that exercise physiology professionals use **risk stratification** strategies to categorize clients as apparently healthy (low risk), possibly at risk (moderate risk), or at higher risk. The ACSM Risk Stratification Categories are based on health risk factors, like those you learned about in Chapter 1, as well as the presence or absence of chronic disease. The ACSM also provides detailed strategies to help you determine the appropriate guidelines to follow for safely testing or assessing the physical abilities of your clients and whether you need to include or consult medical supervision for exercise prescription or exercise testing, or both.

Figure 2.1 provides a summary of a basic and minimum level of health risk screening that, as an exercise professional, you should consider conducting before developing exercise prescriptions or exercise testing that involves vigorous intensity exercise for your clients. The Physical Activity

risk stratification Strategies to categorize clients as apparently healthy (low risk), possibly at risk (moderate risk), or at higher risk.

Laurent Renault/Shutterstock.com

PAR-Q & YOU

(A Questionnaire for People Aged 15 to 69)

Regular physical activity is fun and healthy, and increasingly more people are starting to become more active every day. Being more active is very safe for most people. However, some people should check with their doctor before they start becoming much more physically active.

If you are planning to become much more physically active than you are now, start by answering the seven questions in the box below. If you are between the ages of 15 and 69, the PAR-Q will tell you if you should check with your doctor before you start. If you are over 69 years of age, and you are not used to being very active, check with your doctor.

Common sense is your best guide when you answer these questions. Please read the questions carefully and answer each one honestly: check YES or NO.

YES	NO	
☐	☐	1. Has your doctor ever said that you have a heart condition <u>and</u> that you should only do physical activity recommended by a doctor?
☐	☐	2. Do you feel pain in your chest when you do physical activity?
☐	☐	3. In the past month, have you had chest pain when you were not doing physical activity?
☐	☐	4. Do you lose your balance because of dizziness or do you ever lose consciousness?
☐	☐	5. Do you have a bone or joint problem (for example, back, knee or hip) that could be made worse by a change in your physical activity?
☐	☐	6. Is your doctor currently prescribing drugs (for example, water pills) for your blood pressure or heart condition?
☐	☐	7. Do you know of <u>any other reason</u> why you should not do physical activity?

If you answered

YES to one or more questions

Talk with your doctor by phone or in person BEFORE you start becoming much more physically active or BEFORE you have a fitness appraisal. Tell your doctor about the PAR-Q and which questions you answered YES.

• You may be able to do any activity you want — as long as you start slowly and build up gradually. Or, you may need to restrict your activities to those which are safe for you. Talk with your doctor about the kinds of activities you wish to participate in and follow his/her advice.

• Find out which community programs are safe and helpful for you.

NO to all questions

If you answered NO honestly to <u>all</u> PAR-Q questions, you can be reasonably sure that you can:

• start becoming much more physically active – begin slowly and build up gradually. This is the safest and easiest way to go.

• take part in a fitness appraisal – this is an excellent way to determine your basic fitness so that you can plan the best way for you to live actively. It is also highly recommended that you have your blood pressure evaluated. If your reading is over 144/94, talk with your doctor before you start becoming much more physically active.

DELAY BECOMING MUCH MORE ACTIVE:
• if you are not feeling well because of a temporary illness such as a cold or a fever – wait until you feel better; or
• if you are or may be pregnant – talk to your doctor before you start becoming more active.

PLEASE NOTE: If your health changes so that you then answer YES to any of the above questions, tell your fitness or health professional. Ask whether you should change your physical activity plan.

<u>Informed Use of the PAR-Q</u>: The Canadian Society for Exercise Physiology, Health Canada, and their agents assume no liability for persons who undertake physical activity, and if in doubt after completing this questionnaire, consult your doctor prior to physical activity.

No changes permitted. You are encouraged to photocopy the PAR-Q but only if you use the entire form.

NOTE: If the PAR-Q is being given to a person before he or she participates in a physical activity program or a fitness appraisal, this section may be used for legal or administrative purposes.

"I have read, understood and completed this questionnaire. Any questions I had were answered to my full satisfaction."

NAME _____

SIGNATURE _____ DATE _____

SIGNATURE OF PARENT _____ WITNESS _____
or GUARDIAN (for participants under the age of majority)

Note: This physical activity clearance is valid for a maximum of 12 months from the date it is completed and becomes invalid if your condition changes so that you would answer YES to any of the seven questions.

FIGURE 2.1 Physical Activity Readiness Questionnaire (PAR-Q) and you. (From Canadian Society for Exercise Physiology. Sample found online at: http://uwfitness.uwaterloo.ca/PDF/par-q.pdf.)

Readiness Questionnaire (PAR-Q), developed by the Canadian Society of Exercise Physiology in 2002, provides basic questions that can be used for self-guided, as well as supervised, exercise programming. As shown in the PAR-Q, if clients respond with a "yes" answer to any of the seven questions, they should consult their physician (or delay becoming more active) before exercising harder or undergoing exercise test screening.

More comprehensive health risk evaluations, which are often required in medically supervised programs, can be found via web links listed at the end of this chapter.

HOTLINK *For more information about the ACSM Guidelines for Exercise Testing and Prescription, visit* **www.acsm.org.**

The Science and Art of Prescribing Physical Activity and Exercise

FITT Frequency, intensity, time, and type of exercise.

frequency How often you work.

intensity How hard you work.

time or duration How long you work.

type The specific type or mode of physical activity or exercise you choose.

goal setting/reality A needs analysis based on specific individual characteristics.

inherent ability Analyzing the genetic or heredity traits of the individual as related to exercise.

intrinsic motivation Encouraging motivation from the client to reinforce positive feedback.

client education Educating clients about goals/outcomes so they can perform more effectively and resist injuries or rehabilitate more effectively.

overload/progression Changing the FITT to improve physiological adaptations.

specificity Understanding the specific physiological adaptations that occur because of the specific demands applied.

special situations Adjusting the exercise program or exercise prescription based on illness, disability, medications, and so on.

trainability Evaluating the rate at which an individual improves for a specific FITT.

periodization A systematic approach to altering program variables (like FITT), which improves training efficiency and specificity, allowing for general adaptations and a decrease in the likelihood of overtraining.

overtraining Engaging in intensities, durations, and frequencies of an exercise program that results in negative physiological effects, which, if continued, have been found to cause clinical depression and overuse injuries such as stress fractures.

detraining The loss of positive physiological effects of participating in a program of exercise after a client stops participating.

restoration Enhancing recovery from a program of exercise.

adherence Developing the client's ability to stick to a program of exercise.

Developing a program (plan) of exercise or exercise prescriptions involves applying both the "science" of exercise physiology and the "art" of exercise physiology. The science is based on the results of thousands of research studies that have reported the significant benefits of following a program of exercise, or exercise prescriptions, designed around specific parameters of frequency, intensity, time, and type (or **FITT**) of exercise.

The "art" of developing an exercise prescription program is based on the application of the empirical experience you have gained personally and from the scientific reports and opinions of experts in the field. However, the exercise programs or exercise prescriptions that you develop will need to account for individual factors such as age, sex, health status, fitness levels, and the goals of the individual. As you gain experience in the field of exercise physiology, you will become more comfortable and successful at developing programs and prescriptions, because you will get more opportunities to apply exercise science principles and learn more about the art of applying these principles.

Applying FITT Principles

The science of writing and developing exercise programs and prescriptions is largely based on the FITT formula, which consists of the following components:

- **Frequency:** how often you work
- **Intensity:** how hard you work
- **Time or duration:** how long you work
- **Type:** the specific type or mode of physical activity or exercise you choose

The art of writing and developing exercise programs and exercise prescriptions primarily involves a consideration of the following factors:

- **Goal setting/reality:** a needs analysis based on specific individual characteristics

- **Inherent ability:** analyzing the genetic or heredity traits of the individual as related to exercise
- **Intrinsic motivation:** encouraging motivation from the client to reinforce positive feedback
- **Client education:** educating clients about goals/outcomes so they can perform more effectively and resist injuries or rehabilitate more effectively
- **Overload/Progression:** changing the FITT to improve physiological adaptations
- **Specificity:** understanding the specific physiological adaptations that occur because of specific demands applied
- **Special Situations:** adjusting the exercise program or exercise prescription based on illness, disability, medications, and so on
- **Trainability:** evaluating the rate at which an individual improves for a specific FITT
- **Periodization:** refers to a systematic approach to altering program variables (like FITT), which improves training efficiency and specificity, allowing for general adaptations and a decrease in the likelihood of overtraining
- **Overtraining:** engaging in intensities, durations, and frequencies of an exercise program that result in negative physiological effects, which, if continued, have been found to cause clinical depression and overuse injuries such as stress fractures
- **Detraining:** the loss of positive physiological effects of participating in a program of exercise after a client stops participating
- **Restoration:** enhancing recovery from a program of exercise
- **Adherence:** developing the client's ability to stick to a program of exercise

The principles of the actual exercise training program are discussed later in this chapter after you have learned more about FITT concepts in the following section.

Components of FITT

To help you learn to apply the FITT concepts to develop an effective exercise program or exercise prescription, we approach the FITT concept by discussing the components in the following order:

1. Type (or mode)
2. Intensity
3. Time (or duration)
4. Frequency

The physiological concepts discussed in the remainder of this chapter are developed further in Chapters 4 through 14.

Type (or mode)

The type of exercise that individuals participate in can be categorized in the following general and specific physiological categories.

General Physical Activity Categories

The general physical activity categories are anaerobic (nonoxidative), aerobic (oxidative), anaerobic and aerobic, static exercise (isometric), and dynamic exercise.

Anaerobic (nonoxidative): Activities that depend heavily on metabolic reactions (or bioenergetics) in muscle cells that do not require oxygen. Anaerobic activities do not allow individuals to reach a true steady state (as you learned in Chapter 1). Anaerobic activities include sprints, many specific sport drills, weight lifting and weight training, as well as other short-term, high-intensity (or explosive) muscle power activities, such as shot put, discus, or hammer throw.

Aerobic (oxidative): Activities that depend heavily on metabolic reactions in muscle cells that do require large amounts of oxygen and allow the individual to reach steady state. Aerobic activities include walking, jogging, swimming, cycling, rowing, and cross country skiing, as well as other longer term, moderate- to high-intensity activities. It is important to remember that some aerobic activities require a minimal amount of sport-specific skills on the part of the participant, whereas others require higher levels of sport-specific skills. For example, walking, hiking, or jogging do not require high levels of skill, whereas participation in swimming, cycling, skiing, and rowing requires higher levels of sport-specific skills.

Anaerobic and Aerobic: Many exercise activities that individuals participate in are both aerobic and anaerobic in nature—for example, tennis, racquetball, Association Football (or Soccer), rugby, field hockey, or lacrosse. All of these activities have components of a program of **"interval training"**, as well as requiring high levels of sport-specific skills.

Interval training activities require participation in a high-intensity (anaerobic) bout of activity followed by participation in a lower intensity (aerobic) bout of activity, or vice versa. Optimizing an interval type training program requires developing an appropriate work–rest interval between the work bouts of the individual training session and between each training session to enable the training adaptations to occur. In Chapters 7 and 8, you will learn more about the cardiovascular adaptations that occur in response to a specific program of exercise.

Static exercise (isometric): Another general category of exercise that relies primarily on nonoxidative energy pathways. A static exercise contraction includes an increase in force generated over a very limited range of motion (ROM). These concepts are described in more detail in Chapter 3.

Dynamic exercise: Activities that depend mostly on oxidative energy pathways involving concentric (shortening) and eccentric (lengthening) muscle contractions that produce work. These concepts are described in more detail in Chapter 3.

interval training Participation in a high-intensity (anaerobic) bout of activity followed by participation in a lower intensity (aerobic) bout of activity, or vice versa.

anaerobic (nonoxidative) Activities that depend heavily on metabolic reactions (or bioenergetics) in muscle cells that do not require oxygen.

static exercise (isometric) A static exercise contraction includes an increase in force generated over a very limited range of motion (ROM).

aerobic (oxidative) Activities that depend heavily on metabolic reactions in muscle cells that do require large amounts of oxygen and allow the individual to reach steady state.

dynamic exercise Activities that depend mostly on oxidative energy pathways involving concentric (shortening) and eccentric (lengthening) muscle contractions that produce work.

Specific Physical Activity Categories

The specific physical activity categories are anaerobic power (peak anaerobic power), anaerobic capacity (mean anaerobic power), aerobic power, and aerobic capacity.

Anaerobic power (peak anaerobic power): Activities that last for less than 10 seconds performed at high intensity with limited amounts of oxygen available to the working muscles. For example, a world-class 100-meter sprinter may only take one breath during the race. Anaerobic power activities might include sprints, **plyometric** movements (quick, powerful muscular movements where the muscle is prestretched before contractions like jumping, resistance ball drills, among others), or resistance training (for example, weight training).

Anaerobic capacity (mean anaerobic power): High-intensity activities that last for longer than 10 seconds and may last up to 2 to 3 minutes. These types of activities depend on the individual's ability to continue using anaerobic energy sources because of a rate limitation in oxygen delivery. These activities include 100- to 800-meter sprints, plyometric drills, sport-specific drills, and other muscular power activities.

Aerobic power: Activities that last 3 to 15 minutes and also require a large delivery of oxygen to be available to the working muscles. These types of activities stress an individual's $\dot{V}O_2$ max (oxygen uptake) and their maximal ability to use oxygen without generating an oxygen debt (see Chapter 7 for more). Aerobic power activities might include running the mile for time, brisk walking up a steep, long hill, and other demanding cardiovascular activities such as running, bicycling, or rowing for 10 to 15 minutes.

Aerobic capacity: Activities that last longer than 15 to 20 minutes and require large amounts of oxygen to be delivered to the working muscles.

These types of activities also stress an individual's ability to work at a high percentage of their $\dot{V}O_2$ max, and also require a maximal ability to use oxygen without generating an oxygen debt (see Chapter 10 for more information). Aerobic capacity activities include cardiorespiratory endurance activities such as running 3 miles, Tour de France bicycling, and participating in a marathon or triathlon.

> Describe three examples of exercises that are primarily anaerobic or dependent on nonoxidative energy pathways? Then name three primarily aerobic exercise activities and three exercise activities that are more equally matched between oxidative and nonoxidative energy demands.

Spectrum of Energy Demands

Table 2.1 contains a variety of common physical activities and exercises that require varying amounts of anaerobic and aerobic energy pathway contributions (percentages) based on estimated metabolic requirements. Figure 2.2 further illustrates the concept of the contributions of the various energy pathways (phosphagens or ATP/CP, anaerobic glycolysis, and aerobic) to exercise. You can use the **spectrum of energy demands** to set up exercise training programs that develop the specific metabolic and physiological adaptations that are required to optimize specific exercise performances.

For example, soccer (two 45-minute halves) is a sport that requires 60 to 70 percent anaerobic (sprinting and specific sport

---

anaerobic power (peak anaerobic power) Activities lasting < 10 seconds performed at high intensity with limited amounts of oxygen available to the working muscles.

plyometric Movements (quick, powerful muscular movements where the muscle is pre-stretched prior to contractions like jumping, resistance ball drills, etc.) or resistance training such as weight training.

anaerobic capacity (mean anaerobic power) High-intensity activities that last for longer than 10 seconds and may last up to 2–3 minutes.

aerobic power Activities that last 3–15 minutes and also require a large delivery of oxygen to be available to the working muscles.

aerobic capacity ($\dot{V}O_2$ max or oxygen uptake) Activities that last longer than 15–20 minutes and require large amounts of oxygen to be delivered to the working muscles.

spectrum of energy demands Continuum that contains a variety of common physical activities and exercises that require varying amounts of anaerobic and aerobic energy pathway contributions (percentages) based on estimated metabolic requirements.

TABLE 2.1 Spectrum of Energy Demands

	Primarily Aerobic (Oxidative) Demands	Mixed	Primarily Anaerobic (Nonoxidative) Demands
Sample physical activities and exercises	Marathon Triathlon Stage of Tour de France	Boxing 800-meter run 200-meter swim Chopping wood Carrying 20 pounds upstairs	100-meter sprint Jumping rope Shoveling heavy snow
Aerobic (percent)	100	50	very low
Anaerobic (percent)	very low	50	100
Time	2–3 hours	2–3 minutes	1–5 seconds

(© Cengage Learning 2013)

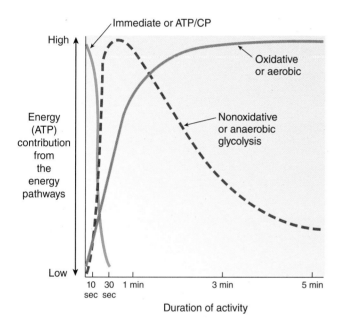

FIGURE 2.2 **Contributions of energy pathways to physical activities and exercise.**
(From Hoeger, W. W. K., and S. A. Hoeger. 2010. Figure 3.13 in *Lifetime physical fitness & wellness*, 11th ed. Belmont, CA: Brooks/Cole-Cengage Learning.)

skills) and 30 to 40 percent aerobic (continuous movement) energy contributions for most participants. However, goalies would primarily participate in activities that require mostly anaerobic exercise (sprinting, blocking, and kicking). Therefore, soccer coaches who are working with highly skilled, competitive athletes would be wise to vary their exercise training programs based on the specific energy requirements by position versus a general training program stressing the specific energy demands of the sport. Chapters 3 through 10 provide a more in-depth understanding of the energy production and physiological requirements in responding to the nonoxidative and oxidative components of a program of exercise.

Intensity

The intensity of exercise can be determined in a variety of ways depending on whether the physical activity is categorized as more oxidative or nonoxidative in nature. Intensity of exercise is the most important variable relative to the amount of caloric expenditure per minute, hour, day, or week of the FITT variables described in this section.

Intensities are often classified in absolute (energy or work required to do an activity without accounting for the physiological capacity of an individual) or relative (takes into account a person's exercise capacity like a percentage of their aerobic power [$\dot{V}O_2$ max]) terms.

Absolute intensity can be expressed as kcal/min, **metabolic equivalents (METs),** or like walking 3 miles/hour or jogging at 6 miles/hour (see discussion of methods to determine intensity for more details). For resistance exercise, absolute intensity is expressed as the amount of weight lifted or force exerted (for example, pounds, kilograms). Absolute intensity also can be classified into various categories, for example, light, moderate, hard, and very hard.

Relative intensity might be expressed as a percentage of a client's aerobic power ($\dot{V}O_2$ max) or $\dot{V}O_2$ reserve ($\dot{V}O_2$ max – resting $\dot{V}O_2$), as a percentage of a person's measured heart rate or heart rate reserve (maximum heart rate – resting heart rate [RHR]), as a perceived exertion rating (how hard a client feels he or she is working from light to very hard), or as a percentage of 1 repetition maximum (maximum one can lift in one trial).

The intensity of exercise has traditionally been expressed in relative terms (for example, 60–70 percent of $\dot{V}O_2$ max) since the 1970s. However, in nearly all large prospective observational studies, exercise intensities are expressed in absolute terms without accounting for each client's exercise capacity. To allow for the comparison of the dose–response data of exercise on functional health, fitness, and performance, you should learn the concept presented in Table 2.2, which shows how the absolute intensity (for example, moderate intensity) varies inversely to the maximal oxygen uptake (or $\dot{V}O_2$ max) of a client.

Figure 2.3 shows that for a highly fit client ($\dot{V}O_2$ max of 14 METs) who walks at 3 miles/hour, the client's relative intensity is 24 percent of max (light), but for someone who has a 4 MET $\dot{V}O_2$ max, the relative intensity is 83 percent of max, or hard. For those with a low aerobic capacity (4 METs), walking at 4 miles/hour (requiring a 5 MET absolute intensity) exceeds their aerobic capacity, and they can maintain the pace only for limited amounts of time because of the higher anaerobic energy costs of the activity.

For aerobic/dynamic activities such as walking, jogging, swimming, and cycling, intensity can be determined by using one of the following methods based on required intensity.

● TABLE 2.2 Classifications of Physical Activity and Exercise Intensity

				Endurance Type Activity								
				Intensity (METs and % $\dot{V}O_2$ max) in Healthy Adults Differing in $\dot{V}O_2$ max								
	Relative Intensity			Resistance Type Exercise								
Intensity	% $\dot{V}O_2R^*$ % HRR	% HR max[†]	RPE[‡]	$\dot{V}O_2$ max = 12 METs (METs)	$\dot{V}O_2$ max = 12 METs [% $\dot{V}O_2$ max)[§]	$\dot{V}O_2$ max = 10 METs (METs)	$\dot{V}O_2$ max = 10 METs (% $\dot{V}O_2$ max)	$\dot{V}O_2$ max = 8 METs (METs)	$\dot{V}O_2$ max = 8 METs (% $\dot{V}O_2$ max)	$\dot{V}O_2$ max = 5 METs (METs)	$\dot{V}O_2$ max = 5 METs (% $\dot{V}O_2$ max)	Relative Intensity (% 1RM)[¶]
Very light	<20	<50	<10	<3.2	<27	<2.8	<28	<2.4	<30	<1.8	<36	<30
Light	20–39	50–63	10–11	3.2–5.3	27–44	2.8–4.5	28–45	2.4–3.7	30–47	1.8–2.5	36–51	30–49
Moderate	40–59	64–76	12–13	5.4–7.5	45–62	4.6–6.3	46–63	3.8–5.1	48–64	2.6–3.3	52–67	50–69
Hard	60–84	77–93	14–16	7.6–10.2	63–85	6.4–8.6	64–86	5.2–6.9	65–86	3.4–4.3	68–87	70–84
Very hard	≥85	≥94	17–19	≥10.3	≥86	≥8.7	≥87	≥7.0	≥87	≥4.4	≥88	≥85
Maximal	100	100	20	12	100	10	100	8	100	5	100	100

*% $\dot{V}O_2R$ = percent of oxygen uptake reserve; % HRR = percent of heart rate reserve.
[†]% HR max = 0.7305 (% $\dot{V}O_2$ max) + 29.95; values based on 10-MET group.
[‡]Borg rating of perceived exertion 6–20 scale.
[§]% $\dot{V}O_2$ max = [(100% − % $\dot{V}O_2R$) METmax^{-1}] + % $\dot{V}O_2R$.
[¶]RM = repetitions maximum, the greatest weight that can be moved once in good form.
Adapted from Howley, E. 2001. Type of activity: resistance, aerobic and leisure versus occupational physical activity. *Med. Sci. Sports Exerc.* 33(6 Suppl):S364–S369.

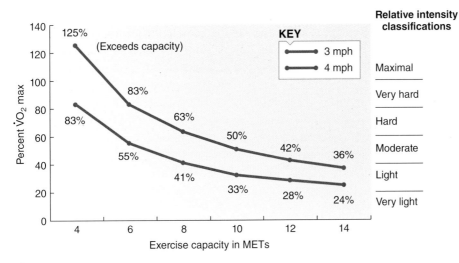

Aerobic/Dynamic Activity Intensity Determination Methods

Percentage of Maximum Heart Rate

The **percentage of maximum heart rate (% MHR)** method uses the simple prediction of maximum heart rate (MHR): 220 − age × percentage of intensity desired. For example, if the goal is to work at 50 to 70 percent of MHR and the person is 25 years old, you would have: 220 − 25 = 195 × 0.5 and 195 × 0.7 or a target heart rate (THR) between 97.5 and ~100 beats per minute (bpm) to 136.5 and 140 bpm. The error involved with predicting MHR using this method is, on average, ±10 beats, but varies greatly with age and can produce errors for other intensity recommendations (see percentage of maximum heart rate reserve [% HHR] and % $\dot{V}O_2$ max sections later in this chapter) that use MHR as a calculation factor. Another popular and more precise method (less error of predicting MHR) is achieved by using the following equation: MHR = 209 − 0.7 × age. The percentage of MHR method described earlier works best for beginning exercisers or those who are at higher health risk because it is more conservative and yields lower intensities than the other methods described later.

HOTLINK *For more information about exercise prescription and ACSM certifications, visit* **www .acsm.org**.

Percentage of Maximum Heart Rate Reserve

The **percentage of maximum heart rate reserve (% HHR)** method also uses the simple prediction of maximum heart rate (MHR) as 220 − age, but then requires that resting heart rate (RHR) be considered in the following equation: MHR reserve = MHR − RHR; then THR = (MHR − RHR) × (desired percentage) + RHR. For a 25-year-old with an RHR of 70 and who works at 50 to 70 percent of HHR, you would have: THR = (195 − 70) × 0.5 + 70 = 112.5 or ~115 bpm and THR = (195 − 70) × 0.7 = 157.5 or ~160 bpm for a THR range (or zone) of 115 to 160 bpm. This calculation is sometimes called the *Karvonen formula,* because Dr. Martti J. Karvonen authored the original publication identifying the efficacy of the formula. This method is often used by personal trainers and coaches to help clients determine a THR zone and specific training intensities to acquire individual goals.

Percentage of Maximal Oxygen Uptake

The **percentage of maximal oxygen uptake (%$\dot{V}O_2$ max)** method uses a simple percentage calculation from an individual's measured, or estimated, $\dot{V}O_2$ max. For example, if the goal is to train at 70 percent of $\dot{V}O_2$ max and the person's $\dot{V}O_2$ max is 50 ml·kg^{-1}·min^{-1} (or ~14 METs), you would use the calculation: 50 ml/kg/min × 0.7 = 35 ml·kg^{-1}·min^{-1} (or 10 METs). The sim-

kilocalories/minute (kcal/min) Method that requires you be able to accurately measure or estimate your client's $\dot{V}O_2$ max (or peak $\dot{V}O_2$) and then use the following conversion factor: 1 liter of oxygen consumed is approximately equal to 5 kcal/min.

ple way of achieving this training (target $\dot{V}O_2$ [T$\dot{V}O_2$] of 35 ml·kg^{-1}·min^{-1} [or 10 METs]) is to again use the linear relationship between heart rate and oxygen uptake ($\dot{V}O_2$), and refer back to your $\dot{V}O_2$ maximal exercise test and relate the heart rate measured at the 70 percent $\dot{V}O_2$ max to use as the training heart rate. The method described earlier works best when you can accurately measure or estimate your client's $\dot{V}O_2$ max (or peak $\dot{V}O_2$). This method is popular in clinical and athletic performance settings (see Chapters 8 and 10 for more information about $\dot{V}O_2$ max or peak $\dot{V}O_2$).

Metabolic Equivalents

The METs method is based on the concept of identifying the work intensity as the metabolic equivalents, expressed in METs, where the resting metabolic rate is defined as 1 MET.

In healthy adults, 1 MET = 3.5 ml·kg^{-1}·min^{-1}. Hence for any activity above rest, the metabolic energy used can be expressed as a multiple of the resting energy. For example, an activity that requires three times the metabolic energy to perform will be identified as costing 3×1 MET = 3 METs. Usually a percentage of the maximal METs achieved on a maximal exercise test evaluation is used to determine an initial or follow-up exercise training intensity. For example, if an individual had achieved a workload of 10 METs at maximal effort during the test, to have the person train at 50 percent of his or her maximum, you can help the person select activities that require a 5 MET level. You can also use the linear relationship between heart rate and $\dot{V}O_2$ to predict the heart rate needed to work at 5 METs. The terms *MET-minutes* (exercising at 5 METs for 20 minutes equals 100 MET-minutes) and *MET-hours* (working at 5 METs for 2.5 hours equals 12.5 MET-hours of exercise) are also used in the *2008 Physical Activity Guidelines for Americans* to help identify the total volume of exercise completed. A basic recommendation is that all adults acquire between 500 and 1000 MET-minutes for various health benefits or between 8.3 and 16.6 MET-hours per week.

lactate threshold (LT) Method that requires that you be able to accurately measure or estimate your client's lactate threshold (LT)—the point at which the body recruits greater percentages of intermediate and fast twitch muscle fibers via anaerobic metabolic pathways, and the accumulation of lactic acid occurs when the lactate clearance becomes less than the lactate production.

ventilatory threshold (Tvent) When the minute ventilation increases exponentially above a threshold workload, or $\dot{V}O_2$, at which point there is an extra stimulus from the central and peripheral chemoreceptors that are sensitive to arterial carbon dioxide (CO_2) and hydrogen ion concentration (pH) to increase ventilation.

Kilocalories per Minute (or per Hour)

The **kilocalories/minute** (kcal/min; or per hour) method requires that you be able to accurately measure or estimate your client's $\dot{V}O_2$ max (or peak $\dot{V}O_2$) and then use the following conversion factor: 1 liter of oxygen consumed is approximately equal to 5 kcal/min. For example, if you wanted your client, who weighs 70 kilograms (kg), to work at 25 ml·kg^{-1}·min^{-1} (7 METs), you could calculate his caloric expenditure as follows: 25 ml·kg^{-1}·min^{-1} × weight/kg × 1000 = oxygen uptake in liters/min or 25 × 70/1000 = 1.75 liters. Then, by conversion to kcal/min, you would have 1.75 liters/min × 5 kcal/min = 8.75 kcal/min, or 525 kcal/hour (8.75 × 60). The method described earlier is probably most effective for clients who are engaged in weight loss (>5 percent of body weight loss) or weight maintenance (< ±3 percent of body weight) programs.

Lactate Threshold

The **lactate threshold (LT)** method requires that you be able to accurately measure or estimate your client's LT—the point at which the body recruits greater percentages of intermediate and fast twitch muscle fibers via anaerobic metabolic pathways, and the accumulation of lactic acid occurs when the lactate clearance becomes less than the lactate production (see Chapter 10 for a more detailed description of the LT). Although many exercise physiologists consider this method as the best predictor for determining aerobic exercise performance, it is more complex and usually limited to use with clinical and athletic performance settings. For example, healthy, aerobically untrained individuals can typically perform exercise at 50 percent of their LT, whereas healthy, aerobically trained individuals can typically work at 75 to 90 percent of their LT. Again, to actually predict the training workload, one needs to identify the LT in relation to the individual's heart rate measured during a progressive increase in workload maximal exercise stress test (see Chapter 10).

Ventilatory Threshold

The **ventilatory threshold (Tvent)** method requires that you be able to accurately measure or estimate your client's ventilatory and respiratory gas exchange response to a progressive increase in workload exercise test to maximum. The Tvent is identified as the workload at which an exponential increase in ventilation occurs. This method is challenging to measure and determine without sophisticated laboratory equipment and is usually limited to use in clinical and athletic performance settings. For example, healthy, aerobically untrained individuals can typically perform exercise at 50 percent of their Tvent, whereas healthy, aerobically trained individuals can typically work at 75 percent of their Tvent.

Rating of Perceived Exertion Scales

The **rating of perceived exertion (RPE)** scales method requires your clients to rate "how hard" they are working during exercise. Figure 2.4 illustrates scales developed by Dr. Gunnar Borg to estimate intensity based on people's overall awareness of their body cues such as how hard they are breathing, their heart rate, how much muscle discomfort they have, and so on.

The perceived exertion scale (RPE) assigns a numerical value to different levels of perceived exertion. A rating of "6" from Figure 2.4 (using the 6–20 scale) would be "no exertion at all," similar to being at rest, whereas a rating of "20" would indicate working at one's maximum level of exertion. In the development of the scale, it was decided that a heart rate of 60 bpm was equivalent to an RPE score of "6," a heart rate of 70 bpm = "7," and so on up to a heart rate of 200 bpm being equivalent to an RPE score of "20." This rating scale appears to be valid for 90 percent of the population, regardless of an individual's fitness.

If you were exercising with a heart rate of 100 bpm, what would you expect your RPE to be?

Notably, of all the physiological variables that appear to be self-monitored by elite endurance athletes during their train-

rating of perceived exertion (RPE) Method that requires your clients to rate "how hard" they are working during exercise.

Category and Category-Ratio Scales for Ratings of Perceived Exertion*

Category scale	Category-ratio scale†		
6	0	Nothing at all	"No I"
7 Very, very light	0.3		
8	0.5	Extremely weak	Just noticeable
9 Very light	0.7		
10	1	Very weak	
11 Fairly light	1.5		
12	2	Weak	Light
13 Somewhat hard	2.5		
14	3	Moderate	
15 Hard	4		
16	5	Strong	Heavy
17 Very hard	6		
18	7	Very strong	
19 Very, very hard	8		
20	9		
	10	Extremely strong	"Strongest I"
	11		
	•	Absolute maximum	Highest possible

*Copyright Gunnar Borg. Reproduced with permission. For correct usage of the Borg scales, it is necessary to follow the administration and instructions given in Borg G. Borg's Perceived Exertion and Pain Scales. Champaign, IL; Human Kinetics, 1998.

†Note: On the Category-ratio scale, "I" represents intensity.

FIGURE 2.4 Borg ratings of perceived exertion scales. (From Borg, G. Psychological Bases of Physical Exertion, in *Medicine and Science in Sports and Exercise,* 14:377–81, 1982. Used by permission.)

ing and competition endurance events, ventilation is primarily linked to perception of effort. Ventilation provides an internal cue to the "perception center" of the brain. Hence it is the ventilation's link to the individual's RPE that appears to be linked to the actual intensity of exercise. This ventilation helps recreational joggers identify when they are working too hard.

For example, one piece of advice Dr. William P. Morgan, the renowned psychobiologist of exercise, used to tell the recreational jogger was, "If you could hold a conversation while running, you were working below your Tvent, and if you could only muster up a 'grunt' in response, you were working above your Tvent." This relationship is so strong that it is now being used by cardiac rehabilitation exercise leaders so that the patient can monitor his or her own intensity of work by using the RPE scale. The method described earlier works best for the client with successful participation experience in regular exercise. This method requires that your clients understand that the intensity of exercise that can be sustained is highly dependent on how they feel. The RPE (0–10+) scale shown in Figure 2.4 is best used for rating occupational tasks or exercise involving more static muscle contractions.

Talk Test

A final method for monitoring intensity of primarily aerobic activities is the simple **"talk test,"** or the ability of your client to carry on a conversation during exercise (obviously this would not apply to some activities like swimming). This method is based on the more complex Tvent method described previously. For example, if your client can talk with only slight discomfort during his or her exercise sessions, then he or she is probably working at an RPE of between 11 and 16 (light to vigorous; refer back to Figure 2.4). If your client cannot carry on a conversation during exercise sessions, he or she is probably working harder than is necessary—unless trying to achieve an athletic goal.

Anaerobic/Static Activity Determination Methods

Anaerobic/static exercise usually involves three different types of physical activity:

1. Resistance work such as machine or free weights, elastic bands, or moving one's own body weight
2. Sprints or agility drills
3. Plyometric activities

The following methods are commonly used to determine intensity for activities such as weight lifting, sprinting, and plyometrics:

1 repetition max (1RM or 5RM, 10RM): This method is based on the weight lifting concept of determining what your client can lift maximally in one lift such as a standard bench press lift. For example, a 20-year-old healthy man can, on average, lift his body weight, whereas a healthy woman of the same age would usually be able to lift approximately 60 percent of her body weight.

Because determining a 1RM can be challenging for a beginning lifter or an elderly client, it often is easier to determine a 5RM (a weight that can be lifted 5 times maximum) or 10RM (a weight that can be lifted 10 times maximum). If you have the performance of a client's 5RM or 10RM, you can estimate that client's 1RM by a variety of methods (see Chapter 3 for more information on neuromuscular training). A 5RM performance usually represents 85 percent of a client's 1RM, whereas a 10RM performance represents about 75 percent of a 1RM.

Percent of maximal speed: Coaches who have their athletes perform sprint drills often use this method. The intensity of sprint drills might be set at approximately 90 percent of an athlete's maximal 40- or 100-yard dash speed.

Volume of workload: This method is also often used by coaches when their

talk test Method for monitoring intensity that evaluates the ability of your client to carry on a conversation during exercise.

1 repetition maximum (1 RM) Method of monitoring intensity based on the weight lifting concept of determining what your client can lift maximally in one lift such as a standard bench press lift.

percent of maximal speed Method of monitoring intensity often used by coaches who have their athletes run at a percentage of their maximal speed (like 90%).

volume of workload Another method often used by coaches when their athletes perform plyometric exercises that include a sport-specific FITT.

athletes perform plyometric exercises. Typically, plyometric exercises are sport-specific, and you should refer to sport-specific literature (like that from reliable sources on the Internet) to determine the intensity for these activities. Generally, however, plyometrics should be performed at high intensities (≥90 percent of maximum effort) no more than twice a week, and with the number of repetitions for each exercise governed by the total volume of work (or FITT) that does not interfere with the individual's recovery (restoration).

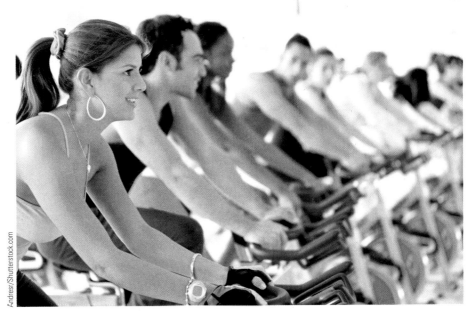
Andresr/Shutterstock.com

HOTLINK *For more information about exercise prescription and ACSM certifications, search* http://www.acsm.org, http://www.nsca-lift.org, *or the commercial websites at* http://www.exrx.net, http://www.brianmac.co.uk, *or* http://www.topendsports.com.

Time (or Duration)

The time (duration) of exercise can be determined depending on whether the physical activity is categorized as more aerobic or anaerobic in nature and based on the client's goals. Table 2.3 provides some general recommendations for determining the duration of various types of exercise.

Frequency

The frequency of exercise can be determined depending on whether the physical activity is categorized as more aerobic or anaerobic in nature and based on the client's goals. Table 2.4 provides some general recommendations for determining the frequency of various types of exercise activities.

● **TABLE 2.3 Time (Duration) General Recommendations**

Type of Activity	Health/Fitness	Medicine	Athletics	Rehabilitation
Aerobic	20–60 minutes	20–30 minutes	20–120 minutes	Specific to the injury
Anaerobic	20–30 minutes	20–30 minutes	20–120 minutes	Specific to the injury
Aerobic/ Anaerobic	Specific to goals	Specific to goals	Specific to goals	Specific to goals

The duration or number of minutes of exercise can be acquired continuously or accumulated in several bouts per day with a preferred minimum of 10 minutes per bout.

● **TABLE 2.4 Frequency General Recommendations**

Type of Activity	Health/Fitness	Medicine	Athletics	Rehabilitation
Aerobic	3–5 days	3–5 days	5–7 days	Specific to the injury
Anaerobic	2–3 days	2–3 days	3–4 days	Specific to the injury
Aerobic/ Anaerobic	Specific to goals	Specific to goals	Specific to goals	Specific to goals

The duration of minutes of exercise should be accumulated over several days per week with a preferred minimum participation rate of 3 to 5 days.

The Art of Applying Specific Exercise Principles

In this section, you will learn how to apply various exercise principles. The way in which you apply each of the exercise principles should be based on your client's goals and needs for developing health/fitness, medicine, athletic performance, or rehabilitation. For example, Figure 2.5 illustrates an example of how intensity, duration, and frequency (volume of training) might be optimized for aerobic training (achieving training zone) to move from being sedentary to obtaining basic functional health and beyond. As the volume of training increases, so do the adverse risks of exercise, such as orthopedic injuries, cardiovascular risks, and lowered immune responses. This model was developed by M. J. Karvonen in the 1950s (Karvonen et al. 1957) when he trained six male students ages 20 to 23 at various intensities, durations, and frequencies. Notice in Figure 2.5 that although there is a window that highlights a zone of optimal improvement, benefits can be gained at all levels of intensities, durations, and frequencies. In fact, the *Physical Activity Guidelines Advisory Committee Report of 2008* supports this concept that some physical activity is better than none and too much leads to problems like increased risks for orthopedic injuries, upper respiratory infections, and depressed immune function. Thus, your clients' fitness outcomes will vary based on how you design their exercise programs.

Training Principles

Goal Setting/Reality Principle

The goal setting/reality principle involves setting realistic and obtainable goals for your clients based on their needs (health/fitness, medicine, athletics, or rehabilitation). You should use the concepts outlined in the Stages of Change model described in Chapter 1 to guide you in helping clients set and adjust their exercise goals. An athletic application of this principle might involve coaching an athlete to understand his or her realistic chances of performing as a starter versus a successful substitute performer.

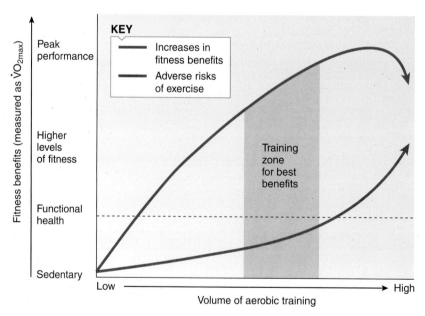

Functional health = *2008 Physical Activity Guidelines for Americans* (Adults; 150 minutes per week)

FIGURE 2.5 Achieving the benefits of training. (© Cengage Learning 2013)

Inherent Ability Principle

The inherent ability principle involves the impact that genetics plays in developing your client's health/fitness and athletic ability. Recent studies suggest that an individual's genetics accounts for between 20 and 60 percent of many health/fitness- and athletic-related performance variables. Although the genetics of your client may predetermine how much they can improve with training, one can still achieve significant improvements (positive overall impact on epigenetic markers as you learned in Chapter 1) if they are provided with quality exercise prescriptions.

Intrinsic Motivation Principle

The intrinsic motivation principle refers to the importance of internal, or intrinsic, motivation on the ability of your client to achieve exercise success. Although many exercise professionals believe that they are important individual motivators for their clients' eventual success, in reality, they are only providing a positive environment for their clients, who must become intrinsically motivated to achieve true personal success and self-responsibility for their exercise behaviors.

Client Education Model Principle

The client education model principle refers to the need to encourage clients to become better educated about their own health/fitness, medicine, athletics, and rehabilitation issues. To be a successful exercise physiologist and health/fitness professional, you must become a good educator and teach your clients based on effective models that motivate them and mentally reinforce positive training principles. For example, Figure 2.6 illustrates an example of an educational model that might be used for a middle-school client who is sedentary but needs to become involved in a regular exercise program.

Physical Assessment Principle

The physical assessment principle refers to the need for you to evaluate the physical abilities of your clients based on their goals and needs before you design their program. The depth of your evaluation will need to be individually based (although you will often work with a team or group of clients), and the results should be shared with your clients for future goal setting, as well as for reviewing barriers to success. Physical assessments are valuable for col-

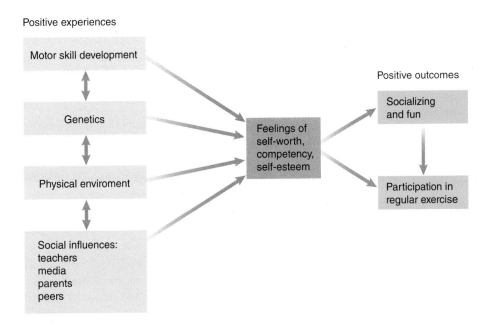

FIGURE 2.6 Client education model (young teen model). (© Cengage Learning 2013)

lecting baseline fitness data and provide an important reference for any future injury rehabilitation needs.

Overload/Progression Principle

The overload/progression principle refers to the need to determine when and how to change the FITT of training. The overload principle suggests that improvements occur by imposing new and higher training demands on your clients to ensure that they are successfully adapting to training (**overcompensation**). Obviously, adaptations do not always occur, so you must learn that it is unwise and often disastrous to change all parts of the FITT at one time. Although empirical evidence is available to use for sport-specific adjustments to overload, you should consider many variables before you change a client's FITT. For example, factors to consider might be whether your client is trying to maintain a current level of fitness or trying to improve one aspect more than another. As you become more familiar with each client and his or her adaptive response to a program of exercise, you will become better at your art. Figure 2.7 illustrates the general aspects of the overload/progression principle.

Specificity Principle

The specificity principle refers to the consistent observation that specific adapta-

tions occur based on the specific neuromuscular demands designed into the program of exercise. When you design an exercise program for a client, you should think specifically about how he or she will need to train. For example, if your client is engaged in a resistance training program, you should provide guidelines on such specifics as what load (force) is needed, repetition to recovery time (duration), the cadence of movement (velocity), the range of motion required, and exercise type. This principle is also often referred to as the SAID principle, or specific adaptations to imposed demands, and provides the basis for the periodization principle (see later in this chapter).

Special Situations Principle

The special situations principle refers to the need to recognize when to change or modify an exercise program based on new challenges or changing situations. For example, these special situations may include injury, illness, medications, lack of recovery, or symptoms of overtraining. These special situations will allow you to educate yourself and your client about the individual adaptations and limitations that occur with the revised exercise program.

Trainability Principle

The trainability principle refers to one's ability to adapt to training stimuli. Trainability involves both genetic ability, in terms of rate of adaptation and maximum potential for adaptation. Figure 2.8 illustrates the various rates and levels of trainability or adaptation that your clients might achieve. The red line represents a curve of improvement that many exercise professionals expect to see; however, there are numerous variations in progression. For some, small improvements occur very early or very late; others will see large early improvements, which then may plateau. This **training plateau** is a normal period during training when little, if any, improvement occurs. It is important for exercise professionals to be able to recognize this phe-

overcompensation The overload principle where improvements occur by imposing new and higher training demands on your client to ensure that they are successfully adapting to training.

training plateau Normal period of time during training when little, if any, improvement occurs.

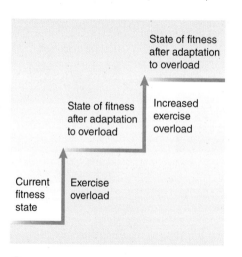

FIGURE 2.7 Overload principle (overcompensation). (From Hales, D. 2009. Figure 5.3 in *An invitation to health.* Belmont, CA: Brooks/Cole-Cengage Learning.)

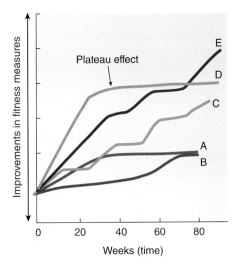

A–E = different individuals

FIGURE 2.8 Trainability principle and plateau effect. (© Cengage Learning 2013)

nomenon so that they can help their clients stay motivated and engaged in their exercise programs, particularly if they have achieved basic functional health status, rather than getting bored and "giving up" their training (becoming sedentary). You will need to change your client's exercise program to break through training plateaus by using the periodization principle that is described next.

Periodization Principle

The periodization principle refers to a systematic approach to altering program variables (for example, FITT), which improves training efficiency and specificity, allowing for general adaptations, and decreasing the chances of overtraining. Figure 2.9 illustrates typical stages of periodization or progress in fitness levels from being sedentary over 40 weeks of participation. Based on the behavioral change model (you will need to keep assessing the amount of change between each stage) from Chapter 1, a client might have an initial stage of 6 to 8 weeks, an improvement stage of 9 to 30 weeks, and a maintenance phase beginning with week 31.

In another example, a periodization plan for an elite athlete might include an overall seasonal plan. Within the seasonal plan or macrocycle, you might include mesocycles (~3-month goals) and microcycles (~4- to 6-week goals) and periods (1–4 weeks) of "active rest" (recreational exercise and weight maintenance without a competition focus) to optimize the training process. You probably experienced the periodization in your own sports participation, if your coach had different training processes and goals

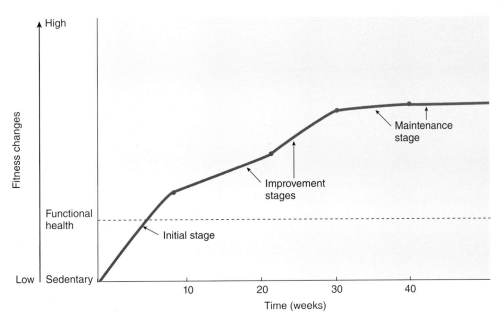

Functional health = *2008 Physical Activity Guidlines for Americans* (Adults; 150 minutes per week)

FIGURE 2.9 Periodization principle (an example). (© Cengage Learning 2013)

overreaching Planned acute over-training that lasts no more than 2–3 weeks.

overuse Participating in too much exercise, where an individual cannot adapt to the workload, often leading to injuries and addictive behaviors.

for preseason, in season, and off-season. Emerging research also supports undulating and non-linear volume periodization programs as methods to further enhance performance. Periodization is influenced by several factors:

- The client's initial fitness level—usually the less fit person will make the greatest initial gains
- The client's trainability level
- The rate at which overload is changed
- The client's specific short- and long-term goals

HOTLINK *For more information about programs of periodization like linear, general to specific, undulating, and so forth, see* **http://www.nsca-lift.org**.

Overtraining Principle

The overtraining principle refers to the negative effects that can occur if your client is too active or exercises too much. These negative effects can produce abnormal physical and psychological stresses on your body. Overtraining is associated with increased **overuse** injuries (overdoing it and causing muscle/skeletal problems) and addictive behaviors (for example, believing you will lose fitness if you miss a day of conditioning). It is important to recognize the symptoms of overtraining. These symptoms include:

- Chronic fatigue—feeling tired all the time, especially after just starting a training program or overloading the body; going too fast, too soon, too often!
- Constant muscle soreness—continues day after day without much relief
- Insomnia—feeling exhausted but cannot sleep
- Rapid weight loss—unusual and probably caused by decreased appetite with increased exercise
- Elevated morning resting pulse rate—many physiologists suggest this is a marker of overtraining if ~10 beats above normal resting values
- Mental stress or burnout—loss of interest
- Addictive personality disorder

Overtraining can occur over a planned "acute" (that is, short, also called **overreaching**) period, or it can be "chronic" (longer period of time). An example of acute overtraining is two-a-day or three-a-day practices that an athlete might do for 2 to 3 weeks in the preseason for football or volleyball. In this case, the acute overtraining is scheduled to be an intense learning and practice period for sports preparation. This type of overtraining can last only 2 or 3 weeks, because most athletes would burn out and increase their overuse injury rate if they continued to overload themselves at these high levels.

Chronic overtraining is more serious than acute overtraining. Chronic overtraining occurs over several weeks or months and often leads to serious mental burnout distress. It is important to recognize the symptoms of overtraining early in a personal fitness program before your client burns out. Most people will not recover from chronic overtraining by just taking a few days off from their personal fitness programs. It can require several weeks or months to recover from chronic overtraining, and it may require special counseling for someone who is prone to an addictive behavior pattern.

Detraining Principle

The detraining principle refers to the loss of health or physiological training benefits that have resulted from a regular program of exercise. For example, if your clients get ill and have to remain in bed for several days with no activity, you will notice that they are weaker when they restart exercising. Figure 2.10 illustrates a normal training cycle and the positive changes in a physiological variable, as well as the detraining changes that occur when training stops. Figure 2.10 also illustrates that once training is resumed, the clients' pretraining fitness levels are regained slowly over time. See Chapters 3 and 8 for more details on specific detraining responses for muscular strength, muscular endurance, and cardiorespiratory endurance.

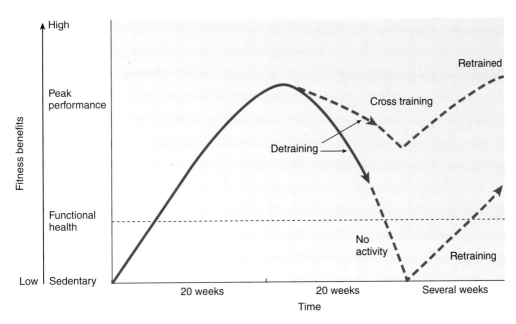

Functional health = 2008 Physical Activity Guidlines for Americans (Adults; 150 minutes per week)

● FIGURE 2.10 **Theory of detraining and retraining.** (© Cengage Learning 2013)

Most of the benefits of exercise—that is, improved functional health, enhanced self-esteem, reduced stress—become progressively diminished over time if your client undergoes an extended period of detraining. It is important to recognize that the benefits may be lost at different rates depending on the individual characteristics of the client. For example, if your clients detrain by reducing their aerobic workouts for 4 weeks, you may notice that their cardiovascular fitness level has declined significantly, whereas their strength may not have decreased by the same degree. You should also realize that clients do not lose their fitness benefits in a day or two, or even three. Because of this, it is always a good idea to have clients take off a day or two, especially if they are unusually tired, sick, or have significant conflicts of schedule. In fact, you should schedule rest/recovery days for your clients as part of their normal exercise plan.

You may also find that it is beneficial to have clients "cross-train" (that is, vary activities and exercises day to day) to prevent or slow the effects of detraining, particularly if they are injured. Your clients can rest their injury while maintaining the majority of the fitness benefits. However, it is important to minimize periods of detraining to maximize the benefits of your clients' exercise programs.

Restoration Principle

The restoration principle refers to optimizing recovery from exercise. The speed at which your clients can recover is dependent on their FITT and other individual factors, such as the following:

- Age—the older clients are, the more slowly they will recover
- Experience—the more experienced clients are, the more quickly they will recover
- Environment—the more extreme the environmental conditions, the slower the recovery
- Amount of sleep—clients need 8 to 10 hours of sleep to speed recovery
- Nutrition
- Fluids

High-performance individuals often have to recover within 24 hours to be ready for their next bout of exercise. If your clients exercise only every other day, they probably will be able to recover more fully

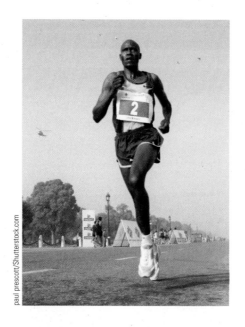

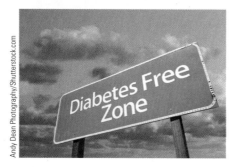

people stop participating in exercise for a variety of reasons. Factors that have a negative impact on adherence include:

- Lack of time
- Poor trainability
- High percentage of body fat
- Unrealistic exercise goals or expectations
- Lack of accurate knowledge about exercise
- Low perceived competency with exercise
- Fear of overtraining
- Past negative experiences with exercise

By understanding some of the factors that might interfere with adherence to an exercise program, you can increase your client's odds for achieving success. In fact, before you design any exercise program, you should consider the likelihood that your client can adhere to the training regimen you want to design. This will help you develop your art of applying the exercise science principles to effectively plan an individual's exercise program.

taper A planned segment of time in a periodization plan where an individual in training reduces the frequency and/or volume of training while maintaining high intensities to achieve a peaking of performance, usually for competition.

than a high-performance person who is usually training every day. One of the most common conditioning mistakes that you can make is to not allow your clients to recover fully from their exercise. Another important factor that can help high-performance individuals improve is to allow them to **taper** or reduce their training volume (maintain intensity, while reducing frequency and or duration) a week to two weeks prior to a major competition to allow for peaking.

HOTLINK See Chapter 12 for a detailed discussion of restoration considerations.

Adherence Principle

The adherence principle refers to the ability of your clients to continue, or stick to, their exercise program. Unfortunately, many

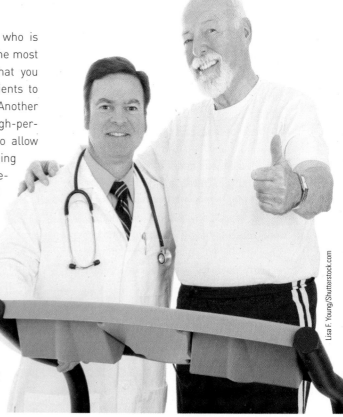

in*Practice*

Examples of Exercise Prescriptions

It is important to understand some practical examples of how you will be using a program of exercise related to your area of interest. The following questions/recommendations for exercise programming are based on the most current understanding of the link between the science and art of exercise physiology, an understanding that continues to evolve.

What does an exercise program look like for promoting good health in a 25-year-old healthy man?

Health/Fitness: One example might include the following based on a maintenance phase plan from the Behavioral Change Model explained in Chapter 1:

Walk 2 miles in 30 minutes 5 days per week; perform 8 to 10 resistance training exercises for at least 1 to 3 sets of 10 repetitions, 2 times per week. Perform 5 to 6 flexibility exercises during both a warm-up and cool-down period associated with your walking and resistance training sessions.

What does an exercise program look like for the control of type 2 diabetes in an otherwise healthy 25-year-old woman?

Medicine: One example might include the following based on an action phase plan from the behavioral change model explained in Chapter 1:

Begin by trying to walk at least 5 days per week for 30 minutes continuously or do three 10-minute bouts per day. Strive to accumulate 150 minutes of exercise each week. Also try to perform resistance training exercises (1 to 3 sets of 8 to 10 with 10 repetitions) at least 2 days per week. Regularly monitor blood sugar concentrations and blood pressure, practice good foot care (to prevent neuropathy or nerve damage), and eat healthy foods.

What does a program of exercise look like for a training session designed to improve the $\dot{V}O_2$ max (see Chapters 8 and 10 for more on $\dot{V}O_2$ max) in a 25-year-old cross-country collegiate runner?

Athletic Performance: One example might include the following for a runner with a best time of 15:00 minutes for 5 kilometers:

Warm-up could include 2 miles of slow jogging . Then run 10×400 meters at 73 seconds/lap with 150 seconds of jogging between each 400-meter bout. The cool-down could include 1 mile of slow jogging and 10 to 15 minutes of dynamic stretching (mobility exercises).

What does a program of exercise look like for a 45-year-old post-myocardial infarction patient in a phase II cardiac rehabilitation program?

Rehabilitation: One example might include:

Intensity: heart rate (HR) of 120 bpm or $HR_{rest} + 20$ beats or to tolerance with symptoms

Time (duration): begin with intermittent bouts of 3 to 5 minutes as tolerated, use an exercise-to-rest time ratio of $2:1$

Frequency: initially 3 to 4 times per day and as duration increases, 2 times per day until patient can perform continuously for 20 to 30 minutes daily (or most days)

Progression: reevaluate patient and change FITT after 6 weeks

CONCEPTS, challenges, & controversies

Can You Be Fat, Fit, and Healthy?

According to research conducted by Dr. Steve N. Blair, professor at the University of South Carolina, the answer is "Yes, you can" based on his current and past research at the Cooper Institute in Dallas, Texas. Blair suggests that a person's health and longevity lie beyond body mass index (BMI; body weight [in kilograms]/height [in square meters]) values and the person's looks. Individuals can be healthy but not meet the standards for healthy status as measured by BMI and other assessments. How can that be? The answer, according to Blair, is related to how much regular exercise an individual performs. If an individual can walk briskly (4 miles/hour, a fast shopping walk) for 30 to 40 minutes, that person probably has a reasonable amount of fitness for functional health. Even if individuals do not lose much weight by participating in regular exercise (although it can help control weight), they can improve their heart health, strengthen their bones, sleep better, and boost their mood. Although some researchers have challenged Blair's research findings, he makes a strong case that supports the importance of regular dosages of exercise for all. The results of the Nurses' Health Study, which has been conducted for more than 20 years, suggests that being moderately active and moderately overweight was better than being inactive. However, maintaining a normal weight, exercising, and not smoking are associated with higher levels of functional health (as measured by cardiorespiratory levels) across the adult life span. In any case, it is likely that you will hear a lot more about the topic of "fit and fat" in the future.

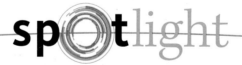

An Expert on Training Principles for Exercise: Jack T. Daniels, Ph.D.

Jack T. Daniels, Ph.D., grew up in California and earned his undergraduate degree from the University of Montana, his master's degree from the University of Oklahoma, a Certificate from the Royal Gymnastics and Sport High School in Stockholm, Sweden, and his Ph.D. in Exercise Physiology from the University of Wisconsin. Daniels taught and served as an associate professor at several universities including Oklahoma City University, the University of Texas, the University of Hawaii, the University of New Hampshire, Arizona State University, and SUNY Cortland (NY).

An athlete himself, Daniels earned silver and bronze Olympic medals and a bronze World Championship medal in the modern pentathlon event, which includes pistol shooting, horse-back obstacle course, swimming, and cross-country running. Daniels is a former doctoral student of Dr. Bruno Balke and became an expert in altitude training before the 1968 Mexico City Olympic Games. His altitude experiences allowed him to become an altitude consultant for the U.S. Olympic Track and Field team in the Mexico City Olympics and he also spent 1 year as the head coach of Peru's National Track Team.

Daniels has more than 30 years of experience as a track and cross-country coach. He also worked three summers for Sport Canada and was a color commentator for CBC television at the 1976 Montreal Olympics. He has coached 30 individual NCAA National Champions, as well as 8 NCAA National Team Champions and 130 All-Americans. He has also coached five U.S. team Olympians. He was named the NCAA Cross Country "Coach of the Century" (1900–2000), has been the "National Coach of the Year" three times, and was named the "World's Best Coach" by *Runner's World Magazine.*

Daniels has also been recognized for his scientific expertise in training by authoring five books on training, including the best-selling *Daniels' Running Formula,* and more than 50 articles in scientific journals on both running and training.

He is frequently asked to speak at coaching clinics around the country. He also spent 6 years as the research director for exercise physiology at Nike, Inc. and was a "Team Nike" honoree in 2003. Daniels recently served as head distance coach at the University of Northern Arizona Center for High Altitude Training in Flagstaff, Arizona, and is now working as the Brevard (North Carolina) College cross-country and track and field coach.

Chapter Summary

- In this chapter, you learned that the general principles of designing a program of exercise can be applied to all populations and individuals; only the specific ingredients need to be changed.

- Developing a program of exercise involves applying both the "science" of exercise physiology and the "art" of exercise physiology. The science you will use is based on the results of hundreds to thousands of research studies that have reported the significant benefits of following a program of exercise based on specific FITTs.

- Use the following exercise principles when developing the art of exercise: goal setting/reality, inherent ability, intrinsic motivation, education models, overload/progression, specificity, special situations, trainability, periodization, overtraining, detraining, restoration, and adherence.

- The general categories for designing different types of exercise programs include aerobic (oxidative), anaerobic (nonoxidative), both aerobic and anaerobic, static, and dynamic exercises.

- The specific categories for types of exercise to be included in a program of exercise include anaerobic power (peak anaerobic power), anaerobic capacity (mean peak anaerobic power), aerobic power, and aerobic capacity.

- There are several methods to determine the aerobic intensity of the exercise in the program of exercise for your clients, including percentage of maximum heart rate (% MHR), percentage of maximum heart rate reserve (% HHR), percentage of $\dot{V}O_2$ max, metabolic equivalents (METs), kcal/min or kcal/hour, lactate threshold (LT), ventilatory threshold (Tvent), rating of perceived exertion scales (RPE), and the talk test.

- There are several methods for determining the anaerobic intensity of exercise programs for your clients, including 1RM, 5RM, 10RM; percentage of maximal speed; and/or sport-specific volume (such as for plyometrics).

- The time (duration) of the exercise program can be determined depending on whether the physical activity is categorized as more aerobic or anaerobic in nature, and based on the client's goals for developing health/fitness, medicine, athletic performance, or rehabilitation needs.

- The frequency of the exercise program also can be determined depending on whether the physical activity is categorized as more aerobic or anaerobic in nature and based on the client's goals for developing health/fitness, medicine, athletic performance, or rehabilitation needs.

Exercise Physiology Reality

 CENGAGE brain.com To reinforce the exercise physiology concepts presented in this chapter, complete the laboratory exercises for Chapter 2. To access labs and other course materials for this text, please visit www.cengagebrain.com.

See the preface on page xiii for details. Once you complete the exercises, have your instructor evaluate your prescriptions. Remember to use your lab experience to help guide you toward future success in exercise physiology.

Exercise Physiology Web Links

Access the following websites for further study of topics covered in this chapter:

- Find updates and quick links to these and other exercise physiology–related sites at our website. To access the course materials and companion resources for this text, please visit www.cengagebrain.com. See the preface on page xiii for details.

- Search for further information about exercise and exercise prescription at the Centers for Disease Control and Prevention (CDC) website: http://www.cdc.gov

- Search for information about exercise prescription and the American College of Sports Medicine (ACSM) at: http://www.acsm.org

Search for information about exercise prescription and the National Strength and Conditioning Association at: http://www.nsca-lift.org

- Search for more information about exercise prescription at: http://www.fitness.gov

- Search for more information about exercise prescription at the U.S. Government health information site: http://www.health.gov/paguidelines

- Search for more information about exercise prescription at the commercial websites: http://www.exrx.net, http://www.brianmac.co.uk, or http://www.topendsports.com

Study Questions

Review the Warm-Up Pre-Test questions you were asked to answer prior to reading Chapter 2. Test yourself once more to determine what you know now that you have completed the chapter.

The questions that follow will help you review this chapter. You will find the answers in the discussions on the pages provided.

1. Define the term *FITT* and how it influences the exercise prescription for your clients. *p. 42*

2. Why is the development of the exercise prescriptions both an art and a science? *pp. 39–42*

3. Why should your clients undergo health risk screening before participation in exercise programs? *pp. 40–41*

4. Define the following terms: goal setting/reality, inherent ability, intrinsic motivation, education models, overload/progression, specificity, special situations, trainability,

periodization, overtraining, detraining, restoration, and adherence. *p. 42*

5. What is the difference between aerobic and anaerobic physical activities? *p. 43*

6. What is the difference between static and dynamic physical activities? *p. 43*

7. Provide one example of a physical activity for each of the following: anaerobic power, anaerobic capacity, aerobic power, and anaerobic capacity. *p. 44*

8. List four ways to determine the intensity of aerobic training intensity. *pp. 45–50*

9. List two ways to determine the intensity of anaerobic training intensity? *pp. 50–51*

10. List two factors that you can use to determine the time (duration) and frequency of exercise for your clients. *p. 51*

Selected References

American College of Sports Medicine. 1978. Position statement on the recommended quantity and quality of exercise for developing fitness in healthy adults. *Med. Sci. Sports Exerc.* 10:vii–X.

American College of Sports Medicine. 1990. Position Stand: The recommended quantity and quality of exercise for developing and maintaining cardiorespiratory and muscular fitness in healthy adults. *Med. Sci. Sports Exerc.* 22:265–274.

American College of Sports Medicine. 1998. Position Stand: The recommended quantity and quality of exercise for developing and maintaining cardiorespiratory and muscular fitness and flexibility in healthy adults. *Med. Sci. Sports Exerc.* 30:975–991.

American College of Sports Medicine. 1998. Position Stand: Exercise and type 2 diabetes. *Med. Sci. Sports Exerc.* 975–991.

American College of Sports Medicine. 2001. Position Stand: Appropriate intervention strategies for weight loss and prevention of weight regain for adults. *Med. Sci. Sports Exerc.* 33:2145–2156.

American College of Sports Medicine. 2002. Position Stand: Progression models in resistance training for healthy adults. *Med. Sci. Sports Exerc.* 34:364–380.

American College of Sports Medicine. 2004. Position Stand: Exercise and hypertension. *Med. Sci. Sports Exerc.* 36:533–553.

American College of Sports Medicine. 2004. Position Stand: Physical activity and bone health. *Med. Sci. Sports Exerc.* 36:1985–1996.

American College of Sports Medicine. 2011. *ACSM's guidelines for exercise testing and prescription*, 8th ed. Philadelphia: Lippincott Williams & Wilkins.

Fulton, J., M. Garg, D. A. Galuska, K. T. Rattay, and C. J. Caspersen. 2004. Public health and clinical recommendations for physical activity and physical fitness: Special emphasis on overweight youth. *Sports Med.* 34(9): 581–599.

Karvonen, M. J., E. Kentala, and O. Mustala. 1957. The effects of training on heart rate; a longitudinal study. *Ann. Med. Exp. Biol. Fenn.* 35:307–315.

Physical Activity Guidelines Advisory Committee. 2008. *Physical activity guidelines advisory committee report, 2008.* Washington, DC: U.S. Department of Health and Human Services. Retrieved from www.health.gov/paguidelines

Tanaka, H., K. D. Monahan, and D. R. Seals. 2001. Age-predicted maximal heart rate revisited. *J. Am. Coll. Cardiol.* 37:153–156.

U.S. Department of Health and Human Services. 1996. *Physical activity and health: A report of the Surgeon General.* Atlanta, GA: U.S. Department of Health and Human Services, Centers for Disease Control and Prevention, National Center for Chronic Disease Prevention and Health Promotion.

U.S. Department of Health and Human Services, Public Health Service, Centers for Disease Control and Prevention, National Center for Chronic Disease Prevention and Health Promotion, Division of Nutrition and Physical Activity. 1999. *Promoting physical activity: A guide for community action.* Champaign, IL: Human Kinetics.

U.S. Department of Health and Human Services, Public Health Service, Centers for Disease Control and Prevention, National Center for Chronic Disease Prevention and Health Promotion, Division of Nutrition and Physical Activity. 2010. *Promoting physical activity: A guide for community action*, 2nd ed., edited by D. R. Brown, G. W. Heath, and S. L. Martin. Champaign, IL: Human Kinetics.

Neuromuscular Responses and Adaptations to Exercise

CHAPTER

3

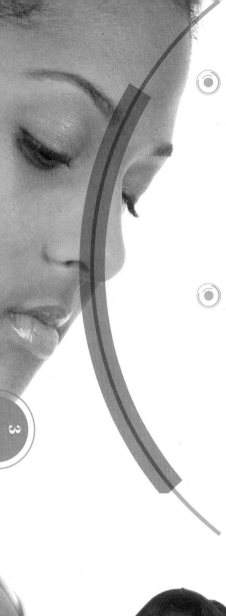

Warm-Up

CENGAGE **brain**.com

What do you already know about neuromuscular responses and adaptations to exercise?

- Use the following Pre-Test or the online evaluation tools for Chapter 3 to determine how much you already know. To access the course materials and companion resources for this text, please visit **www.cengagebrain.com**. See the preface on page xiii for details.

- Need more review? Let the online assessments, animations, and tutorials for Chapter 3 help prepare you for class.

Pre-Test

1. Which nerves carry impulses to the skeletal muscles?

2. The _____ are receptors in connective tissue capsules located between muscle fibers.

3. The _____ respond to tension within the muscle by inhibiting the agonist muscles and facilitating the antagonist muscles during contraction.

4. What is the recording of the electrical activity of skeletal muscle during muscle contraction?

5. Which term refers to a muscle contraction that develops force but the length of the muscle does not change?

6. What is the technique of training to use the storage of muscle energy?

7. Which muscle fibers are associated with being slow twitch and highly oxidative?

8. Which term refers to the increase in the size of muscle fibers?

9. During the first 4 to 6 weeks of a weight (resistance) training program, the gains in strength are primarily due to _____ adaptations.

10. Which type of resistance machines is designed to train a group of muscles at the same speed throughout their complete range of motion?

1. efferent; 2. muscle spindles; 3. Golgi tendon organs; 4. EMG; 5. isometric (static); 6. plyometric exercise; 7. type I; 8. hypertrophy; 9. neural; 10. isokinetic

What You Will Learn in This Chapter

- The basic physiologic concepts concerning neuromuscular responses and adaptations to exercise

- Strategies to improve exercise performance by optimizing neuromuscular responses and specific adaptations to training

- The concepts of neuromuscular integration to optimize exercise

- Basic terminology related to neuromuscular responses and adaptations to exercise

QUICKSTART!

Do you remember studying skeletal muscles and how they contract? If so, what were the differences between isometric (static), concentric, eccentric, and isokinetic muscle contractions? What advice can you give clients who want to optimize their weight (resistance) training program?

Introduction to Neuromuscular Responses and Adaptations to Exercise

Current research of exercise physiology once again focuses on skeletal muscle. The reasons for this renewed interest is not that the scientists have found a new formula for improving exercise performance but that the skeletal muscle's health underlies many diseases, such as type 2 diabetes, cardiovascular disorders, and brain function. In this chapter, it is important that you develop an understanding of how the muscles' ability to function is integrated with functional health of all the major organ systems of the body. For example, it is only recently that the muscle has been identified to act as an endocrine organ that secretes myokines that are transported by the circulation to regulate adipose tissue, brain function, and muscle function. Therefore, we cannot achieve optimal health without having healthy skeletal muscles.

Neuromuscular Integration

The skeletal muscles require an external signal in the form of an action potential emanating in the motor cortex linked via spinal axons to the alpha motor neuron in the spinal cord, which exits the ventral roots of the spinal cord and is connected to a motor unit of the muscle to excite the muscle to contract. As these motor signals are sent from the brain to the muscles to activate contraction, there is a parallel signaling system arising from the cortex, which activates the cardiovascular system and is known as "**central command**." The effects of this parallel neural signaling are explained in more detail in Chapter 7. The sensory receptors (muscle spindles and Golgi tendon organs) located within the skeletal muscle provide sensory feedback to the brain to enable modification of the strength of contraction.

HOTLINK *See Chapter 7 for a more detailed discussion of central command.*

Communication between nerves and muscles (**neuromuscular integration**) is dependent on the presence of a voltage difference across their membranes and the ability to generate action potentials.

Efferent **somatic nerves (axons)** that directly control the muscles are called **motor neurons (nerves)**. Action potential signals from the activated **cell bodies** within the **motor cortex** travel via their individual **axons (motor neurons)** with myelin sheaths within the spinal cord and exit through the **ventral (front)** root of the spinal cord.

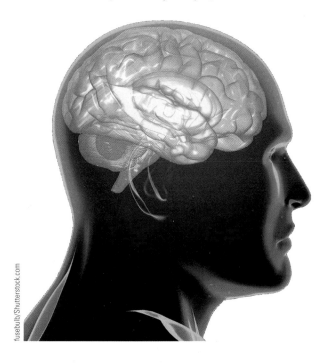

fusebulb/Shutterstock.com

central command A concept that requires there to be a feed-forward set of neural signals emanating from the motor cortex that, in parallel, activate cardiovascular control centers in the brainstem. This activation rapidly withdraws parasympathetic control of the heart, increasing the heart rate, and at the same time increases sympathetic outflow to the heart and vasculature, increasing heart rate and regulating the sympathetic outflow to alter the vasomotor function of the blood vessels to ultimately regulate blood pressure.

neuromuscular integration The communication between nerves and muscles.

somatic nerves (axons) Peripheral nerves that control skeletal muscles.

motor neurons (nerves) The axons that possess a motor function that enclose the nucleus.

cell bodies The body of the nerve cell.

motor cortex The outer layer of the brain that contains the cell bodies and axons of the motor nerves.

axons (motor neurons) The individual motor neurons.

ventral (front) The anatomical front of a structure.

After exiting the spinal cord, the individual axons divide and lose their myelin sheaths as they near the muscle and innervate (connected to) the muscle at a **neuromuscular junction**. The nerves are connected via the neuromuscular junction to the muscle fibers in a ratio of one axon branch fiber to one muscle cell, that is, in a single muscle fiber (see Table 3.1 and Figure 3.1).

The action potentials arrive at the neuromuscular junction and, through a number of complex electrochemical mechanisms (Figure 3.2), cause the muscles to contract.

A number of areas of the brain are involved in controlling how our muscles contract and relax. These areas include the motor cortex (primary, premotor, and somatosensory), the basal nuclei, the thalamus, the brainstem, and the spinal cord (see Figure 3.3).

For example, without the efferent neural signals arising from the motor cortex of the brain signaling the skeletal muscles to contract and the afferent neural signals from the muscle to the brain providing sensory feedback information regarding the muscle's function, the coordinated mechanisms of oxygen delivery to the muscle and energy transduction to provide the bioenergetics of contraction (that is, movement) would not occur.

In this chapter, you will learn how the muscle contracts and the physical principles involved in the generation of muscular force for the different types of muscular contraction. The adaptations of the muscle to both weight and dynamic exercise training are described.

Integration of the Motor Nerves with the Muscle Is Required for Muscle Contraction and Relaxation

In reviewing the anatomy and physiology of the nervous system, you need to have an understanding of the following:

- **Anatomy of the central nervous system (CNS):** The CNS consists of the brain and the spinal cord. The brain has six major areas: the cerebrum (outer gray matter is the cerebral cortex and the central core, or white matter, is the medullary substance containing the basal nuclei; see Figure 3.3), cerebellum, diencephalon, midbrain, pons, and medulla.

- **Spinal cord:** The spinal cord is divided into two areas: the central gray areas and the surrounding white matter. Afferent nerve fibers carrying sensory information from the periphery enter the spinal cord via the dorsal (back) side, and motor nerves leave the spinal cord on the ventral (front) side (see Figure 3.1).

◉ TABLE 3.1 Somatic Nervous System

Feature	Somatic Nervous System
Site of origin	Ventral horn of spinal cord for most; those supplying muscles in head originate in brain
Number of neurons from origin in central nervous system to effector organ	Single neuron (motor neuron)
Organs innervated	Skeletal muscle
Type of innervation	Effector organs innervated only by motor neurons
Neurotransmitter at effector organs	Only acetylcholine
Effects on effector organs	Stimulation only (inhibition possible only centrally through inhibitory postsynaptic potential on dendrites and cell body of motor neuron)
Types of control	Subject to voluntary control; much activity subconsciously coordinated
Higher centers involved in control	Spinal cord, motor cortex, basal nuclei, cerebellum, brainstem

Adapted from Sherwood, L. 2010. Table 7.6 in *Human physiology*, 7th ed. Belmont, CA: Brooks/Cole-Cengage Learning.

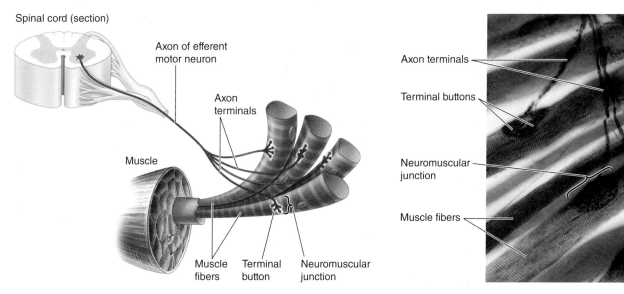

Spinal cord (section)

Axon of efferent motor neuron

Axon terminals

Muscle

Muscle fibers

Terminal button

Neuromuscular junction

Axon terminals

Terminal buttons

Neuromuscular junction

Muscle fibers

Ed Reschke/photolibrary.com

F I G U R E 3.1 Motor neuron innervating skeletal muscle cells. The cell body of a motor neuron originates in the ventral horn of the spinal cord. The axon (somatic efferent fiber) exists through the ventral root and travels through a spinal nerve to the skeletal muscle it innervates. When the axon reaches a skeletal muscle, it divides into many axon terminals, each of which forms a neuromuscular junction with a single muscle cell (muscle fiber). The axon terminal within a neuromuscular junction further divides into fine branches, each of which ends in an enlarged terminal button. Note that the muscle fibers innervated by a single axon terminal are dispersed throughout the muscle, but for simplicity, they are grouped together in this figure. (From Sherwood, L. 2010. Figure 7.4 in *Human physiology,* 7th ed. Belmont, CA: Brooks/Cole-Cengage Learning.)

- **Muscle spindles:** Muscle spindles are made of two types of sensory receptors in connective tissue capsules located between muscle fibers. The primary sensor monitors dynamic changes in muscle length, and the secondary sensor sends signals to the CNS concerning its tonic length. When dynamic increases in length are sensed, the spindle sends afferent signals that synapse at the spinal cord with a motor neuron, resulting in a reflex contraction of the muscle. This is generally termed the *stretch reflex.* When the static length of the muscle is stretched by an increased load, the secondary sensor sends an afferent signal to the CNS, which sends a reflex increase in motor neuron impulses to increase the strength of the tonic contraction (see Figure 3.4).

- **Golgi tendon organs:** Golgi tendon organs respond to tension within the muscle by inhibiting the agonist muscles and facilitating the antagonist muscles during contraction (see Figure 3.4).

- **Corticospinal tracts:** Corticospinal tracts connect the motor cortex to the alpha

motor neurons (motor nerve) via the pyramidal tracts.

- **Neural reflexes:** These reflexes involve four components: a receptor located in the muscle, the gamma afferent neurons arising from the receptor and synapse in the gray matter of the spinal cord, the alpha motor neurons exiting from the cell bodies within the spinal cord, and the muscle fibers of the motor unit (see Figure 3.5).

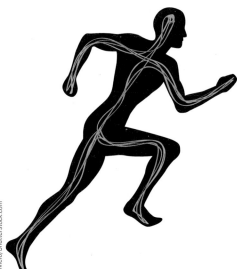

B. Melo/Shutterstock.com

muscle spindles Receptors in connective tissue capsules located between muscle fibers.

neural reflexes Involve four components: a receptor located in the muscle, the gamma afferent neurons arising from the receptor and synapse in the gray matter of the spinal cord, the alpha motor neurons exiting from the cell bodies within the spinal cord, and the muscle fibers of the motor unit.

Golgi tendon organs Respond to tension within the muscle by inhibiting the agonist muscles and facilitating the antagonist muscles during contraction.

corticospinal tracts Connect the motor cortex to the alpha motor neurons (motor nerve) via the pyramidal tracts.

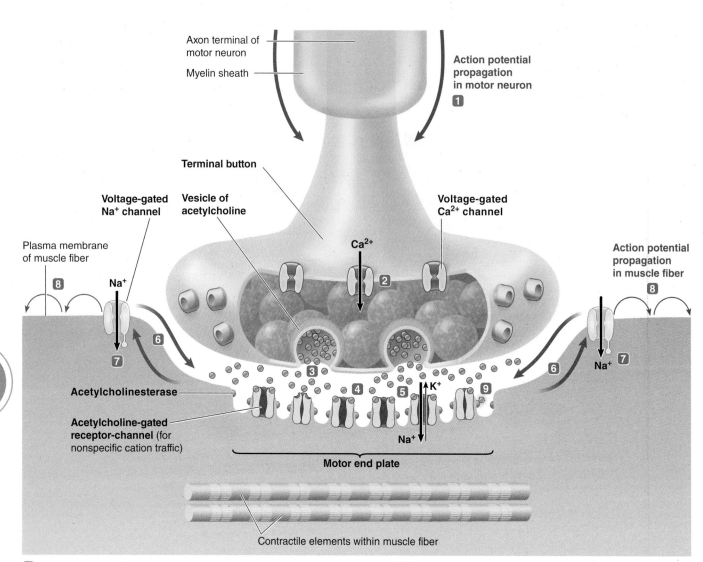

Axon terminal of motor neuron

Myelin sheath

Action potential propagation in motor neuron 1

Terminal button

Voltage-gated Na⁺ channel

Vesicle of acetylcholine

Voltage-gated Ca²⁺ channel

Plasma membrane of muscle fiber 8

Ca^{2+}

Action potential propagation in muscle fiber 8

Na^+

7 6

Na^+

3

4 5

K^+

Na^+

9

6

Na^+ 7

Acetylcholinesterase

Acetylcholine-gated receptor-channel (for nonspecific cation traffic)

Motor end plate

Contractile elements within muscle fiber

1 An action potential in a motor neuron is propagated to the axon terminal (terminal button).

2 This local action potential triggers the opening of voltage-gated Ca^{2+} channels and the subsequent entry of Ca^{2+} into the terminal button.

3 Ca^{2+} triggers the release of acetylcholine (ACh) by exocytosis from a portion of the vesicles.

4 ACh diffuses across the space separating the nerve and muscle cells and binds with receptor-channels specific for it on the motor end plate of the muscle cell membrane.

5 This binding brings about the opening of these nonspecific cation channels, leading to a relatively large movement of Na^+ into the muscle cell compared to a smaller movement of K^+ outward.

6 The result is an end-plate potential. Local current flow occurs between the depolarized end plate and the adjacent membrane.

7 This local current flow opens voltage-gated Na^+ channels in the adjacent membrane.

8 The resultant Na^+ entry reduces the potential to threshold, initiating an action potential, which is propagated throughout the muscle fiber.

9 ACh is subsequently destroyed by acetylcholinesterase, an enzyme located on the motor end-plate membrane, terminating the muscle cell's response.

FIGURE 3.2 Events at a neuromuscular junction. (From Sherwood, L. 2010. Figure 7.5 in *Human physiology.* 7th ed. Belmont, CA: Brooks/Cole-Cengage Learning.)

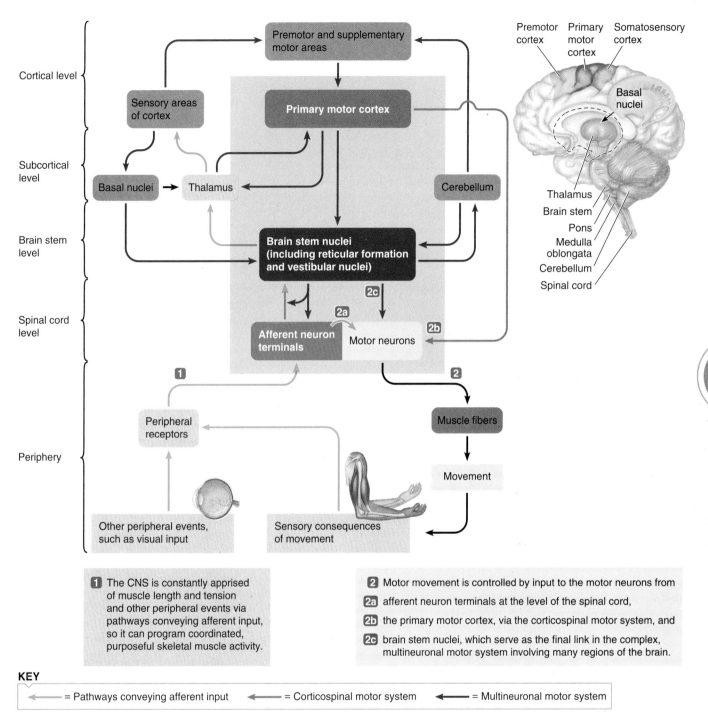

Cortical level

Premotor and supplementary motor areas

Sensory areas of cortex

Primary motor cortex

Subcortical level

Basal nuclei → Thalamus

Cerebellum

Brain stem level

Brain stem nuclei (including reticular formation and vestibular nuclei)

Spinal cord level

2c

2a

Afferent neuron terminals

2b

Motor neurons

1

2

Periphery

Peripheral receptors

Muscle fibers

Other peripheral events, such as visual input

Sensory consequences of movement

Movement

Premotor cortex

Primary motor cortex

Somatosensory cortex

Basal nuclei

Thalamus
Brain stem
Pons
Medulla oblongata
Cerebellum
Spinal cord

1 The CNS is constantly apprised of muscle length and tension and other peripheral events via pathways conveying afferent input, so it can program coordinated, purposeful skeletal muscle activity.

2 Motor movement is controlled by input to the motor neurons from

2a afferent neuron terminals at the level of the spinal cord,

2b the primary motor cortex, via the corticospinal motor system, and

2c brain stem nuclei, which serve as the final link in the complex, multineuronal motor system involving many regions of the brain.

KEY

⟵ = Pathways conveying afferent input   ⟵ = Corticospinal motor system   ⟵ = Multineuronal motor system

● **FIGURE 3.3 Motor control.** Arrows imply influence, whether excitatory or inhibitory; connections are not necessarily direct but may involve interneurons. (From Sherwood. L. 2010. Figure 8.23 in *Human physiology*, 7th ed. Belmont. CA: Brooks/Cole-Cengage Learning.)

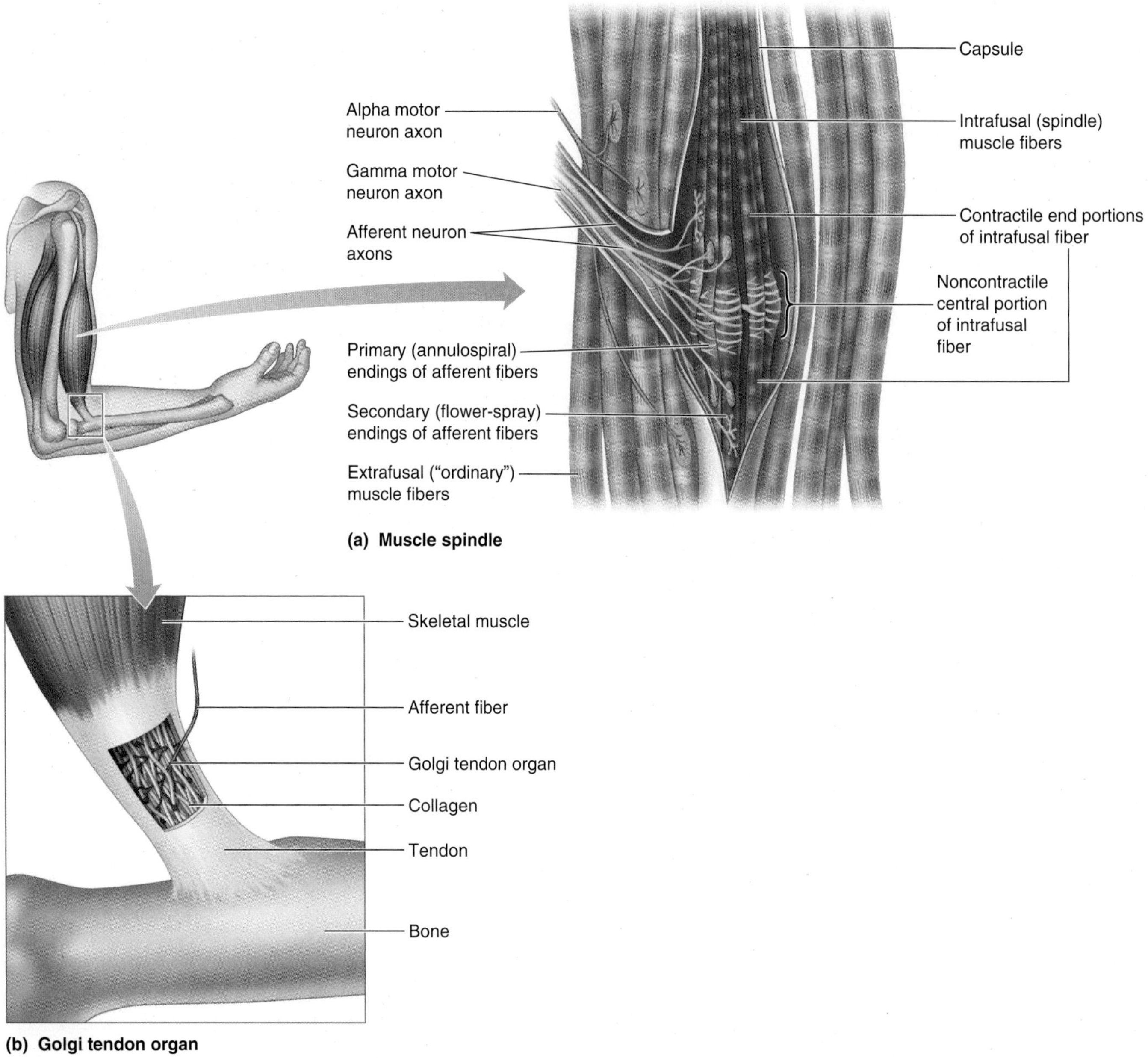

Alpha motor neuron axon

Gamma motor neuron axon

Afferent neuron axons

Capsule

Intrafusal (spindle) muscle fibers

Contractile end portions of intrafusal fiber

Noncontractile central portion of intrafusal fiber

Primary (annulospiral) endings of afferent fibers

Secondary (flower-spray) endings of afferent fibers

Extrafusal ("ordinary") muscle fibers

(a) Muscle spindle

Skeletal muscle

Afferent fiber

Golgi tendon organ

Collagen

Tendon

Bone

(b) Golgi tendon organ

FIGURE 3.4 Muscle receptors (a, b) and muscle spindle function (c). (a) A muscle spindle consists of a collection of specialized intrafusal fibers that lie within a connective tissue capsule parallel to the ordinary extrafusal skeletal muscle fibers. The muscle spindle is innervated by its own gamma motor neuron and is supplied by two types of afferent sensory terminals, the primary (annulospiral) endings and the secondary (flower-spray) endings, both of which are activated by stretch. (b) The Golgi tendon organ is entwined with the collagen fibers in a tendon and monitors changes in muscle tension transmitted to the tendon. (a, b: From Sherwood, L. 2010. Figure 8.24 in *Human physiology,* 7th ed. Belmont, CA: Brooks/Cole-Cengage Learning)

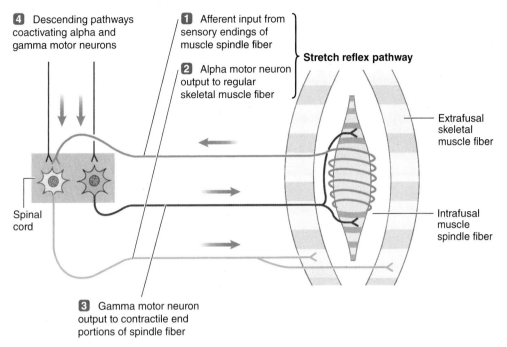

4 Descending pathways coactivating alpha and gamma motor neurons

1 Afferent input from sensory endings of muscle spindle fiber

2 Alpha motor neuron output to regular skeletal muscle fiber

Stretch reflex pathway

Extrafusal skeletal muscle fiber

Intrafusal muscle spindle fiber

Spinal cord

3 Gamma motor neuron output to contractile end portions of spindle fiber

Pathways involved in monosynaptic stretch reflex and coactivation of alpha and gamma motor neurons

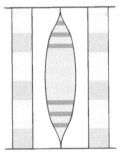 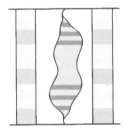 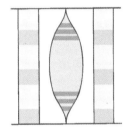

Relaxed muscle; spindle fiber sensitive to stretch of muscle

Contracted muscle in hypothetical situation of no spindle coactivation; slackened spindle fiber not sensitive to stretch of muscle

Contracted muscle in normal situation of spindle coactivation; contracted spindle fiber sensitive to stretch of muscle

(c) Relaxed muscle

Contracted muscle with no spindle coactivation

Contracted muscle with spindle coactivation

⬤ **FIGURE 3.4, cont'd** (C) Muscle spindle function. (From Sherwood, L. 2010. Figure 8.25 in *Human physiology*, 7th ed. Belmont, CA: Brooks/Cole-Cengage Learning.)

Skeletal Muscle Contractions Coordinate the Interaction between Nerves and the Muscles They Innervate

In reviewing the fundamental anatomy and physiology of the skeletal muscle, you need to have an understanding of the following (see Figure 3.6):

• **Structural hierarchy:** Muscles are made up of muscle fascicles (or bundles), muscle fibers (or cells), and the myofilaments of actin and myosin arranged as a series of sarcomeres that provide the striated (striped) appearance. The muscle fiber is surrounded by a double membrane: the inner membrane is the plasma membrane and the outer membrane is the basement membrane. The satellite (stem) cells are located between the two membranes.

structural hierarchy In this case, the structure and branches of skeletal muscles.

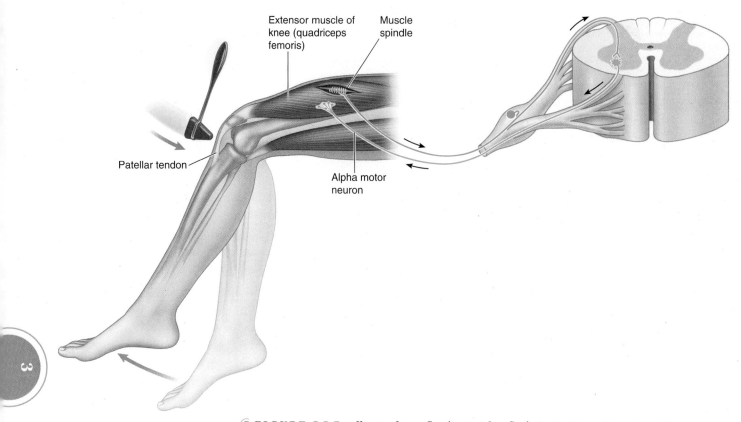

Extensor muscle of
knee (quadriceps
femoris)

Muscle
spindle

Patellar tendon

Alpha motor
neuron

FIGURE 3.5 Patellar tendon reflex (a stretch reflex). Tapping the patellar tendon with a rubber mallet stretches the muscle spindles in the quadriceps femoris muscle. The resultant monosynaptic stretch reflex results in contraction of this extensor muscle, causing the characteristic knee-jerk response. (From Sherwood, L. 2010. Figure 8.26 in *Human physiology,* 7th ed. Belmont, CA: Brooks/Cole-Cengage Learning.)

myotendinous junction The junction between the bones and tendons.

muscle fibers (or cells) Fibers composed of myofibrils.

sarcomeres The smallest contractile units in the muscle fibers.

- **Myotendinous junction:** The tendons are attached at one end to the bone and at the other end are connected to the end of the muscle fibers in a specialized structure. This joining of the muscle and the tendon is known as the myotendinous junction. This specialized junction enables the forces generated by the muscle's contractions to be applied to the bones and results in movement.

- **Muscle fibers or muscle cells:** These are composed of numerous 1-micrometer-diameter myofibrils, which range in number from 50 per muscle fiber in the newborn to approximately 2,000 in the untrained adult. During growth, the number of myofibrils within the muscle fiber is the main factor in the increase in muscle size, or hypertrophy.

- **Sarcomeres:** When viewed with a light microscope, the myofibrils within the muscle fiber appear striated. The striations result from the different light properties associated with the actin and myosin proteins that make up each individual sarcomere. It is the interaction between the contractile and regulatory proteins of the individual sarcomeres that enable contraction.

A controversy exists as to whether the increase in muscle size from weight training is a result of an increase in the number of the myofibrils within the muscle fiber (hypertrophy; that is, increase in diameter of the fiber) only, or whether there is also an increase in the number of muscle fibers (that is, hyperplasia). This controversy will be addressed in more detail in the Training Adaptations of Neuromuscular Contractions section later in this chapter.

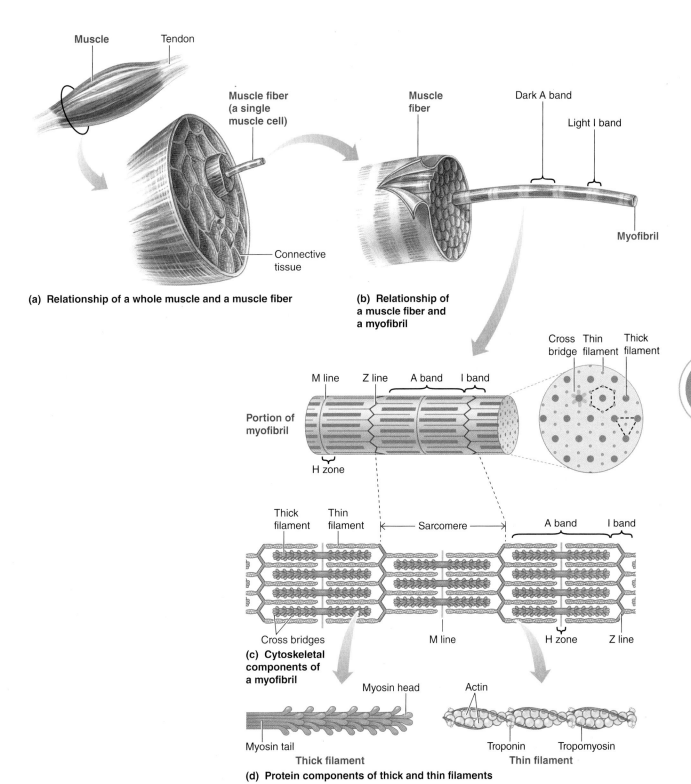

(a) Relationship of a whole muscle and a muscle fiber

(b) Relationship of a muscle fiber and a myofibril

(c) Cytoskeletal components of a myofibril

(d) Protein components of thick and thin filaments

● **F I G U R E 3.6 Levels of organization in a skeletal muscle.** Note in the cross section of a myofibril in part (c) that each thick filament is surrounded by six thin filaments, and each thin filament is surrounded by three thick filaments. (From Sherwood, L. 2010. Figure 8.2 in *Human physiology*, 7th ed. Belmont. CA: Brooks/Cole-Cengage Learning.)

- **Sliding filament and cross-bridge cycling theory of contraction:** This theory describes how the fixed-length filaments of actin and myosin move in relation to each other to shorten the length of the sarcomere, that is, contraction. Because the sarcomeres within the myofibril are connected in series with each other, the muscle fiber also contracts. The cross-bridge cycle is a repetitive, four-step cycle of biochemical and physical events that attaches myosin to actin using adenosine triphosphate (ATP) and its breakdown to ADP + Pi + E, where ADP represents adenosine diphosphate, Pi represents inorganic phosphate, and E represents energy.

- **Oxygen delivery:** Oxygen is delivered to the muscles in the arterial blood via the systemic circulation, which branches from the large arteries to arterioles to capillaries as described in Chapter 7. The blood enters the capillaries of the microcirculation, or as more generally termed, the muscle's *capillary bed*. The capillary bed is the location at which the diffusion of O_2 and the transport of metabolic substrates from the arterial blood enter the myofibers of the muscle, and is also where the excretion of metabolites and diffusion of CO_2 out of the muscle into the blood (venous) is accomplished. Facilitation of these exchanges is a property of the architecture of the microcirculation because the capillaries intertwine with the muscle fibers. The venous blood travels via the venules out of the microcirculation into the small and large veins back to the heart (see Figure 3.7).

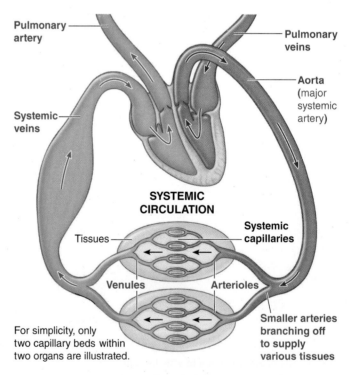

⊙ FIGURE 3.7 Basic organization of the cardiovascular system. Arteries progressively branch as they carry blood from the heart to the organs. A separate small arterial branch delivers blood to each of the various organs. As a small artery enters the organ it is supplying, it branches into arterioles, which further branch into an extensive network of capillaries. The capillaries rejoin to form venules, which further unite to form small veins that leave the organ. The small veins progressively merge as they carry blood back to the heart. (From Sherwood, L. 2010. Figure 10.4 in *Human physiology.* 7th ed. Belmont, CA: Brooks/Cole-Cengage Learning.)

inRETROSPECT

Increases in Blood Flow from Rest to Exercise

Whether all the capillaries in resting muscle have blood flow has been difficult to resolve because of some inherent limitations in measurement techniques. Initially, it was accepted that the increase in muscle blood flow associated with exercise is accomplished, in part, by recruitment of dormant (non–red blood cell flowing) capillaries (N. B. August Krogh was awarded the Nobel Prize for Physiology and Medicine in 1920 for identifying the mechanism of blood vessel recruitment in contracting muscle). However, the compelling weight of more recent work in a range of experimental and physiologic models suggests that the increase in flow from rest to exercise occurs in most capillaries of the muscle because few dormant capillaries are in resting muscle. The historical, and any current, identification of the presence of dormant capillaries in resting muscle is now thought to be a measurement artifact. This concept is counter to Krogh's Nobel Prize award findings.

However, it is noted in Chapter 9 that the lung was also identified (by Krogh) to use recruitment of dormant capillaries to increase pulmonary blood flow during exercise. The situation in the lung, however, is very different from skeletal muscle because of the very low perfusion pressure toward the apices of the upright lung and also the lack of structural support for capillaries in the lung. Therefore, recruitment of the dormant capillaries occurs because of the increase in pulmonary perfusion pressures at the apex of the lung as the intensity of exercise increases. In the resting muscle, each of the capillaries is tethered to the myocytes, which resist, or prevent, collapse even when intravascular pressures fall to very low values.

In addition to reviewing the earlier fundamentals of the skeletal muscle, the bones provide the structure to which the muscles are attached and are the foundation of joints and levers through which the muscle contractions enable movement. In cases where there is congenital misalignment of the muscle attachment to the bone, uncoordinated muscle movements may result, such as is seen in children with cerebral palsy. Often these cases require orthopedic surgery to correct the misalignment while the cerebral palsy patient is young.

Previously, it was thought that the only purpose of bones was to provide the structure by which the muscles were attached and that their role in exercise was minimal. Similar to the soft tissues of muscles, tendons, and ligaments, the weight-bearing bones have been found to be plastic and become thicker and develop greater tensile strength in response to dynamic exercise training. In addition, the bone's response to static (resistance) exercise is found to increase thickness and tensile strength of the bones being exercised regardless of their weight-bearing function. Furthermore, the consequence of chronic exposure to microgravity, a condition of weightlessness or diminished gravitational stress on the skeleton, such as during spaceflight or long-term bed rest, is bone loss, or atrophy, leading to osteoporosis. In extreme conditions, this may result in osteoporotic fractures. The prospect of osteoporotic fractures is one of great concern to humans undergoing long-duration spaceflight and to the nursing care of the elderly who genereally take to their bed when residing in long-term care facilities for the rest of their lives.

HOTLINK *See Chapters 12 and 13 for more details about nutrition and the female athlete triad and possible eating disorders, which are related to bone mineral loss and the development of premature osteoporosis.*

The response of bone to exercise training and detraining is fast becoming a specialized area of exercise physiology and clinical rehabilitation. The exercise physiology of bone's adaptation has become so specialized that it requires separate attention.

Muscle Contraction

There are three types of muscle action:

1. **Isometric**, or **static**, contraction is when the muscle develops force but its length does not change.

2. **Concentric** contraction is when the muscle develops force by causing the length of the muscle to shorten.

3. **Eccentric** contraction is when the muscle develops force and the external force causes the muscle to lengthen.

The Length–Tension Relationship Defines the Amount of Force the Muscle Can Develop

In isolated muscle experiments, it has been demonstrated that the greatest force generated by a skeletal muscle occurs at its optimal length (l_o). The optimal length of a muscle is defined when there is an optimal degree of overlap between the thin (actin) and thick (myosin) filaments of the sarcomeres. This is the point at which the greatest potential for force production via the cross-bridge cycling mechanisms exists. This fundamental length–tension relationship identified in isolated muscle experiments is also apparent in the intact human muscle (see Figure 3.8).

The data in Figure 3.8 indicate that the isometric force is maximal when activated at a muscle length 20 percent greater than its equilibrium length (that is, unattached and unstimulated).

When the muscle is attached by its tendons to the bones in a resting position, it exhibits a moderate tension, because at

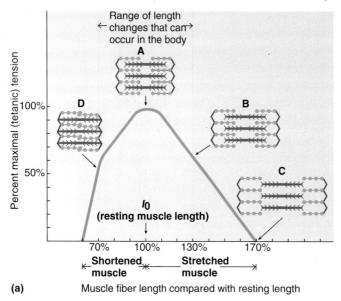

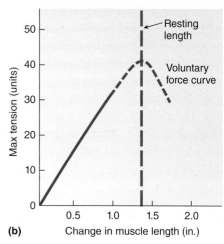

(a) Muscle fiber length compared with resting length

(b) Change in muscle length (in.)

FIGURE 3.8 Length–tension relationship (a) and isometric force–length curve of a human triceps muscle (b). (a) Maximal tetanic contraction can be achieved when a muscle fiber is at its optimal length (l_o) before the onset of contraction, because this is the point of optimal overlap of thick-filament cross bridges and thin-filament cross-bridge binding sites (point A). The percentage of maximal tetanic contraction that can be achieved decreases when the muscle fiber is longer or shorter than l_o before contraction. When it is longer, fewer thin-filament binding sites are accessible for binding with thick-filament cross bridges, but the thin filaments are pulled out from between the thick filaments (points B and C). When the fiber is shorter, fewer thin-filament binding sites are exposed to thick-filament cross bridges because the thin filaments overlap (point D). Also, further shortening and tension development are impeded as the thick filaments become forced against the Z lines (point D). In the body, the resting muscle length is at l_o. Furthermore, because of restrictions imposed by skeletal attachments, muscles cannot vary beyond 30% of their l_o in either direction (the range screened in light green). At the outer limits of this range, muscle still can achieve about 50% of the maximal tetanic contraction. (b) The voluntary force curve was calculated from the difference between a predicted total force curve and a passive force curve. (a: From Sherwood, L. 2010. Figure 8.19 in *Human physiology*. 7th ed. Belmont, CA: Brooks/Cole-Cengage Learning.)

FIGURE 3.9 Schematic representation of the lever lengths of the elbow with the hand holding a weight against gravity at 90° (a), 120° (b), and 45° (c). Note that the length of the weight lever (L) is much greater than the length of the muscle lever (L₁). However, the length of the muscle of b > a > c, and the muscle length in (a) is at its optimum length. (Cengage Learning 2013)

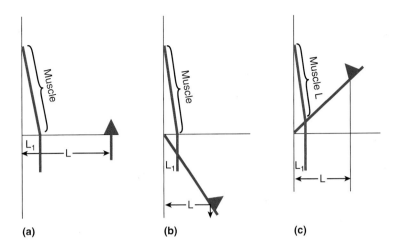

(a)   (b)   (c)

rest it is stretched beyond its equilibrium length. Therefore, in the resting human, the muscle length is near its optimum length—that is, the optimal position for producing maximal isometric tension. Therefore, from the length–tension relationship, the maximal tension a muscle can generate occurs when the length of the muscle is 20 percent longer than its equilibrium length.

between muscle groups makes it difficult in real life to predict the position and length of a specific muscle group that will result in the group's greatest force of contraction.

(What is a muscle's equilibrium length?)

(What does the word *synergy* mean?)

However, the maximal isometric tension that any muscle fiber can generate is dependent on the relative length of the muscle fiber at the time it contracts. The relative length of the muscle in relation to its equilibrium length is affected by the position of the muscle's attachment to its levers, or bones (see Figure 3.9).

Figure 3.9 shows that during elbow flexion and extension exercise, the triceps and biceps are anatomically located differently but collaborate in performing a given movement by having one group contract and the other groups relax. Hence the muscle groups are acting synergistically and the forces on each of the levers change with position of the limb. The synergism

The Force–Velocity Relationship Describes the Power a Muscle Can Generate during an Isometric Contraction

Measurements of the force generated by a muscle against its velocity of contraction identifies that its greatest isometric force occurs when the muscle is not shortening and the muscle generates zero isometric force at its maximal velocity of contraction (see Figure 3.10).

FIGURE 3.10 The force–velocity relationship is hyperbolic in nature in that greater loads produce slower speeds but greater tensions. The effect of strength training is to increase maximum isometric tension, but not maximum velocity. However, a weight-trained muscle moves a given load at a greater velocity. (From Brooks. G.A.. T. D. Fahey. and K. M. Baldwin. 2005. Figure 17-28 in *Exercise physiology: Human bioenergetics and its applications*, 4th ed. New York: McGraw-Hill.)

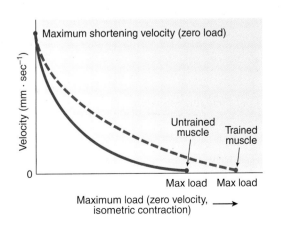

Because the velocity (or speed) of shortening (contraction) affects the force generated by the muscle, the maximal power (force × distance per unit of time) that can be generated by the muscle occurs at 25 to 30 percent of the maximal velocity of shortening. A strength training program increases the maximal isometric force but does not increase the maximal velocity of shortening (see Figure 3.10). However, you should note that the stronger muscle can move a given submaximal load faster.

Because activities of everyday life or athletics rarely involve only isolated muscle activity, our review of the isolated muscle function as a model of neuromuscular integration should be viewed with the understanding that during exercise, groups of muscles contract and relax synergistically. However, the fundamental mechanisms involved in muscle contraction and relaxation are invariant for trained and untrained neuromuscular function.

Isokinetics

The relationship between power and the velocity of shortening is important in evaluating an exercise training program of strength or endurance. If a post-training strength test is performed at a slower velocity of shortening than the pretraining test, you may erroneously conclude that the individual's strength has improved when it has not. Concerns regarding these types of errors resulted in the development of a machine that tested muscle strength at the same speed—the isokinetic (that is, same speed) loading dynamometer (**isokinetics**). Subsequently, these machines have been adapted for use in rehabilitation in an effort to train a group of muscles at the same speed throughout their complete range of motion.

Electromyography

By using electrodes on the surface, or needle electrodes placed in the belly of the skeletal muscle, it is possible to measure and integrate the electrical activity of the active action potentials of the muscle dur-

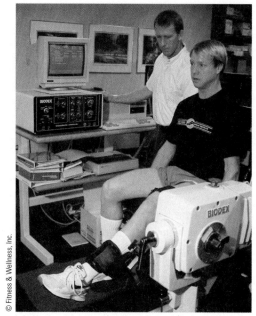

© Fitness & Wellness, Inc.

In isokinetic training, the speed of muscle contraction is constant.

ing its contraction. A linear relation between the force of the contraction and the amount of **electromyographic (EMG)** activity has been demonstrated. The amount of EMG activity is greater during shortening (concentric or positive) contractions than during lengthening (eccentric or negative) contractions (see Figure 3.11).

These responses indicate that the amount of muscle excitation required to produce a given force at the same velocity is less during stretching than during shortening, or when described another way, if the muscle contracts at a constant force, the electrical activity increases linearly with the velocity of shortening but decreases linearly with the velocity of lengthening. It is important to note that the electrical activity (that is, the integrated EMG activity) is the same in maximal contractions at different speeds of contraction. This suggests that during maximal contractions, the number of muscle fibers recruited is the same regardless of the speed of contraction, and it does not matter whether the contraction is isometric (static), concentric (shortens), or eccentric (lengthens).

The electrical activity, or the integrated EMG activity, increases linearly with the

isokinetics A dynamic muscle contraction (**concentric** or **eccentric**) that is accomplished at the same speed of contraction throughout the complete contraction.

electromyographic (EMG) This type of recording is obtained by using electrodes on the surface of or needle electrodes placed in the belly of the skeletal muscle. It measures and integrates the electrical activity of the active action potentials of the muscle. During its contraction, a linear relation between the force of the contraction and the amount of electromyographic **(EMG)** activity has been demonstrated. The amount of EMG activity is greater during shortening (**concentric** or positive) contractions than during lengthening (**eccentric** or negative) contractions.

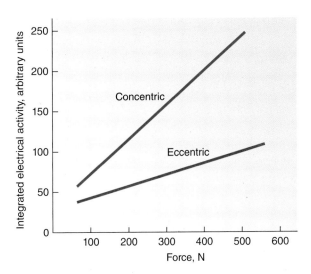

FIGURE 3.11 **The reaction between integrated electrical activity and force in the human calf muscles.** Recordings were made during shortening at constant velocity (top) and lengthening at the same velocity (bottom). (Modified from Astrand, P. O., and K. Rodahl, 1970. Figure 2.14 in *Textbook of work physiology: Physiological bases of exercise*, 3rd ed. New York: McGraw-Hill.)

intensity (rate) of the exercise and, therefore, increases linearly with the oxygen uptake. Comparisons between concentric (positive) and eccentric (negative) work indicates that the negative work demands much less oxygen than the positive work at the same given work intensity (see Figure 3.12).

The underlying physical principle that may explain the difference in oxygen up-take between positive (concentric) and negative (eccentric) muscular contractions is related to the changes in potential energy. During concentric muscle contraction, the muscle loses potential energy (that is, kinetic energy) to perform the contraction. Therefore, at the end of the concentric contraction, the muscle has less potential energy than at the beginning. In dynamic exercise, the muscle restores its potential

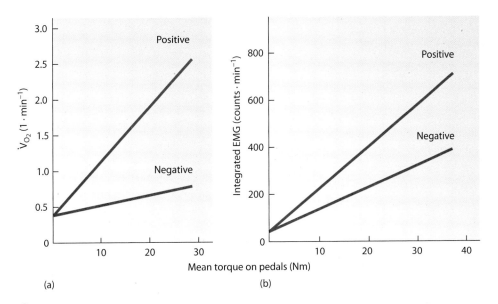

(a)   (b)

FIGURE 3.12 **Relationship between force and oxygen uptake and integrated EMG.** (a) Mean rates of oxygen uptake ($\dot{V}O_2$) and (b) integrated electromyographic recordings obtained in all experiments on the best trained subjects over the course of several months, plotted against the mean torque on the pedals for positive and negative exercise. (Modified from Astrand, P. O., and K. Rodahl, 1970. Figure 2.15 in *Textbook of work physiology: Physiological bases of exercise*, 3rd ed. New York: McGraw-Hill.)

energy during the relaxation phase of the contraction when the muscle is lengthening and the kinetic energy is added back to the muscle. During eccentric muscle contraction, the muscle action gains the kinetic energy when it goes from the resting state of potential energy to the end of the lengthening contraction to an increased state of potential energy. Therefore, the oxygen uptake and the integrated EMG activity of an eccentric muscle contraction will be less than a concentric muscle contraction performed at the same intensity of exercise. This finding suggests that eccentric contractions have a greater **mechanical efficiency (ME)**. Unfortunately, demonstration of this physical principle "in vivo," or in a real-life situation, has been difficult to verify because we are unable to account for changes in entropy.

(Can you provide examples of daily activities that use eccentric, or negative, muscle contractions?)

Mechanical Efficiency (ME) and Storage of Energy

In theory, muscle activities requiring lengthening contractions should result in increases in potential energy, which when released would make us stronger, faster, and have greater endurance. However, in practice, prolonged activities involving eccentric muscle contractions result in muscle soreness because of release of inflammatory cytokines and edema (swelling), and do not appear to improve our athletic performance.

The ME of a muscle can be calculated as a ratio of the external work (W) performed divided by the extra energy (E) required to perform the work above the resting energy (e). This ratio is expressed as a percentage and is summarized in the following equation:

$$ME = W / E - e \times 100$$

Calculations of ME for cycling and running suggest that the human's muscle machinery is 20 to 25 percent efficient. This means that 75 to 80 percent of the energy generated by the bioenergetic reactions of metabolism (see Chapters 4 and 5) to perform the work is added to the body as heat.

Work is measured as a product of force (F) times distance (D):

$$W = F \times D$$

In an isometric contraction where the muscle does not change length, no external work is performed, hence a physical measurement of ME cannot be obtained even though the $\dot{V}O_2$ is increased above rest. However, for anyone who has performed a maximal isometric voluntary contraction, the idea that you have not performed any physical work is contrary to the feelings of fatigue that you feel at the end of 2 to 3 minutes of the contraction.

A similar problem exists for the exercises that produce work partially by anaerobic bioenergetic processes, and the actual energy used (aerobic + anaerobic) is unable to be accurately quantified, for example, a 100-meter sprint. In the 100-meter sprint, the work performed can be accurately assessed, but the energy required to perform the work is unable to be accurately quantified, thereby making any calculation of ME a guesstimate.

In the 1970s, it was noticed that at running speeds of 6 to 7 meters/sec, the shortening contractions of the muscles accounted for the power output of the muscles; that is, the power output followed the power–velocity profile of the muscle (see Figure 3.13). It was expected that when the speed of shortening exceeded one third of the maximal speed of shortening, the maximal power output of the muscles would decrease; however, it was noticed that elite sprinters were able to increase the power at speeds greater than 6 to 7 meters/sec. This phenomenon was explained by the fact that the extensor muscles of the leg were activated before the foot impacts the ground. At foot strike it was theorized that the decrease in velocity of the exten-

mechanical efficiency (ME) ME of a muscle can be calculated as a ratio of the external work (W) performed divided by the extra Energy (E) required to perform the work above the resting energy (e). This ratio is expressed as a percentage and is summarized in the following equation: ME = W/ E − e × 100.

sor muscles released kinetic energy to be stored in the series elastic elements of the muscle fibers. This stored energy was released to be used during contraction of the muscle (see Figure 3.13).

It was surprising to note that not all good sprinters were able to use this extra power, suggesting that perhaps there was a technique to storing and releasing the energy during sprint running or there was some genetic polymorphism that resulted in a specific individual signaling pathway to facilitate storage of the kinetic energy? This increase in power output resulted in an increase in ME, and in some cases, at high running speeds ME was calculated to be 60 to 70 percent. However, in subsequent experiments, it was documented that when activated muscles were forcibly stretched, the kinetic energy was stored as potential energy in the series of elastic elements of the muscles. If the stretch was immediately followed by a shortening, this stored energy was released. The release of the stored energy increased the ME and the

power output of the muscles. The time between the stretch of the active muscle and its shortening was found to be critical in maximizing its effects. High jumpers, long jumpers, triple jumpers, gymnasts, and circus acrobats had been using this technique of energy storage for years before it was identified. The technique of training to use this storage of energy is known as **plyometric exercise training**. Plyometric exercise training involves repeated rapid stretching and contracting of muscles.

Motor Unit

The **motor unit** is the body's fundamental structural unit that functionally integrates the neural activity with skeletal muscle contraction (see Figure 3.14).

The motor unit consists of a cell body in the CNS attached to the alpha motor neuron, which, in turn, innervates a number of muscle fibers. The distribution of muscle fibers of a given motor unit within its muscle is such that the fibers next to each other

plyometric exercise training This involves repeated, rapid stretching and contracting of muscles that, when the activated muscles are stretched, the kinetic energy is stored as potential energy in the series of elastic elements of the muscles.

motor unit The body's fundamental structural unit that functionally integrates the neural activity with that of the skeletal muscle contraction.

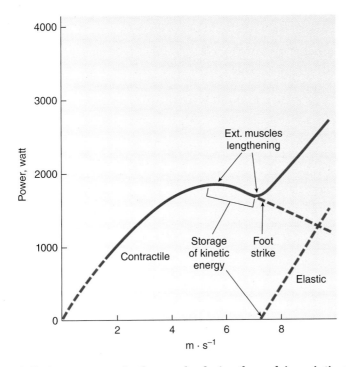

● **FIGURE 3.13** **Average power by the muscles during the push in sprinting as a function of speed.** (Source: Cavagna, G. A., Komarek, L., and Mazzoleni, S.: The Mechanics of Sprint Running. *Journal of Physiology*. 217:709, 1971. Used by permission of Wiley.)

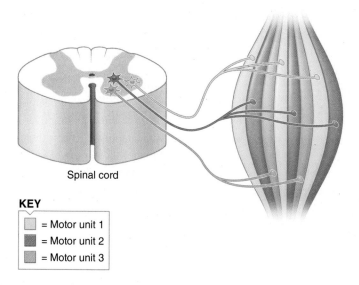

Spinal cord

KEY

☐ = Motor unit 1
■ = Motor unit 2
▨ = Motor unit 3

● **FIGURE 3.14 Motor units in a skeletal muscle.** (From Sherwood, L. 2010. Figure 8.16 in *Human physiology*, 7th ed. Belmont, CA: Brooks/Cole-Cengage Learning.)

recruitment As the required force and speed of contraction increases, the number of slow motor units increases, as does the frequency of their use, until the force requirement increases to a level that causes a further recruitment of the motor units with larger cell bodies (soma) until maximal force output is achieved.

arise from different motor units. When the action potential within a single alpha motor neuron is propagated to its motor unit, acetylcholine (ACh) is released into the motor end plate (or neuromuscular junction; see Figure 3.2) and all the muscle fibers within the motor unit are stimulated to contract. Relaxation of the muscle fibers requires that the release of ACh be reduced or stopped.

In many surgeries in which the patient's muscles are partially or fully paralyzed, pharmacologic derivatives of the drug curare (the drug used to coat the tip of the hunting arrows of some South American natives), which binds to the nicotinic receptors of the neuromuscular junction and prevents acetylcholine (ACh) from stimulating the receptors to contract the muscles (see Figure 3.2).

Notably, the number of muscle fibers per motor unit is related to the type of activity the muscle performs. For example, finger muscles requiring fine dexterous movements have relatively few muscle fibers per unit (100 fibers/unit) compared with a thigh muscle requiring bulk muscle action that has a large number of muscle fibers per motor unit (1,000 fibers/unit). Each motor unit is composed of only one kind (or type) of fiber.

It has been found that the smaller the soma (that is, the neuron cell body located in the CNS; see Figure 3.3), the slower the motor unit but the easier it is to trigger an action potential that transmits to the muscle fiber resulting in a contraction. The slow motor units are the first to be activated at the onset of a contraction and, as the force of the contraction increases, the number of motor units increases; this is called **recruitment** (see Figure 3.15).

As the required force and speed of contraction increases, the number of slow motor units increases, as well as the frequency of their use, until the force requirement increases to a level that causes further recruitment of the motor units with larger cell bodies (soma) until maximal force output is achieved. The motor units with the larger cell bodies are the fast-fatigable and fast fatigue-resistant motor units.

An example of this pattern of recruitment becomes apparent when you transfer from rest to a slow jog to a moderate running speed to an all-out sprint. This requires an incremental increase in the leg muscles' force production, which can be achieved only by recruitment of more and more motor units starting with recruitment of the small and progressing to recruitment of the large motor units (see

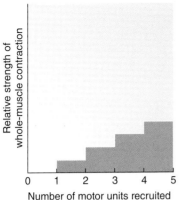

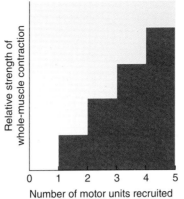

(a) Recruitment of small motor units

(b) Recruitment of large motor units

⬤ **FIGURE 3.15 Comparison of motor unit recruitment in skeletal muscles with small motor units and muscles with large motor units.** (a) Small incremental increases in strength of contraction during motor unit recruitment in muscles with small motor units because only a few additional fibers are called into play as each motor unit is recruited. (b) Large incremental increases in strength of contraction occur during motor unit recruitment in muscles with large motor units, because so many additional fibers are stimulated with recruitment of each additional motor unit. (From Sherwood, L. 2010. Figure 8.17 in *Human physiology*, 7th ed. Belmont, CA: Brooks/Cole-Cengage Learning.)

Figure 3.15). The link between motor unit recruitment and muscle fiber types should become evident in the following section describing muscle fiber types.

Muscle Fiber Types

Historically there are two main methods of describing, or typing, a muscle fiber: (a) histochemistry and immunocytochemistry, and (b) physiologic contraction times. However, because differences in physiologic contraction times of the muscle fibers are qualitatively associated with different histochemical stains and immunocytochemical reactions, more generalized terms, such as *slow* and *fast twitch*, *type I* and *type II*, and *oxidative* and *glycolytic fibers* are commonly used. For example, it is not unusual to hear someone refer to a woman, or man, sprinter as being made of "all white or fast-twitch" muscle, and an endurance athlete as being made of "all red or slow-twitch" muscle. Clearly, the term *all* is an exaggeration, and it is more accurate to say that a combination of the slow- and fast-twitch fibers is the genetic norm. However, in the late 1970s, muscle biopsy studies associated a sprinter as having

more fast-twitch (white) fibers than slow-twitch (red) fibers, and that the endurance runner had more red fibers than white fibers (see Figure 3.16).

Histochemistry and Immunocytochemistry

Muscle biopsy samples are obtained from the muscle of interest and after incubation with various stains or substrates (**histochemistry**) or reactions between specific protein isoforms (a slight structural variation of the same protein) and its antibody (**immunocytochemistry**). Light microscopy, electron microscopy, or other imaging techniques, such as confocal or fluorescence microscopy, are used to identify the different fiber types (see Figure 3.17).

Muscle fibers with high activities (concentrations) of myofibrillar ATPase are found to have high velocities of concentric contraction and a "fast" (short) time to peak tension in an isometric contraction. When stained and viewed through a light microscope with histochemical reagents under alkaline conditions, the "fast" fibers appear dark, but under acid conditions they appear light (see Figure 3.17a and 3.17b).

histochemistry The chemistry of identifying living tissues by using different stains that can be identified by light microscopy, electron microscopy. It is used to identify different fiber types.

immunocytochemistry A technique using the chemical reaction that occurs between proteins and its antibodies within a cell and can be identified by imaging techniques, such as confocal or fluorescence microscopy.

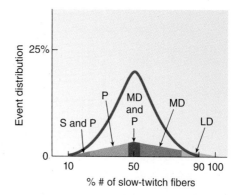

FIGURE 3.16 A complete description of the percentage distribution of the slow-twitch (type I) fibers among long distance (LD), middle distance (MD), power (P; jumpers and throwers), and sprinter (S) male and female athletes. (Modified from Saltins' Biopsy data. B. Saltin, J. Henriksson, E. Nygaard and P. Andersen. Fiber Type and Metabolic Potential of Skeletal Muscles in Man and Endurance Runners in Part VII "Metabolism in Prolonged Exercise" Pages 320–343, published in **The Long Distance Runner: A Definitive Study**, Editor P. Milvy, Published by Urizen Books New York in 1978. Published with Permission from the New York Academy of Sciences from the copyrighted Proceedings of "The Marathon: Physiological, Medical, Epidemiological and Psychological Studies" in *Ann. N.Y. Acad. of Sci.* Vol. 301, 1977.)

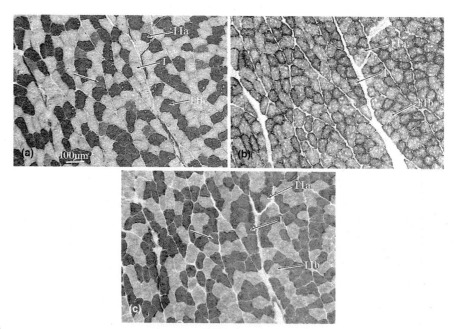

FIGURE 3.17 Serial cross sections of medical gastrocnemius skeletal muscle fibers of a rodent incubated with traditional histochemical procedures. (a) Section was incubated for M-ATPase at pH 10.3. Fibers that appear dark are high in ATPase values—and are often termed *type II* or *fast twitch*. Fibers low in M-ATPase are *type I* or *slow twitch*, and appear to be light. (b) The very same muscle fibers (the next serial section) are incubated for M-ATPase under acid conditions (that is, pH 4.3). The response of the fibers is reversed from that of alkaline conditions. Thus, the high ATPase fast-twitch fibers now appear light; whereas the slow type I fibers appear dark. (c) The same fibers from the next serial section, which has been incubated for the oxidative enzyme succinate dehydrogenase (SDH). High SDH is visualized in the darker areas of fibers, whereas low SDH is seen as a light fiber. Type I fibers are of high SDH, whereas type II fibers can be either high (type IIa) or low (type IIb). Some fibers do not reverse the intensity of M-ATPase when pH is changed from alkaline to acid conditions. One such fiber is identified in (a) and (b) by an arrow. Historically, fibers that do not demonstrate "acid reversal" have been designated as "type IIc" fibers. With our evolving understanding of myosin chemistry, it is possible that "IIc" fibers are actually composed of IIx myosin. (Source: Brooks, G. A., Fahey, T. D., and Baldwin, K. M. *Exercise Physiology: Human Bioenergetics and Its Applications,* 4th Edition, 2005, p. 410. Figure 18.15. Used by permission of The McGraw-Hill Companies.)

In contrast, when the muscle fibers are reacted with an oxidative enzyme, such as succinate dehydrogenase, the areas of the fiber with high oxidative capacity and less glycolytic capacity appear dark, whereas the fibers with lower oxidative capacities appear lighter and are more involved in glycolytic metabolism (see Figure 3.17c).

These differences in oxidative capacities together with their concomitant myofibrillar ATPase activities enable the fibers to be classified as **type I**, or slow-twitch, high-oxidative fibers, and **type IIa**, or fast-twitch fibers with a higher oxidative capacity than the **type IIb** or fast-twitch fiber with low oxidative capacity. The type I and IIa fibers appear pinkish red, whereas the type IIb fibers are pale white.

Recently, using immunocytochemistry techniques, it has been found that in the rat there exists a fourth type of muscle fiber, **type IIx**. The type IIx fiber in the rat appears to have high oxidative capacity and resists fatigue. In both animals and humans, slow-twitch fibers are referred to as type I and fast-twitch fibers are referred to as type II. They are sub-classed into IIa and IIx, with the IIx having a faster twitch than the IIa. In rats fast-twitch type II fibers are sub classed into IIa, IIx, and IIb, with the IIb being faster than the IIx and IIa. The classification of fiber types are based on the type of myosin heavy chain gene that is expressed. That is, the slow-twitch type I MHC and the fast-twitch type IIa, IIx, and IIb MHC genes that encode the myosin protein. Humans do not express the IIx myosin at the protein level and, hence, only express the type I, IIa, and IIb fiber types.

Physiologic Contraction Times

Before the biochemical and molecular biologic techniques were perfected, muscle fiber typing relied on identifying differences in time for the muscle fiber to achieve peak

type I A muscle fiber that is classified by **histochemistry** or **immunocytochemistry** as a slow oxidative red fiber. With light microscopy the type I fiber appears pinky-red.

type IIa A fast-twitch fiber with a higher oxidative capacity that also appears pinky red with light microscopy.

type IIb A fast-twitch fiber that has low oxidative capacity and appears pale white in color with light microscopy.

type IIx A muscle fiber that is only in the rat and appears to have high oxidative capacity and resists fatigue.

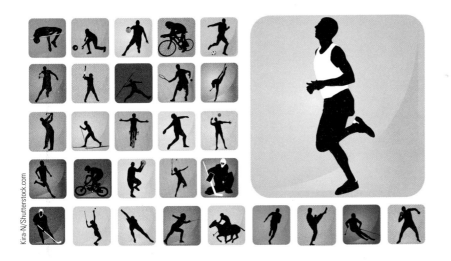

Kira-N/Shutterstock.com

isometric tension. As noted earlier, the type I fibers are known as the slow-twitch fibers and their time to peak tension during a maximal isometric contraction of a human ranges from 80 to 100 milliseconds (msec). The time to peak tension of the type II fibers, or fast-twitch fibers, approximates 40 msec.

> As an exercise science professional, you should attempt to succinctly explain the link between the motor unit recruitment, muscle fiber types, and the EMG recordings that occur when you go from rest to a slow jog, to a moderate-intensity run, and on to an all-out sprint.

Individual Variations

One of the classic discussions fundamental to developmental biology revolves around the concept that "ontology begets phylogeny"—a saying that we understand as, "which comes first, the chicken or the egg?" For the exercise physiologist, these sayings may well be stated as, "is it the genes or the training that makes the athlete?"

In humans, the proportion of slow-twitch fibers in the skeletal muscle ranges from 10 to 95 percent with a balance of fast-twitch fibers of type IIa and IIb. However, in highly trained endurance athletes, the proportion of slow-twitch fibers is generally greater than 70 percent, with the preponderance of type IIb fibers as the balance. In contrast, the power athletes, such as throwers and jumpers, have a greater proportion of the fast-twitch fibers than the slow-twitch fibers and a greater proportion of the type IIb than

the type IIa fast-twitch fiber. The other power athletes, the pure sprinters, have a greater proportion of fast-twitch fibers than slow-twitch fibers, with the majority of the fast-twitch fibers being type IIa (see Figure 3.16).

Muscle Fiber Adaptations: Genetics or Training

Initially, it was thought that as the fiber type was genetically established that the distribution of fiber types identified at birth would provide the individual genetic foundation of their athletic performance. However, recent investigations using rats have documented the ability of a specific electrical stimulation paradigm to change one fiber type to another. These experiments identified a concept of **myoplasticity**—that is, when the exercise training or detraining regimen results in changes in the genetic expression of specific muscle proteins, which, in turn, change one fiber type to another. Indeed, it is these training-induced changes in the muscle proteins that enhance the power generation or the endurance performance capabilities of the muscle.

The underlying question regarding "whether the genes or the training makes the athlete" remains a major debate. The presence of a genetic optimum in one's maximal oxygen uptake is becoming more and more accepted. In addition, the identification of single polymorphisms in proteins or allele deletions in the genes being associated with superior or inferior endurance performance supports the concept that the genes make the athlete. However, the identification that superior endurance performances have been achieved as a result of documented grueling programs of endurance training with a relatively low elite value of maximal oxygen uptake suggests that training adaptations of the skeletal muscle and its metabolic capacities (myoplasticity) and the development of an efficient style of running (running economy

myoplasticity The adaptation that a muscle fiber and its metabolic capacity undergoes as a result of a period of exercise training.

[RE]) are a major component of endurance performance. Endurance athletes require a training program that increases their mitochondrial mass, maximal oxidative capacity, and the development of energy substrate stores to enable the skeletal muscles to contract at a high intensity for long periods.

Training Adaptations of Neuromuscular Contractions

In Chapter 2, you were introduced to the specific principles of aerobic (endurance) and anaerobic (power) training for improvement of athletic or sport-specific performance, or both. This section focuses on the neuromuscular adaptations that occur with a program of exercise training designed to increase strength or endurance performance.

HOTLINK *See Chapter 2 for a review of specific aerobic and anaerobic training principles. See also the following commercial websites for testing calculators for a variety of neuromuscular fitness assessments:* http://www.exrx.net, http://www.brianmac.co.uk, *or* http://www.topendsports.com.

Based on the concept of specificity of training, it was generally thought that to excel at sports requiring a high degree of neuromuscular skill, such as baseball, golf, tennis, shooting a basketball, and so on, you did not need to train for strength and endurance unless the technique itself required it. In all sports and athletics of today, it is highly unlikely that for you or your trainee to excel at an event or sport that you would not devise some program of training that involves strength and endurance.

All athletic events and sports require the participant to generate muscular power; this could be whole-body movement as in running, swimming, jumping, bicycling, rowing, gymnastics, swinging a baseball bat or golf club, or throwing a baseball, javelin, and so on.

The generation of muscular power (force × distance × time) requires the coordination of the muscle's contraction by its neural activation with the release of its energy stores (see Figure 3.18).

Training for Strength Requires You to Use the Overload Principle

Since the time of the ancient Greeks, it has been known that if one progressively increases the work the muscle performs (**overload**), the stronger the muscle becomes. The weight training coach makes use of this overload principle (described in Chapter 2) to plan a training program, which during each training session overloads the specific muscles to be trained and which over years of training progressively increases the training load.

HOTLINK *See the National Strength and Conditioning Association website at:* www.nsca-lift.org. *Using specific keywords, also explore your favorite search engine to find supplemental material describing typical weight-training paradigms, such as pyramid and reverse pyramid programs.*

overload A progressive increase in the work of a muscle or group of muscles (by increases in frequency duration or load) within one period of exercise or over a multiple number of exercise periods.

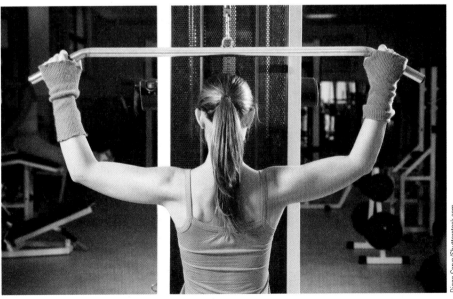

Diego Cervo/Shutterstock.com

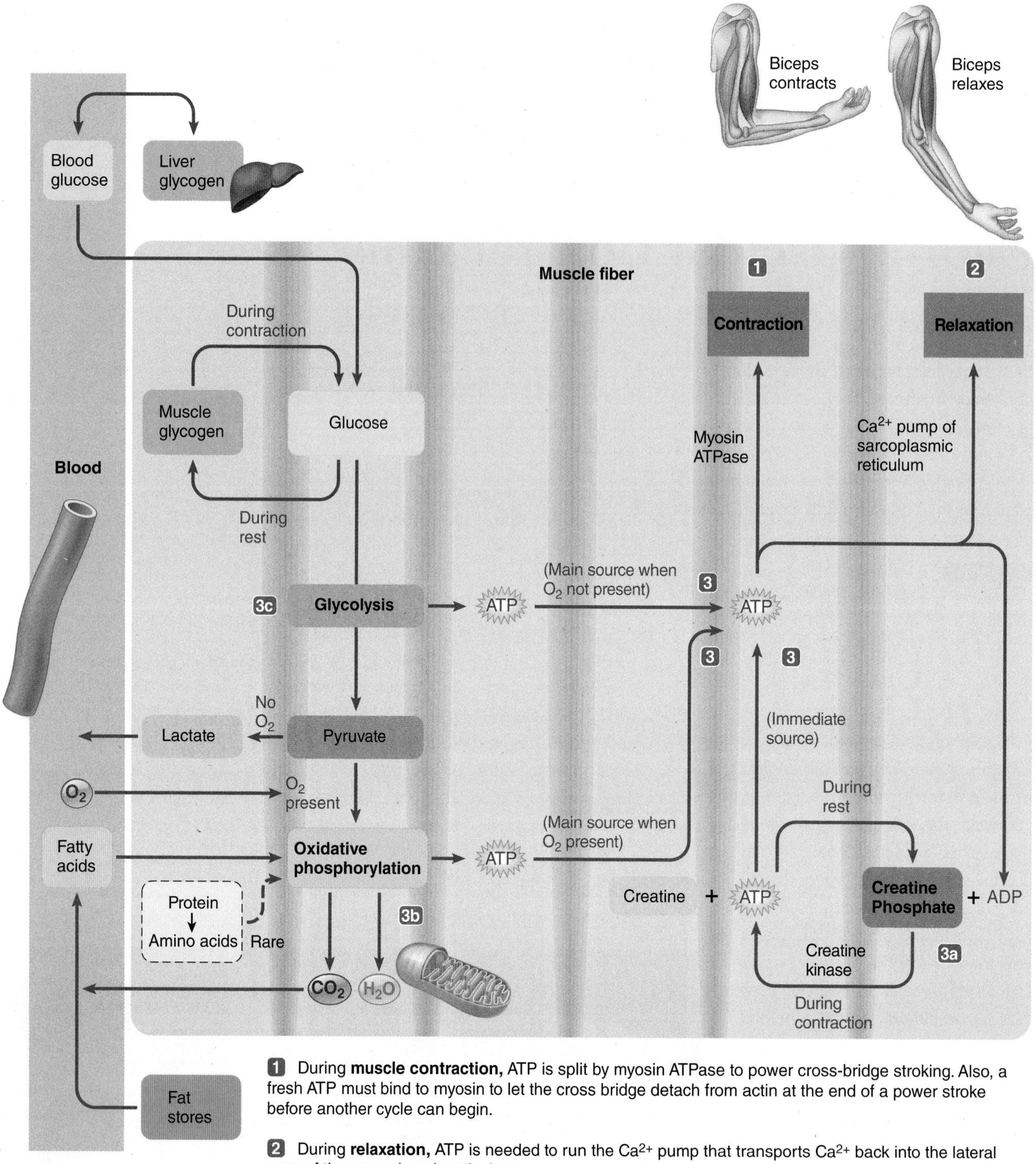

1. During **muscle contraction,** ATP is split by myosin ATPase to power cross-bridge stroking. Also, a fresh ATP must bind to myosin to let the cross bridge detach from actin at the end of a power stroke before another cycle can begin.

2. During **relaxation,** ATP is needed to run the Ca^{2+} pump that transports Ca^{2+} back into the lateral sacs of the sarcoplasmic reticulum.

3. The **metabolic pathways that supply the ATP** needed to accomplish contraction and relaxation are

   3a. transfer of a high-energy phosphate from **creatine phosphate** to ADP (immediate source);

   3b. **oxidative phosphorylation** (the main source when O_2 is present), fueled by glucose derived from muscle glycogen stores or by glucose and fatty acids delivered by the blood; and

   3c. **glycolysis** (the main source when O_2 is not present). Pyruvate, the end product of glycolysis, is converted to lactate when lack of O_2 prevents the pyruvate from being further processed by the oxidative phosphorylation pathway.

FIGURE 3.18 Metabolic pathways producing ATP used during muscle contraction and relaxation. (From Sherwood, L. 2010. Figure 8.22 in *Human physiology,* 7th ed. Belmont, CA: Brooks/Cole-Cengage Learning.)

Overload

In following a training program designed around the important training principle of overload, skeletal muscles increase their size and, as a consequence, their strength. The increase in muscle fiber size (**hypertrophy**) requires an increase in muscle protein accumulation. This can occur if:

1. Protein synthesis increases above protein degradation

2. Protein degradation decreases below protein synthesis

3. A combination of both

An increase in muscle size also occurs if the number of fibers increases (**hyperplasia**).

hypertrophy An increase in muscle fiber size.

hyperplasia An increase in the number of fibers

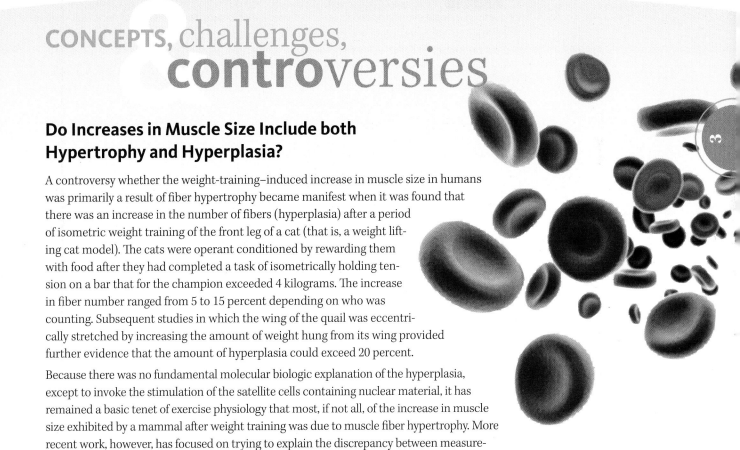

CONCEPTS, challenges, controversies

Do Increases in Muscle Size Include both Hypertrophy and Hyperplasia?

A controversy whether the weight-training–induced increase in muscle size in humans was primarily a result of fiber hypertrophy became manifest when it was found that there was an increase in the number of fibers (hyperplasia) after a period of isometric weight training of the front leg of a cat (that is, a weight lifting cat model). The cats were operant conditioned by rewarding them with food after they had completed a task of isometrically holding tension on a bar that for the champion exceeded 4 kilograms. The increase in fiber number ranged from 5 to 15 percent depending on who was counting. Subsequent studies in which the wing of the quail was eccentrically stretched by increasing the amount of weight hung from its wing provided further evidence that the amount of hyperplasia could exceed 20 percent.

Because there was no fundamental molecular biologic explanation of the hyperplasia, except to invoke the stimulation of the satellite cells containing nuclear material, it has remained a basic tenet of exercise physiology that most, if not all, of the increase in muscle size exhibited by a mammal after weight training was due to muscle fiber hypertrophy. More recent work, however, has focused on trying to explain the discrepancy between measurements of mean fiber cross-sectional area and the anatomical cross-sectional area of humans using magnetic resonance imaging (MRI) measurements of whole muscles of body builders. The discrepancy between the two measures indicated that hypertrophy of the muscle fibers could not account for the observed hypertrophy of the whole muscle. Recently, it has been demonstrated in rats that muscle overload activates, proliferates, differentiates, and fuses the satellite cells. Because this is similar to what happens during the developmental years of mammals, it is thought that the response to the overload results in activation of a developmental gene program. Evidence suggests that the new cells formed in response to the overload principle are formed in the interstitial tissue between the muscle fibers. Current work seeks to determine the important signaling pathways in activating the dormant satellite cells.

In addition, based on the fact that activation of satellite cells is responsible for postnatal muscle growth and new muscle fiber regeneration after injury or atrophy, the discussion has moved to whether muscle hypertrophy is a continuum characterized by the different developmental molecular phases. In other words, the discussion has gone far beyond the presence or absence of a hyperplasia response in the development of muscle hypertrophy and to whether satellite cell activation is fundamental to the molecular process of muscle hypertrophy.

The presence of a mechanism for fiber regeneration, or hyperplasia, in response to over-load weight training in a mammalian muscle has importance to investigators in the clinical fields of physical rehabilitation, neurology, orthopedic surgery, and tissue regeneration. However, it remains accepted dogma to the practicing exercise physiologists, performance and weight-training coaches, and the athletes for whom strength and power are prerequisites for elite performance that increases in muscle size of weight-trained humans is

HOTLINK See Chapter 2 for a review of the overload principle.

Myosin and actin protein accumulation are necessary in both hypertrophy and hyperplasia. The rate of the protein production in a muscle is directly related to the rate of influx of amino acids into the muscle cells. The increased influx of amino acids is directly related to the increase and duration of the muscle's force of contraction. The hypertrophied weight-trained muscle is able to move a submaximal load with a greater velocity of contraction than an untrained muscle. This ability to contract the trained muscle at a faster velocity means that it can generate more power than an untrained muscle (see Figure 3.10).

From this information it should be clear that to strengthen a skeletal muscle, the optimum training stimulus would be to have the muscle contracting as near to maximum tension as possible and at the slowest rate as possible. Many of the elite field event athletes and strength sports (for example, American football and rugby) use this form of weight training to increase their strength during the off-season; then during the preseason period immediately before their competitive season, trainers will have the athletes shift to more event-specific power–speed/strength, plyometric exercise, and skill training programs.

HOTLINK See Chapters 11 and 12 for more information about the role of amino acids in the diet.

Strength and Myoplasticity

Power athletes have little requirement for a large capacity to deliver oxygen, hence their training regimens are focused on increasing their anaerobic capacity and increasing the speed and force of their muscle contractions. This requires the development of contractile proteins and glycogen stores to enable a much greater velocity of shortening than an untrained muscle (see Figure 3.10).

At the beginning of a weight-training program of an inexperienced, untrained individual, a rapid increase in strength occurs. This has been attributed to the repetitive nature of the weight-training program optimizing the recruitment pattern within the motor units and the entrainment of neurologic pathways. This rapid adaptation of neuromotor function is one factor in the specificity of training and provides a rationale for designing a training program requiring repetitive practice of skill movements involving power generation to complete the skill.

Can you think of any athletic event or sport that would benefit from this type of training program?

Specific Adaptations of Fiber Types

If an individual uses only weight-training exercises in a 6-month training program, both type I and type II fibers increase their cross-sectional area. However, the amount of increase in the cross-sectional area of the type II fibers is some 10 percent greater than in the type I fibers (see Figure 3.19).

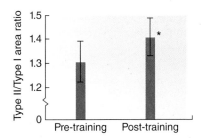

FIGURE 3.19 Figure indicates the increase in type II fiber cross-sectional area as a ratio of the increase in type I cross-sectional area after a 6-month resistance exercise training program. (Adapted from Brooks, G.A., T. D. Fahey, and K. M. Baldwin. 2005. Figure 19.3 in *Exercise physiology: Human bioenergetics and its applications,* 4th ed. New York: McGraw-Hill.)

The increases in the cross-sectional area of the fibers are due to increases in protein content and result in a 2 percent increase in cell volume; however, the increase in cell volume results in 11 and 1 percent decreases in capillary and mitochondrial densities, respectively (see Figure 3.20).

The large decreases in capillary density resulting from fiber hypertrophy without angiogenesis (increase in the number of blood vessels) expands the diffusion distance for oxygen to reach the mitochondrial electron transport chain. These cellular changes result in a reduc-

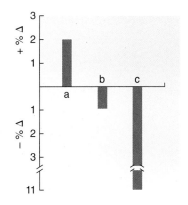

FIGURE 3.20 Percentage change in cytoplasmic volume (a), mitochondria/myofibril ratio (b), and the number of capillaries per square millimeter (c) after a 6-month resistance exercise training program. (© Cengage Learning 2013)

tion in endurance capacity. Therefore, to ameliorate this loss of endurance by the power athletes, many coaches use circuit weight-training programs to maintain endurance while increasing strength.

Summary

Tables 3.2 and 3.3 summarize the neuromuscular and muscle tissue adaptations that occur, respectively, with strength training.

TABLE 3.2 General Neuromuscular Adaptations to Strength (Resistance) Training

- Increases in motor cortex input that allows for greater neural control and increased force production
- Increase in muscle recruitment (more motor units) increasing force production
- Increases in neural firing rates and timing and coordination of recruitment that increases the rate of force production
- Reduction in the inhibitory functions like the Golgi tendon organs allowing for increased force production, motor unit synchronization, and cross-training (education) that helps balance force production between both sides of the body

© Cengage Learning 2013

TABLE 3.3 General Skeletal Muscle Adaptations to Strength (Resistance) Training

- Increases in muscle fiber size and cross-sectional size (muscle mass) that allows for increase in muscular strength
- Increases in myosin heavy chain protein and hypertrophy after early training changes associated with neural adaptations that allow for increases in muscular strength
- No change or decreases in capillary densities and decreases in mitochondrial densities, which are associated with decreased oxidative capacity and reduced changes in aerobic power
- Increases in ATP, creatine phosphate, glycogen stores, fuel mobilization, and anaerobic enzyme activity that allow for improved energy utilization and muscular endurance
- Potential increases in ligament, tendon, collagen, and bone strength with decrease in body fat and increases in lean weight that can enhance functional health and may reduce falls (particularly in the elderly)

© Cengage Learning 2013

Training for Endurance

The athletic event that requires endurance as a fundamental factor to its successful performance usually involves rhythmic muscle contractions that require changes in muscle length and joint movement. This type of muscle movement is termed *dynamic exercise*. Typical events involving dynamic exercise include running, swimming, rowing, and cross-country skiing. During running on level surfaces such as a track, the muscles generate relatively low intramuscular forces. However, during swimming, rowing, bicycling, and cross-country skiing, the rhythmically contracting muscles will need to generate relatively large intramuscular forces at some point in their duty cycle to overcome the event-specific muscular loading. It should be obvious to you that a training program for a specific endurance competition should be based on the repetition of the major muscle groups to be used in that event.

> Why should it be obvious that a training program for a specific endurance competition should be based on the repetition of the major muscle groups to be used in that event?

Endurance exercise training for competition or for health for all ages generally follows the same underlying principles of overload, frequency, intensity, and duration (see Chapter 2). However, if an individual wants to train only for the health benefits of exercise, it follows that once a certain level of health fitness has been achieved, the overload principle of training can be ignored and the frequency, intensity, and duration of the exercise training can be maintained. It is this maintenance of health status that requires us to regularly perform a dynamic exercise training program to prevent the diseases of a sedentary lifestyle associated with the metabolic syndrome (see Chapters 1, 6A, and 6B).

HOTLINK *See the websites for the American Heart Association (http://www.americanheart.org) and American College of Sports Medicine (http://www.acsm.org) for more information about training programs and metabolic syndrome.*

As we become older, the problems associated with overtraining become more prevalent, especially if the trainee has an obsessive/compulsive personality who likes competition and becomes negatively addicted to the training program.

These are not reasons for the many of us after leaving high school, college, and even professional sports to resort to training for a life of being a "couch potato" or spectator. Indeed, once we stop a sport-specific training program, which requires caloric intakes ranging from 3,000 to as much as 12,000 calories or more a day, we have difficulty in adjusting our daily caloric intake to match our more sedentary lifestyle, resulting in us getting fat.

> Is it a myth that exercise-trained hypertrophied muscle turns to fat when we stop our regular exercise training program?

Overloading the Skeletal Muscle during Exercise Is a Requirement for the Muscle to Adapt

In training for specific endurance events, the principles of overload and specificity are usually repetitively combined to entrain the neuromuscular control necessary to maintain the performance of a specific skill during a maximal effort that requires maximal metabolic energy generation. In addition, to perform the activity skillfully during an endurance event that requires the event to be completed in the shortest time possible (for example, cross-country skiing), the capacity of the muscle's metabolic machinery needs to be trained to meet the demands without fatigue.

At the time of the first modern Olympics in 1896 (held in Athens, Greece), it was unlikely that any of the 300 participants from the 15 countries had systematically trained for the events that they had individually entered. Therefore, the winners were probably those who had naturally (genetically) superior skills in the skill events, superior speed and strength in the speed and strength events, and superior endurance in the endurance events. Probably at about the time the athletes became sponsored by their home country and the fame of winning an Olympic Games event became national and international news, the concept of actually training to perform better than the other competitors was begun. Now that professionalism has entered into the lives of athletes and their time is spent in training and competing for ever-increasing rewards, the lives of athletes are focused 100 percent on improving their performance.

At first, endurance exercise training programs were developed by the athlete or coach empirically, and the results were then used as a means to judge whether the training program was successful. The exercise scientist has been playing catch-up to the coaches' development of individualized training programs ever since. Initially, the concept of long, slow distance (LSD) training programs was the first to be used in structuring a training program for the endurance athlete. The addition of "speed-play" (that is, sprinting as fast as one can for approximately 100 meters and then returning to the LSD running) became the fundamental training program for endurance runners from the late 1920s to the present day. A variety of LSD and speed-play training programs continue to be used today, primarily in the pre-competition period of training. In addition, running up hills and down dales of wilderness areas and sand dunes provided the trainee a means of intermittently overloading the system, as well as providing a change of scenery from the monotony of the track. You should understand that

the LSD to modern-day endurance athletes can range from 5 to 8 minutes per mile for 20 miles or more depending on whether they are training hard or light. (I suggest you try to run a mile in 8 minutes to understand what type of exercise workloads these types of training programs involve.) In the 1930s, coaches developed a more specific periodicity of the LSD/speed-play paradigm, and because of its regularity of interspersing speed runs with walking or jogging recovery before repeating the speed run, it became known as **interval training**. Initially, interval training was developed to train the cardiovascular system, and it was based on the idea of using timed speed runs over distances, for example, 100 meters in 12 seconds, 200 meters in 30 seconds, 300 meters in 45 seconds, and 400 meters in 60 to 70 seconds. At completion of the speed run, athletes walked or jogged back to the beginning of the speed run while measuring their heart rate. When their heart rates had recovered to < 120 beats/min, they repeated the speed run and recovery walk/jog/rest paradigm. In one training session, the repetitions of the speed runs and recovery would range from 20 to 40.

HOTLINK *See Chapter 2 to review the basics of the interval training concept.*

A simple calculation of a training program involving 20 repetitions of running 400 meters in 60 seconds, while using a walk/jog recovery until the heart rate was 120 beats/min repeated 3 times in a day, indicates that a heavy training day could extend for periods of 4 to 6 hours.

The distance of the speed runs varied as to what the specific athlete was working on regarding the distance of the events. The modern-day refinement of this training technique is to repeat the speed runs over the distance at a time as a multiple of the athlete's best performance time. For example, in training for breaking the 4-minute mile barrier, Sir Roger Bannister repeated the 440-yard speed runs in 60 seconds.

interval training Based on the idea of using timed speed runs over distances; for example, 100 m in 12 seconds, 200 m in 30 seconds, 300 in 45 seconds, and 400 in 60–70 seconds. At completion of the speed run, the athlete walks or jogs back to the beginning of the speed run while measuring his or her heart rate. When the heart rate recovers to less than 120 beats/min, the athlete repeats the speed run and recovery walk/jog/rest paradigm.

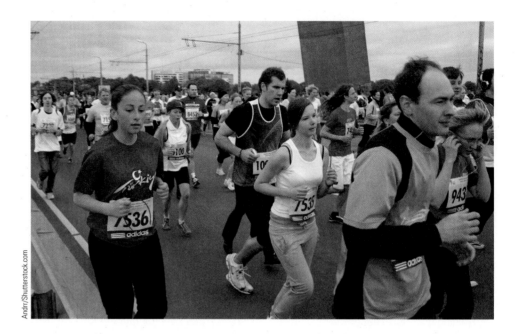

Andrr/Shutterstock.com

These training techniques result in increasing the capacity to deliver oxygen (see Chapters 7, 8, and 9) and improving the capacity of the muscle's metabolic machinery and its neuromuscular coordination. These training techniques are based on the specificity and overload training principles, and are used in improving the performance of running, swimming, bicycling, rowing, and cross-country skiing events, among other sports. In addition, improving one's aerobic capacity is beneficial to those athletes performing sports that require speed and power, as well as endurance, for example, association football (soccer), rugby, ice and field hockey, lacrosse, tennis, and so on. These sports require quick bursts of high-energy output for short periods while the duration of the event can exceed 1 hour. Hence the higher one's aerobic capacity and muscular endurance, the easier it is to recover from the intermittent short time and highly intense bursts of energy output.

Endurance and Myoplasticity

For those of us not interested in competitive events that require a large endurance capacity but who are interested in maintaining their health by living an active lifestyle and preventing the ravages of sedentary lifestyle diseases, a year-round program of LSD activity provides the health benefits of improved cardiorespiratory health and energy balance (that is, keeps the weight off). In contrast, the competitive athlete uses LSD (remember, LSD to a competitive endurance athlete is usually an exercise intensity far above what you and I think of as long slow speeds) and speed-play as an off-season maintenance training program. Before and during the competitive season, the athlete uses the interval training techniques on top of the LSD and speed-play training program in a cyclical manner of peaking, tapering, and recovering throughout the pre-competitive and competitive seasons (see Figure 3.21).

In progressing from a sedentary lifestyle to a progressively more aerobically active lifestyle using an LSD training program, the initial changes in the metabolic capacity of the muscle are greatest over the first 6 months. However, prolonged training beyond 6 months indicates that the cardiovascular system's capacity to deliver oxygen achieves a genetic optimum, whereas the metabolic machinery of the working muscles and neuromuscular coordination continues to improve its function (see Figure 3.18; see also Chapter 8). The major changes occur in the amount of mitochondrial proteins present within

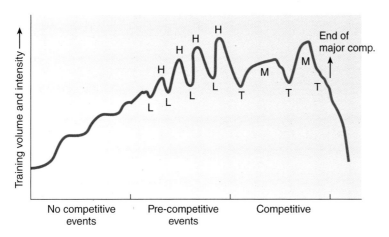

FIGURE 3.21 Example of a year's training schedule. During the off-season, (1) training consists of long, slow distance (LSD) during the pre-competition and (2) training consists of light days (L) LSD and heavy days (H) LSD plus intervals. With taper before first competition, during competitive period, alternate increasing H/L maintenance with taper before actual event. (© Cengage Learning 2013)

the cell (oxidative enzymes, such as succinate dehydrogenase) and the increase in mitochondrial density and capacity (see Figure 3.22).

In terms of endurance performance, it is the increase in the cell's maximal oxidative capacity that appears to be of greater importance than the cardiovascular system's ability to deliver oxygen, as measured by the individual maximal oxygen uptake ($\dot{V}O_2$ max). The elite endurance athlete rarely has a $\dot{V}O_2$ max of less than 70 ml O_2/kg/min, whereas individual elite athletes $\dot{V}O_2$ max values range from 70 to 90 ml O_2/kg/

min, yet there is no performance discrimination. Therefore, it is incorrect to assume that an elite athlete with a higher $\dot{V}O_2$ max tested in the sport-specific activity (for example, running, swimming, cross-country skiing) would best another elite athlete with a lower $\dot{V}O_2$ max when competing.

In addition, interval training further increases oxygen delivery and utilization, but more importantly increases the glycolytic metabolic capacity of the muscle fibers and adapts to higher concentrations of lactic acid production via the lactate shuttle mechanism. This enables the athlete to

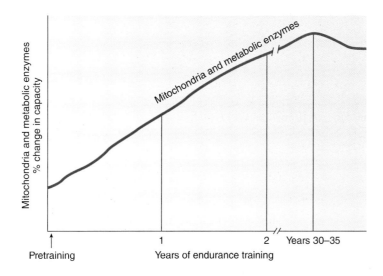

FIGURE 3.22 Schematic representation of changes in mitochondrial density and metabolic enzymes over years of endurance training before 30 to 35 years of age. (© Cengage Learning 2013)

Slow-Twitch Fibers	Various Mitochondrial Enzyme Markers
>90–100	>50–700

© Cengage Learning 2013

meet immediate needs in energy production, such as providing a final kick down the back straight of a 1,500-meter race.

Specific Adaptations and Fiber Type

The maximization of an individual's genetic optimum for aerobic cellular metabolism takes years of endurance training to achieve, and similar to the hypertrophy/hyperplasia controversy, the possibility that endurance exercise training can transform a type IIa or IIb fiber to a type I fiber remains controversial. However, based on rat hind-limb suspension models and rats exposed to spaceflight microgravity, it appears that the most aerobic type IIx fibers become less aerobic and are more metabolically similar to type IIb fibers in the human. In animal experiments in which muscles were chronically stimulated at rates equivalent to LSD training programs, results indicated that some of the type IIb or type IIx fibers had converted to a type I fiber's metabolic profile. For more evidence of the possibility of the training-induced switching of one fiber type to another, see the research biography of Kenneth M. Baldwin, Ph.D., later in this chapter; this biography summarizes the biologic complexity underlying what at first glance appears to be a simple outcome of an exercise training program.

Evidence of similar myoplastic conversion of type IIb to type I fibers metabolic selectivity in humans has been difficult to identify because elite athletes are not always amenable to undergoing repeat muscle biopsies throughout the years of their overload training program that would be required to track the changes in their muscle fiber populations. For example, in 1970 a marathoner had a 50:50 ratio of red and white muscle fibers yet finished 3 seconds behind the bronze medalist in the 1976 Montreal Olympics. Whether his training and competition in the intervening years had changed his muscles' fiber type I distribution was never determined with a follow-up muscle biopsy. However, when muscle biopsy samples obtained from competitive marathoners are compared with sedentary control subjects, the fiber type composition and the mitochondrial oxidative enzyme activities are markedly greater in the marathon runners (see Table 3.4).

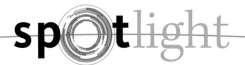

spotlight

An Expert on Neuromuscular Responses to Exercise: Kenneth M. Baldwin, Ph.D.

Dr. Kenneth M. Baldwin received his Ph.D. from the University of Iowa in 1970 and is currently Professor of Physiology and Biophysics at the University of California, Irvine. During Baldwin's 38-year career as an independent investigator, he has become recognized as an international authority on the general topic of cardiac and skeletal muscle plasticity, for example, the muscle's ability to change its phenotype and size in response to a variety of stimuli. The central thrust of his research has focused on the myosin heavy chain (MHC) gene family, which encodes several isoform species of motor proteins that regulate the contraction process. Each of these isoforms comprises the structural backbone of the contractile machinery, and thus regulates the fiber's ability to transduce chemical energy into mechanical force and work.

Therefore, the MHC protein controls the intrinsic contractile properties of each striated muscle fiber. Furthermore, based on the pattern of MHC gene expression across different clusters of skeletal muscle fibers, this diversification of MHC expression defines the functional capability of one muscle versus another.

From a historical perspective dating back about 35 years, it was discovered that the MHC was the primary protein that defined the essence of the fiber typing scheme that delineates fast versus slow muscle fiber types in both the heart and skeletal muscle. It has been long recognized that skeletal muscle is very plastic and can change its metabolic and functional properties in response to a variety of stimuli. A pivotal component of the adaptive process involves the switching of MHC isoforms to remodel the muscle for altered performance depending on the mechanical stimulus imposed. Baldwin's research has focused not only on understanding activity and hormonal factors that derive fiber switching in general, but more importantly on the mechanisms that bring about the actual switching of MHC genes in cardiac and skeletal muscle cells.

It is safe to say that Baldwin, arguably more than any other investigator, has provided more insight concerning: (a) the pattern of expression of these proteins in different types of skeletal muscle, and (b) their adaptive changes in expression in response to a variety of experimental manipulations such as mechanical overload (resistance training), endurance exercise, spaceflight, hormonal (thyroxin and insulin) regulation, and nutritional intervention (caloric restriction and dietary manipulation of carbohydrates). His group defined the plasticity of the MHC gene family and demonstrated that the regulation of these proteins was clearly a pre-translational process; that is, processes that regulate gene expression upstream determine how the protein is actually synthesized.

Practical Summary

To excel at a specific athletic event, or sport, you must follow a training program that involves repetitive movement skills required to complete the event or sport, that is, specificity of training. Most athletic movements require strength, speed, agility, and endurance. Hence your training requires the overload principle designed around manipulating frequency, intensity, and duration of the particular skill necessary to be successful. For example, it would be incongruous to have swimmers or weight lifters train for competition using rowing exercises as a training paradigm. However, regardless of the sport, it has been found beneficial for all athletes in the off-season to develop a base of aerobic and strength conditioning. Those individuals who suddenly see the light and begin exercise training usually after a period of being a "couch potato" or never having attempted to exercise need to be aware, or the exercise trainer needs to make them aware, that the training program must begin slowly and gradually increase the overload, be it for "power" or "endurance." Two of the biggest problems to overcome to ensure compliance of the naive exerciser are muscular fatigue and **delayed onset muscle soreness (DOMS)**.

Multiple Factors Contribute to Muscular Fatigue during Prolonged Exercise

The onset of muscular fatigue during high-intensity and/or prolonged exercise that requires us to stop exercising was initially thought to involve only intrinsic mechanisms within the active skeletal muscle.

(Does lactate cause muscular fatigue?)

Muscular fatigue can be associated with a host of factors that continue to be identified by exercise scientists. It is important for you to understand that muscular fatigue associated with exercise is not usually related to one simple mechanism. Muscular fatigue has been attributed to central (CNS) and peripheral (neuromuscular) factors, as

delayed onset of muscular soreness (DOMS) Usually associated with more severe pain than felt with acute muscle soreness, this occurs 24 to 48 hours following high intensity exercise, especially for the beginning exerciser, or after a period of detraining.

well as individual training status, environmental factors, and changes in homeostasis caused by the following factors: (a) time zone changes off-setting an individual's circadian rhythm from the light/day cycle, (b) lack of sleep, and (c) legal and/or illegal drug use.

Following are some of the commonly reported muscular factors associated with muscular fatigue during exercise:

1. ATP/CP (CP; utilization and resynthesis)

2. Muscle glycogen (depletion and resynthesis)

3. Glucose availability

4. Accumulation or depletion of metabolites (lactate/H^+, $Mg2^+$, ADP, Pi, ammonia [NH_3], Ca^+, and reactive oxygen species)

During the early 2000s a more integrative physiologic model of fatigue has been proposed that involves the peripheral muscular system and CNS, which during heavy-intensity exercise are exacerbated by the respiratory system (see Figure 3.23).

The initial physiologic identification of peripheral muscular fatigue was demonstrated using serial muscle biopsies of the quadriceps muscle during a cycle ergometer ride to exhaustion; that is, the subjects were unable to continue cycling. The end point of cycling was correlated with the fact that the muscle glycogen stores of the quadriceps muscle were also exhausted. However, current investigations have identified that during the progression to physical exhaustion, the subjects' ratings of perceived exertion progressively increased and their neuromuscular coordination decreased. These symptoms indicate the involvement of a progressive increase in **central (neural) fatigue**, which with **transcranial magnetic stimulation** of the

central (neural) fatigue A condition when an individual's Ratings of Perceived Exertion **(RPE)** progressively increases and his or her neuromuscular coordination decreases.

transcranial magnetic stimulation A non-invasive technology that can provide a focused magnetic stimulation of specific areas of the motor cortex.

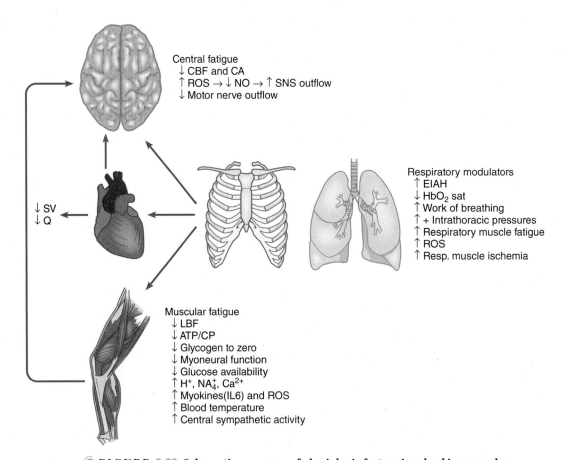

Central fatigue
↓ CBF and CA
↑ ROS → ↓ NO → ↑ SNS outflow
↓ Motor nerve outflow

↓ SV
↓ Q

Respiratory modulators
↑ EIAH
↓ HbO_2 sat
↑ Work of breathing
↑ + Intrathoracic pressures
↑ Respiratory muscle fatigue
↑ ROS
↑ Resp. muscle ischemia

Muscular fatigue
↓ LBF
↓ ATP/CP
↓ Glycogen to zero
↓ Myoneural function
↓ Glucose availability
↑ H^+, NA_4^+, Ca^{2+}
↑ Myokines(IL6) and ROS
↑ Blood temperature
↑ Central sympathetic activity

FIGURE 3.23 Schematic summary of physiologic factors involved in muscular fatigue. (Modified from Dempsey, J. A., M. Amann, L. M. Romer, and J. D. Miller. 2008. Respiratory system determinants of peripheral fatigue and endurance performance. *Med. Sci. Sports Exerc.* 40:457–461.)

motor cortex nerves in humans has been identified to impair motor-neural pathway activation of the muscle up to 4 hours in recovery from a marathon.

The mechanisms underlying central fatigue remain under intense investigation and may be related to exercise-induced arterial hypoxemia (discussed further in Chapter 9) and arterial hemoglobin desaturation (HbO_2), as large as −10 percent, because of a progressive rightward shift in the HbO_2^- dissociation curve associated with metabolic acidosis and increases in blood temperature (Bohr effect discussed in Chapter 9). In addition, the increased work of breathing resulting in respiratory muscle fatigue can also cause HbO_2 desaturation. However, experiments that counteracted the exercise-induced arterial hypoxemia and the decline in HbO_2 did not prolong the onset of muscular fatigue–induced performance time. During heavy-intensity exercise, the ventilation response generates large swings between inspiratory negative and expiratory positive intrathoracic pressures. These oscillations in intrathoracic pressures assist venous return and increase cardiac output during active inspiration but decrease venous return and decrease cardiac output during active expiration. These findings result in the brain and the skeletal muscles being over-perfused and under-perfused, respectively, and result in sustained increases in sympathetic activity and generation of reactive oxygen species. The increase in reactive oxygen species results in a generalized increase in central sympathetic outflow causing sympathetic vasoconstriction in the systemic, pulmonary, and cerebral circulations.

Although all the details of the mechanisms underlying central and peripheral muscular fatigue are yet to be described, it is important for you remember to observe the variability within your clients for the signs of fatigue, and to begin to try and identify the various training and environmental factors that may cause their fatigue. Once you can identify the possible

fatigue factors that affect the individuals, you can more readily educate your clients and develop a training program strategy on how they can minimize the effects of fatigue during competition.

HOTLINK *Review Chapters 4, 5, 6, 11, 12, and 14 for more information about metabolic, nutritional, and environmental factors associated with muscular fatigue; then use your favorite search engine to search for scientific websites that explore the various factors associated with muscular fatigue during exercise.*

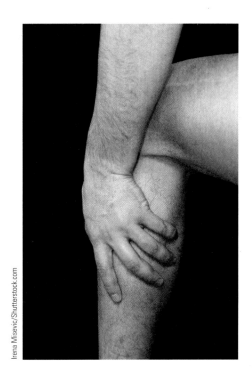

Irena Misevic/Shutterstock.com

Delayed Onset Muscle Soreness Is Linked to Inflammatory Processes

Like muscular fatigue, during exercise, we have all experienced muscle soreness, particularly after exercises to which we are not accustomed. Mild muscle soreness associated with low- to mild-intensity exercise during or immediately afterward is called **acute muscle soreness**. Acute muscle soreness is the pain that lasts for a few minutes to a few hours after the exercise and is related to the accumulation of H^+ and tissue edema (or

acute muscle soreness The feeling of sore muscles immediately after exercise.

swelling) from fluid shifts from blood's plasma to the tissues surrounding active muscle groups. In contrast, DOMS is usually associated with more severe pain than felt with acute muscle soreness, and it occurs 24 to 48 hours after high-intensity exercise, especially for the beginning exerciser or after a period of detraining. Following are some of the activities that result in DOMS:

1. Eccentric muscle contractions, such as running or walking downhill

2. High-intensity exercise that your clients are unaccustomed to that usually results in damage to the muscle structure

3. Overstretching or tearing of muscle connective tissues

Following are some of the commonly reported factors associated with DOMS:

1. Inflammatory reaction of muscles(s)

2. Edema (swelling) after cellular inflammation

3. Secondary chemical damage from cellular inflammation

You can help your clients minimize or prevent the effects of DOMS at the beginning of their exercise training program, whether it be a weight or endurance training program, by having them reduce their eccentric muscle contractions, starting at lower intensities, and using sensible periodization training principles (see Chapter 2). When a client experiences exercise-induced DOMS, they will usually see a temporary reduction in their muscle strength for a few days to a week, after the initial bout of exercise that resulted in DOMS. This is a normal response because of changes in the ability to develop normal muscle excitation-contraction coupling, and it is helpful to educate your clients about this before a DOMS event so that they can anticipate it. You may also remind them that, although the effects of DOMS are uncomfortable, some scientific evidence supports that DOMS associated with increased intensi-

ties of exercise may be an important factor in maximizing the muscle training effect (see Figure 3.24).

Muscle Cramps Remain a Mystery

Another common muscle discomfort problem that a majority of your clients will experience at some time or another is muscle cramping (painful, spasmodic, involuntary muscle contractions). The exact physiologic cause of muscle cramps is unknown, but they are most likely associated with dehydration and disruptions in electrolyte balance and/or carbohydrate stores. Regular conditioning, proper hydration for the environmental conditions (see Chapters 11, 12, and 14), reducing the intensity and duration of the exercise training program at the beginning of the program, and stretching muscle groups prone to cramping are strategies that you can use to encourage your clients to reduce or eliminate the incidence of muscle cramping.

There are health benefits to be accrued in exercise training designed to improve physical performance. However, it is not necessary to be an elite athlete to obtain the health benefits of a regular exercise program. Unfortunately, a lifestyle of sedentary living, overeating (calories in > calories out), television watching, playing video games, and working at a computer has become prevalent among our children and adults. This community acceptance of a life without physical activity has resulted in an epidemic of cardiovascular disease among all ages of the population in the industrialized nations of the world.

The reversal of this epidemic can be achieved only if you the teacher, coach, rehabilitation specialist, exercise leader, personal trainer, exercise scientist, and physicians understand the principles of exercise training, and teach and practice what you preach.

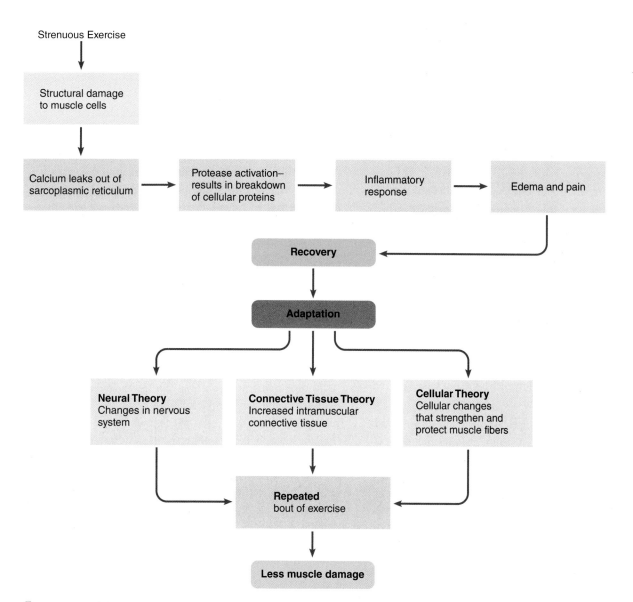

Strenuous Exercise

Structural damage to muscle cells

Calcium leaks out of sarcoplasmic reticulum → Protease activation–results in breakdown of cellular proteins → Inflammatory response → Edema and pain

Recovery

Adaptation

Neural Theory Changes in nervous system

Connective Tissue Theory Increased intramuscular connective tissue

Cellular Theory Cellular changes that strengthen and protect muscle fibers

Repeated bout of exercise

Less muscle damage

FIGURE 3.24 **Flow diagram of the initial onset of delayed onset muscle soreness (DOMS) and theories of adaptation that occur in the recovery period before the next bout of exercise.** (Adapted from Figures 21.4 and 21.5, pages 436 and 437 in *Exercise Physiology* edited by Powers. Scott and Howley, Ed. Copyright © 2004. Reprinted by permission of The McGraw-Hill Companies.)

in*Practice*

Examples of Neuromuscular Responses and Adaptations to Exercise

The following examples are related to neuromuscular responses and adaptations to exercise performance. The considerations for each specific recommendation are based on the most current understanding of the link between exercise and the topics of neuromuscular physiology, which are continuing to evolve.

Health/Fitness: Drew is a 25-year-old college student who has just started a weight-training program at the university recreational sports center. He has been working out for 6 weeks, 3 times per week, by doing 10 different exercises, performing 3 sets of 10 repetitions. He has noticed that he has gotten stronger (can lift more weight, about 10–15 more pounds per exercise) but feels like he has reached a point in the past week where he is not seeing any improvement (he was hoping to see increased hypertrophy, but hasn't). How do you explain his initial exercise progress?

Drew's improvement in strength is quite common, as most of the initial gains seen with resistant training include increased strength via neuromuscular adaptations. Specifically, beginning weight lifters can recruit more motor units in the first 4 to 6 weeks of training, while the changes in muscle size (hypertrophy) do not develop until later in training (about 10–12 weeks or longer). Drew probably needs to change his training routine to see future improvements.

It appears that Drew has hit a plateau in his training, which is normal, but this should be recognized and explained to Drew by his trainer. If you do not help your clients understand this common training response, they most likely will get disappointed with improvements, bored, or both, and quit their exercise routine.

Medicine: Emily is a 26-year-old medical student who has been asked to give a lecture about muscle fatigue to some of her fellow medical school classmates. She has reviewed all of her medical physiology resources regarding neuromuscular responses and adaptations, but she isn't sure how to approach her presentation. How might you help her?

One approach that might help Emily to prepare her talk is to think about how the actual process of neuromuscular contraction is integrated. In other words, initially the brain and spinal cord are involved in voluntary muscle contraction and any factors like lack of motivation or changes in reflex action might cause fatigue and reduce the development of muscle power. This has been referred to as "central muscle fatigue."

"Peripheral muscle fatigue" is often associated with insufficient energy (ATP, CP, etc.); glycogen depletion; increased lactate, which can inhibit calcium release from the endoplasmic reticulum; the accumulation of other metabolic by-products; dehydration; increased muscle heat; and other factors.

It is important for you and Emily to understand that the concept of muscle fatigue is complex, and it is naive to believe that it is as simple as just blaming it on the accumulation of lactate (which is still a common explanation among exercise science practitioners). An effective way to prevent muscle fatigue is to increase our understanding of how to develop appropriate training routines and effective nutritional strategies.

Athletic Performance: Megan is a 24-year-old collegiate distance runner who wants to improve her best 5-kilometer time (19:30). A friend of hers on the track team has told her that she looks inefficient because her running style is more rigid than and not as fluid as one of the faster 5-kilometer runners on the team. Megan has heard that if she can improve her mechanical efficiency (ME), it might help her improve her race time. What advice can you give Megan to enhance her exercise performance?

As you learned earlier, ME is difficult to measure because of the stored elastic energy in muscles. In distance running and other activities such as walking, cycling, and swimming, running economy (RE, the oxygen cost at a given speed) has been used as a measure of running efficiency because it is easier to measure than ME.

Although there is some anecdotal evidence that RE can improve with specific interval training methods (much like drills in team sports), the improvements may be small and yet significant to improvement (30 seconds to 1 minute in Megan's case). Often the observational biomechanics of a runner, for example, may make them appear to be inefficient according to textbook models, yet mature individuals probably have adapted their biomechanics over time, to an efficient movement pattern based on their unique anatomical and gait patterns. Some evidence suggests that changing the form or technique of an athlete actually can make them more inefficient or less economical, at least initially.

Megan probably would be wise to incorporate specific RE training into her program (in consultation with her coach) that includes interval training. Repetitive bouts of intervals that last 30 seconds to 3 minutes in duration should improve her RE by allowing her to recruit fewer motor units at faster paces over time (about 12–30 weeks).

Rehabilitation: Buck is a 25-year-old male collegiate student athletic trainer. He is taking 15 hours of class every semester and working with the football team in the fall and the track team in the spring. Buck is at least 30 pounds overweight, and several of his athletic training colleagues make fun of him behind his back when he has to jog out on the field or track to attend to an athlete. He doesn't seem to be aware that he is not well respected professionally by his colleagues. How can you help Buck out? Why should he be concerned about his physical appearance with regard to his professional acceptance?

One approach might be to have one of Buck's professors make him aware that, as exercise professionals, we should all try to practice what we teach and preach. Although he probably is having a hard time controlling his weight because of the long hours he (and most athletic trainers) is working, he needs to develop a plan that will help him earn and maintain his personal and professional self-respect. He may need to visit with someone who can help him develop a time-management plan that will allow him to incorporate more exercise into his schedule and also develop some new nutritional strategies for effective weight control.

Chapter Summary

- It is important that you review and acquire a working knowledge about neural integration and skeletal muscle contraction to understand how exercise influences homeostasis and steady-state exercise.

- The three types of muscle contraction are isometric (or static), concentric, and eccentric. The response of bone to exercise training and detraining is fast becoming a specialized area of exercise physiology and clinical rehabilitation.

- The synergism between muscle groups makes it difficult in real life to predict the position and length of a specific muscle group that will result in the greatest force of contraction.

- The velocity (or speed) of shortening (contraction) affects the force generated by the muscle; the maximal power (force $\times$ distance per unit of time) that can be generated by the muscle occurs at 25 to 30 percent of the maximal velocity of shortening.

- The electrical activity, or the integrated electromyographic (EMG) activity, increases linearly with the intensity (rate) of the exercise and, therefore, increases linearly with the oxygen uptake.

- The slow motor units are the first to be activated at the onset of a contraction, and as the force of the contraction increases, the number of motor units increases; this is called *recruitment*.

- The differences in oxidative capacities, together with their concomitant myofibrillar-ATPase activities, enable the fibers to be classified as type I, or slow-twitch, high- oxidative fibers and type IIa, or fast-twitch fibers with a higher oxidative capacity than the type IIb, or fast-twitch fiber with low oxidative capacity.

- As an exercise professional, you should see whether you can succinctly explain the link between the motor unit recruitment, muscle fiber types, and the EMG recordings that occur when you go from rest to a slow jog, to a moderate-intensity run, and on to an all-out sprint.

- The increase in muscle fiber size (hypertrophy) requires an increase in muscle protein accumulation. An increase in muscle size also occurs, if the number of fibers increases (hyperplasia).

- The rapid adaptation of neuromotor function is one factor in the specificity of training and provides a rationale for designing a training program that requires repetitive practice of skill movements involving power generation to complete the skill.

Exercise Physiology Reality

CENGAGEbrain To reinforce the exercise physiology concepts presented above, complete the laboratory exercises for Chapter 3. To access labs and other course materials for this text, please visit www.cengagebrain.com. See the pref-ace on page xiii for details. Once you complete the exercises, have your instructor evaluate your prescriptions. Remember to use your lab experience to help guide you toward future success in exercise physiology.

Exercise Physiology Web Links

Access the following websites for further study of topics covered in this chapter:

- Find updates and quick links to sites related to the basics of nutrition for exercise and exercise physiology at our website. To access the course materials and companion resources for this text, please visit www.cengagebrain.com. See the preface on page xiii for details. Search for further information about neuromuscular responses and adaptations to exercise at the governmental publication website: http://www.pubmed.gov.

- Search for information about neuromuscular responses and adaptations to exercise at the American College of Sports Medicine website: http://www.acsm.org.

- Search for more information about neuromuscular responses and adaptations to exercise at the National Strength and Conditioning Association (NSCA) website: http://www.nsca-lift.org.

- Search for more information about training for neuromuscular adaptations at commercial websites, for example: http://www.exrx.net, http://www.brianmac.co.uk, or http://www.topendsports.com.

Study Questions

Review the Warm-Up Pre-Test questions you were asked to answer before reading Chapter 3. Test yourself once more to determine what you know now that you have completed the chapter.

The questions that follow will help you review this chapter. You will find the answers in the discussions on the pages provided.

1. Discuss the anatomy of the CNS including the six major areas of the brain. *pp. 67–71*

2. What are neural reflexes and why are they important to understanding exercise? *pp. 69–74*

3. Discuss six components of the sliding filament theory of muscular contraction. *pp. 73–75*

4. What is the difference between the isometric, concentric, and eccentric muscle contractions? *pp. 78–79*

5. How do you determine the optimal position for muscle contraction that generates maximal muscle tension? *pp. 79–80*

6. Why does negative work require less oxygen than positive work with regard to muscle contraction? Defend your answer. *pp. 80–82*

7. What is mechanical efficiency (ME) and why is it difficult to calculate? *pp. 82–83*

8. How does central command relate to neuromuscular integration? *pp. 67–74*

9. Describe how motor units are recruited to perform work. *pp. 83–85*

10. What are the various fiber types, and how does exercise training influence their ability to change from one type to another? *pp. 83–98*

Selected References

Adams, G., F. Haddad, P. W. Bodell, P. D. Tran, and K. M. Baldwin. 2007. Combined isometric, concentric, and eccentric resistance exercise prevents unloading-induced muscle atrophy in rats. *J. Appl. Physiol.* 103:1644–1654.

Armstrong, R. 1984. Mechanisms of exercise-induced delayed onset muscle soreness: A brief review. *Med. Sci. Sports Exerc.* 16:529–538.

Bailey, D. M. 2004. Regulation of free radical outflow from and isolated muscle bed in exercising humans. *Am. J. Physiol. Heart Circ. Physiol.* 287:H1689–H1699.

Baldwin, K. M., et al. 1972. Respiratory capacity of white red and intermediate muscle, adaptive response to exercise. *Am. J. Physiol.* 222:373–378.

D'Antona, G., et al. 2006. Skeletal muscle hypertrophy and structure and function of skeletal muscle fibers in male body builders. *J. Physiol.* 570:611–627.

Dempsey, J. A., M. Amann, L. M. Romer, and J. D. Miller. 2008. Respiratory system determinants of peripheral fatigue and endurance performance. *Med. Sci. Sports Exerc.* 40:457–461.

Lieber, R. L. 1992. *Skeletal muscle structure and function.* Baltimore: Williams & Wilkins.

McMahon, T. A. 1984. *Muscles, reflexes and locomotion.* Princeton, NJ: Princeton University Press.

Pandorf, C. E., et al. 2006. Dynamics of myosin heavy chain gene regulation in slow skeletal muscle: Role of natural antisense RNA. *J. Biol. Chem.* 281:38330–38342.

Secher, N. H., T. Seifert, and J. J. Van Lieshout. 2008. Cerebral blood flow and metabolism during exercise: Implications for fatigue. *J. Appl. Physiol.* 104:306–314.

Sherwood, L. 2010. *Human physiology: From cells to systems,* 7th ed. Belmont, CA: Brooks/Cole-Cengage Learning.

Tamaki, T., A. Akatsuka, M. Tokunaga, K. Ishige, S. Uchiyama, and T. Shiraishi. 1997. Morphological and biochemical evidence of muscle hyperplasia following weight-lifting rats. *Am. J. Physiol.* 273:C246–C256.

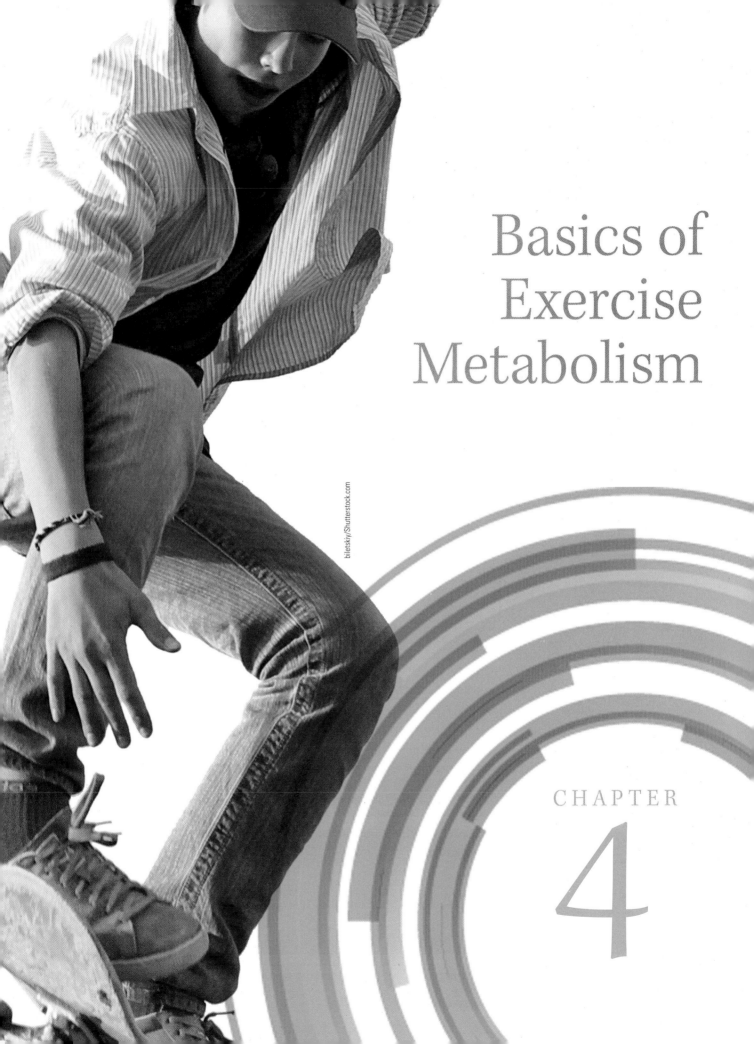

Basics of Exercise Metabolism

CHAPTER

4

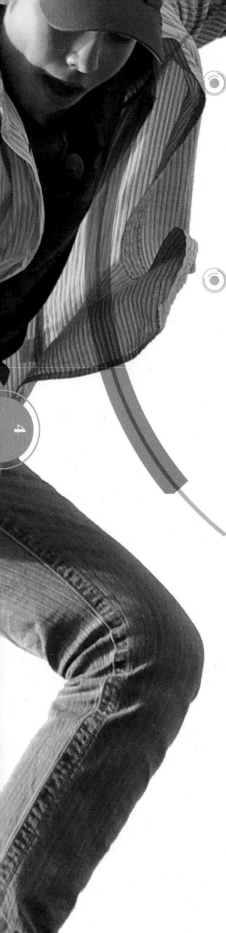

◉ Warm-Up

What do you already know about exercise metabolism?

- Use the following Pre-Test or the online evaluation tools for Chapter 4 to determine how much you already know. To access the course materials and companion resources for this text, please visit www.cengagebrain.com. See the preface on page xiii for details.

- Need more review? Let the online assessments, animations, and tutorials for Chapter 4 help prepare you for class.

◉ Pre-Test

1. Most adenosine triphosphate (ATP) is produced in organelles inside cells called the _____.

2. What process is most ATP normally synthesized by?

3. What are proteins composed of?

4. What is the main source of blood glucose in the fasted state?

5. Glucose enters the muscle cell by _____.

6. What is the most abundant substrate for energy production?

7. Fatty acids are transported in the blood bound to _____.

8. Glycogen stores are used for energy during exercise and replenished during _____.

9. Before metabolism in the mitochondria, glucose and fatty acids undergo chemical reactions in the _____.

10. In healthy people, amino acids are only a minor substrate for _____.

1. mitochondria; 2. oxidative phosphorylation; 3. amino acids joined by amide bonds; 4. liver; 5. transporter-mediated diffusion; 6. triglycerides stored in fat cells; 7. proteins; 8. feeding; 9. cytosol; 10. muscle energy metabolism

What You Will Learn in This Chapter

- The sources of chemical energy
- How chemical energy contained in glucose, fats, and amino acids is converted to a common currency
- The role of key enzymes and organelles in control of energy metabolism

QUICKSTART!

How is energy derived from the foods we eat? What tissues and pathways are involved? What are the conditions that lead to increased needs for energy production?

Introduction to Exercise Metabolism

Your basic nutrition and introductory physiology courses introduced concepts that define how the body converts the foods we eat into the energy we need to sustain physiologic processes. In this chapter, you will learn how metabolism sustains the high rates of energy production needed to exercise. One of the major concepts to learn from this chapter is that the supply of energy to the muscles during exercise can be limited by the rate and amount of oxygen being delivered to the active muscles. The delivery of oxygen is explained in more detail in Chapters 7 to 10. In this chapter, you will learn the key chemical reactions and metabolic pathways that are required to convert carbohydrates and fats into energy necessary to continuously provide energy to muscle, heart, liver, brain, and other tissues during exercise.

Chemical Energy for Exercise

In the resting state, the body requires energy to drive the beating heart, expand the lungs, and maintain electrochemical gradients for membrane transport and for assorted biosynthetic processes. During exercise, the energy requirement of the body undergoes a marked increase. This increase is primarily due to the energy requirement of the muscle contraction and relaxation cycle. Chemical energy to fuel these activities is stored in the foods we eat. These energy-containing foods are carbohydrates, fats, and proteins. Although food consumption occurs intermittently, the body requires energy continuously. To provide chemical energy during a fast, an organism must have the capacity to store nutrients from ingested food for later use.

You learned in previous courses about how ingested food absorbed by the gastrointestinal tract is stored in the body. This process is briefly summarized in this chapter. Carbohydrates are stored predominantly as **glycogen** in muscles and the liver. Fatty acids are stored mainly as **triglycerides**, primarily in adipose tissue. Table 4.1 summarizes the distribution and quantitative importance of body fuel stores.

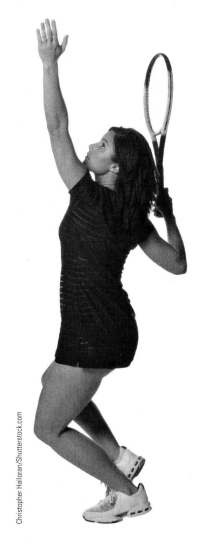

Christopher Halloran/Shutterstock.com

glycogen A molecule that serves as the storage form of glucose. It consists of long polymer chains of glucose and is synthesized and stored mainly in the liver and the muscles.

triglyceride A molecule that serves as the storage form of fat. It consists of glycerol and three fatty acids. It is concentrated in adipose tissue.

TABLE 4.1 Chemical Energy in Overnight-Fasted People (~70 kg)

Tissue	Fuel	Amount (g)	~Energy (Kcal)
Blood	Glucose	4.3	17
	Fatty acids	0.75	7
	Triglycerides	8.00	75
Muscle	Glycogen	350	1,400
	Triglycerides	300	2,700
Liver	Glycogen	100	400
Adipose	Triglycerides	12,000	107,500

© Cengage Learning 2013

Hydrolysis is a chemical process in which a chemical compound is broken down by reaction with water. Hydrolysis reactions result in the breakdown of glycogen to glucose, triglycerides to fatty acids and **glycerol**, and proteins to amino acids. This breakdown allows storage forms to be converted to their smaller constituents that are the immediate reactants of energy-producing pathways. Quantitatively, adipose tissue triglycerides are the primary source of chemical energy. Although glycogen and blood glucose stores are small relative to triglycerides, these fuels are important because the brain relies almost exclusively on carbohydrate metabolism. Protein stores are vast, but they are not utilized for their chemical energy to a great extent, except in specific tissue (for example, intestines) and cell types (for example, macrophages) that use the amino acid glutamine for energy. Branched-chain amino acids are a minor energy substrate in skeletal muscle. Generally, however, protein stores cannot be broken down to yield significant energy without compromising cell function. Figure 4.1 summarizes the major storage (anabolic) and hydrolytic (catabolic) processes of major substrates.

Role of ATP

The **chemical energy** stored in glucose, fatty acids, and amino acids cannot be used until it is transferred to **adenosine triphosphate (ATP)**. ATP is the common energy currency that is used by virtually all energy-requiring processes in the body. Having a common currency of energy has clear regulatory and evolutionary advantages. Energy metabolism is complex. To understand why it is better to have a single currency of energy, you need to imagine the added complexity of a system in which each fuel metabolized generates a different energy currency, and each of the numerous cellular functions used a unique currency. A series of "currency exchange" reactions would be necessary to make the yield from energy-producing pathways compatible with the requirements of energy-consuming pathways. Fortunately, this added layer of complexity is unnecessary because most biochemical systems rely on ATP as the immediate source of energy. Considering the reliance of energy-requiring reactions on ATP, it is clear that the means by which chemical energy is transferred from fuels to ATP is central to metabolism.

ATP contains the purine base adenine and the sugar ribose that is held together by a glycoside bond that together forms the nucleoside adenosine (see Figure 4.2).

One phosphate ester bond and two phosphate anhydride bonds tether the three phosphates (PO_4) and the ribose together. The binding of successive PO_4 results in clustering of negatively charged oxygen (O_2) atoms. These negatively charged atoms repel each other.

Potential energy is the energy stored in a physical system that can be released or converted to other forms of energy. The bonds that maintain the inherently unstable arrangement of negatively charged atoms of ATP have a high potential energy. The energy released when these bonds are broken can drive a wide range of reactions.

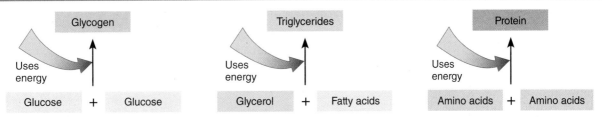

Anabolic reactions include the making of glycogen, triglycerides, and protein; these reactions require differing amounts of energy.

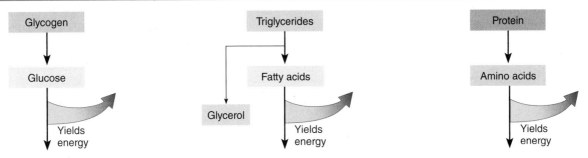

Catabolic reactions include the breakdown of glycogen, triglycerides, and protein; the further catabolism of glucose, glycerol, fatty acids, and amino acids releases differing amounts of energy. Much of the energy released is captured in the bonds of adenosine triphosphate (ATP).

NOTE: You need not memorize a color code to understand the figures in this chapter, but you may find it helpful to know that blue is used for carbohydrates, yellow for fats, and red for proteins.

FIGURE 4.1 Anabolic and catabolic reactions of the major macronutrients. Catabolic reactions include the breakdown of glycogen, triglycerides, and protein; the further catabolism of glucose, glycerol, fatty acids, and amino acids releases differing amounts of energy. Much of the energy released is captured in the bonds of adenosine triphosphate (ATP). (From Whitney, E. N., and S. R. Rolfes. 2010. Figure 7.2 in *Understanding nutrition*, 12th ed. Belmont, CA: Wadsworth Publishing.)

FIGURE 4.2 Adenosine triphosphate is the energy currency of the body. The hydrolysis of a high-energy phosphate bond releases energy that is harnessed to drive physiologic processes. (© Cengage Learning 2013)

On removal of the outermost phosphate group, adenosine diphosphate (ADP) is formed (see Figure 4.3). The energy released is coupled to an energy-requiring process such as contraction of muscle fibers, synthesis of macromolecules, or transport of molecules across membranes. The amount of energy released when the phosphate bond is broken is generally close to that needed by these coupled reactions. As a consequence, little energy is wasted by these biochemical processes (that is, these coupling processes are efficient). The efficiency of these coupled reactions does not reflect the overall efficiency of exercise, which is estimated to be only about 25 to 28 percent. Energy is lost during the metabolic formation of ATP during the breakdown of macronutrients, the generation of contractile force, and in bodily movement even in the absence of a workload.

> How would a greater overall efficiency influence exercise performance?

ATP breaks down rapidly only in the presence of enzymes that catalyze the process—ATPase. The activity of these specific enzymes is regulated, thereby controlling the rate of energy release and the circumstances under which energy is released.

> What is a catalytic process? What would be the consequences of not having specific catalysts controlling ATP breakdown?

HOTLINK *Visit the course materials for Chapter 4 for a detailed animation of enzyme action.*

When ATP is converted to ADP, the ADP is usually immediately recycled in the mitochondria back to ATP. The ATP/ADP cycle turns approximately three times every minute. In response to exercise, the rate of ATP/ADP cycling can increase by 1,000-fold. ATP concentrations in the cell largely remain unchanged, being formed primarily by oxidative processes in the mitochondria only as it is needed. O_2 is not consumed unless ADP and PO_4 are available, and these do not become available until an energy-consuming process hydrolyzes ATP. Energy metabolism is, therefore, mostly self-regulated.

To further discuss the means by which ATP is produced, we must return to the utilization of fuels. We know that **glucose** and **fatty acids** are the primary fuels, and the energy currency they deal in is ATP. The mechanisms that convert the chemical energy contained in these macronutrients to ATP involve a series of reactions compartmentalized within the cell (that is, the cytosol or mitochondria) that result in fuel oxidation. These reactions are catalyzed by enzymes and require coenzymes (NAD^+, FAD^+) and substrates.

glucose A simple sugar that can be derived from diet or formed in the body. Cells use it as a primary source of energy.

fatty acids Comprised of unbranched carbon chains, they contain a terminal carboxylic acid. They can be consumed from the diet or synthesized in the body and are an abundant source of energy.

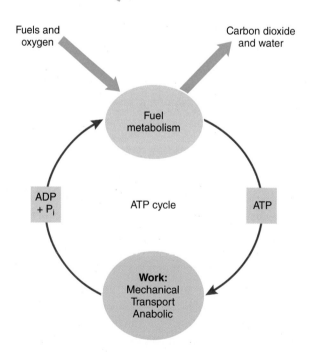

FIGURE 4.3 The ATP cycle couples energy to cellular work. The ATP cycle is the means by which chemical energy is converted to mechanical, transport, and anabolic work. (© Cengage Learning 2013)

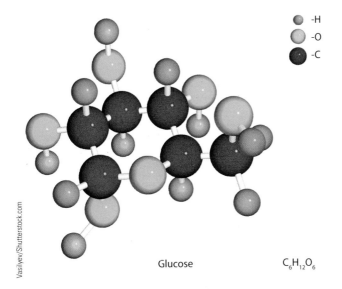

-H
-O
-C

Glucose $C_6H_{12}O_6$

Vasilyev/Shutterstock.com

Extracting Chemical Energy from Glucose

Glucose enters the cell via one of a family of transport proteins (**GLUT4** is the primary transporter in skeletal muscle), after which it is phosphorylated by a hexokinase. Hexokinase I and II are the primary isozymes in skeletal muscle. **Glycolysis** is the sequence of reactions or pathway that results in the conversion of the phosphorylated six-carbon glucose molecule to two three-carbon pyruvate molecules (see Figure 4.4).

In all, two ATP molecules are required to "prime glucose" in the glycolytic pathway. This investment in energy yields a small net production of ATP by substrate phosphorylation. The pyruvate formed is reduced by lactate dehydrogenase to lactate under anaerobic conditions (that is, the absence of adequate O_2), which is exported out of the cell. **Nicotinamide adenine dinucleotide** is a coenzyme that is converted to its reduced form (**NADH**) in the glycolytic pathway. The conversion of pyruvate to lactate results in the conversion of this co-enzyme back to its oxidized form (**NAD+**). Glycolysis would cease without the regeneration of NAD+, because it is an essential coenzyme.

HOTLINK *Visit the course materials for Chapter 4 for detailed animation of metabolic reaction stages.*

In the presence of adequate O_2, two fundamental features of glycolysis change. First, pyruvate in most cells is further metabolized via the **tricarboxylic acid (TCA) cycle**. Second, the electrons of cytoplasmic NADH are shuttled into the mitochondria with the result that electrons are provided into the electron transport chain and NAD+ is regenerated in the cytosol. Aerobic glycolysis generates substantially more ATP per mole of glucose than anaerobic glycolysis does. The utility of glycolysis to muscle rests with the fact that the rate of ATP production is approximately 100 times faster than ATP production from fuel oxidation in mitochondria, and it does so without O_2.

(What type of metabolic pathway does a sprinter use during the race?)

The phosphorylation reactions catalyzed by **hexokinase** and **phosphofructokinase-1 (PFK-1)** are nonequilibrium reactions that are under allosteric control, that is, noncovalent binding of an enzyme by a modifier other than at its active site. Regulation of

GLUT4 A protein that transports glucose into muscle and other specialized cell types (heart and adipose tissue). GLUT4 is regulated by stimuli that result in its incorporation into the cell membrane.

glycolysis The metabolic pathway that results in the conversion of glucose to pyruvate. It results in a small energy yield.

NADH A reducing agent that donates electrons for various reactions, including those that drive the formation of ATP.

tricarboxylic acid (TCA) cycle A series of enzyme catalyzed reactions in the mitochondria of living cells that result in the chemical conversion of carbohydrates, fats, and protein into carbon dioxide and water. NADH formed in these reactions contributes electrons to the electron transport chain, leading to the formation of ATP.

hexokinase This enzyme catalyzes the conversion of glucose to glucose 6-phosphate inside the cytosolic compartment of the cell.

phosphofructokinase-1 (PFK-1) This enzyme catalyzes an important regulatory step of glycolysis, the conversion of fructose 6-phosphate and ATP to fructose 1,6-bisphosphate and ADP. It is sensitively controlled by allosteric regulation.

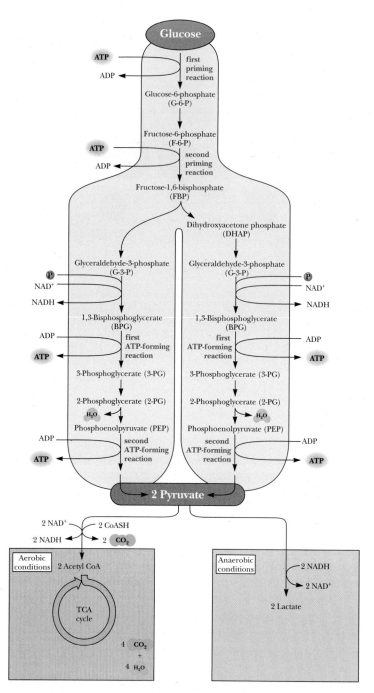

○FIGURE 4.4 Reactions involved in glucose carbon flux during its breakdown.
(a) Pyruvate produced in glycolysis is oxidized in (b) the tricarboxylic acid (TCA) cycle or (c) converted to lactate. ADP, adenosine triphosphate; ATP, adenosine triphosphate; CoA, coenzyme A; GDP, guanosine diphosphate; GTP, guanosine triphosphate; P_i, phosphate ion; NADH, reduced nicotinamide adenine dinucleotide; NAD$^+$, oxidized nicotinamide adenine dinucleotide; FADH$_2$, reduced flavin adenine dinucleotide. (From Garrett, R. H., and C. M. Grisham. 2008. Figures 19.1a and 19.1b in *Biochemistry*, 4th ed. Belmont, CA: Brooks/Cole-Cengage Learning.)

hexokinase may be important in determining the rate of glucose uptake from the blood. However, it is not the major control point in glycolytic flux because large amounts of substrate for glycolysis are derived from the breakdown of glycogen and bypass the hexokinase reaction. Of course,

hexokinase may increase in importance when muscle glycogen is reduced. The most significant reaction in the control of glycolytic flux is catalyzed by PFK-1. PFK-1 contains four subunits and exists in two conformational states that are in equilibrium.

ATP is both a substrate and an allosteric inhibitor of PFK-1. Each subunit has two ATP-binding sites, a substrate site and an inhibitor site. The substrate site binds ATP equally well in either conformation. ATP binds the inhibitor site with highest affinity in one conformation and fructose 6-phosphate (F6P), which is the other substrate for PFK-1, binds preferentially to the other conformation. At high ATP concentrations, the inhibitor site becomes occupied, shifting the equilibrium of PFK-1 conformation so that the binding affinity of PFK-1 to F6P is decreased. The inhibition of PFK-1 by ATP is overcome by AMP, which stabilizes the enzyme conformation that binds F6P with the higher affinity. The most important allosteric regulator of PFK-1, and hence glycolysis, is the metabolite fructose 2,6-bisphosphate (F2,6BP). The concentration of F2,6BP is determined by the phosphorylation/dephosphorylation activity of the bifunctional enzyme phosphofructokinase-2/fructose-2,6-bisphosphatase (PFK-2/F-2,6-BPase).

A point mutation is a single base substitution in the DNA sequence that encodes a protein, which can change the means by which a protein is regulated or prevent its normal function. How would a mutation that reduces PFK-1 activity in muscle affect the metabolic response to exercise?

The next step for extracting chemical energy from glucose is more energy-efficient. In the presence of sufficient O_2, the pyruvate produced during glycolysis diffuses across the mitochondrial double membrane entering the mitochondrial matrix in most tissues (see Figure 4.5).

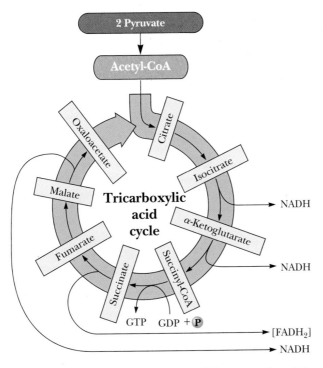

● **FIGURE 4.5 Intermediates of the TCA cycle and the generation of electrons for the electron transport chain.** Electrons liberated in the TCA cycle flow through the electron-transport chain and drive the synthesis of adenosine triphosphate (ATP) in oxidative phosphorylation. In eukaryotic cells, this overall process occurs in mitochondria. ATP, adenosine triphosphate; P_i, phosphate ion; NADH, reduced nicotinamide adenine dinucleotide; NAD^+, oxidized nicotinamide adenine dinucleotide; $FADH_2$, reduced flavin adenine dinucleotide; e^-, electrons; H^+ protons, O_2, oxygen molecule; H_2O, water. (From Garrett, R. H., and C. M. Grisham. 2008. Figure 19.1c in *Biochemistry.* 4th ed. Belmont, CA: Brooks/Cole-Cengage Learning.)

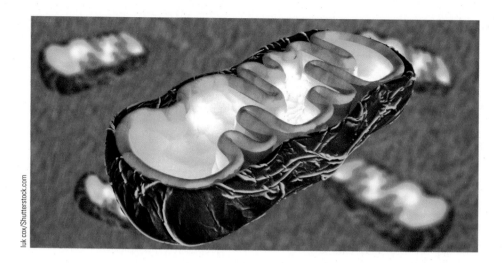

luk cox/Shutterstock.com

Within the mitochondrial matrix, pyruvate reacts with coenzyme A to form **acetyl coenzyme A (acetyl-CoA)**, with release of CO_2 in a reaction catalyzed by the **pyruvate dehydrogenase complex (PDH)**. Acetyl-CoA is broken down in the TCA cycle, producing **CO_2**, reduced NAD^+, reduced **flavin adenine dinucleotide ($FADH_2$)**, and ATP in a series of eight reactions, five of which are energy producing. These reactions are illustrated in Figure 4.5.

Complete oxidation of one molecule of pyruvate requires one turn of the TCA cycle. Because one molecule of glucose is metabolized to two molecules of pyruvate, it then requires two turns of the TCA cycle to be completely oxidized. The two turns produce 6 NADH, 2 $FADH_2$, 2 ATP, and 4 CO_2 molecules. The CO_2 diffuses from the cells to the blood and diffuses from the blood into the air expired from the lungs. The energy yield from glycolysis and the TCA cycle is only a small fraction of the total energy yield by oxidation of glucose. A total of 4 ATP molecules are produced from glucose at the level of substrate phosphorylation in these pathways. However, 10 NADH and 2 $FADH_2$ molecules are formed. Electrons associated with these reduced coenzymes drive a series of reactions in the inner mitochondrial membrane known as the **electron transport chain**. Most of the ATP produced in the presence of O_2 is made using the reactions of the electron transport chain and the enzyme **ATP synthase**.

Carbon flux through the TCA cycle is regulated at several steps. The provision of acetyl-CoA for the TCA cycle is determined by glycolytic flux, the cell redox state (that is, ratio of NADH to NAD^+), and the activation state of PDH. PDH is also subject to feedback inhibition by acetyl-CoA, and its activation state is determined by the phosphorylation state of the enzyme. Substrate availability and product feedback inhibition are also important in regulation of other reactions that comprise the TCA cycle. In particular, the flux through the citrate synthase step is dependent on oxaloacetate availability, and the activity of this enzyme is inhibited by citrate. Cell redox state, calcium concentration, and ADP/ATP also exert regulation on steps of the TCA cycle.

What would be the metabolic consequences during exercise of a mutation that causes a reduction in PDH activity?

Extracting Chemical Energy from Free Fatty Acids

Three fatty acids and a glycerol molecule are mobilized from triglyceride stores by a process known as **lipolysis**. Although the three-carbon glycerol molecule can enter the glycolytic/gluconeogenic pathway in fat, kidney, and liver, little, if any, is metabolized in skeletal muscle. Free fatty acids (FFA) released by lipolysis are readily oxidized by contracting muscle with the transfer of chemical energy to NADH and FADH₂. The carbon chain length and the degree to which those carbons are saturated with hydrogen atoms determine the energy yield from the oxidation of FFA. The process of extracting chemical energy begins with the activation of FFA by reaction with CoA to form an acyl-CoA in the cytoplasm. This process requires an ATP molecule, so it is not without cost. After activation, the acyl-

CoA is exchanged for carnitine by a reaction catalyzed by carnitine-palmitoyltransferase (CPT) I. The acyl-carnitine formed is transported to the inside of the mitochondrion where it reacts with acetyl-CoA in a process catalyzed by CPT II. The acyl-CoA that is formed is a substrate for oxidative processes (see Figure 4.6a).

HOTLINK *Visit the course materials for Chapter 4 for detailed animation of mitochondrial chemiosmosis.*

Mitochondrial fatty acid oxidation occurs through the sequential removal of two-carbon fragments by oxidation of the acyl-CoA molecule. This sequential removal of two carbon fragments occurs in the beta-oxidation pathway (see Figure 4.6b). With the removal of a two-carbon fragment is the formation of 1 NADH, 1 FADH₂, and 1 acetyl-CoA mol-

lipolysis The means by which triglycerides are mobilized to fatty acids and glycerol.

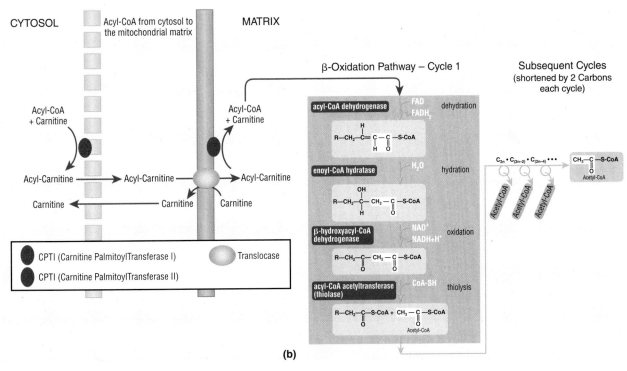

(a)   (b)

FIGURE 4.6 Fatty acids are transported into mitochondria as acyl-carnitine and undergo metabolism in the beta-oxidation pathway. A. After activation to an acyl-coenzyme (CoA) the CoA is exchanged for carnitine by carnitine-palmitoyltransferase I. The fatty-carnitine is then transported to the inside of the mitochondrion, where a reversal exchange takes place through the action of carnitine-palmitoyltransferase II. Once inside the mitochondrion, the fatty-CoA is a substrate for the beta-oxidation pathway. B. In the beta-oxidation pathway the acyl-CoA undergoes enzyme catalyzed dehydration, hydration, oxidation, and thiolysis reactions. Each cycle results in the production of FADH₂ and NADH+H which are substrates for the electron transport cycle and shortens the acyl-CoA by two carbons with the formation of acetyl-CoA. Acetyl-CoA is a substrate for the TCA cycle.

ecule. The acetyl-CoA then enters the TCA cycle, where it is further oxidized to CO_2 with the generation of 3 NADH, 1 $FADH_2$, and 1 ATP molecule. The NADH and $FADH_2$ generated during the complete oxidation of fat donate electrons to the electron transport chain for the production of ATP. Fat oxidation is regulated primarily by the availability of FFA resulting from adipose tissue lipolysis. Enzymes within the muscle are also impor-

tant sites of regulation for fat oxidation. This is described in detail in Chapter 5.

The oxidation of fatty acids yields significantly more energy per carbon atom than does the oxidation of carbohydrates. The net result of the oxidation of 1 mole oleic acid (an 18-carbon fatty acid) is that 146 moles ATP is formed (2 mole equivalents are used during the activation of the fatty acid), as compared with 114 moles from an equivalent number of glucose carbon atoms.

Turning Chemical Energy Extracted from Free Fatty Acids and Glucose into ATP

Quantitatively, production of ATP by substrate phosphorylation in glycolysis, fat oxidation, and the TCA cycle is small. The NADH and $FADH_2$ formed when fat and carbohydrates are oxidized in the mitochondrial matrix are the substrates for the electron transport chain. Most of the

chemical energy of foods is converted to ATP by the reactions of the electron transport chain and **oxidative phosphorylation** (see Figure 4.7). NADH and $FADH_2$ donate electrons that are transferred to and shuttled between a series of proteins that span the inner mitochondrial membrane.

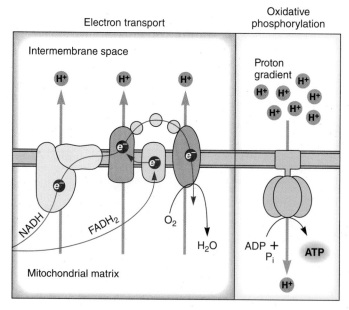

FIGURE 4.7 Reactions of the electron transport chain and the coupling of the protein gradient to ATP synthesis. Electrons are liberated in this oxidation flow through the electron-transport chain and drive the synthesis of adenosine triphosphate (ATP) in oxidative phosphorylation. In eukaryotic cells, this overall process occurs in mitochondria. ATP, adenosine triphosphate; P_i, phosphate ion; NADH, reduced nicotinamide adenine dinucleotide; NAD^+, oxidized nicotinamide adenine dinucleotide; $FADH_2$, reduced flavin adenine dinucleotide, e⁻, electrons; H^+ protons, O_2, oxygen molecule; H_2O, water. (From Garrett, R. H., and C. M. Grisham. 2008. Figure 19.1c in *Biochemistry*, 4th ed. Belmont, CA: Brooks/Cole-Cengage Learning.)

O_2 is the terminal electron acceptor, combining with H^+ ions to produce water. The shuttling of electrons by the electron transport chain results in translocation of protons outward from the matrix across the inner mitochondrial membrane. The result is a proton gradient across the inner mitochondrial membrane. How does this proton gradient act to reattach ADP to PO_4? The resulting electrochemical gradient leads to a stream of protons that drives the molecular machine, ATP synthase. This enzyme couples the channeling of protons across the inner mitochondrial membrane to the synthesis of ATP from ADP and PO_4. ATP synthase contains a pore that permits the flow of protons down an electrochemical gradient. This flow of protons causes conformational changes in catalytic ATP synthase subunits that results in them binding ADP and PO_4, and joining them to form ATP. This enzyme functions much like a molecular water wheel that harnesses the flow of

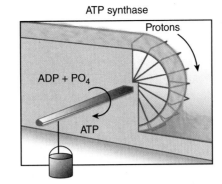

ATP synthase

Protons

ADP + PO_4

ATP

● **FIGURE 4.8** **ATP synthase is a molecular machine.** Adenosine triphosphate (ATP) synthase harnesses the energy from the flow of proteins across the inner mitochondrial membrane much like a water wheel captures the energy from moving water and uses it to provide kinetic energy. ADP, adenosine diphosphate. (© Cengage Learning 2013)

protons to build ATP molecules (see Figure 4.8).

HOTLINK *Visit the course materials for Chapter 4 for detailed animation of electron transfer and oxidative phosphorylation.*

CONCEPTS, challenges, controversies

Reactive Oxygen Species: "A Riddle, Wrapped in a Mystery, Inside an Enigma"

Reactive oxygen species (ROS), to borrow a line from Sir Winston Churchill, are, indeed, "a riddle, wrapped in a mystery, inside an enigma." The formation of ROS and then the biologic impact of their formation during a variety of conditions including muscular work comprise a complex puzzle. In the previous section, the importance of the electron transport chain in creating a proton gradient across the inner mitochondrial membrane is described. Electrons, even under normal circumstances, leak at relatively low rates from specific complexes (complexes I and III) and bind to "ground state oxygen" to form a superoxide anion, the parent molecule of all ROS. Under most situations, superoxide is reduced to form hydrogen peroxide, but it can also react with nitric oxide to form peroxynitrite, another form of ROS. It can also oxidize lipids, DNA, and proteins by a mechanism that is generally nonspecific. Exercise results in a marked increase in flux through the electron transport chain and oxygen utilization by mitochondria. Exercise also increases ROS production, which was initially thought to be due to the increase in respiratory activity. However, it now seems unlikely that mitochondria are the source of ROS during exercise. The electron transport chain and oxidative phosphorylation are very efficient during exercise, and there appear to be no more ROS formed in the mitochondria during exercise than at rest. Rather, it seems that membrane-bound NAPDH oxidases outside the mitochondria are the source of ROS during exercise. ROS production is increased in disease conditions, such as disuse atrophy and diabetes. The source of ROS production (for example, mitochondria or NAPDH oxidase) is likely to be dependent on the physiologic or pathophysiologic state. For example, diabetes is a disease state characterized by an increase in ROS that appears to be largely of mitochondrial origin.

The consequences of ROS formation are also complex. Inappropriately excessive ROS formation is thought to be part of the aging process and contributes negatively to disease states by causing oxidative stress. ROS can cause inflammation and inappropriate oxidation or nitrosylation of DNA, lipids, and proteins, resulting in cellular dysfunction. In contrast, ROS formation, particularly H_2O_2, produced under physiologic conditions is a vital signaling molecule that has been implicated in accelerated glucose transport and increased expression of transcription factors, such as nuclear factor-kappa B (NF-κB) and peroxisome proliferator-activated receptor-gamma coactivator-1α (PGC-1α). Both are necessary for muscle adaptations. NF-κB is a key mediator of the inflammatory response, and PGC-1α is important in mitochondrial biogenesis. Our understanding of the actions of ROS is in a very early stage. ROS in health and disease stands to be a very important area of research for years to come.

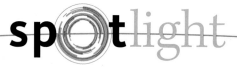

Olympian and Expert on Cellular and Subcellular Bioenergetics: Britton Chance

Britton Chance, Ph.D., was born in Wilkes-Barre, Pennsylvania, in 1913. As a young man, he spent summers sailing, and as a teenager, he invented an auto-steering device to help ships maintain the appropriate course. His love of sailing and intense competitive spirit eventually helped him make the U.S. yacht Olympic team, and he won a gold medal in the 1952 Olympics.

Dr. Chance received his Bachelor's of Science and Master's of Science degrees (chemistry) from the University of Pennsylvania in 1935 and 1936. He earned two Ph.D. degrees, one in physical chemistry from the University of Pennsylvania in 1940 and another in biology and physiology (Sc.D.) from Cambridge University in 1942. He received several honorary M.D. and D.Sc. degrees during his academic research career. He served as the Eldridge Reeves Johnson Professor Emeritus of Biochemistry and Biophysics and Physical Chemistry and Radiologic Physics at the School of Medicine at Pennsylvania at the time of his death in 2010 and as the President of Medical Diagnostic Research Foundation (MDRF) in Philadelphia, Pennsylvania.

Chance's research interests include biochemical, biophysical, and medical topics that include his discovery of the enzyme substrate compounds of peroxidase and the mechanical differential analyzer solutions of the Michaelis–Menten equations. Dr. Chance invented the now standard stopped flow device to measure the existence of the enzyme-substrate complex in enzyme reaction. In later years, while retaining his interest in those fields, he also focused on metabolic control phenomena in living tissues as studied by noninvasive techniques such as phosphorous nuclear magnetic resonance (NMR) and optical spectroscopy and fluorometry. He conducted a wide range of studies of enzyme-substrate compounds of catalases and peroxidases, and with an ingenious optical method, he discovered the NADH and flavin components of the respiratory chain. His studies carried out in vitro (in the test tube) and in vivo (in organisms) formed the basis for the development of sensitive spectrophotometric methods. The Chance dual-wavelength spectrophotometer continues to be widely used.

Dr. Chance progressed from animals to the first human NMR subject studies (using a 1.5-tesla magnet). This technology has led to the diagnosis and treatment of mitochondrial diseases. Chance's research has led to the development of near-infrared spectroscopy and imaging for real-time metabolic studies of the brain (hematoma), breast (cancer), skeletal muscle (metabolic monitoring), and cardiac muscle (hypoxia).

in*Practice*

Examples of Energy Metabolism and Exercise

The following sections provide practical examples of how energy metabolism and exercise are related to your area of interest.

Health/Fitness: By understanding energy metabolism, you can help your clients understand the importance of consuming the appropriate amount of carbohydrates (glucose) as a percentage of total calories (50–60 percent) they consume daily. You can also help them understand that when they try to go on a medically unsupervised low- carbohydrate diet, they may feel too tired to engage in regular exercise because of low glucose/glycogen stores. In addition, you can educate your clients about the need for them to consume 25 to 30 percent of their total calories in the form of fat to meet their extra energy needs from free fatty acids. You can also share with them that when they try to reduce their dietary fat intake to less than 25 percent, they may reduce their levels of steroid hormones, which could actually hinder optimal performance.

Medicine: McArdle disease is a metabolic disease that influences energy metabolism because of a deficiency of the muscle enzyme myophosphorylase that results in the inability of a patient's muscle to break down glycogen effectively. The disease is genetic and rare (1/100,000 births), but it causes muscle weakness and places patients at high risk for myoglobinuria (myoglobin in the patient's urine) and rhabdomyolysis (skeletal muscle breakdown). These conditions can lead to significant muscle injury and kidney damage. Health and fitness professionals need to understand that clients with McArdle disease will fatigue quickly, even with low-intensity programs of exercise, because they cannot meet their ATP needs efficiently, and thus can get chronic muscle soreness, with longer than normal recovery periods of 24 to 48 hours.

Athletic Performance: Coaches who understand energy metabolism can help their athletes optimize their training by identifying the primary energy pathways [the formation of ATP from high energy creatine phosphate (CP), anaerobic glycolysis, aerobic] that are required for a specific physical activity or sport. For example, what energy pathways are stressed for soccer players? If you answered 50 percent anaerobic/50 percent aerobic, you are probably about right. But what about goalies? Goalies would mostly rely on their anaerobic pathways for energy, at least when challenged during a game. One of the primary reasons coaches should want to understand energy metabolism is so that they can develop a training program that can specifically stress the energy pathways in training that will lead to optimal athletic success.

HOTLINK *See Appendix for specific training examples.*

Rehabilitation: It is important for rehabilitation specialists to understand how energy metabolism may limit their client's ability to optimize their exercise rehabilitation. For example, patients with congestive heart failure (CHF) have a reduced ability to provide energy via the aerobic energy pathways. Research has shown that patients with CHF have smaller muscle fibers, higher percentages of fast-twitch fibers, and reduced aerobic enzyme levels. Patients with CHF also have an increased CP/ATP ratio and reduced pH levels as compared with healthy subjects, which may indicate they have an imbalance in the ability to supply energy to do work. Rehabilitation specialists who are aware of these special energy metabolism challenges for patients with CHF can help their clients exercise at their individual capacities while minimizing fatigue.

Chapter Summary

- The chemical energy stored in glucose, fatty acids, and amino acids cannot be used until it is transferred to ATP. ATP is the common energy currency that is used by virtually all energy-requiring processes in the body.

- The means by which chemical energy is transferred from fuels to ATP is central to metabolism. The efficiency and rapidity of this process is a critical determinant of exercise bioenergetics.

- The ATP/ADP cycle turns approximately three times every minute. In response to exercise, the rate of ATP/ADP cycling can increase by 1,000-fold.

- Glucose and fatty acids are the primary fuels, and the energy currency they deal in is ATP. The mechanisms that convert the chemical energy contained in these macronutrients to ATP involve a series of compartmentalized reactions that result in fuel oxidation.

- Energy is extracted from glucose via substrate phosphorylation and oxidative phosphorylation pathways.

- Several limiting factors control the rate of energy extraction from glucose, including enzymes, coenzymes, presence of sufficient oxygen, substrate availability, among others.

- The oxidation of fatty acids yields significantly more energy per carbon atom than does the oxidation of carbohydrates. The net result of the oxidation of 1 mole oleic acid (an 18-carbon fatty acid) is that 146 moles ATP is formed, as compared with 114 moles from an equivalent number of glucose carbon atoms.

- Quantitatively, production of ATP by substrate phosphorylation by the reactions of glycolysis, fat oxidation, and the TCA cycle is small.

- The NADH and $FADH_2$ formed when fat and carbohydrates are oxidized in the mitochondrial matrix are the substrates for the electron transport chain.

- Most of the chemical energy of foods is converted to ATP by the reactions of the electron transport chain and oxidative phosphorylation.

Exercise Physiology Reality

CENGAGE brain.com   To reinforce the exercise physiology concepts presented above, complete the laboratory exercises for Chapter 4. To access labs and other course materials for this text, please visit www.cengagebrain.com. See the preface on page xiii for details. Once you complete the exercises, evaluate your results based on the scales provided and develop a personal plan for successfully completing your exercise physiology course.

Exercise Physiology Web Links

Access the following websites for further study of topics covered in this chapter:

- Find updates and quick links to these and other epidemiology and exercise physiology–related sites at our website. To access the course materials and companion resources for this text, please visit www.cengagebrain.com. See the preface on page xiii for details.

- Search for more information about energy metabolism at the American College of Sports Medicine website: http://www.acsm.org.

- Search for more information about energy metabolism at the Gatorade Sports Science Institute website: http://www.gssiweb.com.

- Search for more information on basics of cell structures and how enzymes work at the How Stuff Works website: http://science.howstuffworks.com/cell.htm.

- Read more about oxidative phosphorylation and view an animation of ATP synthesis in the mitochondria by the enzyme ATP synthase at the Sigma-Aldrich website: http://www.sigmaaldrich.com/Area_of_Interest/Life_Science/Metabolomics/Key_Resources/Metabolic_Pathways/ATP_Synthase.html.

- Search for more information on the enzyme AMP-activated protein kinase at the Medical Biochemistry Page: http://themedicalbiochemistrypage.org/ampk.html.

Study Questions

Review the Warm-Up Pre-Test questions you were asked to answer before reading Chapter 4. Test yourself once more to determine what you know now that you have completed the chapter.

The questions that follow will help you review this chapter. You will find the answers in the discussions on the pages provided.

1. What is the role of chemical energy in ATP formation? *p. 112*

2. Why is ATP important to energy metabolism? *pp. 112–113*

3. Why is the fine control of ATP concentrations important for sustaining muscle contraction? *p. 114*

4. How can energy be extracted from glucose? *pp. 115–118*

5. How can energy be extracted from free fatty acids (FFA)? *pp. 119–120*

6. What role does the anaerobic formation of lactate serve in the cell? *p. 115*

7. Why is feedback control of pathways of energy metabolism important? *pp. 115–118*

8. What role do intramitochondrial electrochemical gradients play in ATP formation? *pp. 120–121*

9. Why might the enzyme PFK-1 be important during exercise? *pp. 115–116*

10. How would metabolic pathways inside and outside the mitochondria be affected by a deficiency in oxygen availability? *p. 116*

Selected References

Anderson, E. J., M. E. Lustig, K. E. Boyle, T. L. Woodlief, D. A. Kane, C. T. Lin, J. W. Price, 3rd, L. Kang, P. S. Rabinovitch, H. H. Szeto, J. A. Houmard, R. N. Cortright, D. H. Wasserman, and P. D. Neufer. 2009. Mitochondrial H2O2 emission and cellular redox state link excess fat intake to insulin resistance in both rodents and humans. *J. Clin. Invest.* 119:573–581.

Boyer, P. D. 1997. The ATP synthase—a splendid molecular machine. *Annu. Rev. Biochem.* 66:717–749.

Hardie, D. G., and K. Sakamoto. 2006. AMPK: A key sensor of fuel and energy status in skeletal muscle. *Physiology* (Bethesda) 21:48–60.

Kresge, N., Simoni, R. D., and R. L. Hill. 2004. Britton Chance: Olympian and developer of stop-flow methods. *J. Biol. Chem.* 279(50):10.

Powers, S. K., E. E. Talbert, and P. J. Adhihetty. 2011. Reactive oxygen and nitrogen species as intracellular signals in skeletal muscle. *J. Physiol.* 589(Pt 9):2129–2138.

Ruderman, N. B., K. Tornheim, and M. N. Goodman. 1995. Fuel homeostasis and intermediary metabolism of carbohydrate, fat, and protein. In *Principles and practice of endocrinology and metabolism,* 2nd ed., edited by K. L. Becker. Philadelphia: JB Lippincott, pp. 1174–1187.

Weibel, E. R., and H. Hoppeler. 2005. Exercise-induced maximal metabolic rate scales with muscle aerobic capacity. *J. Exp. Biol.* 208(Pt 9):1635–1644.

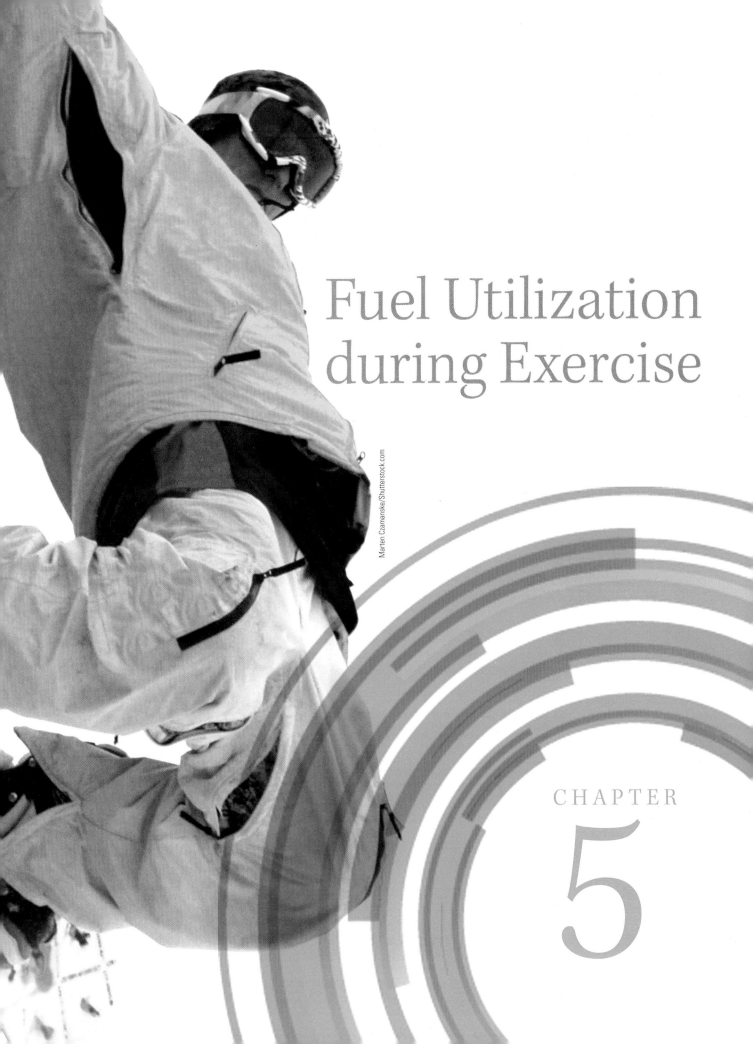

Fuel Utilization during Exercise

CHAPTER

5

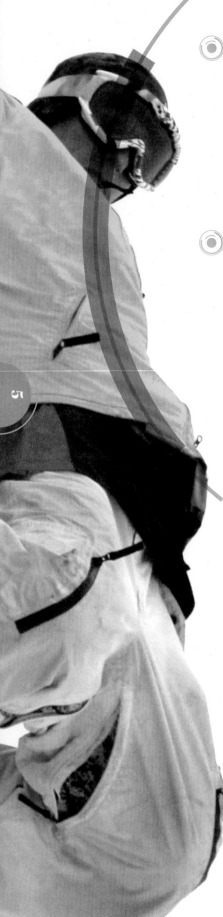

Warm-Up

CENGAGEbrain

What do you already know about fuel utilization during exercise?

- Use the following Pre-Test or the online evaluation tools for Chapter 5 to determine how much you already know. To access the course materials and companion resources for this text, please visit **www.cengagebrain.com**. See the preface on page xiii for details.

- Need more review? Let the online assessments, animations, and tutorials for Chapter 5 help prepare you for class.

Pre-Test

1. The ratio of CO_2 expired to O_2 inspired can be used to estimate the oxidation of _____ and _____.

2. The Fick principle is that the amount of a substance taken up from or released into the circulation per unit time equals the _____ level of the substance minus the _____ level multiplied by the blood flow.

3. Fat is mobilized from the _____ tissue and glucose is mobilized from the _____ in individuals who have fasted.

4. Arterial blood glucose concentrations are closely _____ in healthy people.

5. What is the largest source of stored fuel?

6. Fatty acids can be defined by _____ length and the number of _____ bonds.

7. In the resting state, the primary user of glucose is the _____, whereas during exercise, it is the _____.

8. Energy can be produced from glucose both with and without _____.

9. Amino acids usually contribute only a small fraction to _____.

10. Energy for long-distance exercise comes mainly from _____, and energy for high-intensity exercise comes mainly from _____.

1. carbohydrates; fats; 2. arterial; venous; 3. adipose; liver; 4. regulated; 5. triglycerides; 6. carbon chain; double; 7. brain; muscle; 8. oxygen; 9. energy metabolism; 10. fats; carbohydrates

What You Will Learn in This Chapter

- Ways that fuel utilization can be measured in the laboratory
- Patterns of fuel utilization during exercise and the factors that affect it
- Physiologic objectives of fuel utilization

QUICKSTART!

Ordinarily, a blend of different substrates fuels the working muscle. How is the optimal grade of fuel influenced by the duration and intensity of exercise? How can the inability to use certain fuels limit exercise tolerance?

Introduction to Fuel Utilization during Exercise

The foundation for our current knowledge of fuel utilization can be found in the work of three pioneering figures in the field of chemistry: Joseph Priestly, Antoine Lavoisier, and Pierre-Simon Laplace. Joseph Priestly was born in England in 1733. He was raised in England, where he began his adult life as a theologian. His life dramatically shifted course after meeting Benjamin Franklin, who, in 1766, was visiting England to talk about his experiments identifying electricity. Priestley, who had never had a formal course in any of the fundamental sciences, used his observations and his inquiring mind to logically deduce the presence of many fundamental chemicals. In 1767, he identified that carbon, or graphite (in his day), could conduct electricity. In 1772 and 1773, he identified that a "heavy gas" was consumed by plants and that plants sustained life by producing "dephlogisticated air." This observation was the first description of the process later known as *photosynthesis*.

Antoine Lavoisier was executed via the guillotine in 1794, after the French Revolution, because he was viewed as a member of the French elite. His untimely death cut short the life of a uniquely qualified scientist. He confirmed many of the observations of Priestly and disproved others. He developed the system of "chemical nomenclature" in 1789, which is used today and forms the basis for the development of the periodic table. Based on this system of nomenclature, Lavoisier named Priestley's "heavy gas" carbon dioxide and "dephlogisticated air" oxygen. Finally, Lavoisier established the law of conservation of mass, and based on his wanting to identify all the products of a chemical reaction as a substance, he listed the light and heat emitted from a reaction as substances and named them "light" and "caloric," respectively.

The works of Priestley and Lavoisier were fundamental to the development of the field of fuel metabolism. It remained for the work of another renowned scientist by the name of Pierre-Simon Laplace to place these findings in the context of the energetics of metabolism. In the 1780s, Laplace, a renowned mathematician and astrophysicist, addressed the question of providing a quantifiable value to the heat of a chemical reaction. He used a calorimeter to estimate the heat evolved per unit of carbon dioxide produced in a reaction involving oxygen. He reported the value as calories. Notably, these discoveries are the fundamental basis of our current investigations into the human body's energy metabolism at rest and during exercise and disease.

The intent of this brief history of the discovery of oxygen and carbon dioxide and their link to caloric expenditure is for you to understand that some of the fundamental discoveries in exercise physiology were made by individuals who are regarded as giants in the fields of chemistry and physics and their use of the scientific method. The scientific method has been used in quantifying the energy, or calories, provided to the human body's tissues by the metabolism of different foods.

HOTLINK *See Chapter 1 for a review of the scientific method.*

Quantitative Measurements of Fuel Metabolism

Patterns of fuel utilization have been comprehensively described under a variety of exercise conditions and nutritional states using net exchange of **energy substrates** across a tissue bed, isotopic methods that trace the metabolic breakdown of specific

energy substrates In a biological system, these are nutrients that yield ATP.

arteriovenous difference technique This uses the amount of a molecule entering and leaving an organ or tissue bed to calculate the production or release of a molecule.

isotopic approaches These have many applications. Isotopes are used in exercise physiology research to calculate the flux of energy substrates in and out of the bloodstream.

indirect calorimetry A method by which the oxidation of carbohydrates and fats are calculated from the rate of uptake of O_2 and the rate of production of CO_2. Accurate application of this method requires an estimate of protein oxidation.

pulmonary gas exchange The movement of O_2 from the environment to the pulmonary circulation and the movement of CO_2 from the pulmonary circulation to the environment. The process requires bulk flow of air into the lungs and diffusion of gases between air and blood.

muscle biopsy A muscle sample obtained to measure the composition of muscle.

5

substrates, gas exchange between the lungs and environment, and muscle biopsies. The material presented in this chapter and chapters that follow are based on what has been learned using several approaches for measuring fuel metabolism, including the **arteriovenous difference technique**, **isotopic approaches**, **indirect calorimetry** using **pulmonary gas exchange**, and **muscle biopsy**.

Arteriovenous Difference Technique

The net substrate balance across a tissue bed or limb is calculated as the difference in vascular substrate inflow and outflow to a region of interest by application of Fick principle. Mathematically, this is expressed as $\dot{Q} \times [A] - \dot{Q} \times [V]$, where $\dot{Q}$ is blood flow in liters per minute (L/min), and [A] and [V] are the arterial and venous substrate concentrations in micromoles per liter (μmol/L), respectively. This technique is relatively invasive, requiring simultaneous sampling of arterial and venous blood, and measurement of blood flow through the region of interest. Scandinavian researchers have used this technique extensively to describe substrate utilization during exercise.

Isotopic Approaches

Isotopes of a given element have identical chemical properties but slightly different physical properties that allow them to be distinguished analytically from their common form. For most elements, both stable and radioactive isotopes are known. Specific amino acids, carbohydrates, and **free fatty acids (FFA)** can be synthesized and injected intravenously or ingested to trace the movement of these substrates in and out of the blood and their metabolism in tissues. The two main applications of isotopes in exercise physiology are: (a) tracing the inflow and outflow of a substrate or metabolite from the vascular space, and (b) following the conversion of a substrate through its metabolic pathway into an end product. Isotopic methods can be combined with arteriovenous difference methods to trace the activity of a specific tissue pathway. The weakness of isotopic methods is the assumption that the distribution and clearance of the endogenous molecule is the same as that of the isotope.

free fatty acids Blood fatty acids that are associated with albumin via nonpolar interactions.

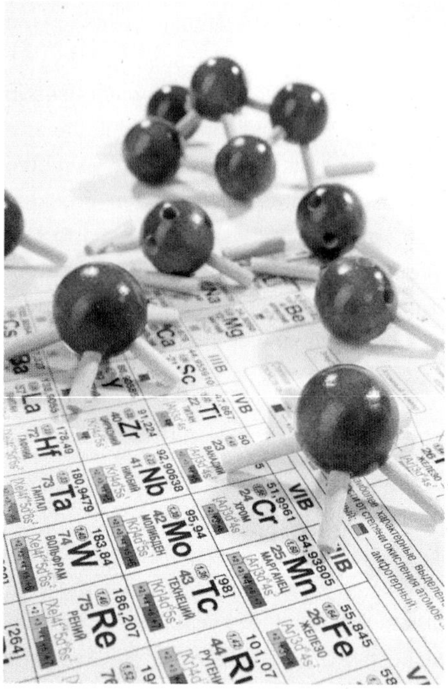

Shebeko/Shutterstock.com

Indirect Calorimetry Using Pulmonary Gas Exchange

Pulmonary CO_2 output and O_2 uptake are measured to estimate the oxidation of carbohydrate and lipid and the energy expenditure using the calorimetric properties of these compounds. The stoichiometry of CO_2 produced and O_2 used in the cellular oxidation of carbohydrate and lipid are reflected under steady-state conditions in the exchange of pulmonary gases. The ratio of CO_2 produced and O_2 used by the body (respiratory quotient [RQ]) is used to estimate carbohydrate and lipid utilization. The kilojoules (kJ) of energy released per liter of O_2 consumed for carbohydrate (15.44 kJ per gram glucose) and lipid (39.12 kJ per gram fat) are treated as constants to calculate energy expenditure. The optimal value of the constants used in the calculation will vary based on the types of sugars and fat that are oxidized. These constants can also be expressed in calories or kilo-calories, as defined by Laplace. There are approximately 4.185 kJ per kilocalorie. The basic stoichiometry for glucose and a representative FFA (palmitate) is:

$$\text{Glucose: } C_6H_{12}O_6 + 6O_2 \rightarrow$$
$$6CO_2 + 6H_2O + \text{energy}$$

Thus, the RQ for glucose is: $6CO_2/6O_2 = 1$.

$$\text{Palmitic acid: } C_{16}H_{32}O_2 + 23O_2 \rightarrow$$
$$16CO_2 + 16H_2O + \text{energy}$$

Thus, the RQ for palmitic acid is: $16CO_2/23O_2 = 0.696$.

The strength of indirect calorimetry is that it is noninvasive, requiring neither blood nor tissue. The calculations of energy expenditure and substrate oxidation require that protein oxidation be estimated or assumed. The usual means of estimation is from urinary nitrogen excretion. Accuracy of this technique is limited if CO_2 produced in the cell is not expired from the lungs (for example, used as a substrate in other pathways or stored in the body as bicarbonate). Acidosis or hyperventilation can also limit the accuracy of this method.

HOTLINK *See Chapter 10 for more information on respiratory quotient (RQ) and respiratory exchange ratio.*

Muscle Biopsy

Muscle biopsies are taken using a fine needle usually from the vastus lateralis. Serial biopsies can be taken to measure changes in muscle glycogen or metabolites over time. Regulation of metabolic pathways can be assessed from a biopsy sample by measuring the expression or covalent modification of an enzyme. Muscle biopsies have provided considerable insight into exercise metabolism and performance. This technique is limited by its invasiveness and the assessment of enzyme activities outside the native subcellular environment.

In addition to the techniques described earlier, spectroscopic methods have also been used to study metabolism during or after exercise. Its applications have been considerably less because of the evolving nature of the technology, the requirement of expensive equipment, and the need to minimize motion artifact in the spectra. The method of choice depends on the substrates or pathways of interest, exercise conditions, and the degree of invasiveness permitted or reasonable in an experiment. It is important to recognize that all methods for assessing metabolism are most reliable when the body is in a dynamic steady state, where the concentrations of substrates and products are relatively constant.

HOTLINK *See the Muscle Biopsy section of the Neuromuscular Disease Center of Washington University website (http://www.neuro.wustl.edu/neuromuscular/lab/mbiopsy.htm) for more information.*

(Which method(s) would be most effective for studying the metabolic regulation of the liver during exercise?)

Three Principles of Substrate Utilization during Exercise

It is well-documented that the increased energy demand of exercise necessitates an accelerated flow of fuels that can be used for ATP (adenosine triphosphate) production from storage sites to the energy-producing pathways in the contracting muscle. The contribution of each substrate (that is, carbohydrate, fat, protein) to the metabolic demand of the working muscle depends on different factors relating to subject characteristics (for example, fitness, nutritional state, specific health deficits) and exercise conditions (for example, high altitude, temperature extremes). Factors that affect fuel utilization during exercise are summarized in Table 5.1.

The most important determinants of the type and amount of fuel used, however, are the exercise duration and intensity. The impact of these two primary exercise variables is such that with increasing exercise duration at mild-to-moderate intensities, more fat is used, and with more strenuous exercise intensities, more carbohydrates are used. Substrate metabolism during exercise has three objectives:

1. Maintain glucose homeostasis
2. Metabolize the most efficient substrate
3. Spare muscle glycogen

Failure to accomplish any of these objectives will impair work performance, ultimately leading to the inability to exercise further.

Preserving Glucose Homeostasis

The first objective of substrate metabolism is to maintain glucose homeostasis, and the primary reason for this is that the brain is reliant on glucose metabolism for energy except under unusual conditions. Therefore, blood glucose must be tightly regulated. Exercise presents a challenge to the control system that maintains blood glucose constant. The Harvard Fatigue Laboratory was a leading center for the study of exercise in the 1930s. It was there that the elegant nature of this control system was first demonstrated. Professor D. B. Dill and colleagues demonstrated that despite a marked increase in carbohydrate oxidation, blood glucose homeostasis was generally maintained constant in healthy subjects during light- to moderate-intensity exercise. The inference from these studies was that the rate at which glucose was released from the liver into the blood under these conditions matched the rate of increase in glucose uptake by the working muscle. Scandinavian researchers later used arteriovenous differences to confirm this finding directly by measuring the rate of entry of glucose into the blood from the splanchnic bed (the anatomic region defined by gut, spleen, pancreas, and liver) and comparing it with the rate that blood glucose is utilized by the legs during cycling.

Blood glucose homeostasis may be compromised under certain exercise conditions. For example, the response to high-intensity exercise takes on characteristics of the stress response as described by Walter B. Cannon in 1932. That is, the stress hormone responses, such as norepinephrine, epinephrine, and cortisol, are excessive and glucose concentrations in the blood increase because it is no longer closely regulated. However, in prolonged exercise (about >90 minutes), mild hypoglycemia is common and can become severe. Ingestion of glucose can correct or prevent the decrease in blood glucose and, in some instances, increase the capacity for prolonged exercise. Blood glucose responses during light- to moderate-intensity types of exercise and to more extreme types of exercise (for example, very heavy or prolonged) are summarized in Figure 5.1.

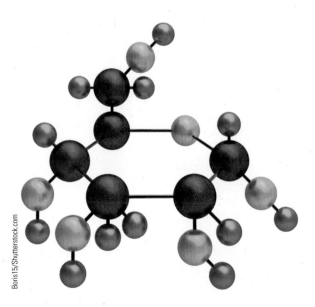

Boris15/Shutterstock.com

(What are the challenges
to maintaining glucose
homeostasis at rest
versus steady-state
exercise?)

Metabolizing the Most Efficient Substrate

The second objective of substrate metabolism is metabolizing the most efficient substrate, because depending on the intensity of exercise, the fuel used results in different rates and amounts of energy yield. For example, the energy yield for carbohydrate and fat has different stoichiometries (see Table 5.2).

During heavy exercise, the need is for the most *metabolically-efficient* (more ATP per O_2) fuel, whereas during light exercise, which can be maintained for a long time, the need is for the most *storage-efficient* (more ATP per substrate mass) fuel.

The reasons for these intensity-related differences in fuel utilization are that during heavy exercises, ATP utilization is more rapid and O_2 supply can be limiting. Under these conditions, it has been found that carbohydrate is more metabolically efficient than is fat and better suits the needs of heavy exercise. The main reason for carbohydrate being more metabolically efficient is that carbohydrate is broken down without O_2 to produce ATP from glycolysis in the muscle cytoplasm, a process that occurs at a much higher rate than mitochondrial ATP production by oxidative phosphorylation. Utilization of both blood glucose and muscle glycogen increases with exercise intensity, with the increments being largest at high work rates (see Figures 5.2 and 5.3).

In contrast, fat is the most storage-efficient fuel and is used preferentially during light exercise that can potentially be sustained for long intervals. Under these circumstances, speed and efficiency of ATP formation are secondary to fuel storage efficiency. Differences in the degree of saturation of free fatty acids and glucose carbons predict that twice the energy can be gained from the oxidation of triglycerides than an equal quantity of glycogen. Fats are immiscible with water and stored in pure form. Glycogen is less economi-

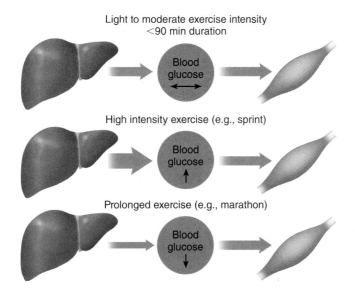

● FIGURE 5.1 Regulation of blood glucose during exercise: role of intensity and duration. The liver release of glucose into the blood is normally increased to match the increased uptake of glucose from the blood by the working muscles (top). However, under extreme exercise conditions and in certain disease states, blood glucose homeostasis may be lost. Blood glucose response to high-intensity exercise (middle); blood glucose response during the latter stage of prolonged exercise (bottom). (© Cengage Learning 2013)

TABLE 5.2 Efficiencies of Energy Metabolism from Carbohydrate and Free Fatty Acids Metabolism in Relation to Exercise Intensity and Duration

Metabolic Efficiency

Carbohydrates (CHO) are preferred during high-intensity exercises because its metabolism yields more energy per liter of O_2 than fat metabolism.

	kcal/L O_2
Anaerobic glycolysis	Energy is produced with no O_2 required
Complete CHO oxidation	5.05
Fat oxidation	4.74

Storage Efficiency

Fat is preferred during prolonged exercise because its metabolism provides more energy per unit mass than CHO metabolism.

	kcal/g fuel
CHO oxidation	4.10
Fat oxidation	9.45

Fats are stored in the absence of H_2O, enhancing storage efficiency.

© Cengage Learning 2013

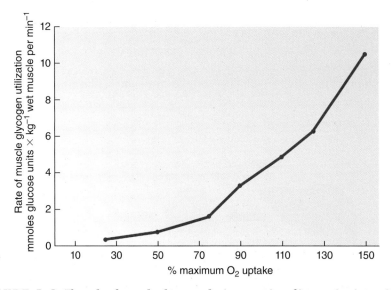

FIGURE 5.2 The role of muscle glycogen during exercise of increasing intensities.
Rates of muscle glycogen utilization with increasing workout intensity expressed as percent maximum oxygen uptake. Data were calculated by muscle biopsies from the vastus lateralis of exercising human subjects. (Adapted from B. Saltin, and J. Karlsson. 1971. Glycogen usage during work of varied intensity. In *Muscle metabolism during exercise*, edited by B. Pernow and B. Saltin. New York: Plenum Press, pp. 289–299.)

cal to store because it forms bonds with water. Indeed, the rapid weight loss that initially occurs with the low-carbohydrate diets is a result of the breakdown of the stored glycogen molecules and the release of its bound water, which is subsequently excreted from the body as urine. The economy of fat storage is recognized in nature by the disposition of fat in fish and birds before their migratory seasons. Table 5.3 summarizes the metabolism of glucose and free fatty acids.

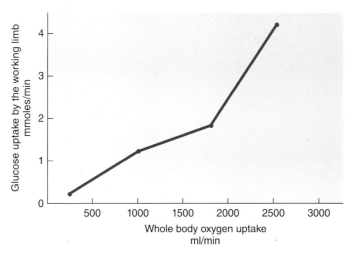

FIGURE 5.3 The role of muscle glucose uptake during exercise of increasing intensities. Rates of glucose uptake by the working leg of human subjects during cycling at different work intensities expressed as whole-body oxygen uptake. Leg glucose uptake was measured using the arteriovenous difference technique. (Modified from Wahren, J., P. Felig, G. Ahlborg, and L. Jorfeldt. 1971. Glucose metabolism during leg exercise in man. *J. Clin. Invest.* 50(12):2715–2725.)

TABLE 5.3 Overview of Cellular Energy Metabolism from Glucose and Free Fatty Acids

Reaction	Substance Processed	Location	Energy Yield (per glucose	End Products Available for Further Energy Extraction molecule processed)	Need for Oxygen
Glycolysis	Glucose	Cytosol	2 molecules of ATP	2 pyruvic acid molecules	No; anaerobic
Tricarboxylic acid cycle	Acetyl-CoA, which is derived from pyruvic acid, the end product of glycolysis and beta-oxidation of acyl-CoA derived from free fatty acids	Mitochondrial matrix	2 molecules of ATP	8 NADH and 2 FADH$_2$ hydrogen carrier molecules	Yes, derived from molecules involved in tricarboxylic acid cycle reactions
Electron transport chain	High-energy electrons stored in hydrogen atoms in the hydrogen carrier molecules NADH and FADH$_2$ derived from tricarboxylic acid cycle reactions	Mitochondrial inner-membrane cristae	32 molecules of ATP	None	Yes, derived from molecular oxygen acquired from breathing

Cytosol

Mitochondrial inner-membrane cristae

Mitochondrial matrix

The mitochondrion is exaggerated and other intracellular components are omitted for better visualization.

Modified from Sherwood, L. 2010. Table 2.2 in *Human physiology*, 7th ed. Belmont, CA: Brooks/Cole-Cengage Learning.

carbohydrate loading The ingestion of a high carbohydrate diet to maximize glycogen stores.

glycogen depletion Results from prolonged fasting or long distance exercise. Low levels of glycogen correspond to exercise fatigue.

gluconeogenesis The pathway, primarily in the liver, that converts lactate, pyruvate, glycerol, and amino acids into glucose. It is important in sustaining blood glucose in a fast or during prolonged exercise.

(If you were asked to design a program of moderate-to-vigorous physical activity for weight loss, what intensity of exercise would you use?)

Sparing Glycogen Stores

The third objective of substrate metabolism is to spare glycogen. The ability for healthy subjects to perform heavy exercise is limited by the cardiovascular system and possibly, in some cases, by the lungs. **Glycogen depletion** is a likely cause of fatigue during prolonged exercise. There is a close relationship between depletion of muscle glycogen stores and time to exhaustion during moderate exercise. Maintaining a high-carbohydrate diet that promotes glycogen stores increases the ca-

pacity to perform prolonged exercise. Whether it is glycogen depletion itself or something closely associated with glycogen depletion that causes exhaustion is difficult to say. The close relationship between glycogen stores and exercise endurance is the basis of the practice of **"carbohydrate loading"** before a long race such as a marathon (see Concepts, Challenges, & Controversies Feature). Means of preserving muscle glycogen are accelerated with increasing exercise duration. Figure 5.4 illustrates the reliance of the working limb on blood-borne and intramuscular fuels as exercise duration progresses. The processes involved can be classified as processes that increase the utilization of FFA by working muscle and processes that increase recycling of carbons into glucose by **gluconeogenesis** in the liver (see Figure 5.5).

Rob Stark/Shutterstock.com

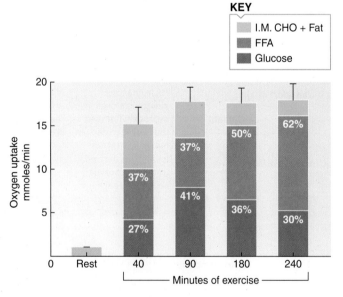

KEY
- I.M. CHO + Fat
- FFA
- Glucose

FIGURE 5.4 Relationship of fuel utilization to exercise duration. Contributions of blood free fatty acids (FFA) and blood glucose to the total oxygen uptake of the working limb determined using the arteriovenous difference technique. The assumption is that these fuels are completely oxidized by muscle when they are taken up from the blood. The rate of oxidation of intramuscular (I.M.) stores (primarily muscle glycogen) is the leg oxygen uptake, which cannot be accounted for by uptake of fuels from the blood. (From Felig, P., and J. Wahren. 1975. Fuel homeostasis in exercise. *N. Engl. J. Med.* 293:1078–1084.)

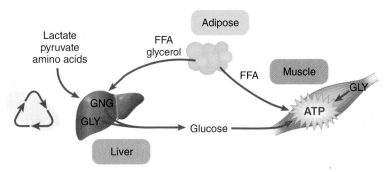

Other fuels are utilized to spare glycogen during
prolonged exercise thereby delaying exhaustion

As exercise duration increases:
• More energy is derived from fats and less from glycogen.
• Amino acid, glycerol, lactate, and pyruvate carbons are
  recycled into glucose.

FIGURE 5.5 **Metabolic pathways for conserving muscle glycogen.** During the latter stages of prolonged exercise, the mobilization of free fatty acids (FFA) and the channeling of metabolites and amino acids into glucose by the gluconeogenic pathway are increased. These pathways can sustain the metabolic requirement of working muscles whereas sparing glycogen stores. The increase in gluconeogenesis is due to increased delivery of substrates for gluconeogenesis to the liver, an increased extraction of these substrates by the liver, and stimulation of the gluconeogenic pathway within the liver. Carbons for gluconeogenesis are derived from lactate, pyruvate, glycerol, and certain amino acids (mainly alanine and glutamine). FFA metabolism is not only critical to the energy requirement of muscle, but also supplies the energy required for gluconeogenesis by the liver. ATP, adenosine triphosphate. (© Cengage Learning 2013)

The former is driven primarily by an increase in lipolysis and FFA concentrations. The latter is determined by the rate that substrates for the gluconeogenic pathway (glycerol, lactate, pyruvate, and amino acids) are delivered to, extracted by, and converted to glucose within the liver. **Branched-chain amino acid** and **ketone body** oxidation are also increased with prolonged exercise and may play a small part in sparing muscle glycogen.

> Which sports drink would be most effective in delaying exhaustion during a marathon?

branched-chain amino acid An amino acid having a side-chain with a branch (a carbon atom bound to more than two other carbon atoms). There are three branched-chain amino acids. They are the essential amino acids: leucine, isoleucine, and valine.

ketone body A water soluble byproduct of fat oxidation in the liver. There are three ketone bodies: acetone, acetoacetate, and beta-hydroxybutyrate. They achieve their highest concentrations when liver fatty acid oxidation is high, as it is during a fast or prolonged exercise. Ketone bodies can be oxidized in the heart and brain.

The Give and Take of Fuel Metabolism during Exercise

All three objectives of substrate metabolism are generally achieved during light-to-moderate exercise of 90 minutes or less, as long as subjects are healthy. One objective is compromised to achieve another when a person attempts to test his or her exercise limits. For example, during heavy exercise, muscle glycogen and blood glucose are used at high rates because of the requirement for a metabolically efficient fuel. High rates of muscle glycogen utilization cannot be sustained without depleting their stores. The liver can normally replenish blood glucose as it is used. As the duration of exercise increases, the liver glycogen becomes depleted, and because **gluconeogenesis** alone is inadequate at maintaining the blood glucose concentration constant, hypoglycemia may result.

What Ensures the Coordinated Mobilization and Utilization of Fuels during Exercise?

It is clear that fuels for energy metabolism are not released in an uncontrolled manner like water gushing forth from a breached levee. Chemical energy stored within glycogen and triglycerides is prudently dispensed in accordance with the three objectives of fuel utilization. How are the needs of the muscle transmitted to the liver and adipose tissue, signaling the release of glucose and lipid stores? This chapter considers the mobilization and use of fuels when the only sources of energy are those stored in the body. "How does feeding influence substrate utilization?" and "What are the signals that control fuel metabolism?" are questions for which you need to know the answers. The complex processes involved in these questions are the topic of Chapter 6.

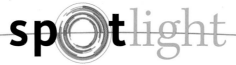

spotlight

An Expert on the Integrated Physiology of Fuel Metabolism during Exercise: Bengt Saltin, M.D., Ph.D.

Although Denmark is geographically small, it is difficult to find a locale that has played a larger role in driving advancements in human physiology. The research of Panum, Bohr, Krogh, Hasselbalch, Lindhard, Christensen, Asmussen, Nielsen, Astrand, and others of the Danish tradition comprise a body of work that has defined much of what is now known of the workings of the human body. Considering the seminal contributions of Swedish scientists to human physiology, it is only fitting that it be a Swede working in Denmark who has been instrumental in the perpetuation of this rich tradition in human physiology. Bengt Saltin received his M.D. in 1962 and Ph.D. in 1964 in Stockholm. He was then appointed to the faculty in the Department of Exercise Physiology at Stockholm's renowned Karolinska Institute. In 1973, he was appointed Professor of Human Physiology at the University of Copenhagen. Beginning in 1993, Saltin was named founding Director of the Copenhagen Muscle Research Center.

Dr. Saltin, like his predecessors August Krogh, who won the Nobel Prize in 1920 for his work on the diffusion of oxygen from capillaries to skeletal muscle, and Erik Howhu

Christensen, has used an integrated approach to better understand human physiology. Saltin was trained as a cardiovascular physiologist and his initial work dealt with cardiovascular exercise capacity and the environment. His authoritative knowledge of the cardiovascular system proved to be key in his subsequent work examining metabolic limitations of the working muscle. Saltin recognized that muscle work capacity could not be understood without understanding the effectiveness of the vessels that perfuse it. A combination of techniques that permit measurements of metabolite concentrations in the muscle vascular, interstitial, and cellular compartments allowed Saltin to delineate factors that limit exercise performance in health and disease. These metabolite measurements were accompanied by assessments of fuel fluxes and enzyme activities to provide a mechanistic framework for metabolic limitations with exercise and extended disuse. His contributions to human physiology and skeletal muscle metabolism include: (a) the effects of exercise training, (b) the complications of extended bed rest, (c) the interaction of human physiology and the environment, and (d) genetic determinants of exercise performance. Saltin's body of work forms a template that continues to drive the field of exercise physiology.

Saltin has laid a foundation that will allow for the rich tradition of human physiology in Denmark to continue well into the future. The presence of accomplished physiologists such as Drs. M. Kjaer, B. Klarlund Pedersen, and E. A. Richter ensure that Denmark will remain an international center for human physiology for many years to come.

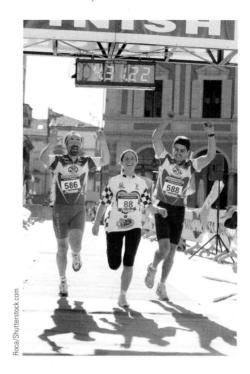

Roca/Shutterstock.com

CONCEPTS, challenges, controversies

Topping Off the Tank

Kenya's Geoffrey Mutai ran 26.2 miles faster than anyone in history when he won the Boston Marathon in 2011. The difference in Mutai's first place time of 2:03:02 and countryman Moses Mosop's second place time of 2:03:06 was less than 0.1 percent. Indeed, it is often the narrowest of margins that separates the best. This reality has prompted athletes to explore ways to get the extra edge through practices involving nutrition as well as physical training. Some dietary practices used by athletes are based more on superstition or intuition rather than science. The nutritional practice of carbohydrate loading may make that small difference over a long race like a marathon. The scientific basis of carbohydrate loading is founded within the rich history of human exercise physiology in Scandinavia. In a classic study published in 1939, E. H. Christensen and O. Hansen of Denmark showed that dietary macronutrient content was a key determinant of exercise endurance. These scientists had volunteers consume three different diets, each for 1 week. Diets contained low, moderate, or high percentages of carbohydrate.

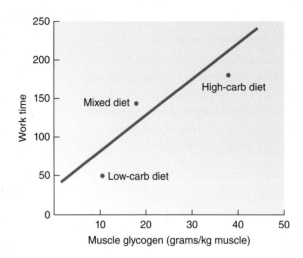

●FIGURE 5.6 **The relationship of muscle glycogen stores to exercise endurance.** There is a tight relationship between pre-exercise muscle glycogen and exercise time to exhaustion. Subjects consumed a low-carbohydrate/high-fat diet, a mixed diet, and a high-carbohydrate/low-fat diet for 1 week before exercise. (Modified from Bergstrom, J., L. Hermansen, E. Hultman, and B. Saltin. 1967. Diet, muscle glycogen and physical performance. *Acta. Physiol. Scand.* 71:140–150.)

After 1 week on each diet, subjects exercised to exhaustion on a bicycle. The results showed a remarkably strong direct relationship between the amount of carbohydrate in the diet and time to exhaustion. The endurance times were approximately 80, 120, and 240 minutes after 1 week of the low-, moderate-, and high-carbohydrate diets, respectively. Swedish scientists in the 1960s applied a percutaneous needle biopsy method for obtaining muscle tissue to extend earlier work by showing that pre-exercise muscle glycogen content was directly related to time to exhaustion (see Figure 5.6). It was also demonstrated by these scientists that pre-exercise muscle glycogen and, therefore, endurance time could be increased by a diet high in carbohydrate. The importance of muscle glycogen for exercise endurance was reinforced by the observation that exhaustion usually coincides with critically low muscle glycogen content. These observations led to a quest to devise the optimal pre-race regimen for expanding muscle glycogen levels. The general principle used by most of these protocols is that if one consumes a diet high in carbohydrates after a period of muscle glycogen depletion, higher than normal muscle glycogen content can be obtained. The strategy of first depleting muscle glycogen, then consuming a high-carbohydrate diet leads to a supercompensation of glycogen stores.

HOTLINK *See the Carbohydrate Loading section of the Nicholas Institute of Sports Medicine and Athletic Trauma website (**http://www.nismat.org/nutricor/carbohydrate.html**) for more information on diet and carbohydrates.*

Do glycogen supercompensation protocols improve exercise endurance? Indeed, these protocols do increase the storage of muscle glycogen, and there is strong evidence that these protocols improve exercise performance. However, glycogen supercompensation does not increase the intensity with which an athlete can work; rather, it increases the time over which moderate exercise can be sustained. It makes sense that depletion of muscle glycogen would limit exercise endurance and delaying glycogen depletion would increase it. It is important to recognize, though, that factors that closely parallel muscle glycogen depletion can contribute to fatigue. Liver glycogen stores decrease and blood glucose concentration declines coincident with low muscle glycogen. These events probably together conspire to cause fatigue during endurance exercise.

One common glycogen repletion protocol uses a 3-day depletion phase, during which training remains intense but carbohydrate intake is reduced, and a 3-day loading phase of a high-carbohydrate (about 75 percent) diet and light or no exercise. Because of the discomfort and fatigue associated with combining intense exercise and low-carbohydrate intake, some athletes have opted to de-emphasize the depletion phase or limit it to a single bout of glycogen-depleting exercise before the start of the loading phase.

There is no doubt that nutrient intake is an important component of exercise performance. This recognition has spawned research activity and the thriving sports supplements industry.

in*Practice*
Examples of Fuel Utilization during Exercise

The following text provides practical examples of how fuel utilization and programs of moderate exercise are related to your area of interest.

Health/Fitness: By understanding fuel utilization, you can help reinforce the concepts from Chapters 4, 11, and 12 (nutrition) to assist your clients in understanding that carbohydrate (glucose) metabolism is necessary to optimize exercise performance. You can help your clients understand how to maintain glucose homeostasis to avoid hypoglycemia and meet their individual exercise program's energy needs. You will also be able to explain to clients why carbohydrate is more metabolically efficient than fat to use during exercise, and that fat is the most storage-efficient fuel. The knowledge you gain about fuel utilization during a program of exercise can help you explain to clients why it is difficult to lose weight and maintain the weight loss without adjusting both caloric intake and caloric expenditure.

Medicine: By understanding fuel utilization, physicians and other healthcare professionals can help those patients in medical weight-loss programs understand why they will need to adjust their dietary habits and how their new habits can improve fuel utilization. For example, in many hospital-based wellness weight-loss programs for obese adults, such as that at the Methodist Hospital in Houston, Texas, patients engage in three 12-week steps. For the first 12 weeks, patients undergo medically supervised fasting and usually see significant weight loss, as one might expect. During the second 12-week period, patients return to consuming normal food and practice behavior intervention, with and without wellness coaching as needed. At 24 weeks, patients move to the maintenance phase of the program and are on their own with regard to weight control, but they can contact a health professional for counseling as needed.

Athletic Performance: Future coaches must understand fuel utilization if they are going optimize the training of their athletes. As the earlier Concepts, Challenges, & Controversies feature highlighted, knowing how to properly fuel up for competition may often mean the difference between winning and losing or having enough energy to compete effectively. For example, how do you think you might use what you know about fuel utilization to make a recommendation to a starting collegiate basketball player concerning his pregame meal? Would it matter with regard to performance whether he consumed more carbohydrates than fats and protein, or should he consume lots of protein in his last meal before competition for more energy? If you have competed as an athlete, did you have a high-quality fuel utilization pregame meal? Why or why not? How might you change what your coach recommended to you to improve performance?

Rehabilitation: By understanding fuel utilization, physical therapists, athletic trainers, and other healthcare professionals can help those with diabetes understand the basics of controlling their blood glucose concentrations. The understanding of the use of insulin supplementation (if necessary) for physically active individuals with diabetes and its effects on blood glucose concentrations must be closely monitored to avoid insulin shock or diabetic coma. To prevent insulin shock (severe hypoglycemia), you will need to monitor the diabetic client's insulin dose and understand that a program of moderate-to-vigorous physical activity has its own insulin effect, which means the dose of supplemental insulin will have to be modified to the individual as she adapts to increased levels of physical activity. To prevent diabetic coma (ketoacidosis), you will need to understand that the client has a lack of insulin and needs to achieve better baseline glucose control before participating in exercise of moderate-to-vigorous physical activity.

HOTLINK *See Chapter 6B for more details on diabetes.*

Chapter Summary

- Fuel utilization can be measured in a variety of ways, including arteriovenous difference techniques, isotopic techniques, indirect calorimetry via pulmonary gas exchange, and muscle biopsy techniques.

- It is well documented that the increased energy demand of exercise necessitates an accelerated flow of energy substrates from storage sites to the energy-producing pathways in the contracting muscle.

- The contribution of each substrate (that is, carbohydrate, fat, protein) to the metabolic demand of the working muscle depends on different factors relating to subject characteristics (for example, fitness, nutritional state, specific health deficits) and exercise conditions (for example, high altitude, temperature extremes).

- The impact of duration and intensity of a program of exercise is such that with increasing exercise duration, more fat is used, and with more strenuous exercise, more carbohydrates are used.

- Substrate metabolism during exercise has three objectives: (a) maintain glucose homeostasis, (b) metabolize the most efficient substrate, and (c) spare muscle glycogen.

- Ingestion of glucose can correct or prevent the decrease in blood glucose and, in some instances, increase the capacity for prolonged exercise.

- Carbohydrate is more metabolically efficient than is fat and better suits the needs of heavy exercise.

- Fat is the most storage-efficient fuel and is used preferentially during light exercise that can potentially be sustained for long intervals.

- Glycogen depletion is a likely cause of fatigue during prolonged exercise. There is a close relationship between depletion of muscle glycogen stores and time to exhaustion during moderate exercise.

- It is clear that fuels for energy metabolism are not released in an uncontrolled manner like water gushing forth from a breached levee. Chemical energy stored within glycogen and triglycerides is prudently dispensed in accordance with the three objectives of fuel utilization.

Exercise Physiology Reality

CENGAGEbrain   To reinforce the exercise physiology concepts presented above, complete the laboratory exercises for Chapter 5. To access labs and other course materials for this text, please visit www.cengagebrain.com. See the preface on page xiii for details. Once you complete the exercises, evaluate your results based on the scales provided and develop a personal plan for successfully applying the concepts you have learned.

Exercise Physiology Web Links

Access the following websites for further study of topics covered in this chapter:

- Find updates and quick links to fuel utilization and exercise physiology–related sites at ourwebsite. To access the course materials and companion resources for this text, please visit www.cengagebrain.com. See the preface on page xiii for details.

- Search for more information about fuel utilization at the American College of Sports Medicine site at: http://www.acsm.org.

- Search for more information about fuel utilization at the Gatorade Sports Science Institute website at: http://www.gssiweb.com.

- Search for more information on glucose homeostasis at Glucose Homeostasis and Starvation at: http://chemistry.gravitywaves.com/CHE452/24_Glucose%20Homeostas.htm.

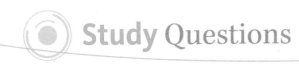

Study Questions

Review the Warm-Up Pre-Test questions you were asked to answer before reading Chapter 5. Test yourself once more to determine what you know now that you have completed the chapter.

The questions that follow will help you review this chapter. You will find the answers in the discussions on the pages provided.

1. How can fuel utilization be measured scientifically? *p. 130*

2. What is the muscle biopsy technique and how does it work? *p. 131*

3. What are the three principles of substrate utilization? *p. 132*

4. How can glucose homeostasis be preserved? *p. 132*

5. What determines whether carbohydrate or fat is primarily used during exercise? *p. 133*

6. What is the relationship between glycogen depletion and fatigue in prolonged exercise? *p. 136*

7. How does the liver help replenish blood glucose? *p. 136*

8. Which fuel type (carbohydrates or fats) provide the muscle with more ATP per carbon atom contained of the fuel? *pp. 133–134*

9. What are ways that the body can spare muscle glycogen? *p. 137*

10. How is ATP produced in mammalian cells when metabolism is anaerobic? *p. 134*

Selected References

Bergstrom, J., L. Hermansen, E. Hultman, and B. Saltin. 1967. Diet, muscle glycogen and physical performance. *Acta. Physiol. Scand.* 71:140–150.

Hawley, J. A., E. J. Schabort, T. D. Noakes, and S. C. Dennis. 1997. Carbohydrate-loading and exercise performance. An update. *Sports Med.* 24(2): 73–81.

Hellsten, Y., and B. Saltin. 2010. The legacy of the Copenhagen School: In the footsteps of Lindhard and Krogh. *Acta. Physiol. (Oxf).* 199(4):347–348.

Hultman, E. 1995. Fuel selection, muscle fibre. *Proc. Nutr. Soc.* 54(1):107–121.

Joyner, M. J. 2011. Into the real world: physiological insights from elite marathoners. *Med. Sci. Sports Exerc.* 43(4): 656–64.

Kiens, B. 2006. Skeletal muscle lipid metabolism in exercise and insulin resistance. *Physiol. Rev.* 86(1):205–243.

Spriet, L. L., and M. J. Watt. 2003. Regulatory mechanisms in the interaction between carbohydrate and lipid oxidation during exercise. *Acta. Physiol. Scand.* 178(4):443–452.

Wasserman, D. H. 2009. Solomon A. Berson Award Lecture: Four grams of glucose. *Am. J. Physiol.* 296(1):E11–E21.

Wasserman, D. H., and A. Cherrington. 1996. Regulation of extrahepatic fuel sources during exercise. In *The American Physiological Society Handbook of Physiology—Integration of Motor, Circulatory, Respiratory, and Metabolic Control during Exercise,* edited by L. B. Rowell and J. T. Shepherd. Rockville, MD: Waverly Press, pp. 1036–1074.

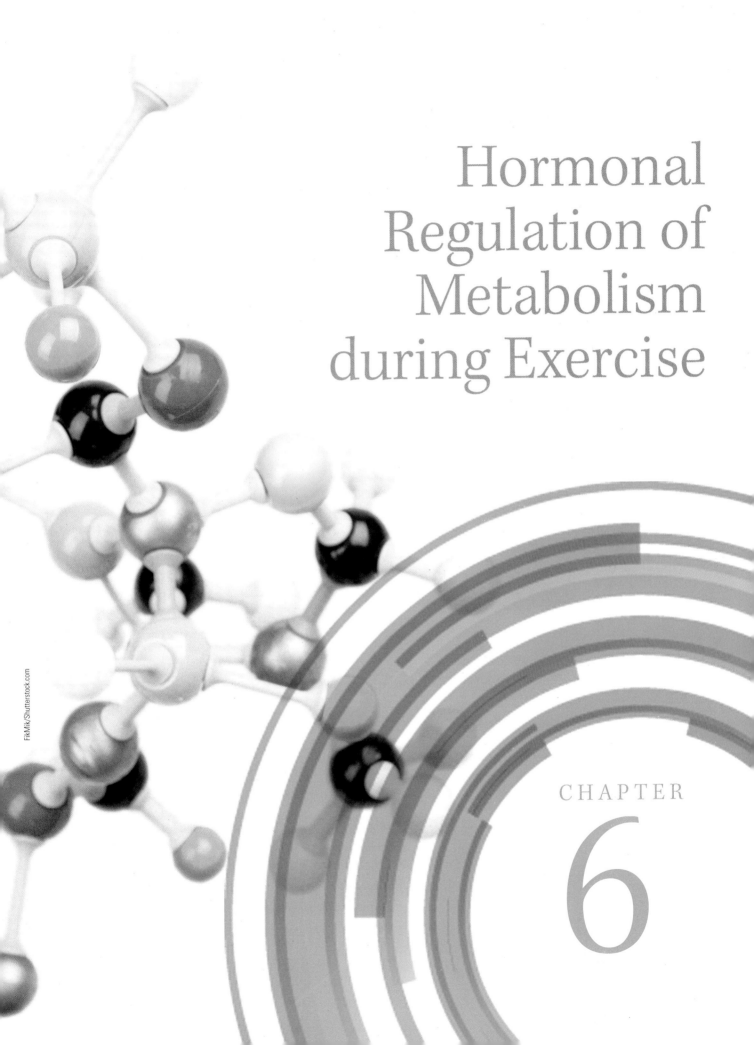

Hormonal Regulation of Metabolism during Exercise

CHAPTER

6

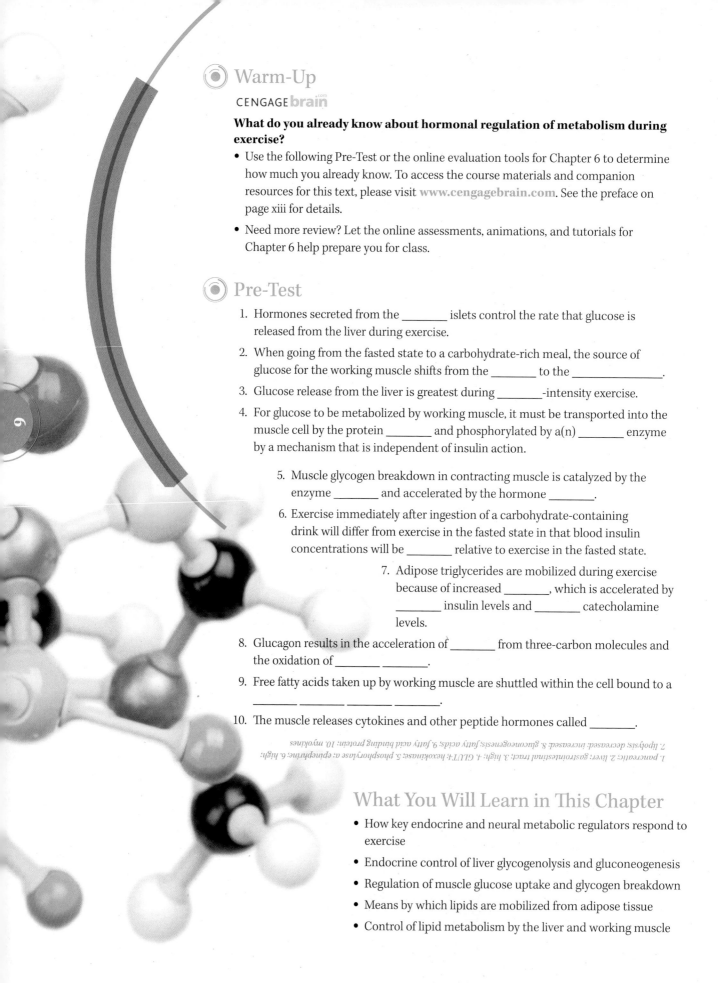

Warm-Up

CENGAGE **brain**

What do you already know about hormonal regulation of metabolism during exercise?

- Use the following Pre-Test or the online evaluation tools for Chapter 6 to determine how much you already know. To access the course materials and companion resources for this text, please visit **www.cengagebrain.com**. See the preface on page xiii for details.

- Need more review? Let the online assessments, animations, and tutorials for Chapter 6 help prepare you for class.

Pre-Test

1. Hormones secreted from the _____ islets control the rate that glucose is released from the liver during exercise.

2. When going from the fasted state to a carbohydrate-rich meal, the source of glucose for the working muscle shifts from the _____ to the _____.

3. Glucose release from the liver is greatest during _____-intensity exercise.

4. For glucose to be metabolized by working muscle, it must be transported into the muscle cell by the protein _____ and phosphorylated by a(n) _____ enzyme by a mechanism that is independent of insulin action.

5. Muscle glycogen breakdown in contracting muscle is catalyzed by the enzyme _____ and accelerated by the hormone _____.

6. Exercise immediately after ingestion of a carbohydrate-containing drink will differ from exercise in the fasted state in that blood insulin concentrations will be _____ relative to exercise in the fasted state.

7. Adipose triglycerides are mobilized during exercise because of increased _____, which is accelerated by _____ insulin levels and _____ catecholamine levels.

8. Glucagon results in the acceleration of _____ from three-carbon molecules and the oxidation of _____ _____.

9. Free fatty acids taken up by working muscle are shuttled within the cell bound to a _____ _____ _____ _____.

10. The muscle releases cytokines and other peptide hormones called _____.

1. pancreatic; 2. liver; gastrointestinal tract; 3. high; 4. GLUT4; hexokinase; 5. phosphorylase α: epinephrine; 6. high; 7. lipolysis; decreased; increased; 8. gluconeogenesis; fatty acids; 9. fatty acid binding protein; 10. myokines

What You Will Learn in This Chapter

- How key endocrine and neural metabolic regulators respond to exercise
- Endocrine control of liver glycogenolysis and gluconeogenesis
- Regulation of muscle glucose uptake and glycogen breakdown
- Means by which lipids are mobilized from adipose tissue
- Control of lipid metabolism by the liver and working muscle

QUICKSTART!

How does exercise affect hormones and sympathetic nerves involved in energy metabolism? What signals the liver to produce more glucose during exercise? What factors control how blood glucose, free fatty acids, and muscle glycogen are used during exercise? What signals result in the mobilization of free fatty acids from adipose tissue?

Introduction to Hormonal Regulation of Metabolism during Exercise

Chapter 5 discussed the importance of carbohydrates and lipid as fuel during exercise. With regard to the metabolism of carbohydrates, the roles of gluconeogenesis in the liver and glycogen mobilization from the liver and muscle were described. Two important factors are clear. First, carbohydrate utilization is increased with exercise at rates directly proportional to the exercise intensity. Second, carbohydrate stores are limited and can be depleted with prolonged exercise. Two important factors also define the role of lipid metabolism during exercise. Fats are efficiently stored as triglycerides in adipocytes and are in great abundance. Second, the energetic benefits

of fat metabolism can be reaped only when oxygen is readily abundant. The endocrine and autonomic nervous responses are key to the regulation of carbohydrate and lipid metabolism during exercise.

The goal of this chapter is to discuss the regulation of the mobilization and utilization of carbohydrate and lipid stores during exercise. Because of the important roles of the endocrine and sympathetic nervous responses to exercise, such a discussion must begin with an overview of how these regulatory factors respond to exercise.

HOTLINK *Visit the course materials for Chapter 6 for a review of the endocrine system.*

Responses of Hormones Involved in Metabolic Regulation

Hormones are released from endocrine glands into the blood, where they regulate events such as metabolism, blood pressure, energy and fluid balances, ionic composition of bodily fluids, growth, and reproduction. In this chapter, we focus on those hormones that involve the regulation of metabolism during exercise. Other aspects of the endocrine system will be discussed later in the context of the systems they regulate.

The importance of the endocrine system in metabolic regulation was recognized almost immediately after the concept of a hormone as a bloodborne messenger was introduced. Since that time, the metabolic role of the endocrine system has been studied extensively. The development of sensitive hormone assays since the 1960s has been instrumental in describing the endocrine response to exercise. Measurements of increased circulating **norepinephrine**, which

hormones Chemicals released by a cell or a gland in one part of the body that sends out messages that are transmitted through the blood to target cells in other parts of the organism. Hormones act through specific receptors.

norepinephrine A catecholamine with multiple roles including as a hormone and a neurotransmitter. It is also called noradrenalin.

sympathetic activity The rate of release of sympathetic neurotransmitter (usually norepinephrine) from sympathetic nerves of the autonomic nervous system.

insulin A hormone released from pancreatic islet beta cells that lowers blood glucose by stimulating its uptake from the blood into muscle, liver, and fat and suppressing the release of glucose from the liver into the blood.

glucagon A hormone released from pancreatic islet alpha cells that stimulates glucose release, fat oxidation, and ureagenesis by the liver. It counters the glucose lowering effect of insulin.

catecholamines Released from the adrenal medulla and sympathetic nerves in response to exercise or stressful conditions. These include norepinephrine, epinephrine, and dopamine.

growth hormone (GH) A peptide hormone secreted from the anterior pituitary. It is regulated by a number of stimuli, including exercise. It is postulated to be involved with adaptations to regular physical activity.

thyroid hormone Releases hormones triidothyronine and thyroxine that participate in the control of how the body uses energy and makes proteins and controls how sensitive the body is to other hormones.

adrenocorticotropic hormone (ACTH) A polypeptide hormone produced and secreted by the anterior pituitary gland. It acts through receptors on the adrenal cortex to promote the synthesis and secretion of gluco- and mineralo-corticoids. ACTH release is increased by exercise.

beta-endorphin A peptide neurotransmitter in both the central and peripheral nervous systems. It also may have an endocrine function. It is formed from the same precursor gene as ACTH (pro-opiomelanocortin). Its levels may increase with exercise.

gastrointestinal hormones Constitute a group of hormones secreted by enteroendocrine cells in the stomach, pancreas, and small intestine. These control digestive function, but they have also been implicated in systemic metabolic regulation and in control of feeding centers in the brain.

renin A peptide hormone released by the kidney that acts as an enzyme to cleave angiotensinogen to angiotensin I, which is then converted to angiotensin II. Angiotensin II constricts blood vessels and stimulates the release of antidiuretic hormone and aldosterone.

is released primarily from sympathetic nerves, and direct measurements of nerve activity, indicate that **sympathetic activity** is also affected by exercise. These hormonal and neural responses are generally more pronounced with increased exercise duration and intensity. Other factors such as age, nutritional status, and fitness level are also important in determining the responses of the endocrine and sympathetic nervous systems to exercise. Exercise in the fasted state is characterized by a decrease in arterial **insulin**, an increase or no detectable change in arterial **glucagon**, and increases in arterial **catecholamine**, **growth hormone (GH)**, **thyroid hormone**, **adrenocorticotropic hormone (ACTH)**, **beta-endorphin**, **gastrointestinal hormones**, **renin**, **cortisol**, and **gonadal hormones**, among others. An important characteristic of the endocrine response to exercise is that it synergizes with other stimuli. For example, the catecholamines, glucagon, and cortisol are generally stimulated synergistically by exercise in the presence of hypoglycemia or hypoxia. The absorption of nutrients from the gastrointestinal tract alters many of the hormonal responses to exercise. The pre-

cise effects depend on size, content, and timing of the meal with respect to exercise.

Despite the characterization of the arterial hormone responses to exercise, two major issues have made it difficult to assess the actions of these key regulators. The first is that measurements of arterial and venous blood hormone and neurotransmitter concentrations do not always reflect those at their sites of action. The second component of the endocrine and autonomic nervous responses to exercise that has not been well defined is the signal or signals that initiate these responses. It has been postulated that small changes in blood glucose, neural or chemical feedback originating from the working muscle, and/or feedforward mechanisms originating in the brain may be involved. These putative mechanisms are illustrated in Figure 6.1.

Hormones such as GH and the gonadal hormones do not participate in the metabolic response during exercise, but they may contribute to the long-term metabolic adaptations. The role of the endocrine system in an adaptive capacity is complex and is likely to involve the interaction of a variety of hormones and paracrine factors.

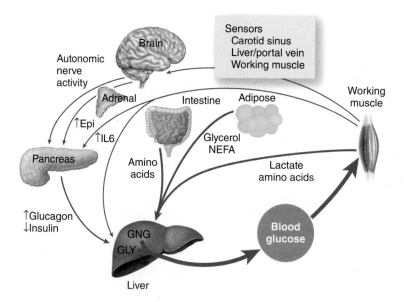

FIGURE 6.1 Signals and substrates implicated in control of glucose fluxes during exercise. The metabolic demands of working muscle require an increase in the uptake of glucose from the blood. A coordinated neural and hormonal response stimulates the liver to accelerate its release of glucose. The neural and sensory mechanisms that initiate these signals still remain to be clearly defined. Amino acids and various metabolites are recycled back to glucose in the liver by the gluconeogenic pathway. (© Cengage Learning 2013)

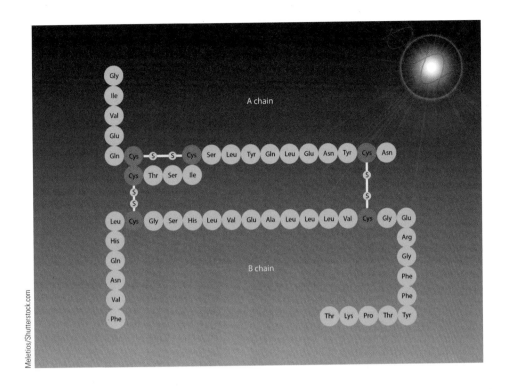

A chain

B chain

gonadal hormones Steroid hormones made in the ovaries or testes. These hormones have diverse actions. In addition to those involved with development, they have synthetic and metabolic actions.

cortisol A steroid hormone, or a glucocorticoid, that is released from the adrenal cortex in response to strenuous exercise. It has effects that can accelerate glucose, fat, and protein metabolism. It also suppresses the immune system.

Insulin

The hormone insulin when unopposed decreases blood glucose by inhibiting the release of glucose from the liver and stimulating glucose uptake by muscle, fat, and liver. Insulin is secreted from **beta cells** of the islets of Langerhans of the pancreas. The hormones secreted by the islets enter pancreatic veins that drain into the hepatic portal vein. The hepatic portal vein perfuses the liver before it enters the vena cava. Blood flow through the portal vein comprises the majority of the total hepatic blood perfusing the liver. Thus, secretions from the pancreatic islets are ideally suited to control liver function. Because the liver extracts about 50 percent of the insulin with which it is presented, arterial levels are much less than those at the liver. For this reason, changes in insulin secretion will lead to smaller changes in arterial insulin levels. The reduction in insulin levels with exercise is due to a decrease in beta-cell secretion (Figure 6.2). The magnitude of the decline in insulin levels is directly related to exercise duration. A decline in plasma insulin levels of up to about 50 percent is present after 2 hours of moderate exercise in fasted subjects.

What causes the decrease in insulin secretion with exercise? Regulation of the pancreatic secretions is complex, because they are under the control of nutrients, hormones, and the autonomic nerves that innervate them. It is notable that sympathetic nerve activity and circulating catecholamine concentrations both increase in response to exercise. When norepinephrine reacts with alpha-adrenergic receptors on the beta cells, insulin secretion is suppressed. The suppression in circulating insulin levels may be, at least in part, caused by the interaction of norepinephrine with this receptor type on the beta cell. Neural input to the pancreas has been proposed to comprise a component of the effector system that regulates the pancreatic hormone response to exercise.

Circulating glucose particularly during exercise sensitively regulates insulin secretion. It is possible that a decrease in insulin secretion during exercise is a result of small decrements in blood glucose acting on the beta cell either directly or via the sympathetic nervous system. The decline in insulin level is attenuated by high-intensity exercise that results in an increase in circulating glucose. Besides the pancreas, cells sensitive to glucose are

beta cells Endocrine cells located in the islets of Langerhans that secrete insulin.

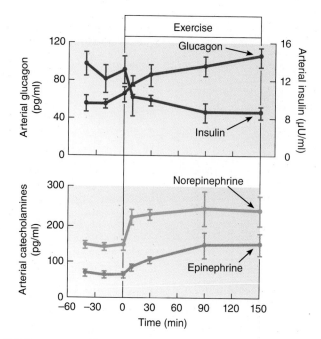

FIGURE 6.2 Responses of key glucoregulatory hormones to prolonged moderate-intensity exercise. Plasma insulin level declines gradually, whereas glucagon, epinephrine, and norepinephrine levels increase. (© Cengage Learning 2013)

located in the portal vein, liver, brain, and carotid bodies that monitor glucose concentrations or oscillatory patterns in the bloodstream. Neural networks are in place to transmit glucose-related signals to the pancreas.

HOTLINK *Visit the course materials for Chapter 6 for more information about glucose and glucagon.*

Glucagon

The hormone glucagon is released by the alpha cells of the islets of Langerhans. Glucagon is the most potent hormone in the body at stimulating glucose release from the liver. Like insulin, glucagon is carried by pancreatic venous drainage to the hepatic portal vein that perfuses the liver (Figure 6.3). Perfusing the liver with pancreatic venous drainage is efficient for regulation of glucose output from the liver because it permits glucagon to have rapid and potent effects on the liver without the need for excessive glucagon secretion and high arterial levels.

This is an efficient arrangement physiologically, but it adds a degree of difficulty to the assessment of changes in glucagon

secretion. This is because increases in glucagon at the liver (that is, in the portal venous blood) are not strictly reflected by concentrations in the systemic circulation from which blood is sampled. Increases in arterial and peripheral venous glucagon levels are often small or undetectable in humans after short- or moderate-duration exercise (less than about 45 minutes). A decrease in peripheral glucagon levels may even occur during high-intensity exercise. Exercise longer than 1 hour generally results in an unequivocal increase. However, studies in the laboratory with animals with indwelling arterial and portal vein catheters show that arterial glucagon levels greatly underestimate the levels to which the liver is exposed (Figure 6.4). Studies in humans suggest that increases in glucagon secretion are approximately fourfold during moderate exercise. The reason that increases in glucagon release and portal vein glucagon do not translate into proportional increases in arterial concentrations is an increased hepatic extraction of glucagon by the liver.

As is likely the case with the exercise-induced decline in insulin, an exercise-induced increase in glucagon is, at least

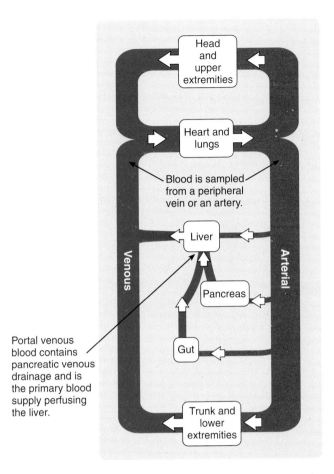

FIGURE 6.3 Minimal overview of the circulation. Peripheral venous and arterial glucagon underestimates the concentration to which the liver is exposed in the portal vein. Blood vessels that are red reflect that they contain oxygenated arterial blood. Blood vessels that are blue reflect that they contain deoxygenated venous blood. (© Cengage Learning 2013)

in part, due to **adrenergic stimulation**. Several lines of evidence support the possibility that adrenergic drive stimulates glucagon release during exercise. First, both alpha- and beta-adrenergic receptors stimulate glucagon release from pancreatic **alpha cells**, and **alpha- and beta-adrenergic receptor** blockade attenuate the increment in arterial glucagon during

exercise in animal models. In addition, during prolonged exercise, a decrease in blood glucose is probably an important stimulus. The view that glucose is an important determinant of the glucagon response to exercise is supported by the demonstration that the increase in glucagon is abolished when glucose is ingested before or during exercise.

adrenergic stimulation The stimulation of adrenergic receptors by the catecholamines. This is increased in many cell types during exercise. Effects of adrenergic stimulation are cell type-dependent.

alpha cells Endocrine cells located in the islet of Langerhans that secrete glucagon.

alpha- and beta-adrenergic receptors The two major types of adrenergic receptors. They bind to and are activated by the catecholamines.

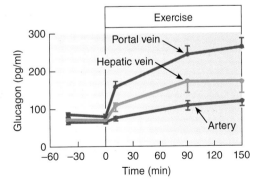

FIGURE 6.4 Glucagon concentrations in the artery, portal vein, and hepatic vein, during rest and moderate exercise. (Wasserman, D. H., D. B. Lacy, and D. P. Bracy. 1993. Relationship of arterial to portal vein immunoreactive glucagon during experience. *J. Appl. Physiol.* 75:724–729.)

Responses of Hormones Involved in Metabolic Regulation **151**

Catecholamine

Epinephrine secretion from the adrenal medulla increases with exercise, resulting in increased circulating levels of this hormone. The magnitude of this increase is directly related to the duration and intensity of exercise. Epinephrine may increase by approximately twofold after 30 minutes of moderate exercise (60 percent of the maximum O_2 uptake) and by approximately 10-fold after 3 hours. The relationship between exercise intensity and epinephrine response is such that increments in work rate greater than about 50 percent of the maximum O_2 uptake are far greater than similar increments constrained to be less than this work rate. During exhaustive exercise at 100 percent maximum O_2 uptake, epinephrine can increase by as much as 10-fold to 20-fold!

Norepinephrine is also released from the adrenal medulla. Nevertheless, the more important sources of norepinephrine are the sympathetic nerve endings, which result in very high levels in sympathetic synaptic clefts. Exercise increases sympathetic nerve activity to major fuel depots (liver, muscle, adipose tissue). As is the case with the response of epinephrine to exercise, the norepinephrine response is also directly related to exercise duration and intensity. Norepinephrine responds differently from epinephrine in two ways: It is both more rapid and more marked at low work rates. The signal for the increase in norepinephrine concentrations during exercise may relate to neural feedback from the cardiovascular system or a feedforward emanating from the brainstem. Epinephrine is more sensitive to metabolic stressors such as a decrement in blood glucose. It may also be increased by a feedforward signal. Arterial norepinephrine, which is the most common readout of sympathetic activity, does not reflect those at the synaptic cleft nor can it provide information related to the specific tissue beds affected.

Cortisol

Corticotropin-releasing factor released by the hypothalamus triggers ACTH secretion from the anterior pituitary gland. ACTH then increases cortisol secretion from the adrenal cortex. It circulates primarily bound to the protein, cortisol-binding globulin, which is produced in the liver. The cortisol concentration in the blood is determined by the circulating cortisol-binding globulin level, as well as adrenal cortical secretion. This hypothalamic pituitary adrenal axis is activated by exercise and leads to an increase in cortisol if it is of sufficient duration (>15 minutes). Cortisol concentrations are associated with circadian oscillations and meal-associated changes, which will influence the response to exercise.

Growth Hormone

GH is secreted by the anterior pituitary gland in a pulsatile manner. Its secretion is regulated by the hypothalamic peptides growth hormone-releasing hormone (GHRH), somatostatin, and ghrelin. GHRH stimulates GH synthesis and secretion, somatostatin inhibits GH release, and ghrelin increases GH release directly. GH secretion changes throughout the life span with maximal GH secretion during the adolescent years, after which it declines. In addition to age-related events, circulating GH is determined by factors such as a person's sex, nutrition, sleep, body composition, stress, gonadal steroids, insulin, and fitness. Aerobic exercise is a potent stimulus to GH release. GH secretion is directly related to exercise intensity.

Cytokines

A number of **cytokines** (for example, IL-4, IL-6, IL-10, IL-12) are released during exercise. Of these, interleukin-6 (IL-6) is generally the first cytokine to respond to exercise and its response is the most marked, increasing by as much as 100-fold. In addition to anti-inflammatory effects, IL-6 may also have metabolic effects. Pioneering work on IL-6 showed that one important source of IL-6 is the working muscle. IL-6 mRNA in skeletal muscle and its release from skeletal muscle may increase dramatically with exercise. It has been suggested that

cytokines Encompass a large and diverse family of protein or glycoprotein regulators produced throughout the body by cells of diverse embryological origin. Responsiveness to exercise and their actions are dependent on the individual member of this broad family of molecules.

IL-6 may be one mechanism by which the metabolic state of working muscle is conveyed to other organs. Cytokines and other novel hormones released by muscle have been termed **myokines**. In addition to the ILs, other myokines include brain-derived neurotrophic factor, leukemia inhibitory factor, fibroblast growth factor 21 (FGF21), and follistatin-like 1. Although a number of potential roles for the myokines have been proposed, their precise role and regulation are largely unknown and remain the topic of intensive investigations.

Adipokines and Adipose-Derived Hormones

A number of cytokines are also released by adipocytes. These are called **adipokines** and include tumor necrosis factor-alpha, visfatin, IL-6, plasminogen activator inhibitor-1, and retinol-binding protein 4. As noted earlier, IL-6 may play a role in the response to exercise. However, the source of this IL-6 is probably skeletal muscle. Leptin, adiponectin, and resistin are adipose-derived hormones that are important in regulation of body weight control and metabolism. The circulating concentrations of adipokines and adipose-derived hormones vary with fat mass, which, of course, may decrease with regular physical activity. However, there does not generally appear to be a large change in the release of these proteins from adipose tissue in response to a bout of exercise.

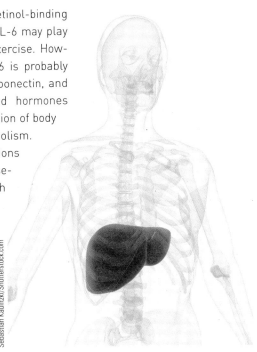

Sebastian Kaulitzki/Shutterstock.com

Regulation of Glucose Release from the Liver

Exercise-induced increments in hepatic **glycogenolysis** and **gluconeogenesis** normally approximate the rate of muscle glucose utilization, and as noted in Chapter 5, euglycemia (normal blood sugar) is maintained within narrow limits. The importance of this coupling process is illustrated by the precipitous decline in circulating glucose, which would result if hepatic glucose production did not increase in synchrony with glucose utilization. Glucose utilization may increase by 3 mg/(kg·min) in response to just moderate-intensity exercise. If the liver did not respond to the exercise stimulus, blood glucose levels would decrease at a rate of approximately 1.5 mg/dl every minute, and overt hypoglycemia would be present in just 30 minutes.

The rate of glycogenolysis in the liver is determined by the degree of activation of the enzyme, phosphorylase *a*. Phosphorylase *a* is activated by phosphorylation of the inactive enzyme, phosphorylase *b*. Phosphorylase *a* is activated by two basic cascade systems. Glucagon, epinephrine, and several other hormones bind to cell surface receptors that activate the enzyme adenylate cyclase. Adenylate cyclase catalyzes formation of cyclic adenosine monophosphate (cAMP), which activates cAMP-dependent protein kinase, ultimately resulting in an increase in phosphorylase *a*. The second cascade system is initiated by binding of norepinephrine and epinephrine to cell surface alpha-adrenergic receptors and involves an increase in cytosolic calcium ions.

In contrast with glycogenolysis in which stimulation is brought about by signaling mechanisms within the liver, gluconeogenesis is regulated by increased gluconeogenic precursor delivery to the liver and mechanisms that lead to gluconeogenic precursor extraction and conversion to glucose within the liver (see Chapter 5). Exercise stimulates each of these three processes. Increased proteolysis in intestine and skeletal muscle, lipolysis in adipose tissue, and glycolysis in muscle increase amino acid, glycerol, lactate, and pyruvate formation. The result is a greater availability

myokines Molecules released from the muscle that serve an endocrine or paracrine function. It is thought that they transmit a signal related to the metabolic, structural, or inflammatory state of the muscle.

adipokines Protein hormones such as adiponectin and leptin that transmit information related to the size of adipocytes. They act in diverse tissues involved in metabolic regulation. Leptin sensitively inhibits brain feeding centers.

glycogenolysis The enzyme-catalyzed conversion of glycogen polymers to glucose monomers.

gluconeogenesis The pathway, primarily in the liver, that converts lactate, pyruvate, glycerol, and amino acids into glucose. It is important in sustaining blood glucose in a fast or during prolonged exercise.

of precursors for glucose formation in the liver. The extraction of gluconeogenic amino acids such as alanine and glutamine are increased in response to exercise because of activation of amino acid transport systems. Gluconeogenesis is stimulated by exercise as a result of increases in key gluconeogenic enzyme activities within the liver (for example, phosphoenolpyruvate carboxykinase [PEPCK], fructose-1,6-bisphosphatase, glucose 6-phosphatase) and decrease in the activity of the glycolytic enzyme phosphofructokinase (PFK). The mechanism for the increase in liver gluconeogenesis may be, at least in part, caused by increases in the transcription of genes that encode key gluconeogenic enzymes.

The relative contributions of hepatic glycogenolysis and gluconeogenesis are determined by the duration and intensity of exercise and the absorptive state of the subject. The initial increment in hepatic glucose production with exercise occurs almost entirely because of an increase in glycogenolysis. Scandinavian investigators concluded, by summing the splanchnic lactate, pyruvate, glycerol, and amino acid uptakes, that gluconeogenesis does not contribute significantly to the increase in the rate that glucose is released from the liver with short- to moderate-duration light, moderate, or heavy exercise. The increase in gluconeogenesis observed with prolonged exercise plays a key role in delaying the depletion of liver and muscle

glycogen by transforming the energy provided by hepatic fat oxidation to formation of new glucose. At the end of a long race such as a marathon, nearly all the glucose released by the liver is gluconeogenic in origin (see Chapter 5).

The importance of exercise intensity as a determinant of **glucose flux** is illustrated by the increased hepatic glucose output that occurs with more strenuous work. The increase in hepatic glucose production per increase in exercise intensity is greater at work rates above the lactate threshold. It is interesting that impairment in oxygen delivery caused by anemia or breathing air with a reduced fraction of inspired O_2 stimulates glucose production and muscle glucose uptake relative to controls even when the energy requirement is not different. The added increment in glucose production that occurs with heavy exercise is due to an increased rate of liver glycogenolysis. Nevertheless, measurements of gluconeogenic precursor uptake indicate that if heavy exercise can be sustained, gluconeogenesis will become important more rapidly because the finite glycogen stores will deplete at a faster rate and hormonal signals will be greater.

Glucagon and insulin are the two major factors that regulate glucose production from the liver. As is the case in the resting state, it is these hormones that are most important in control of glucose production during exercise (Figure 6.5). Insulin

glucose flux The rate at which glucose enters and leaves the blood. It is accelerated by exercise.

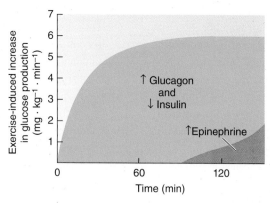

FIGURE 6.5 Contributions of exercise-induced changes in glucagon, insulin, and epinephrine to the increase in glucose production. The exercise-induced increase in glucagon and decrease in insulin are the primary regulators of the accelerated release of glucose from the liver. The increase in glucagon serves to stimulate both gluconeogenesis and glycogenolysis in the liver during exercise. The reduction of insulin during exercise promotes hepatic glycogenolysis. (Wasserman, D. H., and A. D. Cherrington. 1991. Hepatic fuel metabolism during exercise: role and regulation. *Am. J. Physiol.* 260:E811–E824.)

potently suppresses glucose release from the liver. The decline in insulin during exercise reduces this suppressive effect. In the presence of a decrement in insulin, such as is seen with moderate exercise, the liver becomes so sensitive to the effects of glucagon that an increase in glucose production will result with an increase in this hormone that is so small as to be undetectable by conventional assay.

No other biological compound has been shown to approach the potency of glucagon in stimulating glucose production. Although the change in glucagon with exercise may be small or undetectable in peripheral blood, as described earlier, glucagon in the portal vein blood that perfuses the liver is increased dramatically. It has been shown that if one pharmacologically prevents the increase in glucagon during exercise, the increase in glucose production by the liver is attenuated because of impairments in glycogenolysis and gluconeogenesis. If the decline in insulin with exercise is prevented by infusion of insulin, the normal increase in glucagon is only about half as effective as the glycogenolytic response of the liver is inhibited. This is, in fact, what frequently happens in diabetics treated with insulin and why these individuals are subject to hypoglycemia during exercise (see Chapter 68). The increase in glucagon and insulin work in tandem to control most of the increase in glucose released from the liver during moderate exercise. It has also been postulated that IL-6 released from skeletal muscle during exercise plays a small role in stimulating release of glucose from the liver.

There is little or no evidence to suggest that catecholamines directly stimulate glucose release from the liver during exercise. During the latter stages of prolonged exercise, epinephrine may indirectly stimulate gluconeogenesis by enhancing the release of gluconeogenic precursors from muscle and fat. High-intensity exercise is characterized by stresslike norepinephrine and epinephrine concentrations. There appears to be little or no effect of catecholamines on control of glucose release from the liver even under these extreme conditions. Interestingly, glucagon and insulin cannot fully explain the entire increase in glucose production by the liver during high-intensity exercise. It is possible that increased IL-6 or some as yet poorly defined stimulus results in the increased glucose release from the liver during exercise.

Although the acute effects of cortisol are usually considered minimal, they may play a role in the exercise-induced increase in gluconeogenesis. GH is known to increase hepatic gluconeogenesis and may also be a factor during prolonged exercise.

Regulation of Glucose Metabolism by the Working Muscle

Metabolic pathways for converting carbohydrate to ATP were discussed in Chapter 4. In this chapter, we discuss how these processes are regulated during exercise. Metabolism requires that glucose must travel from blood to interstitial space to intracellular space, and then be phosphorylated to glucose 6-phosphate by a hexokinase. Movement of glucose from blood to interstitial space is determined by muscle blood flow, capillary recruitment, and endothelial permeability to glucose. **Sarcolemma GLUT4 concentration** and the intrinsic activity of these transporters determine the capacity for glucose transport from interstitial to intracellular space. The capacity to phosphorylate glucose is determined by the amount of muscle hexokinase, hexokinase compartmentalization within the cell (that is, free cytosolic or associated with mitochondria), and the concentration of hexokinase inhibitors, such as glucose 6-phosphate. Phosphorylation of glucose is irreversible in muscle, so with this reaction, glucose is trapped. Muscle glucose uptake is shown schematically in Figure 6.6 as a three-step process consisting of muscle glucose delivery, membrane transport, and intracellular phosphorylation. Muscle glucose uptake is regulated by and glucose intolerance (such as occurs with diabetes) is due to an alteration in one or more of these three steps.

In sedentary, fasted subjects, muscle receives only 15 to 20 percent of the total cardiac output (see Chapter 7). With exercise, 70 to 85 percent of the cardiac output goes to muscle. This hyperemia increases delivery of glucose (and other nutrients) to muscle. Capillary recruitment is increased by exercise, thereby increasing surface area for diffusion from blood and decreasing diffusion distance to muscle. The increased blood flow and capillary recruitment seen during exercise are dependent on the small molecule, nitric oxide. The activity of the enzyme nitric oxide synthase in endothelial cells is critical to the increase in muscle blood flow with exercise.

> Why are increases in both muscle blood flow and capillary recruitment necessary for effective nutrient exchange?

The most comprehensively studied system involved in muscle glucose uptake is glucose transport. Sarcolemma GLUT4 concentration is low in the basal, fasted state, making the muscle nearly impermeable to glucose. The muscle is a minor consumer of glucose in the basal state but becomes the predominant site of glucose usage during exercise. In response to muscle contraction, GLUT4 is translocated from intracellular storage vesicle to the sarcolemma. This makes the sarcolemma highly permeable to glucose, and it can accommodate the high muscle glucose influx during exercise. Exercise and insulin are the two major stimuli for GLUT4 translocation to the sarcolemma. The cell signaling pathway of contraction-stimulated glucose transport is distinct from that for insulin-stimulated glucose transport. A number of pathways may play a role in contraction-stimulated muscle glucose uptake. Muscle contraction requires cytosolic calcium influx from sarcoplasmic reticulum, which can then act through a number of calcium-sensitive signaling pathways. In particular, there is strong evidence that calcium activation of an enzyme, protein kinase C, may be involved.

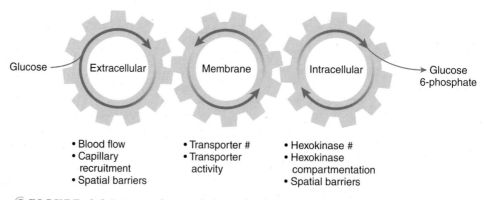

FIGURE 6.6 Integrated control of muscle glucose uptake. Muscle glucose uptake requires three closely coupled steps. Glucose must be delivered to the muscle, transported across the muscle membrane, and phosphorylated inside the muscle cell. Glucose flux during exercise can be regulated at any of these three steps. Listed in the figure are potential regulatory mechanisms. (1998. *Adv. Exp. Med. Biol.* 441:1–16. Review.)

The enzyme **adenosine monophosphate-activated protein kinase (AMPK)** is activated during exercise, presumably as a consequence of direct or indirect effects of adenosine monophosphate (AMP). Activation of AMPK is thought to play a central role in coordination of metabolism in muscles and other tissue. Among other things, pharmacologic activation of AMPK is associated with increased glucose transport in muscle. This has led to the theory that AMPK is key to muscle contraction-induced glucose uptake. Activation of the mitogen-activated protein kinase and nitric oxide synthase pathways may also contribute to contraction-induced muscle glucose uptake. The roles of various signaling pathways during exercise require more investigation to be fully elucidated.

(What is the advantage of having AMP-sensitive regulation of energy metabolism?)

The capacity for glucose phosphorylation, the third step necessary for muscle glucose uptake, may also be increased by exercise. It has been hypothesized that exercise increases glucose phosphorylation capacity by causing the hexokinase II isozyme to bind to mitochondria, where it would have privileged access to ATP, a substrate in the reaction it catalyzes, and be less sensitive to inhibition by glucose 6-phosphate. The latter is notable because changes in glucose 6-phosphate

concentration are a sensitive mechanism by which intracellular metabolism feeds back to regulate glucose uptake by working muscle. Although hexokinase II gene expression is dramatically increased during exercise, time needed for accumulation of the protein is too long for this to be an acute regulatory mechanism.

(What is the regulatory role of hexokinase inhibition by glucose 6-phosphate?)

Once control of muscle glucose delivery, transport, and phosphorylation are considered independently, the issue then becomes how changes in these three steps translate into functional control of muscle glucose uptake (Figure 6.7). This is a difficult problem to address. Studies in animal models have been instrumental in elucidating control of muscle glucose uptake. At rest, the membrane transport step governs the rate of muscle glucose uptake. **GLUT4 translocation** to the sarcolemma is so effectively increased during exercise, however, that the sarcolemma is no longer a major barrier to glucose. Moreover, the marked hyperemia with exercise increases glucose delivery to muscle. The consequence of the dramatic increases in blood flow and sarcolemma glucose permeability is a shift so that glucose phosphorylation becomes the chief barrier to glucose uptake by the muscle.

adenosine monophosphate-activated protein kinase (AMPK) An enzyme that is under covalent and allosteric regulation. It accelerates pathways involved in energy production and decelerates pathways involved in energy consumption.

GLUT4 translocation The movement of the GLUT4 transport protein from intracellular vesicles to the plasma membrane where it facilitates glucose entry into cells. It is increased in response to exercise.

Modulation of Muscle Glucose Uptake during Exercise by the Internal Milieu

The preceding paragraphs describe the basic mechanisms that control muscle glucose uptake during exercise. Hormones and substrates in the circulation can further regulate this response. Following are

some of the means by which circulating factors influence the exercise response.

HOTLINK *Search the Web at sites such as* http://www.nejm.org/doi/full/10.1056/NEJM bkrev39287 *to learn more about hormones and exercise.*

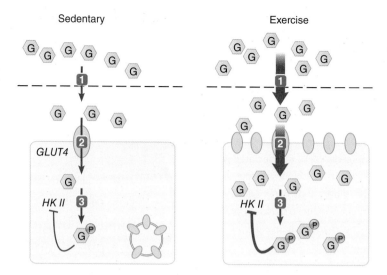

Sedentary

Exercise

FIGURE 6.7 Three steps required for muscle glucose uptake. Exercise makes the muscle membrane more permeable by stimulating the translocation of GLUT4 transport proteins from intracellular storage vesicles to the plasma membrane. The hyperemia that occurs during exercise is important in keeping the supply of glucose to muscle adequate. Feedback inhibition of hexokinase by glucose 6-phosphate serves to regulate the inflow of glucose for metabolism. (© Cengage Learning 2013)

Insulin Sensitivity

Exercise sensitizes the body to the actions of insulin (Figure 6.8). The effects of this increase in insulin action are probably most important in the postprandial state (after eating a meal) and in the intensively treated diabetic state when insulin levels can be higher than those that normally accompany exercise. The primary route of insulin-mediated glucose metabolism at rest is nonoxidative metabolism.

Acute exercise shifts the route of insulin-stimulated glucose disposal so that all the glucose consumed by the muscle is oxidized.

The increased effectiveness of insulin and exercise is due, at least in part, to the increased blood flow to the working muscle and capillary recruitment. These mechanisms increase the exposure of muscle to circulating insulin. Exercise may also increase insulin-stimulated glucose uptake by a mechanism secondary to insulin's suppressive effect on free fatty acid (FFA) availability. The absolute magnitude of the insulin-induced suppression of plasma FFA levels and fat oxidation is greater during exercise. The interaction of circulating FFA concentrations and muscle glucose uptake during exercise is described in the following paragraph (Table 6.1).

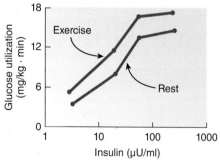

Insulin-stimulated glucose utilization is increased during exercise.

FIGURE 6.8 Exercise increases insulin action during exercise. Glucose utilization during exercise is shown at four different insulin concentrations. Exercise causes a "left shift" in the dose–response curve of glucose utilization to insulin concentration. (© Cengage Learning 2013)

TABLE 6.1 Factors Proposed to Contribute to Increased Insulin Action during Exercise

- Increased blood flow to the working muscle and capillary recruitment increase the exposure of muscle to circulating insulin
- Insulin's suppressive effect on lipolysis increases reliance of muscle on glucose
- Progressive decrease in muscle glycogen

© Cengage Learning 2013

Insulin sensitivity is not only increased during exercise, but also after exercise as well. The increase in sensitivity after exercise is related, in part, to the extent that glycogen has been depleted by exercise. Other factors, however, are clearly involved. The persistent increase in insulin sensitivity can last from hours to days after exercise. This persistence may relate to the exercise duration and intensity, as well as postexercise nutritional factors.

Effect of Circulating Free Fatty Acid Concentrations

Increased FFA concentration can attenuate the increase in muscle glucose uptake during exercise. Sir Phillip Randle and colleagues proposed in 1963 that fats impaired muscle glucose uptake by metabolic feedback resulting from accumulation of metabolic intermediates involved in fat oxidation. This effect of FFA may be prominent in poorly controlled diabetes or during a prolonged fast as FFA levels are increased.

Effect of Adrenergic Stimulation

Glucose uptake by working muscle may also be impaired by adrenergic stimulation. One mechanism for the inhibitory effect of the beta-adrenergic receptor stimulation on muscle glucose uptake is the inhibition of hexokinase secondary to the increase in muscle glucose 6-phosphate resulting from stimulation of muscle glycogenolysis. In addition, metabolic effects caused by catecholamine-stimulated lipolysis may also be a factor.

Effect of Decreased Oxygen Availability

Excessive increments in muscle glucose uptake occur when oxygen availability is limited, such as exercise under anemic conditions, when breathing a hypoxic gas mixture, or at high altitude. This effect occurs even though insulin levels are no higher and catecholamines, which may be antagonistic to glucose uptake, are greater. Hypoxia may stimulate glucose uptake by causing accumulation of AMP and stimulation of AMPK.

insulin sensitivity A variable that defines insulin action. It is increased during and after exercise. It can increase as an adaptive response to long term exercise.

Regulation of Muscle Glycogen Breakdown during Exercise

At the onset of exercise, the enzyme **phosphorylase kinase** catalyzes the phosphorylation of phosphorylase *b*, creating the active form of the enzyme, phosphorylase *a*. The breakdown of muscle glycogen is catalyzed by phosphorylase *a*. Phosphorylase activity is under covalent and allosteric regulation. Moreover, the mass of glycogen in the muscle is a sensitive determinant of carbon flux through this enzyme step. Muscle glycogen breakdown is highest at exercise onset as glycogen phosphorylase *a* is rapidly activated. Rates of glycogenolysis decrease as exercise duration progresses because muscle glycogen mass declines and inhibitors of phosphorylase increase. Glycogen is not only the substrate for phosphorylase, but it is also a positive regulator of the activity of this enzyme. Glycogen is physically associated with phosphorylase, as well as a number of other proteins involved in its metabolism. Glycogen depletion closely parallels the

phosphorylase kinase A serine-/threonine-specific protein kinase that activates glycogen phosphorylase to degrade glycogen.

People with McArdle disease have an inborn deficiency of muscle phosphorylase. How might the metabolic response to exercise be affected by this disorder?

fiber type recruitment. Thus, during light to moderate exercise in which work is accomplished primarily by type I fibers, glycogen depletion will be observed almost exclusively in these type muscle fibers. Type II fibers are recruited with increased exercise intensity and show glycogen depletion at higher work intensities or as exhaustion from prolonged exercise is approached.

It is thought that the initial activation of phosphorylase kinase occurs because of increased cytosolic calcium and binding of epinephrine to the beta-adrenergic receptors on the cell surface. Beta-adrenergic receptor activation stimulates the formation of cAMP, which activates phosphorylase a. Phosphorylase a activity is further regulated by allosteric modifiers that match

glycogen breakdown to energy needs. AMP, adenosine diphosphate (ADP), and inorganic phosphate reflect the energy state of the cell so that increases in their concentrations signal the need for greater fuel metabolism. These by-products of energy metabolism increase phosphorylase a activity and glycogen breakdown. The result is that glucose 6-phosphate is formed, which is then able to enter the glycolytic pathway providing energy for the formation of ATP. Decreased muscle pH, which may occur because of anaerobic glycolysis, inhibits phosphorylase activity, decreasing glycogen breakdown and the availability of substrate for continued flux through the glycolytic pathway.

Regulation of Glycolytic Flux and Carbohydrate Oxidation in Working Muscle

Muscle glucose uptake and glycogen breakdown lead to the formation of glucose 6-phosphate. Because muscle lacks the ability to remove inorganic phosphate from this molecule and produce free glucose, glucose 6-phosphate is trapped in the cell. In the hormonal and intracellular milieu of exercise, glucose 6-phosphate is metabolized in the glycolytic pathway, resulting in formation of pyruvate and production of the reduced form of nicotinamide adenine dinucleotide (NADH) and ATP. This was discussed in detail in Chapter 4. It is important to recognize that flux through the muscle glycolytic pathway is determined by the amount of glucose 6-phosphate and the activity of the enzyme PFK. Glucose 6-phosphate is made more available during exercise because of increased glucose uptake and glycogen breakdown. As is the case with phosphorylase, accumulation of AMP, ADP, calcium, and inorganic phosphate will increase PFK activity. The result of this regulation is an increase in PFK activity and glycolytic flux geared to match the

metabolic demands of muscle. A decrease in pH, such as that which can occur with heavy exercise, will decrease the activity of this enzyme. The pyruvate formed by glycolysis is, in the presence of adequate oxygen supply, metabolized by pyruvate dehydrogenase to acetyl-coenzyme A (CoA) in the mitochondria. During exercise, the major activators of this enzyme are increased calcium and ADP. Pyruvate dehydrogenase is also stimulated by reductions in NADH and acetyl-CoA. Acetyl-CoA is further oxidized in the tricarboxylic acid cycle to CO_2. Reducing equivalents formed in the tricarboxylic acid

> How does allosteric regulation increase glycolytic flux to match the need for energy?

cycle are used in the formation of ATP in the electron transport chain (see Chapter 4).

Heavy exercise is characterized by high rates of glycolytic NADH production that is not quantitatively matched by mitochondrial NADH oxidation. The consequence is that NADH accumulates in the muscle cytosol and the oxidized form of nicotinamide adenine dinucleotide (NAD), an essential cofactor for reactions of glycolysis, declines. Whether it is hypoxia or some other characteristic of heavy exercise that results in the more reduced cytosol (that is, NADH/NAD) is an area of longstanding debate. Certainly any maneuver that impairs O_2 delivery to working muscle will increase NADH/NAD. This causes the equilibrium between pyruvate and lactate to shift so that the lactate is increased in muscle and blood with little or no increase in pyruvate. The enzyme lactate dehydrogenase catalyzes the equilibrium reaction between lactate and pyruvate. Indeed, a hallmark of heavy exercise is an increase in the ratio of lactate to pyruvate. The work rate at which the lactate-to-pyruvate ratio increases is referred to as the anaerobic threshold or the lactate threshold. Scientists have argued whether the muscle is indeed "anaerobic" at this work rate. What is certain is that NADH is not being adequately oxidized to NAD by aerobic means and there is a greater oxidation to NAD by anaerobic means. The work rate at which lactate increases disproportionately to pyruvate is about 50 percent of a person's maximum oxygen uptake.

Ingested Carbohydrates as a Fuel

The carbohydrate stores of the body are finite, and in the fasted state, their depletion represents one factor that is limiting for prolonged exercise. The limitations posed by the exhaustible carbohydrate stores of the body can be circumvented to some extent by carbohydrate ingestion. The important role carbohydrate ingestion can play in exercise tolerance was demonstrated by Dill and colleagues in 1932, when they showed that intermittent glucose feeding (20 grams every hour) increased endurance time in the exercising dog by more than threefold. Since these experiments were conducted, numerous experiments have demonstrated the potential importance of glucose ingestion in exercising humans.

The mechanism by which carbohydrate ingestion delays fatigue is related to an increased availability of glucose to the working muscle and prevention of the effects of a decline in blood glucose. The development of just moderate hypoglycemia may contribute to glycogen depletion by accentuating the exercise-induced increases in glucagon and catecholamines. These hormonal changes, in turn, accelerate glycogen breakdown. The effectiveness with which carbohydrate feeding maintains glucose availability to the working muscle, preventing a decline in glucose, will depend on the amount and form of ingested glucose. Moreover, the timing of glucose ingestion with respect to exercise is a key factor. Finally, duration and intensity of exercise will, to a large extent, determine the contribution of ingested glucose to exercise metabolism.

Factors That Determine Gastrointestinal Absorption of Carbohydrate

Because exercise causes a reduction in gut blood flow, it was thought that ingested glucose might not be absorbed effectively. In fact, it seems that ingested glucose is readily available during submaximal exercise. The effectiveness with which ingested glucose enters the blood is determined, in part, by the time ingested glucose spends in the gastrointestinal tract or its "transit time." The longer the transit time is, the greater the time that is available for gastrointestinal absorption. Exercise causes an increase in intestinal transit time, which may effectively counterbalance the reduction in blood flow to the gut, allowing efficient nutrient absorption.

The precise metabolic availability of ingested carbohydrate will depend on many factors related to the composition and quantity of carbohydrate. In addition, exercise parameters (that is, work rate, duration, modality) will also be important determinants of how readily ingested glucose

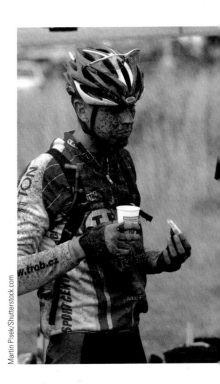

Martin Písek/Shutterstock.com

Sucrose A disaccharide comprised of glucose and fructose.

will be made available. During very light rates of exercise, there is probably little difficulty in delivering adequate amounts of ingested glucose to the working muscle. As exercise intensity increases and glucose oxidation by the working muscle increases, it may no longer be possible to absorb adequate amounts of ingested glucose. As exercise intensity increases to about 50 percent of the maximum oxygen uptake, the oxidation of ingested glucose increases proportionally. Muscle carbohydrate oxidation continues to increase with further increases in exercise intensity; however, oxidation of ingested glucose does not increase further because the rate that glucose is made available from the gastrointestinal tract has become limiting.

One approach for increasing the amount of carbohydrate that enters the blood from the gut is simply to increase the amount of ingested glucose. With this approach, the fraction of the ingested glucose that is made available for metabolism is actually decreased. The decreased percentage of ingested glucose that is oxidized when larger quantities of glucose are consumed suggests that one or more steps involved in the intestinal absorption of glucose have become saturated. This saturation can be circumvented and more carbohydrates can be made available by using different sugar types. A greater percentage of ingested sugar is oxidized during exercise if it is given as a combination of glucose and fructose rather than in one form or the other. It is important to recognize that carbohydrate ingestion may result, in some instances, in a paradoxical decrease in plasma glucose, which is counterproductive for work performance. This typically will occur if glucose ingestion precedes exercise by an interval (about 45 minutes) that causes exercise to coincide with peak postprandial insulin concentrations.

Ingestion of glucose polymers has been frequently employed during exercise. The basis for consuming this form of sugar is that the osmolarity of the ingested solution will be reduced, thereby decreasing the movement of water and electrolytes into the gastrointestinal tract. Once in the small intestine, the glucose polymers are rapidly hydrolyzed to free glucose and absorbed. **Sucrose** ingestion has been used during exercise with similar effectiveness to ingested glucose. This is not surprising because the hydrolysis of this disaccharide leads to the entry of glucose into the circulation.

HOTLINK *See Chapter 12 for more information about the appropriate concentration of carbohydrate recommended for consumption when using commercially available sports drinks to enhance peak athletic performance.*

Effect of Carbohydrate Ingestion on Body Fuel Stores

Carbohydrate ingestion is accompanied by hormonal and metabolic changes that impact on the fuel supply to the working muscle. Carbohydrate ingestion usually slows the rate of decline of circulating glucose that generally occurs with prolonged exercise or leads to an overt increase in circulating glucose. At least two important endocrine changes accompany the increase in glucose availability. The exercise-induced decline in insulin and increase in glucagon are attenuated or eliminated altogether. The higher insulin level will suppress both the mobilization of FFA from adipose tissue and glucose from the liver, whereas a reduction in glucagon will reduce the latter.

Insulin suppresses muscle glycogen breakdown. However, multiple signals act on the working muscle (for example, epinephrine or calcium), and the antiglycogenolytic effects of insulin more often than not are counterbalanced by these. The decreased availability of circulating FFA with glucose ingestion may require continued utilization of muscle glycogen that, in some cases, may offset the effects of insulin and glucose on muscle glycogen breakdown.

Glucose ingestion sensitively reduces liver glycogen breakdown exercise. Furthermore, it inhibits gluconeogenesis during prolonged exercise. The potent effect of carbohydrate ingestion at the liver

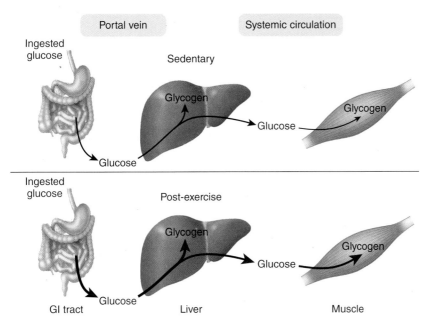

Portal vein   Systemic circulation

Ingested glucose

Sedentary

Glycogen

Glucose

Glycogen

Glucose

Ingested glucose

Post-exercise

Glycogen

Glucose

Glycogen

GI tract   Glucose   Liver   Muscle

● **FIGURE 6.9 Glycogen storage of ingested glucose is increased following exercise.** When glucose is ingested, it exits the gut and is extracted mainly by the liver and skeletal muscle. After exercise, the rate of glucose absorption from the intestine and the uptake of glucose by the liver and muscle are accelerated. The fate of glucose taken up by the liver and muscle after exercise is deposition as glycogen. GI, gastrointestinal. (© Cengage Learning 2013)

is probably mediated, in large part, by the attenuated glucagon response to exercise.

Liver and muscle glucose uptake after ingestion of carbohydrate are both increased after exercise (Figure 6.9). Insulin sensitivity is increased after exercise. The improved ability of the liver and muscle to extract glucose from the blood is due, in part, to this increase in insulin sensitivity. The glucose taken up by the liver, like the glucose taken up by muscle, is largely used to replenish tissue glycogen stores. Glycogen replenishment is facilitated after exercise by an increased capacity for intestinal glucose absorption of ingested glucose.

(How does prior exercise affect the disposition of a mixed meal?)

Free Fatty Acid Mobilization from Adipose Tissue

Free fatty acid (FFA) mobilization from adipose tissue is determined by the activities of two opposing nonequilibrium reactions. These two reactions form a substrate cycle, the rate of which depends on the rate that triglycerides are hydrolyzed to glycerol and FFAs (lipolysis) and the rate at which FFAs are bound to glycerol 3-phosphate by re-**esterification**. Substrate cycling is a mechanism used to cause large changes in substrate flux without extreme activation or inactivation of any one reaction. The function of this substrate cycle during exercise is to amplify the rate that FFAs are mobilized from adipose tissue (Figure 6.10). A substrate cycle formed by two opposing chemical reactions is much like a balance. When a weight is on one end of a balance

esterification The formation of an ester bond between glycerol and a fatty acid. Three ester bonds link fatty acids to the glycerol backbone in triglyceride molecules.

Free Fatty Acid Mobilization from Adipose Tissue **163**

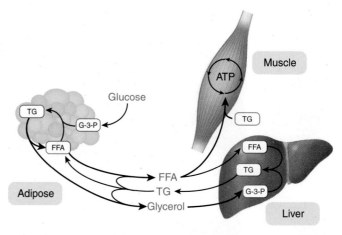

FIGURE 6.10 Substrate cycling between lipolysis and esterification of FFA to glycerol-3-phospate. The availability of free fatty acids (FFA) in blood for uptake by working muscle is largely determined by re-esterification in liver and adipose tissue to triglycerides (TG) and lipolysis of triglycerides in adipose tissue. ATP, adenosine triphosphate; G-3-P, glycerol 3-phoshpate. (© Cengage Learning 2013)

unopposed, force is required to shift the balance. Consider the sensitivity of the balance when objects of equal weight oppose each other on the same balance. Movement of the arm of the balance is considerably more sensitive to the same force under this condition. Figure 6.11 is a schematic of the triglyceride-FFA substrate cycles.

In response to exercise, both limbs of the substrate cycle, lipolysis and re-esterification, are modified in such a way as to increase the flux of FFAs into the blood. The stimulation of lipolysis, however, is considerably more important. The intracellular events that lead to an increase in lipolysis begin with the formation of cAMP. cAMP, in turn, activates a protein kinase that, in turn, activates the enzyme, **hormone-sensitive lipase (HSL)**. HSL catalyzes the hydrolysis of triglycerides to three FFA molecules and one glycerol molecule. This reaction is the chief enzyme control site and, therefore, is of major importance in lipolysis. These reactions are stimulated by catecholamines and inhibited by insulin after interaction with their respective cell surface receptors. Cellular control of lipolysis is illustrated in Figure 6.12. Re-esterification requires the activation of FFAs to acyl-CoA by the enzyme acyl-CoA synthetase and the presence of glycerol 3-phosphate. One aspect of the latter requirement is particularly notable. The adipocyte lacks the enzyme glycerokinase that phosphorylates glycerol and,

as a result, cannot use glycerol released by the complete lipolysis of triglycerides. Glycerol 3-phosphate must instead be derived from glycolysis. NEFA re-esterification in the adipocyte in resting, fasting subjects is

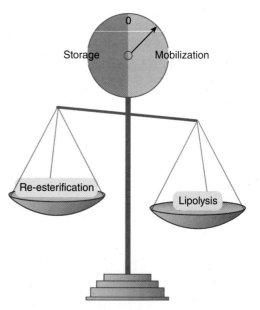

FIGURE 6.11 Exercise shifts the delicate balance of re-esterification and lipolysis so that more FFA are mobilization. Re-esterification and lipolysis form a substrate cycle that allows for sensitive regulation of triglyceride storage and mobilization. Re-esterification requires the activation of fatty acids to acyl-CoA by the enzyme acyl-CoA synthetase and the presence of glycerol 3-phoshpate. Lipolysis is catalyzed by a hormone-sensitive lipase. During exercise in the fasted state, the balance of re-esterification and lipolysis is weighted to lipolysis. (© Cengage Learning 2013)

hormone-sensitive lipase (HSL)
An intracellular neutral lipase that is capable of hydrolyzing a variety of esters.

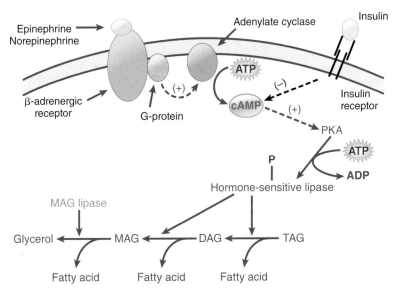

F I G U R E **6.12** **Signaling pathways for activation of hormone-sensitive lipase.** Hormone-sensitive lipase (HSL) catalyzes the breakdown of triglycerides. Epinephrine (or norepinephrine) binds its receptor and, via a G-protein coupled mechanism, leads to the activation of adenylate cyclase. The resultant increase in cyclic adenosine monophosphate (cAMP) activates protein kinase A (PKA), which then phosphorylates and activates HSL. Hormone-sensitive lipase hydrolyzes fatty acids from triacylglycerols (TAG) and diacylglycerols (DAG). The final fatty acid is released from monoacylglycerols (MAG) through the action of monoacylglycerol lipase, an enzyme active in the absence of hormonal stimulation. Activation of the insulin receptor inhibits this pathway, and activation of AMP-dependent protein kinase activates it. ATP, adenosine triphosphate. (© Cengage Learning 2013)

about 20 percent of lipolysis. Thus, there is net flow of FFAs out of the adipocyte. During moderate exercise, re-esterification is reduced to about 10 percent of the lipolytic rate. As a result of this reduction in the ratio of re-esterification to lipolysis, more FFAs leave the cell and are available for metabolism in other tissues, primarily working muscle.

Lipolytic rate and FFA mobilization, as determined by the increase in blood glycerol levels and isotopic techniques, increase with the onset of moderate-intensity exercise. Arterial FFA levels, however, increase gradually. The slow increase in plasma FFA levels reflects an increase in its metabolism by the working muscle. The two main regulators of lipolysis are the stimulatory effects of catecholamines and the inhibitory effects of insulin. The effects of the catecholamines are mediated by beta-adrenergic receptors, and it appears that norepinephrine derived from sympathetic nerves is more important than circulating epinephrine from the adrenal medulla. The mechanism by which norepinephrine stimulates lipolysis is related not

only to an increase in sympathetic nerve activity, but also to an increased effectiveness of beta-adrenergic stimulation. Insulin secretion from the pancreatic beta cells is inhibited in response to exercise. Circulating insulin concentrations decrease and its suppressive effect on adipose tissue FFA release is diminished, resulting in increased mobilization of FFAs. For individuals who exercise after eating a meal rich in glucose or for diabetic patients treated with insulin (see Chapter 6B), the decline in insulin that normally occurs with exercise may be absent. In these cases, the increase in lipolysis and the increase in blood FFAs that normally occur with exercise are reduced and may, in some instances, be completely alleviated.

The role of FFA mobilization during high-intensity exercise is minor. Despite the increased adrenergic drive that is present during high-intensity work, the arterial FFA levels. This is paradoxical in light of the extremely large increase in catecholamine concentrations present during exercise. It has been proposed that the increase in blood lactate that occurs with heavy exercise may serve to reduce blood FFA availability because it is an inhibitor of HSL activity and, as a precursor for glycerol 3-phosphate, promotes re-esterification in adipocytes. It has also been postulated that a reduction in adipose tissue blood flow may contribute to the reduction in circulating FFA levels during exercise.

Lipolysis is not regulated homogenously in all human adipose tissue. Adipose tissue in the femoral and gluteal regions, for example, is less lipolytically active than abdominal adipose tissue. Intra-abdominal depots seem particularly sensitive to lipolytic stimuli and are relatively insensitive to insulin. There also appears to be a significant gender difference in the lipolytic response to exercise. This is evident by a twofold greater release of glycerol from abdominal adipose tissue of women compared with men. The ability to mobilize FFAs during exercise may also be affected by the presence of obesity. For example, women characterized by upper body obesity have a 50 percent reduction in the exercise-induced increase in FFA availability in comparison with women with lower body obesity.

Free Fatty Acid Transport in the Plasma

The means by which fatty acid release is controlled within adipose tissue was discussed in the previous section. How are fatty acids released from adipose tissue transported in the blood? Because of their insolubility in aqueous mediums, fatty acids are transported in the blood bound to **albumin**. Skeletal muscle and heart are the main destinations for fatty acids during exercise. The liver extracts more fatty acids during exercise as well. As described later in this chapter, these fatty acids are oxidized or used in the liver for the synthesis of triglycerides. Triglycerides synthesized in the liver are exported to other tissues in association with proteins, which together with fats form **lipoproteins**. **Chylomicrons** are lipoproteins assembled mainly in the intestinal mucosa from ingested fats.

Lipoproteins are not a significant source of fuel for the working muscle in postabsorptive subjects (supplying <10 percent of the total energy cost). Chylomicrons have a high turnover rate and may obtain levels, in response to a high-fat meal, that permit them to be a significant fuel for working muscle. Triglycerides associated with lipoproteins are hydrolyzed by **lipoprotein lipases** located in the vascular endothelium, making fatty acids available to the tissues they vascularize. Skeletal muscle vasculature is rich in lipoprotein lipase, with vessels associated with oxidative fibers containing more of the enzyme than the nonoxidative, glycolytic fibers.

Fat Metabolism by the Liver: Oxidation and Triglyceride Synthesis

The liver oxidizes FFAs or incorporates them into triglycerides. The pathways involved can be estimated by the dynamics of circulating ketone bodies and lipoproteins, respectively. In fasting, healthy individuals, neither fate provides appreciable amounts of fuel to the working muscle directly. As explained later, the regulation of hepatic fatty acid oxidation and triglyceride synthesis can, nevertheless, have important effects on muscle fuel metabolism by indirect mechanisms.

Liver Fat Oxidation

Ketone bodies (acetone, acetoacetate, and beta-hydroxybutyrate) are produced in the liver and are a reflection of liver fat oxidation. Ketone body formation is a process that involves beta-oxidation of fatty acids with the generation of acetyl-CoA and the synthesis of acetoacetate from two acetyl-CoA molecules. Acetoacetate remains as such, is decarboxylated to acetone, or is reduced to beta-hydroxybutyrate. Regulation of **ketogenesis** can be exerted through effects on the mobilization of FFAs from adipose tissue and delivery to the liver, the extraction of FFAs by the liver, and the conversion of FFAs to ketone bodies within the

albumin The predominant protein in plasma. It maintains osmotic pressure gradient between plasma and the interstitial space. It plays an important role in transport of fatty acids, cations, hormones, and other molecules in the blood.

lipoproteins These are diverse in the body. Important species are assembled from proteins and fat in the liver and used to transport lipids, such as triglycerides and cholesterol, in the blood. Low-density lipoproteins, intermediate-density lipoproteins, and high-density lipoproteins are important lipoproteins in the blood.

chylomicrons Lipoproteins assembled from dietary fat in the intestinal mucosa.

lipoprotein lipase A water soluble enzyme that hydrolyzes triglycerides in lipoproteins, such as those found in chylomicrons and very low-density lipoproteins (VLDL), into two free fatty acids and one monoacylglycerol molecule.

ketogenesis The process by which ketone bodies are produced as a result of fatty acid breakdown in the liver.

liver. Ketogenesis is increased with prolonged exercise because of stimulation of each of these processes. The rates that the liver releases ketone bodies are quantitatively unimportant as a fuel for the working muscle. The significance of ketogenesis is that it is a marker of fat oxidation, a key pathway in providing energy to fuel gluconeogenesis. Increasing FFA availability spares liver glycogen by providing the energy that allows gluconeogenesis to occur.

Any hormone or neurotransmitter that regulates FFA mobilization, hepatic FFA extraction, or intrahepatic fat oxidation may play a role in the regulation of ketogenesis during exercise. Each of these processes required for gluconeogenesis is increased by exercise. Any factor that stimulates FFA mobilization, such as the decline in insulin and the beta-adrenergic effects of the catecholamines, may stimulate ketogenesis. FFA is taken up at a greater rate by the liver during exercise, even at the same rate of FFA delivery to the liver. Thus, some aspect of the exercise response stimulates the extraction of FFAs by the liver. The increased FFA extraction may be because of a direct transport effect or a primary increase in intrahepatic fat oxidation, which effectively "pulls" FFAs into the cell. The increase in blood glucagon that occurs with prolonged exercise stimulates fat oxidation and activates ketogenic enzymes. The AMPK signaling pathway has been implicated as a pivotal step in control of fat oxidation in the liver, as it is in the muscle. AMPK activation in the liver is increased by exercise. The role of AMPK in muscle fatty acid oxidation is described in a following section.

Triglyceride Synthesis

Earlier in this chapter, substrate cycling between triglycerides and FFAs in the adipocyte was discussed. Substrate cycling also occurs at the interorgan level as FFAs mobilized from adipose tissue are released, transported to and extracted by the liver, synthesized into triglyceride, and incorporated into lipoprotein. The fatty acids from these triglycerides will be hydrolyzed and metabolized in various tissues. If these fatty acids form triglycerides in adipose tissue, a substrate cycle will exist. During exercise, modification of this interorgan substrate cycle may be significant in amplifying the rate that FFAs are made available to the working muscle. It has been estimated that about 60 percent of the FFA released from adipose tissue is re-esterified by the liver in resting humans, whereas only about 20 percent is re-esterified during exercise. Inhibition of re-esterification in liver and adipose tissue make more FFAs available to the working muscle. By doing so, it is an important mechanism for increasing total fat oxidation.

Regulation of Muscle Fatty Acid Metabolism

The lipophilic microenvironment of the plasma membrane would seem to allow for efficient FFA passage. Up until recent years, the prevailing view was that movement of FFA into cells occurs by passive diffusion alone, with the rate of diffusion determined by the vascular delivery of FFA. The vascular FFA delivery rate is determined by the circulating FFA concentration and muscle blood flow. There is now compelling evidence, however, that a substantial component of FFA flux across the plasma membrane is protein mediated. Three proteins have been identified as aiding in FFA transport across the plasma membrane: plasma membrane **fatty acid binding protein** (FABPpm), fatty acid translocase (FAT, also called CD36), and the fatty acid transport protein (FATP). The abundance of these proteins is higher in oxidative muscle fibers compared with nonoxidative muscle fibers. The increased capacity for membrane transport matches the higher mitochondrial content of oxidative fibers and the greater ability of oxidative fibers to undertake fatty acid metabolism. It appears that FAT, at least, is a site of regulation during exercise. This protein

fatty acid binding protein A family of carrier proteins for fatty acids and other lipophilic substances. These proteins facilitate the transfer of fatty acids between extracellular space to and within intracellular compartments.

is translocated from an intracellular pool to the plasma membrane in response to muscle contractions and, by doing so, increases the capacity of muscle to extract FFAs.

The question is why should fatty acids, which can almost instantaneously cross the plasma membrane, have such a seemingly elegant transport system for getting inside the membrane? It may be that the membranous proteins are not so important to the actual transport of FFA across the membrane so much as they are critical for coupling to reactions on the inner membrane surface. FFAs that cross the membrane by diffusion must still contend with the aqueous environment they face inside the cell. It may be that these transport proteins facilitate coupling of FFAs to proteins that will allow for efficient FFA mobility and metabolism in the aqueous intracellular compartment.

Once inside the cell, fatty acids are bound to the cytosolic fatty acid binding protein (FABPc) with which they are shuttled to sites of storage or metabolism. An enzyme catalyzes the addition of CoA to the FABPc-bound FFA, priming it for subsequent reactions. The fatty acid bound to CoA is transferred to an acyl-CoA binding protein to form a complex that is a substrate for triglyceride storage or energy production in oxidative pathways described in Chapter 4.

The factors that regulate fatty acid membrane and intracellular transport during exercise are summarized in Figure 6.13. Much of the cellular processes involved remain to be worked out. It is notable that the activation of the enzyme, AMPK, by AMPK kinase and allosteric modifiers (e.g., AMP), stimulates a number of the pathways involved in energy production during exercise, including fatty acid uptake and oxidation. AMPK is increased in the cells of the working muscle. The enzyme acetyl-CoA carboxylase (ACC) stimulates fatty acid synthesis. Malonyl-CoA is formed in the reaction catalyzed by ACC. Malonyl-CoA inhibits CPT I. AMPK phosphorylates and thereby deactivates ACC, leading to decreased malonyl-CoA production and increased acetyl-CoA oxidation in the TCA cycle. Inhibition of ACC, thereby, decreases malonyl-CoA, which releases the inhibition of CPT I. The resulting increase in CPT I activity increases binding of fatty acids to carnitine

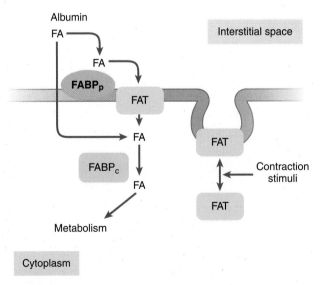

⊙ **FIGURE 6.13 Fatty acid flux into the sarcoplasm.** Fatty acids enter cells by diffusion across the membrane lipid bilayer, or they can be transported across the cell membrane by plasma fatty acid binding protein (FABPp), fatty acid transport protein (FATP), and CD36/fatty acid translocase (FAT). Whereas FABPp and FATP seem to reside in the cell membrane, CD36 is translocated to the membrane from intracellular storage vesicle. Translocation is regulated by adenosine monophosphate kinase (AMPK), insulin, and, perhaps calcium. Contraction stimulates translocation possibly through AMPK or calcium-dependent mechanisms. Fatty acids are shuttled in the cell in conjunction with cytosolic fatty acid binding protein (FABPc). (© Cengage Learning 2013)

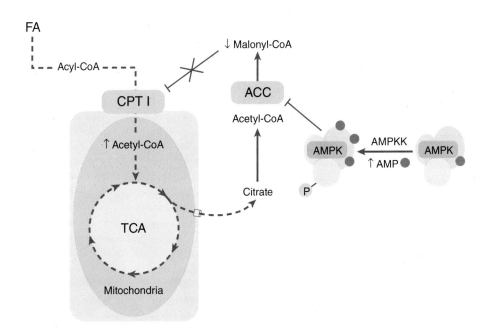

● **F I G U R E** **6.14** **Proposed role of AMPK in the oxidation of fatty acids during exercise.** Activation of AMPK by one or more postulated AMPK protein kinases AMPKK phosphorylates and thereby deactivates acetyl-CoA carboxylase (ACC). AMP binding promotes phosphorylation and inhibits dephosphorylation of AMPK. AMPK activation leads to a decrease in the formation of malonyl-CoA. Malonyl Co-A inhibits CPT I. The reduction in malonyl-CoA decreases its inhibitory effect on CPT I. The resulting increase in CPT I activity increases binding of fatty acids to carnitine and transport into mitochondria where they are oxidized. AMP is depicted by red circles.

and transport into mitochondria where they are oxidized (Figure 6.14). Activation of AMPK also stimulates the utilization of muscle glycogen and glucose. It may be that AMPK is a key hub that is sensitive to and integrates metabolic needs including muscle FFA uptake and metabolism.

Triglycerides are stored in muscle and can be a minor substrate for energy metabolism during exercise, particularly in oxidative muscle fibers. Muscle triglyceride stores may be a quantitatively more important substrate in endurance-trained athletes, because they are markedly increased in these individuals.

Summary of Regulation of Fat Metabolism during Exercise

Fat metabolism during exercise occurs at multiple sites. Signals that control mobilization of triglyceride stores, primarily from adipose tissue, are turned on by activation of an HSL. We learned that circulating glucose concentration is regulated in healthy subjects within narrow limits. Blood FFA concentration is under no such constraints because it can increase by several-fold during

prolonged exercise. The challenge for FFA transport is that its immiscible nature requires protein chaperones to transport them through the blood, facilitate transport across cell membranes, and shuttle them to sites of utilization. Muscle fat oxidation is a quantitatively important pathway for energy production during exercise, particularly exercise of extended duration.

Glucagon: A Well-Kept Secretion

Insulin is a hormone secreted from the beta cells of the islets of Langerhans in the endocrine pancreas. Insulin potently reduces blood glucose by inhibiting the rate that glucose is released from the liver and increasing the rate that glucose is taken up by muscle, liver, and adipose tissue. Insulin deficiency causes diabetes. When insulin was isolated from pancreatic extracts in 1921, it was celebrated as a great medical breakthrough. Indeed, it was one of the great milestones in twentieth-century medicine. Far less attention was given to a potent but transient hyperglycemic effect caused by those same extracts that was observed before the more persistent glucose-reducing effect of insulin. A "hyperglycemic factor" was later isolated, but with considerably less fanfare. This factor was appropriately named *glucagon,* a contraction of the words "glucose" and "agonist."

Little was known about the role of glucagon in health and disease until sensitive immunoassays for protein measurements were developed and applied to glucagon in the 1960s. The response of circulating glucagon to a variety of physiologic conditions, including exercise, was characterized in the years that followed. Defining a functional role for glucagon still required that obstacles be overcome. This was particularly true for the dynamic role of glucagon during exercise.

With the development of pharmacologic tools to control glucagon concentrations and isotopic methods to measure glucose release from the liver, a definitive and potent role for glucagon during exercise has become evident. Glucagon, on either a molar or weight basis, is considerably more potent than any other endogenous compound in stimulating the release of glucose from the liver. Moreover, in the presence of a small decrement in insulin, such as that seen during exercise, the liver becomes so sensitive to the effects of glucagon that an increase in glucose production is clear in the presence of minimal, nearly immeasurable increases in this hormone in peripheral blood.

Glucagon and its islet counterpart insulin are the yin and yang of glucose homeostasis. A loss of function of either one of these hormones has repercussions. The presence of insulin guards against hyperglycemia, and glucagon protects against hypoglycemia. Hypoglycemia in the short term is the far more dangerous condition, and glucagon is the most potent protector against hypoglycemia. Insulin has justifiably received much attention from scientists because of its role in health and diabetes. Although glucagon receives far less attention than its partner from the pancreas, it too is vital to glucose metabolism and plays an important role in sustaining glucose flux during exercise.

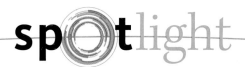

spotlight

An Expert in Immunology, Endocrinology, and Exercise Metabolism: Bente Klarlund Pedersen, M.D., D.Sc.

Chapter 5 highlighted the remarkable contributions of the Danish scientific community. This tradition is well served by the contributions of Dr. Bente Klarlund Pedersen. Pedersen received her M.D. in Copenhagen in 1983. She is currently Professor of Integrative Medicine and a specialist in infectious diseases and internal medicine. She was named the Founding Director of the Danish National Research Foundation's Centre of Inflammation and Metabolism in 2005. The Centre of Inflammation and Metabolism has provided a unique discovery platform for immunology, endocrinology, and the muscle. In the early 1990s, Pedersen began the first systematic studies of exercise as a tool to better understand the immune system. With this began the field of "exercise immunology." It was while looking for a mechanistic explanation for exercise-induced immune changes that she identified an "exercise factor" being released from the contracting skeletal muscle. She identified that the "exercise factor" was interleukin-6 (IL-6). Since then she has gone on to define a number of novel proteins released by working muscle

and termed the expression myokines to describe them. Dr. Pedersen delineated the subcellular production of IL-6 in the skeletal muscle, the secretion of IL-6 from skeletal muscle, and how IL-6 affects other organs. Her research on IL-6 established that skeletal muscle, in addition to causing the mechanics of movement, is an endocrine organ, which transmits regulatory proteins through the circulation. Pedersen's research shows that IL-6 is not simply a proinflammatory cytokine, as had been previously thought. Her work has shown that muscle-derived IL-6 possesses important metabolic properties and has anti-inflammatory effects as well.

Pedersen has advanced the field of exercise physiology in ways that would have never been projected. She has received numerous honors for her research. Her contributions to exercise physiology extend well beyond the laboratory. Dr. Pedersen has been extremely active in promoting general health through exercise. She has served as president for the National Council for Public Health in Denmark.

in*Practice*

Hormonal Regulation of Metabolism during Exercise

The following section provides practical examples of how the regulation of carbohydrate and exercise are related to your area of interest (review the future career table from Chapter 1).

Health/Fitness: By understanding carbohydrate regulation, you can help clients understand how hormones are influenced by regular participation in exercise. The regulation of hormones such as insulin, glucagon, catecholamines, growth hormone, thyroid hormone, adrenocorticotropic hormone, beta-endorphin, gastrointestinal hormones, renin, gonadal hormone levels, and others are all impacted

by acute and chronic bouts of exercise. The up-regulation (increase) of hormones improves skeletal muscle metabolism of carbohydrate and is important in the prevention and treatment of type 2 diabetes.

Medicine: By understanding carbohydrate regulation, physicians and other healthcare professionals can help patients who are metabolically challenged understand how their dietary intake and caloric expenditure behaviors can influence their resting metabolic rate. For example, metabolic studies can be in clinical settings using indirect calorimetry via pulmonary gas exchange techniques that can determine the effects of various interventions on carbohydrate metabolism and regulation (review Chapter 5). This can be achieved by comparing the volume of carbon dioxide produced relative to the amount of oxygen consumed that provides a respiratory exchange ratio between 0.7 and 1.00. A value of 0.7 indicates that fat is primarily being metabolized, whereas a value of 1.00 indicates carbohydrate is the primary fuel of choice. Normally, we use fat and carbohydrates, and the regulation of these fuels is significantly affected by regular bouts of exercise.

Athletic Performance: It is important for coaches to understand carbohydrate regulation during exercise to help their athletes prevent glycogen depletion and hypoglycemia. For example, a trained endurance runner can store approximately 2,000 kilocalories (kcal) energy in the form of carbohydrate (glucose/glycogen). If one assumes that the runner burns about 100 kcal energy per mile run, we could predict that the runner will deplete their carbohydrate stores or "hit the wall/bonk" at approximately the 20-mile mark. This is indeed what happens to many inexperienced marathon runners who do not adjust for carbohydrate regulation during exercise (see carbohydrate-loading example in Chapter 5 for more details).

Rehabilitation: By understanding carbohydrate regulation, physical therapists, athletic trainers, and other healthcare professionals can help clients with type 2 diabetes understand why regular participation in exercise can help control their insulin resistance. Insulin resistance refers to the inability of the beta cells to respond to insulin and, therefore, blood glucose levels remain increased. As increased insulin resistance occurs, it can also cause an up-regulation of sympathetic nervous activity (catecholamines) that may contribute to the development of hypertension in the client as well. Insulin resistance is associated with an increased risk for the development of atherosclerosis and neuropathy (nerve disease). Regular participation in exercise has several positive effects on carbohydrate regulation that can help your clients with type 2 diabetes manage their disease much more effectively.

Chapter Summary

- Exercise is characterized by a coordinated endocrine response that is responsive to metabolic demands.

- Glucagon and insulin secreted from the pancreatic islets are increased and decreased, respectively, with exercise. The responses of these hormones are necessary for the stimulation of liver glycogenolysis and gluconeogenesis.

- Liver gluconeogenesis is controlled by the mobilization of gluconeogenic precursors from the gut, adipose tissue, and muscle and by the activation of gluconeogenic pathways in the liver.

- The endocrine response to exercise is responsive to environmental factors, such as the hypoxia seen with altitude, and nutritional state.

- The decrease in circulating insulin and increase in circulating epinephrine and sympathetic nerve activity act together to accelerate mobilization of muscle glycogen and adipose tissue triglycerides for use in energy production.

- Sympathetic drive and epinephrine release increase with exercise intensity and exercise duration.

- Arterial or systemic venous measurements of glucagon and norepinephrine do not reflect their concentrations at their sites of action as they are released in inaccessible compartments (portal vein and synaptic cleft, respectively) in human subjects.

- Exercise stimulates muscle glucose uptake by a mechanism that is independent of insulin action. Glucose uptake by working muscle is controlled by the rate of glucose delivery to the muscle by the circulation, the rate of transport into the muscle by GLUT4, and the rate of phosphorylation of glucose inside the cell by a hexokinase. Hexokinase is a more significant limitation to muscle glucose uptake during exercise as compared to the resting state.

- Glycogenolysis is catalyzed by the enzyme phosphorylase a. Phosphorylase a activity is increased by exercise due to allosteric modifiers and a signaling cascade that results in its covalent activation.

- Triglyceride breakdown within the adipocyte is catalyzed by a hormone-sensitive lipase. This lipase is activated by cyclic AMP-dependent protein kinase.

- Circulating free fatty acid availability to working muscle is determined by the balance between adipose tissue lipolysis and adipose tissue and liver re-esterification of fatty acids.

- AMP-dependent protein kinase is a key enzyme in channeling fatty acids into energy producing oxidative pathways in both the liver and working muscle.

Exercise Physiology Reality

CENGAGE brain   To reinforce the exercise physiology concepts presented above, complete the laboratory exercises for Chapter 6. To access labs and other course materials for this text, please visit www.cengagebrain.com. See the preface on page xiii for details. Once you complete the exercises, evaluate your results based on the scales provided and develop a personal plan for successfully applying the concepts you have learned once your exercise physiology course is completed.

Exercise Physiology Web Links

Access the following websites for further study of topics covered in this chapter:

- Find updates and quick links to these and other epidemiology and exercise physiology–related sites at our website. To access the course materials and companion resources for this text, please visit www.cengagebrain.com. See the preface on page xiii for details.

- Search for more research about hormonal regulation during exercise at the National Center for Biotechnology Information PubMed website: http://www.pubmed central.nih.gov/.

- Search for more information about hormonal regulation at the American College of Sports Medicine website: http://www.acsm.org.

- Search for more information about hormonal regulation at the Federation of American Societies for Experimental Biology website: http://www.faseb.org.

- Search for more information about hormonal regulation at the Gatorade Sports Science Institute website: http://www.gssiweb.com.

Study Questions

Review the Warm-Up Pre-Test questions you were asked to answer before reading Chapter 6. Test yourself once more to determine what you know now that you have completed the chapter.

The questions that follow will help you review this chapter. You will find the answers in the discussions on the pages provided.

1. What factors determine hormone secretion during exercise? *pp. 147–148*

2. What is the advantage of having the blood draining the pancreas perfuse the liver? *p. 151*

3. How might feedback control act to stimulate hormone release in response to exercise? *p. 148*

4. What role does the decrease in circulating insulin play in control of glucose homeostasis during exercise serve? *p. 154*

5. How is allosteric regulation involved in glycolytic flux during exercise? *p. 160*

6. How is covalent regulation involved in glycogenolysis during exercise? *pp. 159–160*

7. What are the cellular mechanisms by which glucagon binding to its liver cell membrane receptor stimulates the release of glucose from the liver? *pp. 154–155*

8. What role do specialized proteins serve in fatty acid flux during exercise? *p. 167*

9. How does glucose ingestion spare muscle glycogen during exercise? *p. 162*

10. What are mechanisms for mobilization of free fatty acids from adipose tissue triglycerides? *p. 165*

Selected References

Bergstrom, J., L. Hermansen, E. Hultman, and B. Saltin. 1967. Diet, muscle glycogen and physical performance. *Acta. Physiol. Scand.* 71:140–150.

Hawley, J. A., E. J. Schabort, T. D. Noakes, and S. C. Dennis. 1997. Carbohydrate-loading and exercise performance. An update. *Sports Med.* 24(2):73–81.

Hultman, E. 1995. Fuel selection, muscle fibre. *Proc. Nutr. Soc.* 54(1):107–121.

Jensen, M. D. 2003. Fate of fatty acids at rest and during exercise: Regulatory mechanisms. *Acta. Physiol. Scand.* 178(4):385–390.

Kiens, B. 2006. Skeletal muscle lipid metabolism in exercise and insulin resistance. *Physiol. Rev.* 86(1):205–243.

Mandarino, L. J., R. C. Bonadonna, O. P. McGuinness, A. E. Halseth, and D. H. Wasserman. 2001. Regulation of muscle glucose uptake in vivo. Chapter 27 in *The American Physi-ological Society handbook of physiology-endocrine pancreas* (pp. 803–848), edited by L. S. Jefferson. Rockville, MD: Waverly Press.

Pedersen, B. K. 2011. Muscles and their myokines. *J. Exp. Biol.* 214(pt 2):337–346.

Schaffer, J. E. 2002. Fatty acid transport: The roads taken. *Am. J. Physiol.* 282:239–246.

Spriet, L. L., and M. J. Watt. 2003. Regulatory mechanisms in the interaction between carbohydrate and lipid oxidation during exercise. *Acta. Physiol. Scand.* 178(4):443–452.

Wasserman, D. H., and A. Cherrington. 1996. Regulation of extrahepatic fuel sources during exercise. Chapter 23 in *The American Physiological Society handbook of physiology-integration of motor, circulatory, respiratory, and metabolic control during exercise* (pp. 1036–1074), edited by L. B. Rowell and J. T. Shepherd. Rockville, MD: Waverly Press.

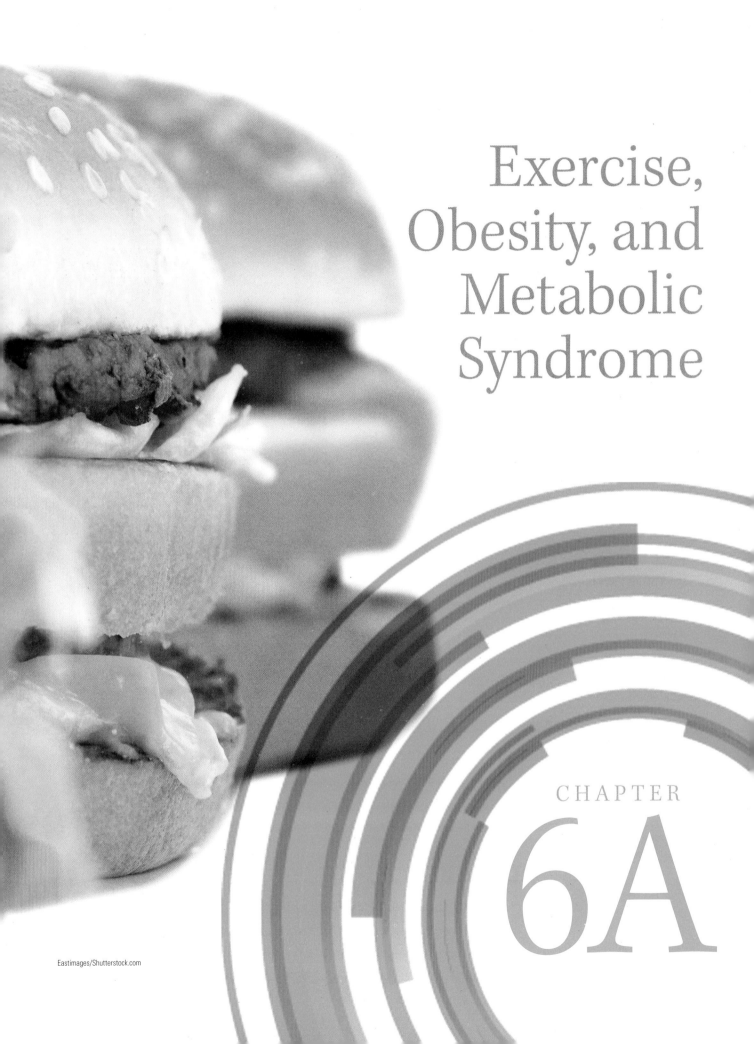

Exercise, Obesity, and Metabolic Syndrome

CHAPTER

6A

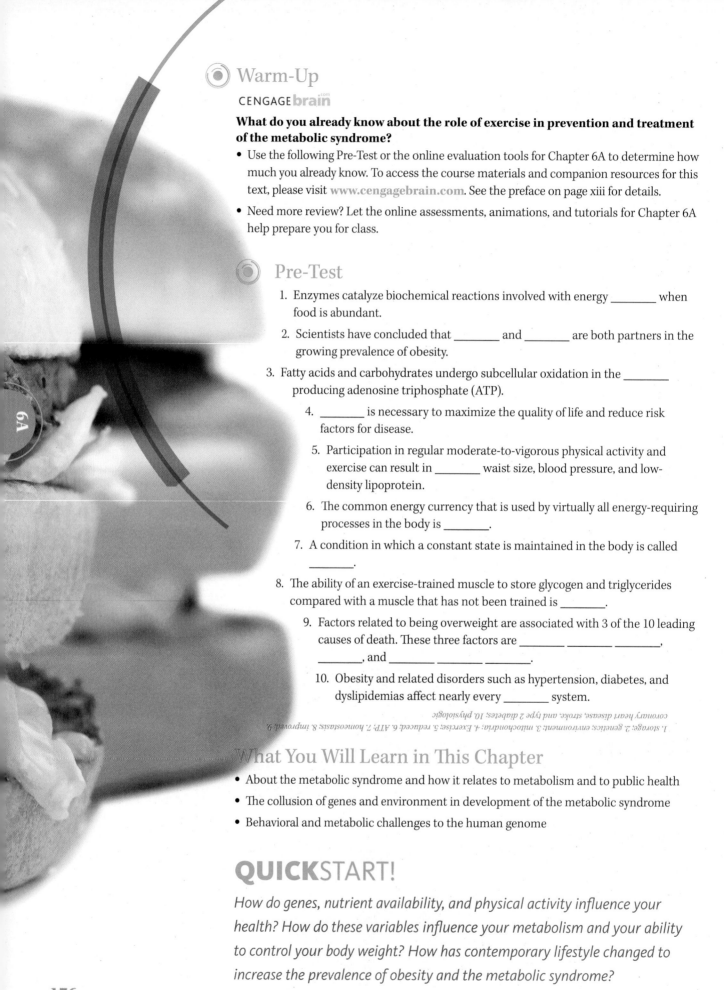

Warm-Up

CENGAGE **brain**

What do you already know about the role of exercise in prevention and treatment of the metabolic syndrome?

- Use the following Pre-Test or the online evaluation tools for Chapter 6A to determine how much you already know. To access the course materials and companion resources for this text, please visit **www.cengagebrain.com**. See the preface on page xiii for details.

- Need more review? Let the online assessments, animations, and tutorials for Chapter 6A help prepare you for class.

Pre-Test

1. Enzymes catalyze biochemical reactions involved with energy _____ when food is abundant.

2. Scientists have concluded that _____ and _____ are both partners in the growing prevalence of obesity.

3. Fatty acids and carbohydrates undergo subcellular oxidation in the _____ producing adenosine triphosphate (ATP).

4. _____ is necessary to maximize the quality of life and reduce risk factors for disease.

5. Participation in regular moderate-to-vigorous physical activity and exercise can result in _____ waist size, blood pressure, and low-density lipoprotein.

6. The common energy currency that is used by virtually all energy-requiring processes in the body is _____.

7. A condition in which a constant state is maintained in the body is called _____.

8. The ability of an exercise-trained muscle to store glycogen and triglycerides compared with a muscle that has not been trained is _____.

9. Factors related to being overweight are associated with 3 of the 10 leading causes of death. These three factors are _____ _____ _____, _____, and _____ _____ _____.

10. Obesity and related disorders such as hypertension, diabetes, and dyslipidemias affect nearly every _____ system.

1. storage; 2. genetics, environment; 3. mitochondria; 4. Exercise; 5. reduced; 6. ATP; 7. homeostasis; 8. improved; 9. coronary heart disease, stroke, and type 2 diabetes; 10. physiologic

What You Will Learn in This Chapter

- About the metabolic syndrome and how it relates to metabolism and to public health
- The collusion of genes and environment in development of the metabolic syndrome
- Behavioral and metabolic challenges to the human genome

QUICKSTART!

How do genes, nutrient availability, and physical activity influence your health? How do these variables influence your metabolism and your ability to control your body weight? How has contemporary lifestyle changed to increase the prevalence of obesity and the metabolic syndrome?

Introduction to Exercise, Obesity, and Metabolic Syndrome

From the moment we begin to exercise, a complex response is initiated. Skeletal muscle contracts due to neural stimulation. In support of muscle contraction fuels are mobilized and oxygen (O_2) is delivered to skeletal muscle for energy-producing reactions. Skeletal muscle is capable of increasing its metabolic rate by a magnitude that exceeds the responsiveness of any other tissue in the body. Contraction can require a 10-fold increase in muscle O_2 and glucose utilization, and a similar rate of carbon dioxide (CO_2) output. Yet, despite the dramatic increase in energy expenditure the concentrations of these molecules in arterial blood generally remain constant.

The need to increase energy expenditure with exercise is an important benefit of exercise. An imbalance between energy expenditure and energy intake (Caloric consumption), so that energy intake exceeds energy expenditure results in weight gain. Increasing energy expenditure by exercise and a healthy diet are the first line of defense against obesity. The reason for the emphasis early in the text is that an imbalance in energy metabolism resulting in obesity is now an epidemic in the United States that continues to worsen (Figure 6A.1). This epidemic is blind to sex (Figure 6A.2) and affects every ethnic group to some extent. Particularly worrisome is the increase in obesity among American children (Figure 6A.3), because they are more apt to be obese adults and have long-standing healthcare needs.

The **obesity syndrome** is a metabolic disorder where energy intake exceeds energy expenditure, causing excess body fat. If trends since the 1970s continue, obesity-related disorders will dominate healthcare needs and healthcare dollars in the future. Obesity and related disorders such as

obesity syndrome The condition of being overweight due to excess fat mass. It is defined as having a BMI >30%.

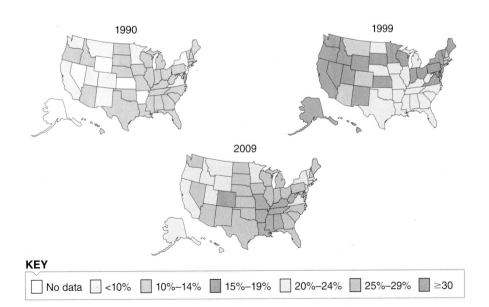

KEY

| No data | <10% | 10%–14% | 15%–19% | 20%–24% | 25%–29% | ≥30 |

● **FIGURE 6A.1 Changes in prevalence of adult obesity.** Data are for ages 18 years and older, based on self-reported weight and height via telephone interview. Obesity is defined as body mass index (BMI) ≥ 30.0. (Data are from Behavioral Risk Factor Surveillance System, National Center for Chronic Disease Prevention and Health Promotion, Centers for Disease Control and Prevention at http://www.cdc.gov/obesity/data/index.html.)

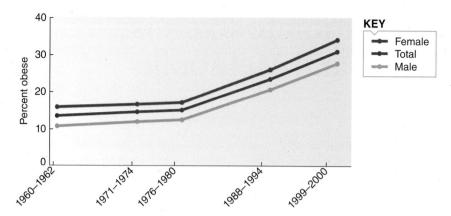

FIGURE 6A.2 Trends in adult obesity. Data are for ages 20 years and older, age-adjusted to the 2000 standard population. Obesity is defined as body mass index (BMI) ≥ 30.0. (Data are from National Health Examination Survey, National Health and Nutrition Examination Surveys I, II, III and 1999–2000, National Center for Health Statistics, Centers for Disease Control and Prevention at http://www.cdc.gov/nchs/nhanes.htm.)

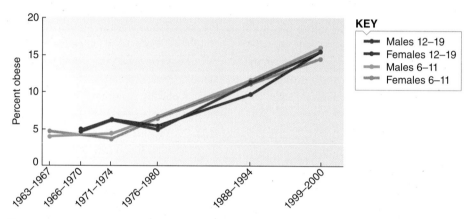

FIGURE 6A.3 Trends in child and adolescent obesity. Overweight is defined as body mass index (BMI) ≥ gender- and weight-specific 95th percentile from the 2000 Centers for Disease Control and Prevention Growth Charts for the United States. (From National Health Examination Surveys II (ages 6–11) and III (ages 12–17), National Health and Nutrition Examination Surveys I, II, III and 1999–2000, National Center for Health Statistics, Centers for Disease Control and Prevention at http://www.cdc.gov/nchs/nhanes.htm.)

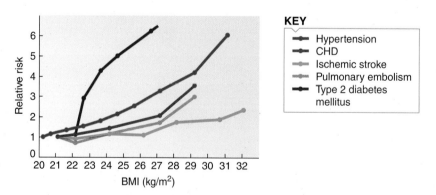

FIGURE 6A.4 Relationship of body mass index (kg/m²) on cardiovascular disease and type 2 diabetes mellitus. (© Cengage Learning 2013)

hypertension, diabetes, and dyslipidemias affect nearly every physiologic system.

The term **metabolic syndrome** has been used to describe the state characterized by the coexistence of multiple pathologies associated with obesity. The two most common of these are central obesity and insulin resistance.

Figure 6A.4 shows the relationship of body mass index to several diseases.

Risk factors that are characteristic of the metabolic syndrome are listed in Table 6A.1. People with the metabolic syndrome are at increased risk for coronary heart disease and other diseases related to plaque buildups in artery walls (for example, stroke and peripheral vascular disease) and type 2 diabetes. The American Heart Association estimated that, in 2006, more than 50 million Americans have the metabolic syndrome. Conditions associated with the metabolic syndrome include physical inactivity combined with excess ingestion of Calories, aging, neuroendocrine imbalance, and genetic predisposition.

What is the relationship between body weight regulation, the rate that we expend energy to support metabolism, and dietary energy intake?

● **TABLE 6A.1 Metabolic Syndrome Is Characterized by the Coexistence of Multiple Metabolic Risk Factors for Cardiovascular Disease**

Abdominal obesity (excessive abdominal fat tissue)
Atherogenic dyslipidemia (high triglycerides, low high-density lipoprotein cholesterol, high low-density lipoprotein cholesterol)
Elevated blood pressure
Insulin resistance or glucose intolerance
Prothrombotic state (for example, high blood fibrinogen or plasminogen activator inhibitor-1)
Proinflammatory state (for example, increased blood C-reactive protein level)

© Cengage Learning 2013

The pathogenesis of the metabolic syndrome is complex and is, as yet, not fully understood. Exercise and diet are the first line of defense for most forms of obesity. Exercise physiologists and healthcare providers who incorporate exercise into their practice are uniquely positioned to engage this growing problem.

HOTLINK *Log on to the Centers for Disease Control and Prevention website to learn about programs for healthy living:* **http://www.cdc.gov/HealthyLiving/**.

The obesity epidemic has resulted because of collusion between genetic factors and environmental factors. How genetic and environmental factors interact in the pathogenesis of obesity will also be considered.

6A

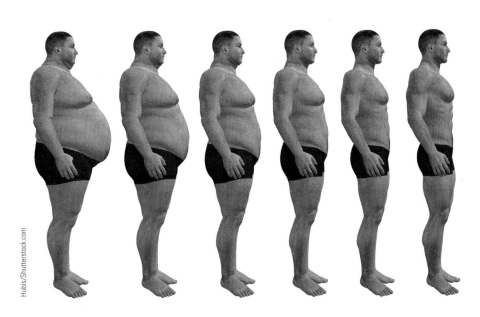

Hubis/Shutterstock.com

Introduction to Exercise, Obesity, and Metabolic Syndrome **179**

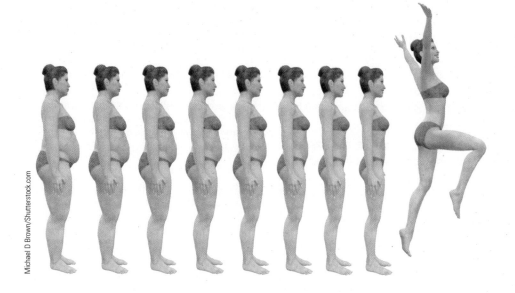

Michael D Brown/Shutterstock.com

The Nature of Adaptations to Regular Exercise

Encapsulated within the response to exercise are signals that cause the body to adapt. These signals cause changes in constituents of the body, making an organism better able to accomplish physical work and maintain homeostasis. Adaptations occur not only in working muscles, but also in the organs and tissues that support their function.

Adaptations fall into the category of those that are due to a change in **protein content** within cells and those that result because of a repartitioning of fuel stores (for example, loss of fat mass). Protein content is determined predominantly by the rate of **gene transcription**. However, changes in **RNA translation** and the degradation of RNA or protein may also, in some cases, play significant roles (Figure 6A.5).

Proteins serve many functions. They catalyze biochemical reactions, maintain cellular or extracellular structural integrity, and cause motion associated with muscle contraction and relaxation. Proteins are also transporters, channels, transcription factors, and hormones.

protein content The abundance and type of proteins that are contained in or surrounding cell or tissue.

gene transcription The formation of mRNA from the gene that encodes it in the nucleus, and to a lesser extent in the mitochondria, of a cell. This is an enzymatic process that is regulated by complex activators and activation sites on the gene.

RNA translation The synthesis of peptide chains from the nucleic acids that comprise mRNA. An enzyme-catalyzed process that has diverse and stringently controlled regulatory sites.

neuroendocrine regulators Molecules that are secreted by nerves or glands to control the functions of an organism.

> What are some proteins that might be increased as an adaptation to oxidative exercise?

A repartitioning of fuel stores resulting in a decrease in fat mass is one of the important adaptations to regular physical activity. Consider again all the pathologic conditions that are associated with obesity (see Figure 6A.4). Exercises that reduce fat mass partner with a good diet to be a formidable prophylactic measure for obesity-associated diseases. Exercise improves insulin's action on target tissue (review Chapter 6), and there is evidence that the effectiveness of other **neuroendocrine regulators** may also be improved (Figure 6A.6).

In addition to being a target tissue for a number of hormones and neural transmitters, it is now well accepted that adipose tissue is an endocrine organ, secreting a number of peptides such as leptin, tumor necrosis factor-alpha,

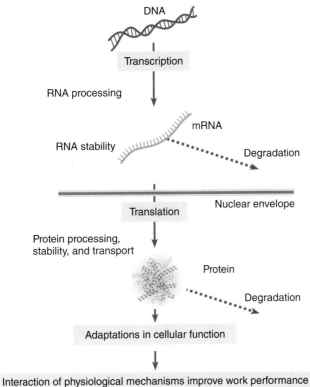

FIGURE 6A.5 Adaptations to physical activity begin with changes at the level of the gene. Adaptations to exercise training are characterized by increased expression of many proteins. This can occur because of transcriptional, translational, and post-translational regulation. Messenger RNA and protein pool sizes are also determined by their rates of degradation. (© Cengage Learning 2013)

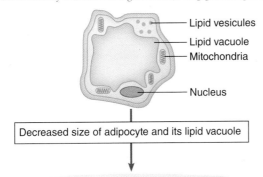

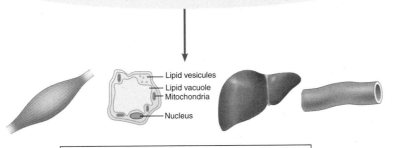

FIGURE 6A.6 A loss in body fat mass often accompanies regular exercise. Physical activity is a valuable tool in countering obesity and the pathologic conditions that associate with it. (© Cengage Learning 2013)

resistin, and adiponectin. The actions of these "adipokines" affect insulin action and influence appetite (see Chapter 6).

Although primary adaptations to regular exercise may be subcellular, the end result is a well-coordinated integration of physiologic mechanisms that leads to an improvement in function of the body to perform work. Let us examine the adaptations to long-distance exercise. Exercise of duration longer than a few minutes requires an increased provision of O_2 (see Chapters 7–10) and metabolic substrates (primarily carbohydrate and fat described in Chapters 4–6) to muscle so that adenosine triphosphate (ATP) for muscle contraction and relaxation is continually replenished. Mitochondria are the site where fatty acids and carbohydrates are oxidized, producing ATP. Mitochondria proliferate in endurance exercise–trained muscle, increasing the structural proteins and enzymes necessary for complete oxidation of macronutrients. This adaptation alone would be of little value in improving the ability to perform prolonged exercise. Fortunately, this adaptation does not occur in isolation. The exercise-trained muscle is better able to: (a) store glycogen and triglycerides, (b) transport glucose and fatty acids from the blood across its membrane into the muscle, and (c) increase in capillary density. These adaptations ensure that delivery of O_2 and substrates to the trained muscle is increased. In addition, the exercise training results in a more efficient heart muscle, thereby enabling the muscle capillaries to be adequately perfused.

The adaptive response to exercise is a well-conserved feature of the human genome and has its roots in our hunter–gatherer ancestry. Moreover, it is highly conserved between species. The ability to adapt to conditions that require high physical activity was an important aspect of survival when humans were foragers, hunters, and the hunted (Figure 6A.7). Systems for adapting to cold, heat, and altitude have also been conserved for millennia. Adaptations to physical activity remain important in the twenty-first century in preserving quality of life and promoting long-term survival. The reasons that physical activity is important in current times, however, is much different than in ancient times, as discussed later in this chapter.

HOTLINK *For a detailed analysis of "obesity genes," see O'Rahilly and Farooqi's article, "Genetics of Obesity":* **http://www.ncbi.nlm.nih.gov/ pmc/articles/PMC1642700/.**

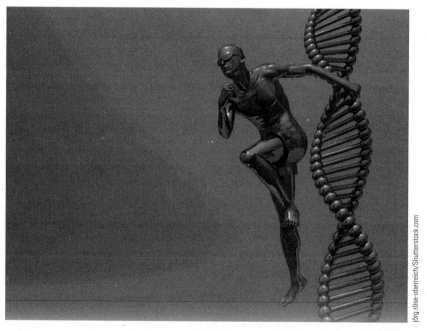

jörg röse-oberreich/Shutterstock.com

● **FIGURE 6A.7** **The human genome is designed for a culture of physical activity.**

The Human Genome in the Age of Fast Food and Screen Time

Present-day Western culture is much different from the culture of our ancestors from whom the human genome evolved. The **human genome** is designed for intermittent feeding, but food is now available on a continuous basis. Moreover, the human genome is designed for a diet lower in fat and sucrose than present-day foods. Foods high in fat (>15%) did not exist in the diet of early humans but is now a standard of fast-food culture in Western societies. Approximately 40% of the calories in a hamburger from the fast-food world are from fat. The result is a conspiracy of genetics and environment so that the metabolic engine we have inherited has fuel requirements that differ from present-day fuel provision, in both quantity and composition. Indeed, scientists have concluded that genetics and environment are both partners in the growing prevalence of obesity.

HOTLINK *To learn about the role of nutrition in the increased prevalence of obesity, see the Food and Agriculture Organization of the United Nations website:* **http://www.fao.org/FOCUS/E/obesity/obes2.htm**.

Genes necessary for food storage have been termed **thrifty genes** because they encode proteins that manage calories so that they are stored and not spent unnecessarily. Examples of thrifty genes are those that encode hormones that promote fuel storage, such as adiponectin released from adipose tissue, and insulin released from pancreatic beta cells. Thrifty genes are also those that encode enzymes that catalyze lipogenesis. These genes contribute to a metabolic network that determines the capacity to store chemical energy as fat.

(Why are genes that previously were essential to our survival now a threat to our quality of life?)

The conspiracy of genes and environments is also felt in the changed physical demands of daily life. The daily caloric requirement of people who hunt and forage for their meals is much higher than that of people who make a living at a desk or in front of a computer. Furthermore, recreation is less about physical activities and increasingly more related to **screen time**. The capacity for physical exercise was necessary for survival in earlier times. As a consequence, *the human genome is designed for a culture of physical activity*. With modern conveniences, comforts, and technology, the activities necessary for survival of our ancestors are no longer a part of our lives. However, maintaining a culture of physical activity is no less essential; indeed, it becomes imperative.

(What specific lifestyle changes would reverse the obesity trend?)

Without regular physical exercise, a mismatch of genome and culture exists that contributes to obesity and the many abnormalities that comprise the metabolic syndrome (see Table 6A.1). Physical exercise is necessary to maximize the quality of life and reduce risk factors for disease.

human genome The nucleic acid sequences that comprise genes that make up chromosomes. Genes encode the proteins that lead to human development and physiological function. Errors or mutations can result in abnormalities or disease.

screen time The compilation of time spent in using computers, video games, and television. This may contribute to decreased physical activity if it is excessive in duration.

thrifty genes The name given to those genes that encode the proteins that are used for nutrient storage. These genes were necessary for survival in hunter and gatherer societies. They are now hypothesized to be a cause of obesity in societies where food is always available.

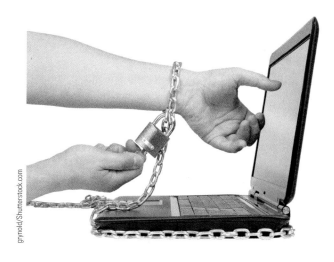

grynold/Shutterstock.com

HOTLINK *For information on how exercise can reduce risk factors for disease, access the American Heart Association website:* **http://www.americanheart.org/presenter.jhtml?identifier=4563**.

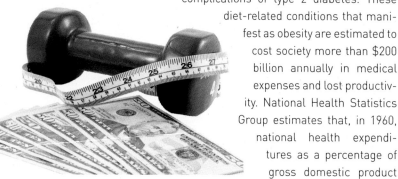

Factors related to being overweight are associated with 3 of the 10 leading causes of death: coronary heart disease, stroke, and complications of type 2 diabetes. These diet-related conditions that manifest as obesity are estimated to cost society more than $200 billion annually in medical expenses and lost productivity. National Health Statistics Group estimates that, in 1960, national health expenditures as a percentage of gross domestic product was 5 percent. In 2006, it was estimated to be nearly 20 percent. Continued increases at this rate will be debilitating to the U.S. economy.

> How can the community you live in, the school you attend, or your workplace be more conducive to an active lifestyle?

HOTLINK *To learn about the impact of physical inactivity on healthcare costs and our society, access the Centers for Disease Control and Prevention website:* **http://www.cdc.gov/obesity/causes/economics.html**.

CONCEPTS, challenges, & controversies

Trouble in Paradise!

In the Pacific Ocean, some 2,900 miles southwest of Hawaii, is the tiny volcanic island of Kosrae, a part of the Federated States of Micronesia. In 1994, American researchers headed by Dr. Jeffrey M. Freidman from Rockefeller University in New York City came to Kosrae to find the genetic and molecular bases for susceptibility to obesity and the metabolic syndrome in humans. Dr. Friedman and his team postulated that body weight is a manifestation of what American geneticist Dr. James V. Neel in 1962 called the "thrifty gene" theory. Dr. Neel theorized that in an environment prone to famine, hunter–gatherers gained a selective advantage if their genes predisposed them to storing fat when food was available. Only those who managed to fatten themselves in advance of lean times lived to pass on these thrifty genes to subsequent generations. When cooking oil, fatty meats, and processed sugars arrived on the island, most adults grew fat. A corollary to the thrifty gene theory is that people who lived in early agricultural societies, such as those in the Fertile Crescent in present-day Iraq, had a steady supply of food from plants and domesticated animals, and thus did not need to store fat. Although once essential for survival, thrifty genes are a liability in present-day societies where there is an abundance of food high in fat. However, thrifty genes did not offer a selective advantage for people thriving in tame climates where food supply was consistently adequate. Populations with this ancestry are now less vulnerable to obesity brought about by Westernization of lifestyle.

Kosrae's genetically isolated population and its abrupt changes in eating habits have made it nearly perfect for examining obesity and other pathologic conditions associated with

Marcus Miranda/Shutterstock.com

6A

the metabolic syndrome. Most of the 8,000 Kosraeans can trace their heritage to a small "founder" population of about 50 people who came from Polynesia about 1,000 years ago. In the mid to late 19th century, Caucasian whalers visited and, in many cases, settled on the island, and so today many Kosraeans can trace their ancestry to both groups. **Kosraeans** were historically active, ate native foods, and were reported to be relatively lean. They lived a near-subsistent life, experiencing frequent droughts and stormy seasons that laid waste to crops. In the years after World War II, most began leading sedentary lifestyles while eating foods supplied by a U.S. aid program that were high in fat content. Subsequently, in just one generation, a disproportionate percentage of people on the island experienced development of obesity and other conditions associated with metabolic syndrome.

Dr. Friedman and colleagues set out to measure islanders' weight, height, and waist size; to document the family history of diseases; and to assess blood chemistry and blood pressure. The researchers also extracted DNA from blood drawn from islanders to search for genes for obesity, heart disease, and diabetes. They determined that more than 80 percent of adult Koraeans are overweight or obese, and diabetes afflicts 1 in 8 adults. With increasing waistlines of the Koraean people are projections of decreased life expectancy. Researchers can scan genomes of the islanders for differences in single base pairs at specific locations, which can then be associated with differences in susceptibility to diseases such as obesity or diabetes. The goal of these studies is to identify a library of genes that correlate with the islanders' predispositions to be fat or lean. Genetic studies of Kosraeans and other genetically non-complex populations (for example, Pima Indians of Southwest United States and Mexico) have confirmed the existence of a strong link between susceptibility to obesity and genetic makeup. Hundreds of genes have been implicated in regulation of feeding behavior and body weight. The likelihood of becoming obese and experiencing development of the metabolic syndrome may depend on the collection of those genes you have inherited.

HOTLINK *To learn more about the impact of industrialization on the metabolic health of the Pima Indians of Arizona, access the National Institute of Diabetes and Digestive and Kidney Diseases website:* **http://diabetes .niddk.nih.gov/dm/pubs/pima/obesity/obesity.htm**.

The ironic twist in this tale of the Kosraeans is that these enduring islanders survived decimation by microbes and the battering of typhoons, only to fall victim to the assault of Westernization on their unassuming traditional culture. Programs supported by the Centers for Disease Control and Prevention to administer programs to reintroduce healthy eating and an active lifestyle to the inhabitants of Kosrae are currently under way.

Successful diet and exercise programs are those in which compliance is not a chore. The Kosrae State College Campus offers innovative programs, such as PE 101: "Surfing," to promote activity that takes advantage of the waves breaking off the island's coral reefs.

Kosraeans Natives of the island of Kosrae that is part of the Federated States of Micronesia in the South Pacific. Their isolation for many centuries resulted in a limited genetic diversity, making them a unique population for studying the genetics of obesity. Obesity and diabetes became highly prevalent among the inhabitants of Kosrae during World War II as military installations imported processed foods rich in fat and sucrose.

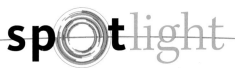

spotlight

An Expert on the Metabolic Dysfunction of Skeletal Muscle in Overweight Humans: Lawrence J. Mandarino, Ph.D.

Few understand the insulin-resistant muscle as well as Dr. Lawrence Mandarino, and no one understands it better. Dr. Mandarino received his Ph.D. in Anthropology from Arizona State in 1978. Considering that we now know that obesity and metabolic syndrome have a major genetic component, his background has proved to be a solid foundation for his research. Dr. Mandarino had an illustrious career studying the insulin-resistant muscle before returning home to Arizona from San Antonio. He is currently Professor of the School of Life Sciences at Arizona State University and Professor of Medicine at the Mayo Clinic Arizona. He is Founding Director of the Mayo/Arizona State University Center for Metabolic and Vascular Biology (CMVB) at Mayo Clinic Arizona and Arizona State University. The CMVB is an interdisciplinary center designed to bring together basic and clinical scientists to understand the mechanisms responsible for insulin resistance, type 2 diabetes mellitus, and cardiovascular disease.

Mandarino's research has had continuous National Institutes of Health support and resulted in numerous publications. Research in the Mandarino laboratory focuses on the molecular mechanisms responsible for insulin resistance in human skeletal muscle. Of particular interest have been the roles of mitochondrial dysfunction and the regulation of insulin receptor substrate-1 function. Experimental systems used to study these issues include a wide variety of techniques, ranging from in vivo methods to assess human metabolic events, such as the euglycemic hyperinsulinemic clamp, muscle biopsies, arterial catheterizations, and use of stable isotopes to assess metabolic rates, to cell culture and molecular biology techniques for addressing questions of insulin signaling.

When Mandarino founded the CMVB in 2005, he did so with a vision. He has developed a comprehensive proteomics laboratory, with modern and highly sensitive mass spectrometers that can be used for a variety of proteomics techniques. This technology has allowed him to identify targets of insulin resistance by sensitive analysis of phosphorylated protein. He has also identified aberrant accumulation of muscle extracellular matrix proteins and potential signaling pathways by which these extracellular proteins influence muscle metabolism and overall contractile function in insulin-resistant states.

The application of sensitive mass spectroscopy to an important clinical problem will be critical in determining the pathogenesis of insulin resistance, type 2 diabetes, and the metabolic syndrome. Moreover, the strategies employed by Mandarino and colleagues will continue to be fruitful in identifying potential therapeutic targets.

in*Practice*

Examples of Metabolic Adaptations to Exercise

This section provides some practical examples of how metabolic adaptations of physiologic systems to exercise are related to your area of interest (review the future career table from Chapter 1).

Health/Fitness: Participation in regular exercise can help repartition fuel stores in the body and allow one to increase the number of Calories expended. Although many other factors contribute to the global obesity epidemic, exercise causes the signals related to cellular metabolism, hormonal regulation, gene expression, cellular organelles, and other processes to adapt in positive ways to help control the storage of body fat. As discussed earlier, the *2008 Physical Activity Guidelines for Americans* (http://www.health.gov/paguidelines) recommends that adults achieve a minimum of 150 minutes of moderate physical activity per week, or 75 minutes of vigorous physical activity per week. For extensive health benefits, adults should achieve 300 minutes of moderate physical activity per week or 150 minutes of vigorous physical activity per week, and add muscle-strengthening activities for all major muscle groups two or more times per week.

Medicine: Participation in regular exercise can help prevent and/or control metabolic syndrome. Clinical evidence suggest that for adults, accumulating a minimum of 150 minutes of exercise per week can positively influence the following metabolic syndrome risk factors (refer to Table 6A.1):

- Decrease in waist (circumference) girth
- Decreases in resting triglyceride levels, reduced low-density lipoprotein cholesterol levels, and higher high-density lipoprotein cholesterol levels
- Lower resting blood pressure
- Improvement in insulin and glucose regulation
- Reduction of thrombotic risk
- Decline of blood C-reactive protein level
- Help achieve and/or maintain functional health

Lifestyle interventions that include physical activity and exercise, and the achievement and/or maintenance of functional health have been shown to be clinically effective (together with medication as prescribed) in disease prevention and treatment programs.

Athletic Performance: Participation in regular high-intensity exercise can help athletes optimize their ability to extract energy from glucose, increase their glycogen storage and mobilization capabilities, and improve their ability to use free fatty acids more effectively, whereas sparing glycogen. For example, interval training programs that require distance runners to work at 90 percent or more of their maximal oxygen uptake ($\dot{V}O_2$ max), for no more than 10 percent of their total training volume (no more than 6 miles out of a 60-mile training week; more can increase risk for injury), can substantially improve metabolic efficiency (produce big changes with a little discomfort).

Rehabilitation: Patients who participate in regular exercise via a cardiac rehabilitation program may get the most benefits from metabolic adaptations that occur in the periphery (skeletal muscles) versus changes in their cardiac output (central component). After a myocardial infarction (heart attack), the potential physiologic adaptations that can occur to cardiac output often are limited because of myocardial damage; therefore, metabolic adaptations can allow the patient to regain the ability to engage in daily personal physical activities again. By exercising in an outpatient or at-home cardiac rehabilitation program, patients can help reduce or manage their cardiovascular and metabolic syndrome risk factors such as hypertension, abnormal lipids, overweight, fasting glucose, fasting insulin, and functional health levels for secondary prevention of another myocardial infarction.

 # Chapter Summary

- In this chapter, you learned about the metabolism of fuels for energy related to the areas of Health/Fitness, Medicine, Athletic Performance, and Rehabilitation.

- The obesity syndrome is a metabolic disorder in which energy intake exceeds energy expenditure.

- Conditions associated with the metabolic syndrome include physical inactivity combined with excess ingestion of calories, aging, neuroendocrine imbalance, and genetic predisposition. The pathogenesis of the metabolic syndrome is complex and is, as yet, not fully understood.

- A repartitioning of fuel stores that results in a decrease in fat mass is one of the important adaptations to regular physical activity.

- Although primary adaptations to regular exercise may be subcellular, the end result is a well-coordinated integration of physiologic mechanisms that leads to an improvement in function of the body to perform work.

- Adenosine triphosphate (ATP) is the common energy currency that is used by virtually all energy-requiring processes in the body.

- Glucose and fatty acids are the primary fuels, and the energy currency they deal in is ATP.

- The human genome is designed for intermittent feeding, but food is now available on a continuous basis.

- Without regular physical exercise, a mismatch of genome and culture exists that contributes to obesity and the many abnormalities that comprise the metabolic syndrome (Table 6A.1). Physical exercise is necessary to maximize the quality of life and reduce risk factors for disease.

 # Exercise Physiology Reality

CENGAGE brain   To reinforce the exercise physiology concepts presented above, complete the laboratory exercises for Chapter 6A. To access labs and other course materials for this text, please visit www.cengagebrain.com. See the preface on page xiii for details. Once you complete the exercises, evaluate your results based on the scales provided and develop a personal plan for successfully completing your exercise physiology course.

 # Exercise Physiology Web Links

Access the following websites for further study of topics covered in this chapter:

- Find updates and quick links to these and other epidemiology and exercise physiology–related sites at our website. To access the course materials and companion resources for this text, please visit www.cengagebrain.com. See the preface on page xiii for details.

- Search for further information about metabolism and metabolic syndrome at the Centers for Disease Control and Prevention (CDC) website: http://www.cdc.gov.

- Search for information about energy metabolism at the American College of Sports Medicine website: http://www.acsm.org.
- Search for more information about cellular physiology in Sherwood's *Human Physiology* text at the Cengage website: http://www.cengagebrain.com.
- Search for more information about metabolic syndrome and the future economic costs of controlling obesity at the U.S. National Health Information Center website: http://www.healthierUS.gov.
- Search for more information about metabolism at the Gatorade Sports Science Institute website: http://www.gssiweb.com.

Study Questions

Review the Warm-Up Pre-Test questions you were asked to answer before reading Chapter 6A. Test yourself once more to determine what you know now that you have completed the chapter.

The questions that follow will help you review this chapter. You will find the answers in the discussions on the pages provided.

1. Define the term *metabolic syndrome* and how it relates to the field of exercise physiology. *p. 179*
2. What roles does protein synthesis play in adaptations to regular exercise? *p. 181*
3. What is the significance of adipokines in regulation of fat mass? *p. 180*
4. Why is ATP synthesis important to energy expenditure? *p. 182*
5. How do mitochondrial adaptations improve the ability to oxidize nutrients? *p. 182*
6. What adaptations to physical activity make the blood better able to use circulating nutrients? *p. 182*
7. How do human genes and our social and physical environments influence food storage? *p. 183*
8. Why are 80 percent of Koraean adults overweight or obese? *p. 184*
9. What are mechanisms by which regular physical exercise might improve the metabolic syndrome? *p. 186*
10. What are examples of "thrifty genes"? *p. 183*

Selected References

Dietz, W. H., and T. N. Robinson. 2005. Overweight children and adolescents. *New Engl. J. Med.* 352:2100–2109.

Grundy, S. M. 2006. Metabolic syndrome: Connecting and reconciling cardiovascular and diabetes worlds. *J. Am. Coll. Cardiol.* 47:1093–1100.

Kraus, W. E., and C. A. Slentz. 2009. Exercise training, lipid regulation, and insulin action: A tangled web of cause and effect. *Obesity* (Silver Spring) 17(Suppl. 3):S21–S26.

Lazar, M. A. 2005. How obesity causes diabetes: Not a tall tale. *Science* 307:373–375.

Lefort, N., Z. Yi, B. Bowen, B. Glancy, E. A. De Filippis, R. Mapes, H. Hwang, C. R. Flynn, W. T. Willis, A. Civitarese, K. Højlund, and L. J. Mandarino. 2009. Proteome profile of functional mitochondria from human skeletal muscle using one-dimensional gel electrophoresis and HPLC-ESI-MS/MS. *J. Proteomics.* 72(6):1046–1060.

Popkin, B. M., Duffey, K., and P. Gordon-Larsen. 2005. Environmental influences on food choice, physical activity and energy balance. *Physiol. Behav.* 86:603–613.

Shmulewitz, D., S. B. Auerbach, T. Lehner, M. L. Blundell, J. D. Winick, L. D. Youngman, V. Skilling, S. C. Heath, J. Ott, M. Stoffel, J. L. Breslow, and J. M. Friedman. 2001. Epidemiology and factor analysis of obesity, type II diabetes, hypertension, and dyslipidemia (syndrome X) on the Island of Kosrae, Federated States of Micronesia. *Hum. Hered.* 51(1–2):8–19.

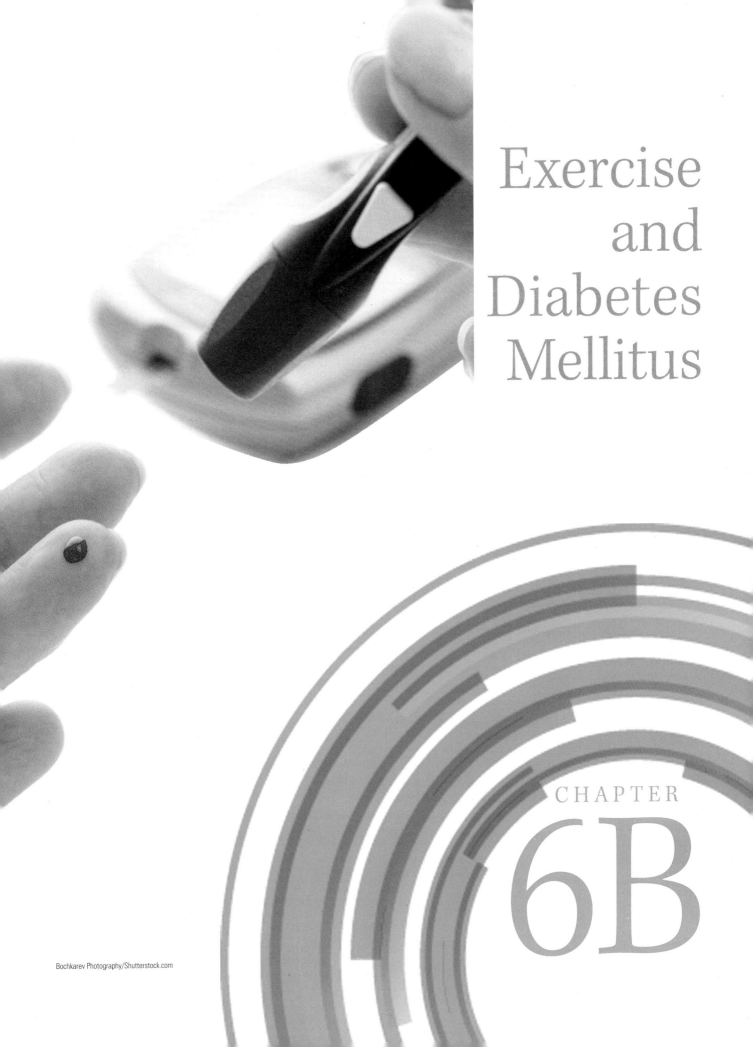

Exercise and Diabetes Mellitus

CHAPTER

6B

Warm-Up

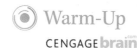

What do you already know about exercise in individuals with diabetes mellitus?

- Use the following Pre-Test or the online evaluation tools for Chapter 6B to determine how much you already know. To access the course materials and companion resources for this text, please visit **www.cengagebrain.com**. See the preface on page xiii for details.

- Need more review? Let the online assessments, animations, and tutorials for Chapter 6B help prepare you for class.

Pre-Test

1. The response to exercise in individuals with diabetes will depend on many factors including whether they are treated with the hormone _____ or by drugs that are taken orally.

2. One bout of strenuous exercise will lead to persistent increases in _____ _____.

3. Regular exercise may be valuable to individuals with diabetes because it decreases risk factors for _____ disease.

4. Intensive insulin therapy designed to maintain blood glucose at normal levels at rest may lead to _____ during and after exercise.

5. The metabolic response to exercise in individuals treated with insulin will be influenced by the time and size of insulin treatment and _____ _____.

6. The likelihood of hypoglycemia during exercise in some individuals with diabetes can be reduced by administering insulin at a site on the body away from the working _____.

7. A short bout of intense exercise may lead to _____ in individuals treated with insulin.

8. Regular exercise in individuals with diabetes is most effective when combined with a healthy _____.

9. If blood glucose level is more than 250 mg/dl and ketone bodies are high, individuals with diabetes could experience a further _____ in these metabolic substrates.

10. Individuals with diabetes may need to avoid certain types of exercise if they have advanced _____ of diabetes.

1. insulin; 2. glucose tolerance; 3. cardiovascular; 4. hypoglycemia; 5. carbohydrate ingestion; 6. muscle; 7. hyperglycemia; 8. diet; 9. increase; 10. complications

What You Will Learn in This Chapter

- Why individuals with diabetes should lead active lifestyles
- How individuals with type 1 and type 2 diabetes respond to exercise
- Special precautions that individuals with diabetes should consider in anticipation of exercise

QUICKSTART!

What makes the response of individuals with diabetes to exercise different? What are important benefits of exercise to individuals with diabetes? What special difficulties might people with diabetes have during acute exercise or a regular program of physical activity?

Introduction to Exercise and Diabetes Mellitus

The effects of exercise on individuals with diabetes were recognized well before the advent of modern medicine. In the writings of one prominent East Indian physician appears the recommendation that people stricken with a disease that had the characteristics and likely was diabetes should exercise if symptoms are mild, but refrain if their case is more severe. That analysis was made in approximately 500 B.C.E. and remained the prevailing view until insulin was discovered in 1921. The clinical use of insulin that followed changed the way that exercise was viewed. Before the age of insulin therapy, **hypoglycemia** was a rarity. The combination of insulin treatment and exercise was shown to result in hypoglycemia if precautions to avoid this dangerous condition were not taken. This is still true today. A major focus of this chapter is on the physiologic bases of insulin-induced hypoglycemia during exercise and precautions that can be taken to avoid it.

With the widespread use of insulin treatment, individuals with diabetes now live longer. With the added longevity that followed the discovery of insulin, the progression of **diabetic complications** became a much more important clinical problem. Many people who treat or live with diabetes advocate the use of exercise because of the positive effects it may have in slowing the development of diabetic complications and improving overall quality of life. There is good reason to promote regular exercise in clients with diabetes.

diabetic complications Cardiovascular, neural, and metabolic impairments that often accompany diabetes. They are far less common and less severe in people who have well-controlled blood sugar levels.

hypoglycemia A fall in blood glucose that is most prevalent in people treated with insulin. Exercise can increase the risk of insulin-induced hypoglycemia. Hypoglycemia may lead to seizure and death in extreme cases.

What Is Diabetes Mellitus?

Diabetes mellitus is a syndrome characterized by diminished or inadequate insulin secretion. Insulin, as discussed in Chapter 6, is a vital controller of many metabolic pathways, including those that maintain glucose homeostasis. Either reduced insulin concentration or insensitivity to insulin can result in increased glucose and free fatty acid levels in the blood. If left untreated, the person with diabetes may become ketoacidotic and comatose. Diabetes can be further defined by its pathogenesis. **Type 1 diabetes** is a disease where the body's immune system attacks and destroys its insulin-producing beta cells of the islets of Langerhans in the endocrine pancreas. Childhood and adolescence is the usual time of onset of type 1 diabetes; however, onset may also occur in adulthood. Approximately 2 million people in the United States have this disease. Currently, no broadly available cure exists for type 1 diabetes, but it is treatable with insulin. Insulin is either injected or delivered by an adjustable pump under the skin. Insulin preparations suitable for ingestion or inhalation are under development. Type 1 diabetes is also called **insulin-dependent diabetes** or juvenile diabetes.

HOTLINK *See Chapters 6 and 6A for more information about insulin.*

Obesity is the most common cause of target tissue (for example, muscle, adipose, liver) resistance to insulin. In many individuals, the pancreas can compensate for insulin resistance by secreting more insulin. In individuals with **type 2 diabetes**, the pancreas cannot secrete enough insulin to compensate for insulin resistance, and high blood glucose and lipid levels result. Obesity and insulin resistance are part of the cluster of symptoms that defines the metabolic syndrome (see Chapter 6A). Approximately 20 million people have been diagnosed with type 2 diabetes in the United States. It is estimated that another

insulin-dependent diabetes Diabetes that requires insulin therapy. All people with type 1 diabetes require insulin therapy and many people with type 2 diabetes.

type 1 diabetes A form of diabetes mellitus that results from autoimmune destruction of insulin-producing beta cells of the pancreas. Hyperglycemia occurs if insulin treatment is inadequate.

type 2 diabetes Usually develops from resistance to the actions of insulin due to excess body fat. Ultimately both type 1 and type 2 are characterized by inadequate pancreatic beta cell insulin response.

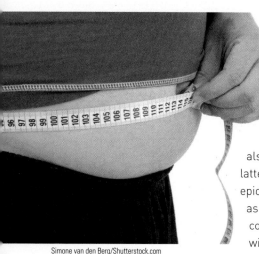

Simone van den Berg/Shutterstock.com

9 million people have the disease but have not been diagnosed and are not receiving treatment for it. Another 79 million people are categorized as prediabetic based on fasting blood glucose and the level of fasting glycosylated hemoglobin. Type 2 diabetes is also called *maturity-onset diabetes*. The latter name is outdated. With the obesity epidemic that is affecting young people, as well as adults, type 2 diabetes is becoming prevalent in children. Individuals with type 2 diabetes may be treated using a number of different drug classes. These drugs increase insulin sensitivity, increase insulin secretion, suppress liver release of glucose, or inhibit the absorption of ingested glucose from the intestine. Symptoms can also be reduced by a change in lifestyle that results in increased physical activity, a diet with lower saturated fat content, and weight loss.

(How does the development of type 1 diabetes differ from type 2 diabetes?)

There are complications common to type 1 and type 2 diabetes that compromise vision (retinopathy), kidney function (nephropathy), heart function (cardiomyopathy), and neural function (neuropathy). In fact, diabetic retinopathy and nephropathy are the most common causes of blindness and kidney disease in the Western world. These complications are microvascular and macrovascular in origin. It is these debilitating complications that ultimately are most significant in diminishing the quality of life in individuals with diabetes.

HOTLINK *See the website for the National Diabetes Education Program:* **http://ndep.nih.gov/** *for more information on the treatment of diabetes and its complications.*

Why Individuals with Diabetes Should Exercise

Individuals with diabetes should exercise for the same reasons that individuals without diabetes should exercise. Regular physical activity can reduce risks factors for cardiovascular disease. Individuals with type I and type 2 diabetes are predisposed to cardiovascular disease (Table 6B.1) and should be even more compelled to incorporate some form of exercise into their lifestyles. Exercise sensitizes the body to insulin and can alleviate symptoms of

insulin resistance or lead to a reduction in the doses of glucose-lowering drugs. Unfortunately, exercise will not improve the diminished beta-cell mass in individuals with type 1 diabetes and in those with type 2 diabetes who have diminished beta-cell function. The ability of exercise to sensitize the body to insulin may alleviate symptoms in those individuals with type 2 diabetes in whom insulin resistance is the primary pathology. The effects of regular exercise in individuals with type 2 diabetes are particularly profound if they are accompanied by weight loss.

TABLE 6B.1 Cardiovascular Disease Risk Factors That Are Potentially Improved by Regular Exercise

- Glucose intolerance
- Hyperinsulinemia
- Hyperlipidemia
- Coagulation abnormalities
- Hypertension
- Obesity

© Cengage Learning 2013

(How might exercise improve quality of life, especially in patients with type 1 or type 2 diabetes?)

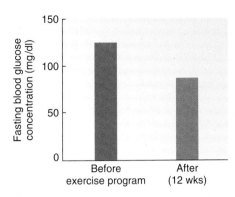

FIGURE 6B.1 The relationship of physical activity to fasting blood glucose in people with type 2 diabetes. A program of regular exercise can result in a reduction of fasting glucose and glycosylated hemoglobin in individuals with type 2 diabetes, both of which are indices of glucose control. (© Cengage Learning 2013)

Because glucose tolerance and insulin resistance are prominent defects in individuals with type 2 diabetes, regular exercise stands to be of great value in this population. Fasting blood glucose concentration is a marker of short-term control of blood glucose, and the glycosylated hemoglobin concentration (specifically hemoglobin A1c) is a marker of long-term regulation of blood glucose. In fact, regular physical activity in individuals with type 2 diabetes may decrease fasting blood glucose and reduce the amount of hemoglobin A1c in the blood, toward normal concentrations (Figure 6B.1). Reduced hemoglobin A1c, in particular, is associated with a delay in the development of the complications of

diabetes. Thus, the ability of regular exercise to reduce hemoglobin A1c in individuals with type 2 diabetes has important implications for the long-term progression of this diabetic syndrome.

> How might exercise be of value to people who are obese, glucose intolerant, and have high fasting serum insulin concentration, but do not yet have diabetes?

One notable feature of the metabolic effects of exercise is that just one strenuous bout of exercise can have persistent effects that last long after its completion. Glucose tolerance is measured by the magnitude of the blood glucose excursion after the ingestion of a drink containing glucose. This is called an *oral glucose tolerance test*. The magnitude of the glucose excursion is directly related to the severity of glucose intolerance. Glucose intolerance caused by insulin resistance is a hallmark of type 2 diabetes. A single bout of exercise can improve glucose tolerance for an extended period after exercise. Figure 6B.2 shows glucose tolerance before

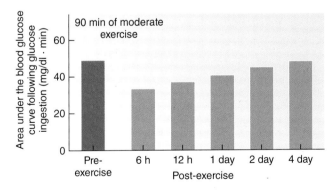

FIGURE 6B.2 Glucose tolerance is increased following exercise. Just one strenuous bout of exercise can have persistent effects that last long after its completion. Glucose tolerance is measured by the blood glucose excursion after ingestion of glucose. The glucose excursion is directly related to glucose intolerance. A single bout of exercise can improve glucose for an extended period after exercise. Glucose tolerance before 90 minutes of strenuous exercise and at different intervals afterward is shown. (© Cengage Learning 2013)

90 minutes of strenuous exercise and at different intervals afterward. Glucose tolerance is improved for up to 2 days after exercise. A part of the persistent effect of exercise on glucose tolerance is related to the glycogen-depletion and an acceleration of glycogen-repletion mechanisms. The persistence of glucose tolerance is also dependent on the intensity and duration of exercise and the dietary carbohydrate content before and after exercise.

HOTLINK *See Chapter 6A for more information about exercise and metabolic syndrome.*

Insulin action can be assessed using a diagnostic test called an *insulin clamp*. An infusion of insulin levels will cause a decline in blood glucose. During an insulin clamp, insulin is infused at a constant rate and glucose is infused in the blood to maintain glucose homeostasis. The glucose infusion rate during an insulin clamp is defined as the glucose disposal rate. The glucose disposal rate is directly proportional to insulin sensitivity. A program of regular exercise leads to a marked improvement in glucose disposal in individuals with type 2 diabetes (Figure 6B.3). Type 2 diabetes is associated with a defect in the ability to store glucose as glycogen. A benefit of regular exercise is that it specifically improves the effectiveness of insulin in stimulating muscle glycogen synthesis from glucose (see Figure 6B.3). The improvement in insulin sensitivity with regular exercise can be traced back to genes that express key proteins for muscle glucose metabolism. Figure 6B.4 shows how regular exercise increases the expression of GLUT4 in the trained muscle. As discussed in Chapters 5 and 6, GLUT4 is the protein required for insulin to stimulate the uptake of glucose by skeletal muscle.

For the reasons described earlier, exercise should be an important part of the lives of individuals with diabetes. However, the impaired regulation of metabolism associated with diabetes leads to challenges specific to those with diabetes.

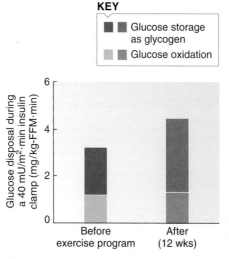

KEY
- Glucose storage as glycogen
- Glucose oxidation

● **FIGURE 6B.3 The effect of physical activity on insulin-stimulated oxidative and non-oxidative glucose disposal.** Glucose disposal during an "insulin clamp" is increased after a 12-week program of regular exercise. The increased glucose disposed of during an insulin clamp after a training program is stored as glycogen. (© Cengage Learning 2013)

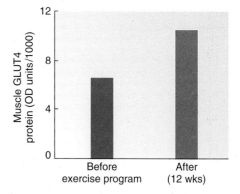

● **FIGURE 6B.4 Skeletal muscle GLUT4 expression with regular physical activity.** The expression of GLUT4 in the trained muscle is increased after a 12-week exercise program. GLUT4 is the protein required for insulin and exercise to stimulate the transport of glucose into skeletal muscle. (Modified from 1993. *Am. J. Physiol.* 264(6 Pt. 1):E855–E862. PMID: 8333511.)

Metabolic Response to Exercise in Individuals with Diabetes

Insulin concentration is an important determinant of the metabolic response to exercise. It is not surprising, therefore, that individuals with diabetes may be characterized by an abnormal response to exercise. Exercise intensity and duration, fitness, nutritional state, and environmental factors are all important in individuals with diabetes, as they are in the general population. In addition, factors relating to blood glucose control, use of insulin or other pharmacologic agents, and temporal relationship to feeding are critical to the metabolic response to exercise in individuals with diabetes. Depending on these factors, exercise may result in a deleterious hyperglycemic response or result in hypoglycemia in individuals with diabetes.

Exercise in Individuals with Type 2 Diabetes Not Treated with Insulin

Individuals with type 2 diabetes maintained on diet therapy alone are able to exercise with no more caution than the individual with normal glucose tolerance, provided that there are no major vascular or neurologic complications. There may be a tendency for hypoglycemia during prolonged exercise when oral hypoglycemic agents are used. Individuals with diabetes who are treated with pharmaceutical agents that work by increasing insulin concentration are particularly apt to become hypoglycemic. For many patients with diabetes, weight loss

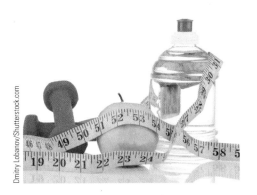

Dmitry Lobanov/Shutterstock.com

is an important aspect of their therapy. For this reason, these individuals may be maintained on a low-calorie diet. Exercise can be sustained during a low-calorie diet provided that an adequate amount of carbohydrates is used to maintain glycogen stores close to normal. The body compensates for a reduction in calories by increasing the hormone response to exercise so that the drive to mobilize substrates is increased. Severe calorie restriction over a period of days can be associated with cardiac arrhythmias and should not be done in conjunction with sustained physical exertion.

Exercise in Individuals with Diabetes Treated with Insulin

The release of insulin from the beta cells of the pancreas is spontaneously regulated in individuals with normal functioning pancreata, in accordance with metabolic needs. The inability of type 1 and some type 2 diabetics to regulate the delivery of insulin into the blood in a similar fashion can seriously compromise their ability to meet the metabolic requirements of exercise. Given the state of current glucose sensing and insulin delivery technology, it is extremely difficult to duplicate the normal metabolic responses in nondiabetics. Frequently, insulin delivery is mismatched to insulin needs, and risk for hypoglycemia or exacerbated **hyperglycemia** can result. The following sections address the problems of overinsulinization and underinsulinization. Figure 6B.5 summarizes the potential repercussions of too much or too little insulin.

The results of the Diabetes Complications Clinical Trials, an assessment of the effects of blood glucose control on the long-term complications of diabetes, demonstrated conclusively that tight glucose control prevents or delays the progression of microvascular complications. Whereas the Diabetes Complications Clinical Trials

hyperglycemia High blood glucose characteristic of diabetes. Can occur transiently with stress or in response to a glucose-rich meal.

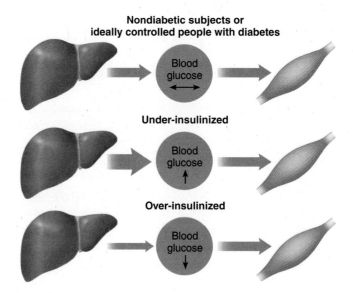

Nondiabetic subjects or ideally controlled people with diabetes

Blood glucose ↔

Under-insulinized

Blood glucose ↑

Over-insulinized

Blood glucose ↓

● FIGURE 6B.5 **Insulin treatment and the regulation of blood glucose in people with diabetes.** Moderate exercise in individuals with diabetes that is ideally controlled and healthy subjects maintain euglycemia during exercise (top). Moderate exercise in individuals with diabetes who are undertreated with insulin will exhibit an increase in blood glucose (middle). Moderate exercise in individuals with diabetes who are overtreated with insulin will exhibit a decline in blood glucose. (Modified from 1979. *Diabetes.* 28(2):147–163. Review. No abstract available. PMID: 369929.)

findings provide a firm basis for advocating tight metabolic control in individuals with diabetes, the move toward more rigorous control creates an added risk for hypoglycemia and is exemplified by the third panel of Figure 6B.5.

Too Much Insulin

All individuals with diabetes treated with subcutaneous insulin injections are over-insulinized at times. If this occurs during exercise, the increases in the release of glucose from liver and free fatty acids from adipose tissue that normally occur are inhibited. Because muscle glucose utilization increases with exercise, the attenuation of glucose release from the liver leads to a decline in circulating glucose (see Figure 6B.5). If the exercise period is sufficiently long, hypoglycemia will eventually result (see Figure 6B.6). Because exercise is one of the main causes of hypoglycemia in individuals treated with insulin, the implementation of treatment regimens designed to achieve tight control requires an understanding of the factors that can increase the risk for hypoglycemia during exercise. Three factors make individuals who require insulin treatment vulnerable to becoming

overinsulinized and hypoglycemic during exercise:

1. The failure of plasma insulin to decrease as it does in nondiabetic subjects with exercise can result in relative overinsulinization. As a result, a dose of insulin appropriate while at rest may be excessive for exercise. A decrease in insulin is essential to the metabolic response to exercise. Individuals maintained on insulin should reduce their insulin dosage in anticipation of exercise or try avoiding exercise during periods of peak insulin action. A reduction in premeal insulin dose may be important for exercise conducted in the postprandial state.

2. The exercise-induced increase in insulin action may lead to a relative overinsulinization in people with diabetes that are treated with insulin if a compensatory decrease in insulin dosage is not made. Because the exercise-induced increase in insulin action can persist for many hours after exercise, subjects treated with insulin who have not made appropriate adjustments in insulin dosage

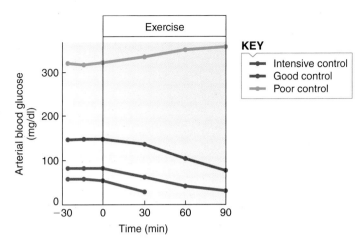

FIGURE 6B.6 The influence of intensive, good, and poor control on the glycemic response to exercise. Blood glucose responses to exercise in individuals with diabetes depend on how well blood glucose is controlled. Intensive control can result in serious hypoglycemia. Ingestion of a simple sugar can be used to counter hypoglycemia. (© Cengage Learning 2013)

risk becoming hypoglycemic long after the cessation of exercise.

3. The absorption of subcutaneously injected insulin can be accelerated by exercise (Figure 6B.7). Injecting away from the site of contraction can minimize this effect. The effect of exercise on insulin absorption can be increased even further if insulin is injected into the muscle, as opposed to the subcutaneous region of the working limb. Thus, extra care must be taken to avoid inadvertent injection into skeletal muscle. Even though precautions need to be made to minimize inappropriately rapid insulin absorption, it is important to realize that hypoglycemia can result

even when insulin mobilization is not accelerated.

In healthy, nondiabetic subjects, there are highly sensitive mechanisms for countering a decline in blood glucose. The hormones glucagon, epinephrine, and cortisol increase with very small changes in blood glucose during exercise and generally prevent overt hypoglycemia. In individuals with diabetes, the response of these hormones to hypoglycemia is often impaired. There are at least two reasons for this defect. The first one is that autonomic nerve dysfunction (that is, neuropathy) that often accompanies diabetes can lead to an impaired sympathetic nerve response to hypoglycemia, thereby increasing the risk for hypoglycemia. The second is that recent hypoglycemic episodes impair the endocrine response to exercise and subsequent episodes of hypoglycemia.

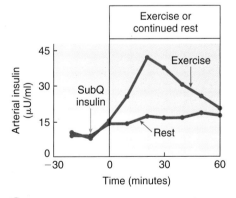

FIGURE 6B.7 The influence of exercise on the absorption of insulin injected subcutaneously. Exercise can accelerate the absorption of insulin in individuals treated by subcutaneous injections, increasing the risk for hypoglycemia. (© Cengage Learning 2013)

What are ways that defective glucagon, catecholamine, and cortisol secretion may contribute to insulin-induced hypoglycemia?

HOTLINK *See Chapter 6 for more information about hormones and exercise.*

There are many ways to manipulate the timing and amount of insulin administration and food intake to best avoid hypoglycemia. It is clear that a reduction in insulin dose in anticipation of exercise decreases the risk for hypoglycemia. This is particularly important in the postprandial state because the extra insulin needed to minimize the glycemic excursion in response to feeding can create insulin levels that, although normal for meal ingestion, are excessive when exercise is added. Individuals with diabetes maintained on intensive insulin therapy using either multiple subcutaneous injections or continuous subcutaneous insulin infusion are particularly vulnerable to becoming hypoglycemic if the insulin injection is given or the infusion is increased within 2 hours before the onset of exercise. Hypoglycemia can be avoided if insulin dosage before the onset of exercise is decreased. This may effectively re-create the decrease in circulating insulin that is normally seen with exercise.

> How might this persistent increase in insulin action be problematic for individuals treated with insulin?

Too Little Insulin

Individuals with diabetes who are dependent on insulin treatment and who have poor metabolic control are hyperglycemic, hyperlipidemic, and ketotic. These markers of metabolic control are worsened by exercise when individuals with diabetes are treated with too little insulin. The blood glucose response in individuals with diabetes under poor control is illustrated in Figure 6B.6. Although glucose fluxes may be normal or accelerated, the mechanism for the response is different in individuals with and without diabetes. A greater fraction of the glucose released by the liver is from gluconeogenesis under insulin-deficient conditions. Muscle glucose utilization occurs even when insulin levels are deficient because the mass-action effect of hyperglycemia overcomes the impaired ability to take up glucose. Nevertheless, a smaller percentage of glucose used in diabetics who are deficient in circulating insulin is fully oxidized because of impaired activity of the key enzyme, pyruvate dehydrogenase. People with diabetes that are not meticulously controlled may also have diminished glycogen stores and increased lipid stores within the muscle. This may, in turn, result in a decrease and an increase, respectively, in the use of these intramuscular stores during moderate exercise. In individuals with diabetes, high-intensity exercise (>80% of maximum oxygen uptake) and resistance exercise often leads to an increase in blood glucose that persists after the completion of exercise even when they are well treated with insulin. Exercise of these types elicits hormone responses that resemble those that occur with stress (for example, high catecholamines, high cortisol). In subjects without diabetes, insulin increases, preventing a marked increase in blood glucose. In individuals with diabetes who require insulin therapy, the stress hormone response is unopposed and blood glucose increases.

> How do circulating insulin concentrations in the individual without diabetes normally differ from those in clients treated with insulin during high-intensity or high-resistance exercise?

Practical Considerations for Adapting Therapy to Physical Activity

Individuals with type 2 diabetes not treated with insulin and without extensive vascular or neurologic complications can generally exercise with no more concern than individuals without diabetes of equal cardiovascular fitness. However, this does depend to some extent on the pharmacologic agents being used. For example, the blood glucose-lowering drug metformin can result in lactic acidosis, which can be worsened further by high-intensity exercise. Also, people with type 1 or type 2 diabetes who are taking insulin should take a number of precautions. Table 6B.2 presents some general guidelines for patients taking insulin. It is impossible, however, to give precise guidelines for diet and insulin therapy that will be suitable for all individuals with diabetes who wish to be physically active. Moreover, the metabolic demands associated with exercise vary depending on the type of exercise. Nevertheless, some general strategies can be applied. Self-monitoring of blood glucose is now routine, with a number of lightweight easily portable devices on the market. Frequent self-monitoring of blood glucose should be conducted so that immediate risks for hypoglycemia or worsened hyperglycemia can be identified. Table 6B.3 describes the value of blood glucose

TABLE 6B.2 Prevention of Hypoglycemia or Hyperglycemia during Exercise

Before exercise
1. Estimate intensity, duration, and the energy expenditure of exercise.
2. Eat a meal 1–3 hours before exercise.

3. Administer insulin in accordance with anticipated requirements.
   a. Administer insulin >1 hour before exercise so that the peak insulin action does not coincide with the exercise period.
   b. Decrease the dose of insulin to compensate for increased insulin action during exercise.

4. Assess metabolic control.
   a. If blood glucose is <5 mmol/L (90 mg/dl), extra calories before exercise will likely be required.
   b. If blood glucose is 5–15 mmol/L (90–270 mg/dl), extra calories may not be required.
   c. If blood glucose is >15 mmol/L (270 mg/dl), delay exercise and measure urine ketones.
     i. If urine ketones are negative, exercise can be performed, and extra calories are not required.
     ii. If urine ketones are positive, take insulin and delay exercise until ketones are negative.

5. Do not use an exercising extremity as an injection site.
During exercise
1. Monitor blood glucose during long sessions.
2. Always replace fluid losses adequately.
3. If required, use supplemental carbohydrate feedings (30–40 g for adults, 15–25 g for children) every 30 minutes during extended periods of exercise.
After exercise
1. Monitor blood glucose, including overnight, if amount of exercise is not habitual.
2. Adjust insulin therapy to decrease immediate and delayed insulin action (intensive therapy regimens provide increased flexibility in adjusting insulin).
3. If required, increase calorie intake for 12–24 hours after activity, depending on the intensity and duration of exercise and risk for hypoglycemia.

Source: Adapted from Tsui, E., and B. Zinman. 1995. Exercise and diabetes: new insights and therapeutic goals. *Endocrinologist* 5:263–271.

TABLE 6B.3 Blood Glucose Monitoring

- Learn the glycemic response to different exercise conditions and in the postexercise state.
- Identify when changes in therapy or food intake are necessary.
- For more extreme sports (for example, skydiving, rock climbing, scuba diving), test blood sugar multiple times before exercise to establish a pattern.

© Cengage Learning 2013

monitoring. Self-monitoring of blood glucose also provides feedback for implementing therapy for subsequent exercise. If, before exercise, blood glucose readings are less than approximately 90 mg/dl, the risk for hypoglycemia is great, and exercise should not be initiated without the ingestion of glucose. If fasting blood glucose is greater than approximately 250 to 300 mg/dl and ketone bodies are present, patients are generally advised to administer insulin and delay exercising. In addition to pre-exercise evaluation, blood glucose monitoring should be performed during and after exercise with the primary purpose of minimizing the risk for hypoglycemia. It is important to consider not only the absolute blood glucose when monitoring, but also the rate at which any change in blood glucose may occur. For example, a glucose level that is stable at 100 mg/dl may reflect a safe situation, whereas a glucose level that is 100 mg/dl is indicative of an imbalance between glucose production and utilization if the preceding glucose measurement was 150 mg/dl. The latter situation would require further attention (that is, glucose ingestion).

The need to reduce the insulin dose before exercise and avoid administrating insulin in the region of the working muscles was emphasized in a previous section. Table 6B.4 lists precautions that can be taken to avoid having too much insulin in the blood during exercise. The precise size of any reduction in insulin depends on many factors that will vary from person to person. For prolonged exercise in the postprandial state, individuals maintained on intermediate- and short-acting insulin may decrease or omit the short-acting insulin, depending on the circumstances. Alternatively, the intermediate-acting dose could be reduced but supplemented with added short-acting insulin later in the day. Some individuals with diabetes are treated by a continuous subcutaneous insulin infusion using a pump, rather than by subcutaneous injection. Individuals using a pump who have the intention of exercising in the postprandial state should reduce the pre-meal insulin bolus. An advantage of using an insulin pump is that it eliminates much of the variability in circulating insulin levels that occurs because of exercise-induced changes in insulin absorption from subcutaneous depots. The reason for the decreased variability in insulin levels with a pump is that the insulin depot is in the device and not in a subcutaneous depot where it is subject to changes in the absorption profile.

Added glucose ingestion before, during, or after exercise may be a more practical alternative to reducing insulin dose in prevention of hypoglycemia. Exercise is often unanticipated, particularly in children. In these instances, the individual may have already committed to an insulin dose. Guidelines for ingestion of carbohydrates in prevention of hypoglycemia are listed in Table 6B.5. Maintaining a source of simple sugar during exercise is an important precaution in individuals with diabetes who are dependent on insulin.

HOTLINK *See Chapter 5 for more information on fuel utilization.*

TABLE 6B.4 Insulin Administration

- Be aware of interval of peak insulin action.
- Reduce the insulin dose if exercise is anticipated.
- Administer away from the working muscles.

© Cengage Learning 2013

TABLE 6B.5 Food Intake

- A source of carbohydrate should be readily available during and after exercise.
- Consume carbohydrates as needed to avoid hypoglycemia.
- Consume complex carbohydrates for prolonged exercise to prevent postexercise hypoglycemia.
- Stay well hydrated to prevent large shifts in blood pressure.

© Cengage Learning 2013

Aside from considerations relating to modifications in insulin delivery and glucose ingestion, such as type of exercise, duration of exercise, and time of exercise, several other considerations are necessary. Exercise that requires repetitive recruitment of large muscle groups, such as running or walking, cycling, or swimming, causes a large and sustained increase in oxygen uptake and is appropriate for obtaining long-term cardiovascular adaptations. A work intensity that elicits an increase to about 50% of an individual's maximum oxygen uptake and an exercise duration of longer than 20 minutes is sufficient to obtain exercise-related adaptation (Table 6B.6). Exercise of extended duration, however, increases the risk for hypoglycemia and should be undertaken with appropriate precautions. Competitive sports frequently require high-intensity exertion. This type of exercise is important not only because of its contribution to fitness, but also because many find it an enjoyable form of physical activity. The time of day that an individual exercises should be considered. The risk for hypoglycemia appears to be lowest if an individual engages in exercise in the morning before the pre-breakfast insulin dose. Insulin levels are usually lowest at this time. Late afternoon or early evening exercise can be hazardous if sufficient precautions are not taken to minimize the risk for hypoglycemia during sleep. This can be done by prudent insulin therapy and a snack before bedtime. Adapting insulin and diet therapy to regular exercise can be achieved if the time of day for exercise and the exercise parameters are consistent. Although this may be a reasonable objective for some adults, the spontaneity of exercise in children and the variety of different sports in which they may participate make this goal difficult to obtain.

The complications of diabetes may introduce unique practical considerations to an exercise regimen. Table 6B.7 lists precautions to take in individuals who have experienced development of diabetes complications. One of the most common complications of diabetes is diabetic neuropathy. Neuropathy means damage to the nerves that run throughout the body, connecting the spinal cord to muscles, skin, blood vessels, and other organs. As a result of peripheral neuropathy, individuals with diabetes may experience a lack of senses in their feet. The consequence of this is that blisters or other sores may be undetected and become seriously infected. This problem can be further exacerbated by poor blood flow to the extremities. Individuals with diabetes who have signs of peripheral neuropathy should avoid exercise that can be difficult on the feet (for example, running on a hard service) and should inspect their feet regularly. Autonomic neuropathy, which is also common in diabetes, affects the nerves that control the heart, regulate blood pressure, and control blood glucose levels. Damage to nerves in the cardiovascular system interferes with the body's ability to adjust blood pressure and heart rate. As a result, blood pressure may drop sharply after exercise, causing light-headedness or fainting. Damage to the nerves that control heart rate can result in tachycardia after exercise. The system

TABLE 6B.6 Characteristics of Exercise That May Delay Progression of Some Complications of Diabetes

Progression of some complications of diabetes is most likely to be delayed by exercise with the following characteristics:

- Is sustained (>20 minutes)
- Involves large muscle group
- Is moderate in intensity (< lactate threshold)

© Cengage Learning 2013

TABLE 6B.7 Individuals with Diabetes Should Take Special Care in Choosing an Exercise Modality

- Avoid exercise that leads to high arterial blood pressures if proliferative retinopathy, nephropathy, or cardiovascular disease is present.
- Autonomic neuropathy may reduce exercise tolerance and cause postexercise hypotension.
- Avoid exercise that causes excessive wear on legs and feet if peripheral neuropathy is present.

© Cengage Learning 2013

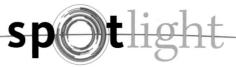

that restores blood glucose levels to normal in response to a decline may be affected by autonomic neuropathy. The consequence of this is a loss of the warning signs of hypoglycemia such as sweating and palpitations. Autonomic neuropathy may also cause impaired glucagon response to hypoglycemia in some individuals with diabetes. The deficient warning signs of hypoglycemia and impaired endocrine response in response to hypoglycemia are particularly serious deficits during exercise in insulin-dependent diabetes as the risk for hypoglycemia is high.

Longstanding diabetic retinopathy (that is, damage to the retina) is a microvascular disease characterized by damage to and closure of blood vessels. In response to this damage, new blood vessels grow in the retina. These new vessels are weak and can leak blood, blocking vision. Hypertension such as that that results from heavy weight lifting can increase leakage from these fragile vessels and lead to a further impairment in vision.

There are clearly circumstances that some individuals with diabetes should avoid, particularly those with longstanding diabetes with advanced complications. The philosophy in dealing with the difficult issue of exercise in individuals with diabetes has changed since the late 1980s. Previously, individuals with diabetes were steered away from different kinds of activities. This may be difficult and undesirable if a person enjoys a particular activity or sport. The more current thought is that the disease should not dictate lifestyle, but diet and therapy used to treat the disease should be adjusted to accommodate lifestyle.

spotlight

An Expert on Diabetes Prevention in the Young: Roberto P. Treviño, M.D.

Roberto P. Treviño grew up in San Antonio, Texas, in the downtown projects (public housing) and graduated from Brackenridge High School. He began his university training at San Antonio College, where he completed his first 30 hours of academics. He graduated with his medical degree from the National Autonomous University of Mexico in Monterrey in 1980, and completed his internal medicine residency at the University of Health Science/Chicago Medical School in 1983. Dr. Treviño is at the forefront of diabetes education and prevention, and was inducted into the Texas Diabetes Institute's Wall of Honor in 2006.

Treviño is the founder and the executive director of the Social and Health Research Center (S&HRC), a non-profit corporation founded in 1993 to study the healthcare needs of the Mexican American community. The primary clinic of the S&HRC is located just a few blocks from where Treviño lived as a youngster and went to high school.

Treviño, via the S&HRC and the San Antonio community, has developed the Bienestar and Neema programs. Studies by the S&HRC have reported significant relationships between diabetes and being overweight, diabetes and low educational attainment, and diabetes and low socioeconomic status.

The Bienestar Health Program is a bilingual school-based health program that aims to decrease dietary fat, increase physical fitness levels, prevent obesity, and prevent diabetes. The Neema Program is modeled after Bienestar but targets African Americans specifically. Both programs are research based and implement kindergarten through middle school learning activities based on social cognitive and capital health theories.

Social cognitive theory helps youths and adolescents understand the interrelationships between individual beliefs and knowledge, with regard to their surrounding social support, to promote positive health behaviors. Social capital theory helps youths and adolescents understand the interrelationships between financial, individual, and social messages that can help them change unhealthy behaviors.

The Bienestar and Neema programs have both been shown to reduce blood glucose levels in youths. Youngsters also learn to improve their health behaviors through four health programs: the Bienestar and Neema Health and P.E. Curricula, the After School Health Club, the Parent and Community Program, and the Cafeteria Program.

Both Bienestar and Neema have received national acclaim, and they have been implemented in several school curriculums in Texas and Mexico. Treviño served as a principal investigator on a national, multicenter, multimillion-dollar diabetes prevention study entitled "HEALTHY," sponsored by the National Institute of Diabetes and Digestive and Kidney Diseases. HEALTHY was conducted to determine whether lifestyle modifications (such as those for adults in the Diabetes Prevention Program) can reduce the diabetes risks for young adolescents. The study population included greater than 50 percent minorities, especially Mexican Americans and African Americans in lower socioeconomic categories. The primary results of the study were published in *the New England Journal of Medicine* ("A School-Based Intervention for Diabetes Risk Reduction," 2010;363:443–453).

in*Practice*

Examples of Exercise and Diabetes

This section provides some practical examples of how providing accurate exercise advice to your clients with diabetes relates to your area of interest (review the future career table from Chapter 1).

Health/Fitness: What lifestyle modification advice would you give an adolescent who is prediabetic (borderline high glucose levels that usually increase over time and age consistent with diabetic levels)? Studies such as the HEALTHY study encourage youths to maintain a healthy body mass index (see Chapter 13 for more information), participate in regular bouts of exercise, and eat healthy (see Chapter 11 for a more detailed discussion). Your client should be encouraged to participate in his school physical education and/or athletic programs as applicable. The client should consult with his physician regularly and educate himself about how to monitor his blood glucose. In addition, contacting and encouraging your client's parents to support his lifestyle modifications can be helpful and optimize his treatment.

Medicine: What lifestyle modification advice would you give an adult client who has type 2 diabetes? Research from the National Diabetes Prevention Program has shown conclusively that adults (regardless of ethnicity) can reduce their risk for diabetes by 58 percent with lifestyle modifications that include eating less fat and fewer calories, exercising for a total of 150 minutes per week, and aiming to lose 7 percent of their body weight with the goal of maintaining the weight loss. It appears that adults older than 60 can achieve even greater diabetes risk factor changes (71 percent reduction) by following the same guidelines.

Athletic Performance: What general recommendations can you give your diabetic athletic client? As discussed in this chapter, many considerations depend on whether your client is taking insulin and whether the client has an implanted insulin pump. However, you should encourage your client to monitor her glucose level regularly, carry a carbohydrate snack with her when exercising, carry medical identification, carry a cellular phone if possible, invest in quality shoe wear, and adjust her dietary and exercise routines appropriately for extreme environmental challenges (heat and cold).

Rehabilitation: What special considerations should you be aware of when treating an elderly diabetic patient? Obviously, you have to contend with the glucose, insulin, and diabetic neuropathy issues discussed in this chapter. In addition, you need to be aware that elderly diabetics are also at an increased risk for cardiovascular disease and stroke because of their age and the microvascular damage that occurs to the eyes, limbs (feet), and kidneys. Diabetes is typically a progressive disease that causes blindness, amputations, and renal failure. You should always assume that your elderly diabetic patient has cardiovascular limitations, in addition to the diabetes, unless it is medically documented otherwise. This assumption will help you adjust the FITT (frequency, intensity, time, and type) appropriately to optimize the benefits of exercise, whereas minimizing the hazards.

CONCEPTS, challenges, &controversies

Eliminating Barriers to Physical Activity and Maximizing Exercise Performance

What do NFL football star Jay Cutler, NBA basketball player Chris Dudley, elite long-distance runner Missy Foy, and five-time Olympic gold medal swimmer Gary Hall, Jr. have in common? They are a few of the great athletes with type 1 diabetes who have excelled at the upper tier of their sport. Two of baseball's icons, third baseman Ron Santo and pitcher Jim "Catfish" Hunter, played their entire major league careers with type 1 diabetes, as did hockey legend Bobby Clarke. Individuals with type 1 diabetes are able to participate in sports, and they can do so at a truly elite level. There is a need, however, to take precautions to avoid hypoglycemia. These may include adjustments in insulin dose and nutrient ingestion, accompanied by frequent blood glucose monitoring.

Diabetes is currently a chronic disease where treatment regimen is determined on a dose-to-dose basis by the individual with the disease. As a result, individuals with diabetes have a very sophisticated knowledge of their disease. A special few have made research into the cause, prevention, and treatment of diabetes a career. Three of these exceptional few share their thoughts on how they prepare for exercise.

Patrick T. Fueger, Ph.D., Assistant Professor, Herman B. Wells Center for Pediatric Research, Indiana University, Indianapolis, IN

I have had type 1 diabetes for more than 20 years and am treated by injection of insulin under my skin. Preventing hypoglycemia is my main concern before, during, and after exercise, especially long exercise sessions such as a bicycling more than 50 miles or running a marathon. I choose to start a moderate exercise session with a blood sugar level of approximately 200 mg/dl. My blood sugar will decline throughout the course of the aerobic exercise session, such that it will be approximately 100 mg/dl by the end of the session. For longer exercise sessions, I might consume additional calories before (such as a chocolate bar) and/or during (such as sports drinks) the exercise. An additional variable that I may manipulate is my insulin regimen before and/or after exercise. Because exercise increases insulin sensitivity, I often reduce my insulin dose by one third for longer exercise sessions. I largely make these adjustments to my insulin dose at dinner because I exercise in the late afternoon. I am careful to document relevant information (for example, blood sugars, insulin doses, time of day, exercise duration and intensity, weather) such that each exercise session becomes a learning experience that will better prepare the person with diabetes for performing exercise safely in the future.

Raul C. Camacho, Ph.D., Research Scientist, Merck Research Laboratories, Rahway, NJ

When I was diagnosed with type 1 diabetes at the age of 5, I also began playing soccer, and have not stopped playing since. Twenty-five years later, I continue to play my favorite sport, in addition to regularly exercising with nightly walks, bicycling, and weight lifting, all to help maintain control of my diabetes, in addition to having fun. I know what my blood glucose is before I start any prolonged exercise (like a full soccer game), and I will eat accordingly such that I anticipate having a little higher blood glucose than is optimal under normal conditions, even after exercise, just to be safe. After a game, and numerous times later in the day, I closely monitor my blood glucose to make sure it does not go too low. Over the past several years, I have learned about the effects of exercise on a body's ability to counter hypoglycemia, whether by letting the rest of the body know about it (increased hypoglycemic symptoms) or actually increasing the blood glucose (increased glucose production), and that these things can actually be attenuated for a day or so after prolonged exercise. Therefore, I continue close monitoring of my blood glucose for at least the next 24 hours. Conversely, in some people (including myself), strenuous exercise (like weight lifting) can sometimes paradoxically cause an increase in blood glucose. Keeping a diligent eye on my blood glucose level can also let me know of these times and, as a result, if I need to take a little more insulin.

Patricia L. Brubaker, Ph.D., Professor and Canada Research Chair, Department of Physiology, University of Toronto, Toronto, Ontario, Canada

I was diagnosed with type 1 diabetes when I was a graduate student, almost 30 years ago. At the time, I was much less active than I am today, having learned since then about the value of exercise to promote glycemic control and cardiovascular health, as well as mental well-being! My normal daily activities now include 60 minutes of dog walking, as well as a 6-kilometer (4-mile) round-trip to work on my bicycle. As these are routine events, I have already programmed a small reduction in my insulin requirements for these activities into my insulin pump. However, I also go to the gym about three times per week, where I do some form of aerobic exercise (that is, elliptical trainer, rowing machine, etc.) for 30 minutes. As I know by experience that my blood sugar may increase immediately after the exercise, but will definitely then fall about 2 to 4 hours later, I take a small amount of sugar (glucose) with the exercise and then monitor my blood sugars and adjust my insulin infusion rate appropriately for at least 8 hours after the exercise. Interestingly, I also played a great deal of squash a few years ago. Being a very competitive sport, my blood sugars always increased significantly during this activity, and I often was required to take insulin rather than glucose after the game to get back to normal. Finally, my main vacation activity is trekking in the mountains, and I have been fortunate enough to travel to the Himalayas on several occasions, as well as to climb Mt. Kilimanjaro. This type of activity provides the additional challenges of high altitude, cold temperatures, and exotic foods, on top of an increased level of exercise (for example, walking for 8–10 hours/day), and it is only through much more frequent glucose monitoring (up to 10 times/day) and appropriate adjustments in my insulin infusion rates that I manage to keep my blood sugars under any reasonable sort of control (and even then, not always).

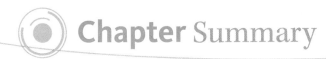

Chapter Summary

- Many people who treat or live with diabetes advocate the use of exercise because of the positive effects it may have in slowing the development of diabetic complications and improving overall quality of life.

- Type 1 diabetes is a disease where the body's immune system attacks and destroys its insulin-producing beta cells of the islets of Langerhans in the endocrine pancreas.

- In individuals with type 2 diabetes, the pancreas cannot secrete enough insulin to compensate for insulin resistance, and high blood glucose and lipid levels result.

- Individuals with diabetes should exercise for the same reasons that individuals without diabetes should exercise. Regular physical activity can reduce risks factors for cardiovascular disease.

- Glucose tolerance is measured by the magnitude of the blood glucose excursion after the ingestion of a drink containing glucose. This is called an oral glucose tolerance test. Exercise causes a persistent improvement in glucose tolerance.

- The improvements in insulin sensitivity with regular exercise can be traced back to genes that express key proteins for muscle glucose metabolism.

- There are many ways to manipulate the timing and amount of insulin administration and food intake to best avoid hypoglycemia. It is clear that a reduction in insulin dose in anticipation of exercise decreases the risk for hypoglycemia.

- Individuals with type 2 diabetes not treated with insulin and without extensive vascular or neurologic complications can generally exercise with no more concern than individuals without diabetes of equal cardiovascular fitness.

- In addition to pre-exercise evaluation, blood glucose monitoring should be performed during and after exercise with the primary purpose of minimizing the risk for hypoglycemia.

- Added glucose ingestion before, during, or after exercise may be a more practical alternative to reducing insulin dose in prevention of hypoglycemia.

Exercise Physiology Reality

CENGAGE brain To reinforce the exercise physiology concepts presented above, complete the laboratory exercises for Chapter 6B. To access labs and other course materials for this text, please visit www.cengagebrain.com. See the preface on page xiii for details. Once you complete the exercises, have your instructor evaluate your prescriptions. Remember to use your lab experience to help guide you toward future success in exercise physiology.

Exercise Physiology Web Links

Access the following websites for further study of topics covered in this chapter:

- Find updates and quick links to these and other diabetes and exercise physiology–related sites at our website. To access the course materials and companion resources for this text, please visit www.cengagebrain.com. See the preface on page xiii for details.

- Search for further information about diabetes at the Centers for Disease Control and Prevention website: http://www.cdc.gov/chronicdisease/resources/publications/AAG/ddt.htm.

- Search for further information on the effect of diet and exercise in the physically active diabetic at the American Diabetes Association website: http://www.diabetes.org/food-and-fitness/.

- Search for further information on exercise and diabetes at the Diabetes Exercise & Sports Association website: http://www.diabetes-exercise.org/.

- Search for further information about exercise and diabetes at the Centers for Disease Control and Prevention (CDC) website: http://www.cdc.gov.

- Search for information about exercise and diabetes at the American College of Sports Medicine website: http://www.acsm.org.

- Search for more information about exercise and diabetes at the President's Council on Fitness, Sports & Nutrition website: http://www.fitness.gov.

- Search for more information about exercise and diabetes at the National Diabetes Education Program (NDEP) website: http://ndep.nih.gov/.

Study Questions

Review the Warm-Up Pre-Test questions you were asked to answer before reading Chapter 6B. Test yourself once more to determine what you know now that you have completed the chapter.

The questions that follow will help you review this chapter. You will find the answers in the discussions on the pages provided.

1. Define the term diabetes mellitus and how it influences exercise and the exercise prescription for people with diabetes. *pp. 191, 199*

2. What is the difference between type 1 and type 2 diabetes? *p. 191*

3. Why is type 2 diabetes associated with lifestyle? *p. 194*

4. Why should individuals with diabetes participate in regular exercise? *p. 192*

5. What are two differences between exercise in individuals with diabetes who are and are not treated with insulin? *p. 195*

6. What precautions should your diabetic clients take to avoid having too much insulin in their blood during exercise? *p. 196*

7. Which general FITT (see Chapter 2) recommendations should you provide your diabetic clients? *p. 42*

8. List three guidelines for added glucose ingestion before, during, or after exercise. *p. 199*

9. Discuss the problems associated with diabetic neuropathy. *pp. 197, 201*

10. What precautions should an active diabetic athlete take before, during, and after exercise? *pp. 199–202*

Selected References

Camacho, R. C., P. Galassetti, S. N. Davis, and D. H. Wasserman. 2005. Glucoregulation during and after exercise. *Exerc. Sports Sci. Rev.* 33(1):17–23.

Crofford, O. B. Diabetes control and complications. *Annu. Rev. Med.* 46:267–279, 1995.

Department of Health, Physical Activity, Health Improvement and Prevention. 2004. *At least five a week: Evidence of the impact of physical activity and its relationship to health: A report from the Chief Medical Officer.* London: Department of Health, Physical Activity, Health Improvement and Prevention.

The HEALTHY Study Group. 2010. A school-based intervention for diabetes risk reduction. *New Engl. J. Med.* 363(5):443–453.

Riddell, M. C., and K. E. Iscoe. 2006. Physical activity, sport, and pediatric diabetes. *Pediatr. Diabetes.* 7:60–70.

Sigal, R. J., G. P. Kenny, D. H. Wasserman, C. Castaneda-Sceppa, and R. D. White. 2006. Physical activity/exercise and type 2 diabetes: A consensus statement from the American Diabetes Association. *Diabetes Care* 29(6):1433–1438.

Sigal, R. J., G. P. Kenny, D. H. Wasserman, and C. Castaneda-Sceppa. 2004. Physical activity/exercise and type 2 diabetes: Technical review. *Diabetes Care* 27(10):2518–2539.

Strong, W. B., R. M. Malina, C. J. Blimkie, S. R. Daniels, R. K. Dishman, B. Gutin, A. C. Hergenroeder, A. Must, P. A. Nixon, J. M. Pivarnik, T. Rowland, S. Trost, and F. Trudeau. Evidence based physical activity for school-age youth. *J. Pediatr.* 146:732–737, 2005.

U.S. Department of Health and Human Services. *Healthy people 2010: Understanding and improving health.* Washington, DC: U.S. Department of Health and Human Services, 2000.

Wasserman, D. H., Z. Shi, and M. Vranic. 2002. Metabolic implications of exercise and physical fitness in physiology and diabetes. Chapter 27 in *Diabetes mellitus: Theory and practice* (pp. 453–480), edited by D. Porte, R. Sherwin, and A. Baron. Stamford, CT: Appleton & Lange.

Wasserman, D. H., S. N. Davis, and B. Zinman. 2001. Fuel homeostasis. Chapter 4 in *The health professionals guide to diabetes and exercise* (pp. 63–100), edited by N. B. Ruderman and J. Devlin. Alexandria, VA: American Diabetes Association.

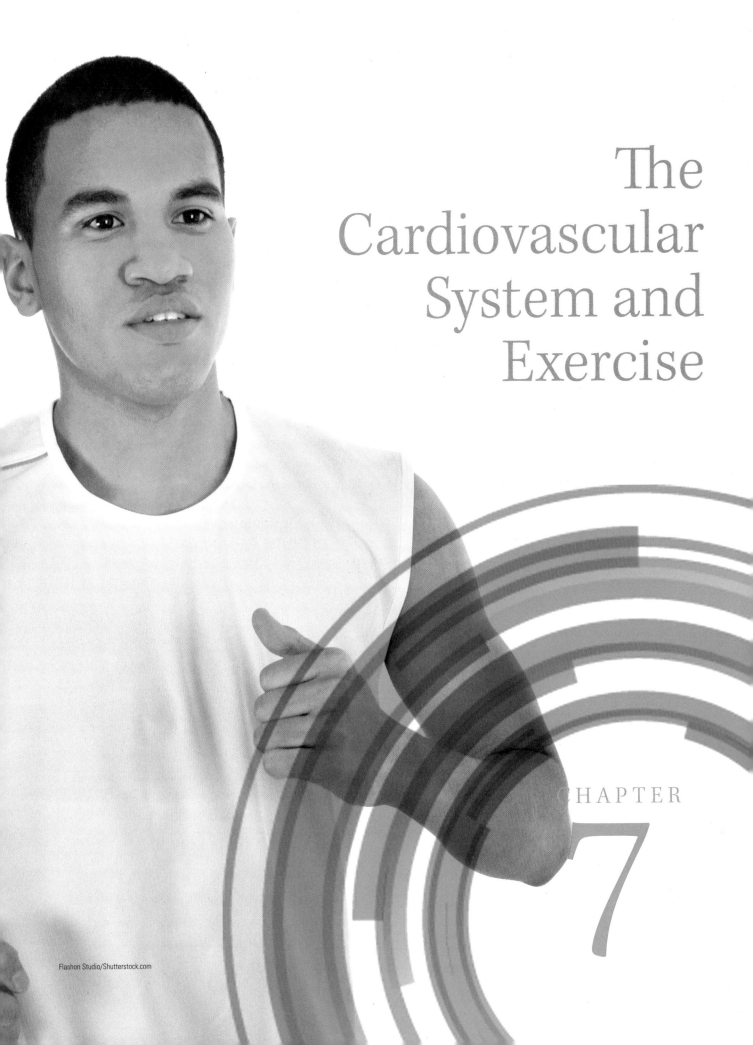

The Cardiovascular System and Exercise

CHAPTER

7

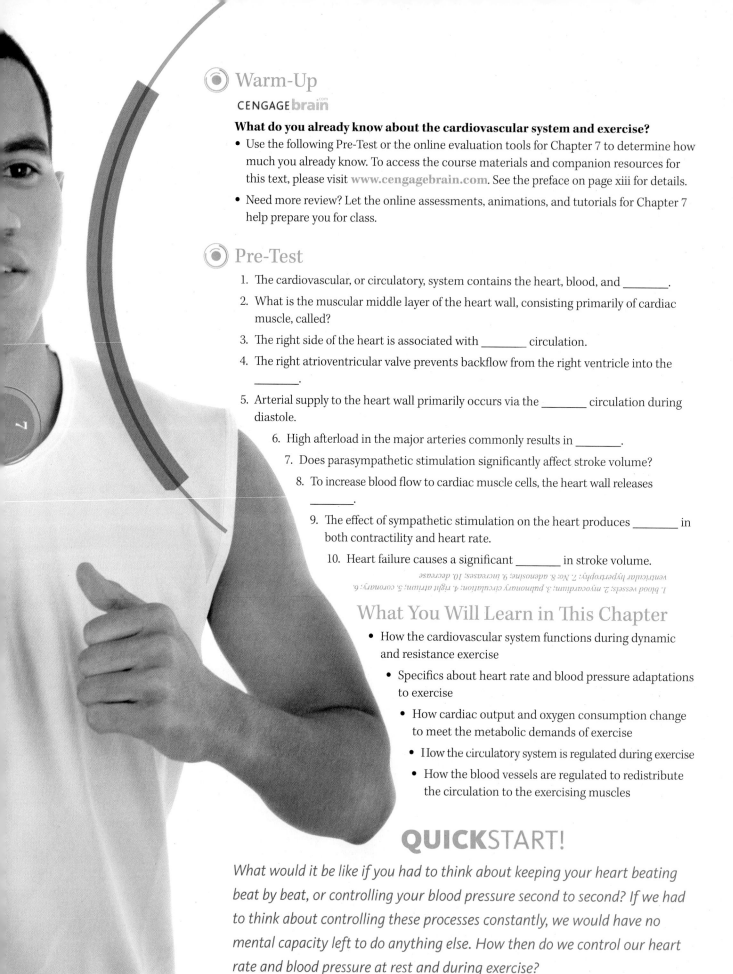

Warm-Up

CENGAGE **brain**

What do you already know about the cardiovascular system and exercise?

- Use the following Pre-Test or the online evaluation tools for Chapter 7 to determine how much you already know. To access the course materials and companion resources for this text, please visit **www.cengagebrain.com**. See the preface on page xiii for details.

- Need more review? Let the online assessments, animations, and tutorials for Chapter 7 help prepare you for class.

Pre-Test

1. The cardiovascular, or circulatory, system contains the heart, blood, and _____.

2. What is the muscular middle layer of the heart wall, consisting primarily of cardiac muscle, called?

3. The right side of the heart is associated with _____ circulation.

4. The right atrioventricular valve prevents backflow from the right ventricle into the _____.

5. Arterial supply to the heart wall primarily occurs via the _____ circulation during diastole.

6. High afterload in the major arteries commonly results in _____.

7. Does parasympathetic stimulation significantly affect stroke volume?

8. To increase blood flow to cardiac muscle cells, the heart wall releases _____.

9. The effect of sympathetic stimulation on the heart produces _____ in both contractility and heart rate.

10. Heart failure causes a significant _____ in stroke volume.

1. blood vessels; 2. myocardium; 3. pulmonary circulation; 4. right atrium; 5. coronary; 6. ventricular hypertrophy; 7. No; 8. adenosine; 9. increases; 10. decrease

What You Will Learn in This Chapter

- How the cardiovascular system functions during dynamic and resistance exercise

- Specifics about heart rate and blood pressure adaptations to exercise

- How cardiac output and oxygen consumption change to meet the metabolic demands of exercise

- How the circulatory system is regulated during exercise

- How the blood vessels are regulated to redistribute the circulation to the exercising muscles

QUICKSTART!

What would it be like if you had to think about keeping your heart beating beat by beat, or controlling your blood pressure second to second? If we had to think about controlling these processes constantly, we would have no mental capacity left to do anything else. How then do we control our heart rate and blood pressure at rest and during exercise?

Introduction to the Cardiovascular System and Exercise

In previous chapters, you learned about the health benefits, disease prevention, clinical rehabilitation, and athletic performance of moderate-to-vigorous intensity exercise. In Chapters 4 and 5, you are told about the physiologic concepts of cellular anaerobic and aerobic metabolism associated with the basics of skeletal muscle function and whole-body activity: The cells must receive oxygen for skeletal muscle contractions to occur over extended periods.

In this chapter, you will learn how:

1. Oxygen in the air is taken up by blood within the pulmonary circulation in the lungs

2. The heart, blood, and blood vessels work together as part of the **cardiovascular system** to deliver oxygen to the tissues of the body

3. This oxygenated or arterial blood is delivered by the pumping action of the heart via the circulatory system to all tissues of the body

4. At the tissues, the oxygen is unloaded from the arterial blood, which enables energy production via aerobic processes within the cell, which, in turn, supports muscle contraction

5. After the arterial blood passes through the active tissues and the oxygen is unloaded, the blood exiting the tissues has reduced oxygen content and an increase in carbon dioxide content, and is termed *venous blood*

6. With the help of the pressure gradient between the left side of the heart and the right side of the heart, as well as the "muscle and respiratory pumps," the venous blood is returned to the right side of the heart to again begin its journey through the lungs to pick up another load of oxygen for delivery to the tissues and unload the carbon dioxide.

This circulatory process is continuous both at rest and during exercise (see Figure 7.1).

To understand the link between the uptake of oxygen and the individual's circulatory capacity to deliver oxygen during **dynamic**, or **aerobic**, **exercise** and **isometric**, or **resistance**, **exercise**, you must first understand the functional capacity of the cardiovascular system, such as how the heart and blood vessels function, as well as how blood pressure and flow are related. To better understand acute responses to exercise, you must also understand the regulatory control mechanisms of the cardiovascular system.

The primary regulator of the circulation is the **autonomic nervous system (ANS)**, which is the principal system involved in the acute response to dynamic exercise. The ANS redistributes blood flow to active tissues away from the inactive tissues, primarily by increasing sympathetic activity to blood vessels, at the same time as it regulates **blood pressure (BP)** (the pressure exerted by blood against the arterial walls). Indeed, during high-intensity aerobic exercise or heavy-resistance exercise, the body is challenged to decide whether it needs to maintain BP or blood flow. In both hot and cold environments, the body is faced with a number of factors that influence its regulation of flow or pressure.

Elevated BP is the result of the heart pumping increased amounts of blood, as well as the vasoconstriction of the inactive vascular beds to redistribute blood flow to the active muscles. Increases in BP require reflex mechanisms to protect the brain from increases in perfusion pressure (the BP) and blood velocity in the cerebral blood vessels. In addition, as the duration and intensity of the exercise increases, metabolites from the exercising muscles and vascular active hormones,

cardiovascular system Consists of the heart and blood vessels that circulate blood to all major organs of the body.

dynamic or aerobic exercise Involves rhythmic contractions that primarily use aerobic energy production.

isometric exercise Involves a static muscle contraction that primarily uses anaerobic energy production.

resistance exercise When the isometric exercise involves some rhythmic dynamic contractions (for example, weight training).

autonomic nervous system (ANS) Includes both the sympathetic and parasympathetic (vagal) nerves.

blood pressure (BP) The pressure exerted by the blood against the blood vessel walls.

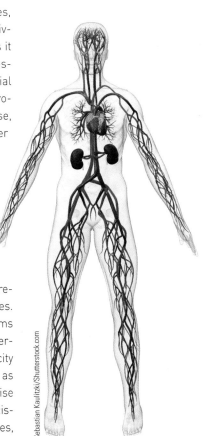

Sebastian Kaulitzki/Shutterstock.com

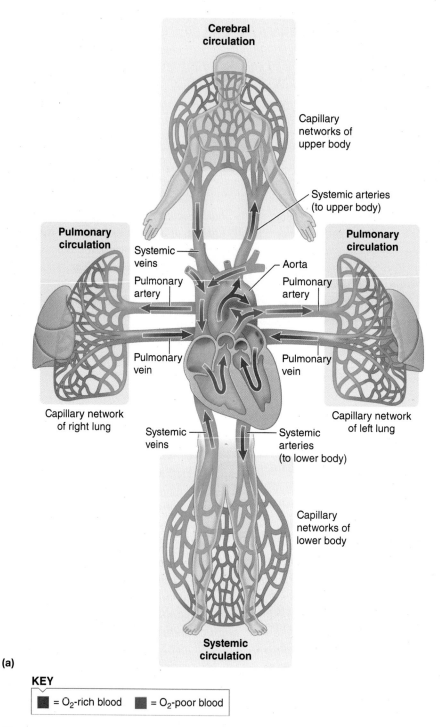

Cerebral
circulation

Capillary
networks of
upper body

Systemic arteries
(to upper body)

**Pulmonary
circulation**

Systemic
veins

Pulmonary
artery

Aorta

Pulmonary
artery

**Pulmonary
circulation**

Pulmonary
vein

Pulmonary
vein

Capillary network
of right lung

Systemic
veins

Systemic
arteries
(to lower body)

Capillary network
of left lung

Capillary
networks of
lower body

**Systemic
circulation**

(a)

KEY

■ = O₂-rich blood   ■ = O₂-poor blood

⬤ **FIGURE 7.1** **(a) The circulatory system consists of two separate vascular loops: the pulmonary circulation, which carries blood between the heart and lungs; and the systemic circulation, which carries blood between the heart and organ systems.** Each of these loops forms a figure eight with the pulmonary circulation simultaneously supplying the right and left lungs and the systemic circulation simultaneously supplying the upper body and lower body. (From Sherwood, L. 2010. Figure 9.1 in *Human physiology*, 7th ed. Belmont, CA: Brooks/Cole-Cengage Learning; and Sherwood, L. 2010.)

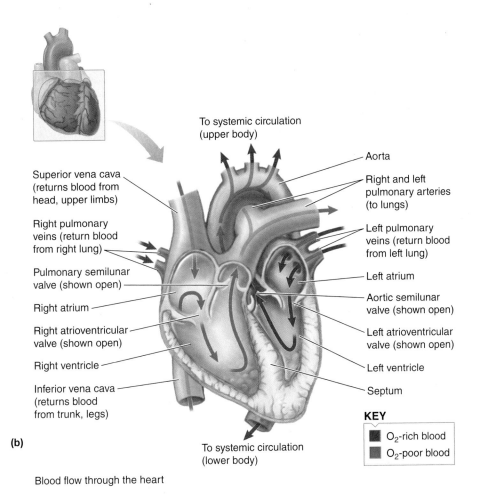

To systemic circulation
(upper body)

Aorta

Right and left
pulmonary arteries
(to lungs)

Superior vena cava
(returns blood from
head, upper limbs)

Right pulmonary
veins (return blood
from right lung)

Left pulmonary
veins (return blood
from left lung)

Pulmonary semilunar
valve (shown open)

Left atrium

Right atrium

Aortic semilunar
valve (shown open)

Right atrioventricular
valve (shown open)

Left atrioventricular
valve (shown open)

Right ventricle

Left ventricle

Inferior vena cava
(returns blood
from trunk, legs)

Septum

(b)

KEY

To systemic circulation
(lower body)

■ O$_2$-rich blood

■ O$_2$-poor blood

Blood flow through the heart

FIGURE 7.1 (b) Blood flow through and pump action of the heart. Arrows indicate the direction of blood flow. All of the heart valves are shown open, which is never the case, to illustrate the direction of blood flow through the heart. The right side of the heart receives O$_2$-poor blood from the systemic circulation and pumps it into the pulmonary circulation. The left side of the heart receives O$_2$-rich blood from the pulmonary circulation and pumps it into the systemic circulation. (Figure 9.2a in *Human physiology.* 7th ed. Belmont, CA: Brooks/Cole-Cengage Learning.)

such as norepinephrine, angiotensin II, and endothelin, become involved in regulating BP and circulatory redistribution.

A similar understanding of acute circulatory responses and the neural control of the circulation during static (isometric) exercise is needed, but because researchers once believed that isometric, or resistance, exercise training had relatively few cardiovascular health benefits, it has received far less attention, and hence less information

is currently available. However, as the age of the population increases, and incidences of falls increase, it is becoming more accepted to use weight training as a means of maintaining neuromuscular and bone health to ensure the ability of the elderly to perform dynamic exercise. Therefore, the use of resistance exercise, or weight training exercise, is becoming a greater part of the health professional's toolkit in preventive health programs.

Overview of the Cardiovascular System

To contrast the workings of the cardiovascular system under conditions of exercise, this section begins with a brief review of the anatomy and physiology of the system at rest. Then the physiologic effects of the two types of exercise, dynamic and isometric (or resistance), are discussed to demonstrate how the cardiovascular system adapts from the homeostasis of rest to the challenge of progressive increases in exercise intensity, or the homeostasis of steady-state exercise.

The Heart Pumps Oxygen-Poor Blood to the Lungs and Oxygen-Rich Blood to the Body

The main organs of the circulatory system are the heart and blood vessels. The heart is a muscle about the size and shape of your fist. Although we think of the heart as one pump, it actually consists of two pumps (see Figure 7.1).

HOTLINK *Visit the course materials for Chapter 7 for a detailed animation of the circulatory system (heart and blood vessels).*

The inferior and superior vena cavae channel the venous blood returned into the right side of the heart via the right atrium, and blood then flows through the right atrioventricular (AV), or tricuspid, valve into the right ventricle, which pumps the blood to the lungs. During the transfer of the venous blood from the right atrium to the right ventricle, the blood is thoroughly mixed, and as it exits the ventricle into the pulmonary artery, a sampling of the blood provides the most accurate measure of venous oxygen content. While circulating the alveoli of the lungs, the blood picks up oxygen, rids itself of carbon dioxide, and is returned to the left side of the heart by the pulmonary vein entering the left atrium. The blood passes from the left atrium across the left AV, or bicuspid (mitral), valve into the left ventricle. The left ventricle pumps the oxygen-rich blood into the systemic circulation to deliver the oxygen to your cells and produce the energy you need to meet the demands of the activities of daily living.

The Heart Is a Pump

In engineering terms, a functional pump requires a simple push/pull piston, which can increase its rate of pumping similar to that of an automobile. An increase in the rate of pumping (acceleration) increases the output of the pump. However, the heart is a dual pump, which increases the rate of pumping by increasing its **heart rate (HR)**. In addition, the heart is able to increase the volume of blood pumped for each heartbeat (**stroke volume [SV]**) by intrinsic changes in the muscle function related to the amount of blood being returned to the heart and sympathetic stimulation. What is extraordinary about the healthy heart's pumping is that the two pumps deliver the same volume of blood during each beat into their respective circulations.

Electrocardiogram

The heart requires an intrinsic neural network that is connected to an external neural system (the ANS), which coordinates the electrical activity of the heart, to ensure that the right and left pumps of the heart pump (beat) synchronously and can speed up and slow down simultaneously. External recordings of the electrical activity of the heart is known as an *electrocardiogram*, and is used for measuring HR and analyzing the patterns of the electrical activity (depolarization and repolarization) for diagnostic purposes.

The flow of electrical depolarization of the cells of the heart is described in

heart rate (HR) The number of times the heart beats (contracts) in one minute.

stroke volume (SV) The volume of blood pumped during one heart beat.

Figure 7.2. Note that the sinoatrial (SA) node initiates a wave of cell depolarization across the atria and down the internodal pathway that connects the SA node to the AV node at the junction of the atria with the ventricles. In the healthy heart, the AV node is the only point of electrical connectivity between the atria and the ventricles, and acts as a gate to funnel the electrical activity from the atria to the ventricle. The AV node has a slight delay in transmission of the depolarization wave in the bundle of His (this delay can be shortened by catecholamines). The bundle of His connects to the Purkinje fibers, and the Purkinje fibers enable the simultaneous spread of the depolarization wave across the left and right ventricles. Depolarization of the cells of the contractile muscle fibers is required to initiate contraction of the muscle. Therefore, by tracking the wave of depolarization and repolarization with the electrocardiograph and knowing the normal time intervals (seconds) between the specific waves (formed by deflections from the isoelectric zero) identified as the P wave, QRS complex, and the T wave, the cardiologist is able to diagnose specific heart conditions (see Figures 7.3 and 7.4) and recommend further evaluations to confirm the diagnoses, if necessary.

In the healthy heart, the electrical depolarization of the heart's muscles and their contraction are linked, but at no time can the heart muscle contract without the muscle being depolarized (see Figure 7.5).

As the HR increases during exercise, because of the increased sympathetic activity and parasympathetic withdrawal, the time to fill the ventricle with the venous return decreases. The volume of venous blood returned for each beat then needs to proportionally increase, and the transmission speed of the electrical activity in the AV node needs to increase to maintain and/or increase the heart's **cardiac output ($\dot{Q}$)**.

The heart beats (contracts) at different rates and is dependent on whether the body is at rest or at work. On average, when resting, the heart beats 72 times per minute. Clinically, within normal limits (WNL) values for resting HR range from 50 to 80 beats/min. However, elite endurance performers have resting HRs ranging from 30 to 40 beats/min. Nonendurance-trained individuals with HRs this low would be clinically diagnosed with sinus bradycardia, or may be in a ventricular escape rhythm

cardiac output ($\dot{Q}$) The volume of blood pumped by the heart in one minute.

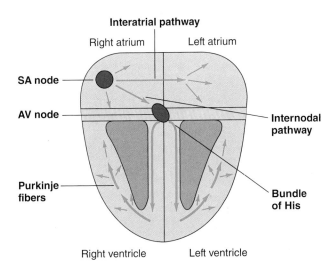

FIGURE 7.2 Spread of cardiac excitation. An action potential initiated at the SA node first spreads throughout both atria. Its spread is facilitated by two specialized atrial conduction pathways, the interatrial and internodal pathways. The AV node is the only point where an action potential can spread from the atria to the ventricles. From the AV node, the action potential spreads rapidly throughout the ventricles, hastened by a specialized ventricular conduction system consisting of the bundle of His and Purkinje fibers. (From Sherwood, L. 2010. Figure 9.14 in *Human physiology.* 7th ed. Belmont, CA: Brooks/Cole-Cengage Learning.)

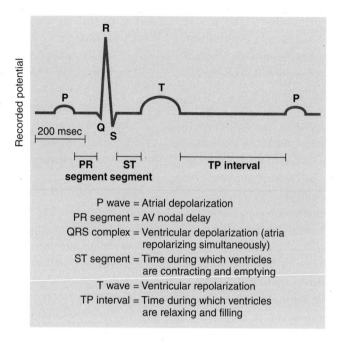

FIGURE 7.3 Electrocardiogram waveforms in lead II. (From Sherwood, L. 2010. Figure 9.19 in *Human physiology,* 7th ed. Belmont, CA: Brooks/Cole-Cengage Learning.)

and usually have symptoms of lightheadedness, dizziness, and fainting. How the athlete's heartbeat remains in sinus rhythm at these very low resting HRs remains a question. During strenuous physical activity, your HR increases because your working muscles need a larger supply of blood with oxygen and other nutrients to meet the demands of the activity. The HR response to exercise is discussed further later in the chapter.

HOTLINK *Visit the course materials for Chapter 7 to view animations on the events associated with the electrocardiograph.*

Arteries Carry Oxygen-Rich Blood to Cells, Whereas Veins Carry Oxygen-Poor Blood Back to the Heart

Blood is carried from the heart via arteries to the capillaries of various tissues, where oxygen and other nutrients are delivered to individual cells. After the physiologic exchange of oxygen and nutrients occurs in the capillaries, blood is returned to the heart via the veins. The systemic circulation consists of the blood flowing from the left ventricle to the right atrium, whereas the pulmonary circulation consists of blood flowing from the right ventricle to the left atrium. Figure 7.1 highlights the differences between the various blood vessels. An artery is a blood vessel that channels blood away from the heart, and a vein is a blood vessel that channels blood toward the heart. The pulmonary artery is the only artery in the body that carries deoxygenated

REDAV/Shutterstock.com

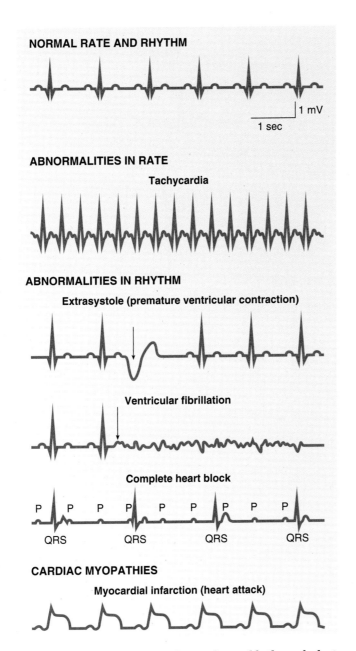

NORMAL RATE AND RHYTHM

1 mV
1 sec

ABNORMALITIES IN RATE

Tachycardia

ABNORMALITIES IN RHYTHM

Extrasystole (premature ventricular contraction)

Ventricular fibrillation

Complete heart block

P P P P P P P P P
QRS   QRS   QRS   QRS

CARDIAC MYOPATHIES

Myocardial infarction (heart attack)

FIGURE 7.4 Representative heart conditions detectable through electrocardiography. (From Sherwood, L. 2010. Figure 9.15 in *Human physiology*, 7th ed. Belmont, CA: Brooks/Cole-Cengage Learning.)

blood, and the pulmonary vein is the only vein that carries oxygenated blood.

One exception to the veins only carrying venous blood is when they are involved in temperature regulation in the heat, and they anastomose (directly join an artery) and bypass the capillary beds. The arteries act as conduits for blood to flow throughout the body to all tissues. However, the conduit artery vessels are connected to arterial resistance vessels, and the resistance vessels vasoconstrict when stretched by an increase in intraluminal pressure and vasodilate in response to a decrease in intraluminal pressure. This mechanism is known as **autoregulation**, and it effectively maintains blood flow relatively constant and is most prominent in the cerebral circulation.

However, the ANS is connected to the arteries and veins, and actively regulates the diameter of the arterial resistance vessels in conjunction with vasoconstrictor regulatory hormones (norepinephrine, angiotensin II, endothelin, among others) and vasodilator hormones and metabolites

autoregulation An intrinsic mechanism that enables a blood vessel to automatically alter its diameter.

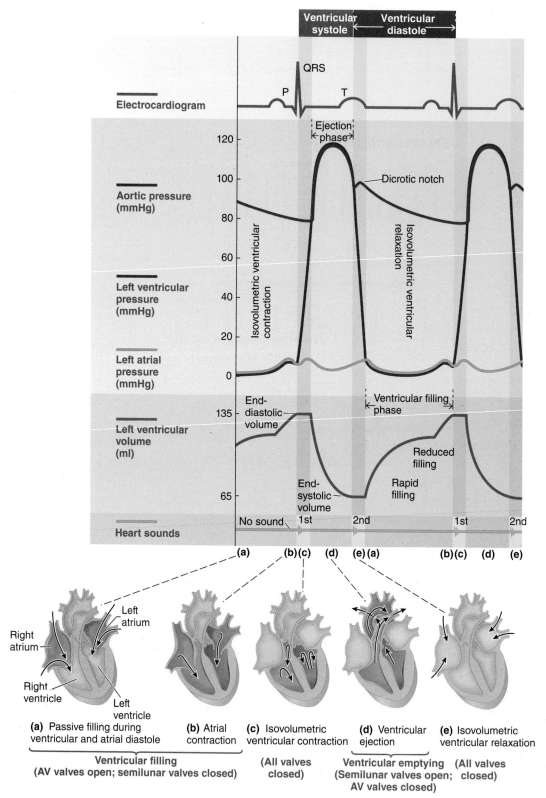

Ventricular systole ⟷ **Ventricular diastole**

Electrocardiogram

QRS

P   T

Ejection phase

Aortic pressure (mmHg)

120

100 — Dicrotic notch

80

Isovolumetric ventricular contraction   Isovolumetric ventricular relaxation

60

Left ventricular pressure (mmHg)

40

20

Left atrial pressure (mmHg)

0

Left ventricular volume (ml)

135 — End-diastolic volume

Ventricular filling phase

Reduced filling

End-systolic volume   Rapid filling

65

Heart sounds

No sound   1st   2nd   1st   2nd

(a)   (b)(c)   (d)   (e)(a)   (b)(c)   (d)   (e)

Left atrium

Right atrium

Right ventricle   Left ventricle

(a) Passive filling during ventricular and atrial diastole

(b) Atrial contraction

(c) Isovolumetric ventricular contraction

(d) Ventricular ejection

(e) Isovolumetric ventricular relaxation

Ventricular filling (AV valves open; semilunar valves closed)

(All valves closed)

Ventricular emptying (Semilunar valves open; AV valves closed)

(All valves closed)

FIGURE 7.5 Cardiac cycle. Graph depicting various events that occur concurrently during the cardiac cycle. Follow each horizontal strip across to see the changes that take place in the electrocardiogram; aortic, ventricular, and atrial pressures; ventricular volume; and heart sounds throughout the cycle. The last half of the diastole (one full cardiac cycle) and another systole are shown for the left side of the heart. Follow each vertical strip downward to see what happens simultaneously with each of these factors during each phase of the cardiac cycle. The sketches of the heart illustrate the flow of O_2-poor (dark blue) and O_2-rich (dark pink) blood in and out of the ventricles during the cardiac cycle. (From Sherwood, L. 2010. Figure 9.16 in *Human physiology*, 7th ed. Belmont, CA: Brooks/Cole-Cengage Learning.)

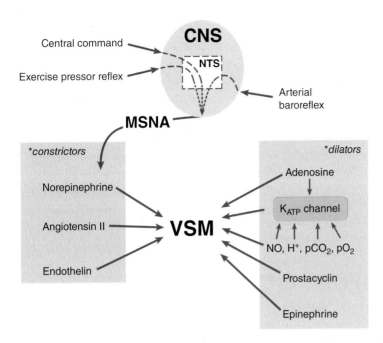

FIGURE 7.6 Schematic model of central and local control of the blood vessels. (© Cengage Learning 2013)

(epinephrine, prostacyclin and nitric oxide [NO], hydrogen ions, adenosine, among others; see Figure 7.6).

When the diameter of an artery is reduced, the blood vessel is vasoconstricted and blood flow decreases, and when the diameter is enlarged, the blood vessel is vasodilated and blood flow increases. The regulation of the blood vessels during exercise is discussed further later in this chapter.

Blood Pressure Is Determined by the Heart Pumping Blood into the Blood Vessels

The heart is the main pump that develops the energy to push blood through the systemic, cerebral, and pulmonary circulations. The amount of energy added to the circulation is reflected in the BP. The BP is similar to a garden hose after turning on the tap: Before turning on the tap, the hose has no pressure inside; but after turning on the tap, the hose fills with water. Because the walls of the hose are restraining the water to flow only inside the hose, the pressure builds up in relation to the amount of water flow and resistance the walls of the

hose impart on the water flow. Thus, BP is determined by how much blood the heart pumps through the blood vessel, as well as the resistance the arterial walls provide against the blood flowing through them.

The BP is measured in terms of systolic, mean, and diastolic pressure. When the heart contracts and pushes blood out into the circulation, the peak pressure measured in the arteries is known as the **systolic blood pressure (SBP)** because it occurs as a result of the peak contraction (systole) of the heart. When the heart relaxes (diastole), no blood flows from the heart into the arteries, and the pressure in the arteries declines to a low point known as the **diastolic blood pressure (DBP)**. The DBP never goes to zero because the next systole, or heart contraction, refills the pulmonary artery and aorta before the blood completely drains from the arteries (see Figure 7.7).

This pressure wave is propagated throughout the arterial tree and at specific anatomic locations. This provides the clinician with both qualitative and quantitative points of reference to judge the adequacy of the circulation in specific limbs or organs of the body. The pressure wave is the rate of change of pressure (dp) per unit change

systolic blood pressure (SBP) The peak pressure exerted by the pressure wave of the blood against the blood vessel walls.

diastolic blood pressure (DBP) The lowest pressure exerted by the pressure wave of the blood against the blood vessel walls.

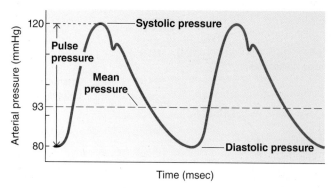

FIGURE 7.7 Arterial blood pressure. The systolic pressure is the peak pressure exerted in the arteries when blood is pumped into them during ventricular systole. The diastolic pressure is the lowest pressure exerted in the arteries when blood is draining off into the vessels downstream during ventricular diastole. The pulse pressure is the difference between systolic and diastolic pressure. The mean pressure is the average pressure throughout the cardiac cycle. (From Sherwood, L. 2010. Figure 10.7 in *Human physiology.* 7th ed. Belmont, CA: Brooks/Cole-Cengage Learning.)

mean blood pressure or mean arterial pressure (MAP) The average pressure exerted by the pressure wave of the blood against the blood vessel walls.

total peripheral resistance (TPR) The total resistance to blood flow within the cardiovascular system.

of time (dt) and reflects the velocity of the blood flow in the vessel. The integration of the pressures over time between the SBP and DBP is the **mean blood pressure**, or **mean arterial pressure (MAP)**. The velocity varies with the **total peripheral resistance (TPR)**, and the resistance is related to the changes in vessel diameter encountered as the blood flows through the circulatory system and to the cardiac output (Q̇). The Q̇ is the amount of blood pumped by the heart in 1 minute (L/min).

In the body, the relationship between pressure, flow, and resistance is expressed as:

$$MAP/\dot{Q} = TPR \qquad [7.1]$$

Example calculation:

Given: MAP = 120 mmHg; Q̇ = 20 L/min

Equation 7.1 is 120/20 = 6 resistance units

HOTLINK *See the American Heart Association website to learn more about within normal limits (WNL) values for blood pressure:* **http://www.americanheart.org/presenter.jhtml?identifier=4450**.

Measuring Blood Pressure

The BP can be measured in two different ways: with a standard cuff or directly through arterial catheterization. The more common method that is usually performed in the physician's office is termed *brachial auscultation*. See Figures 7.7 and 7.8 for a review of BP auscultation.

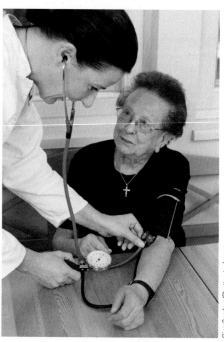

The BP can also be measured directly by catheterizing an artery connected to an electronic pressure transducer to provide a replica of the arterial pressure wave, as depicted in Figure 7.7. It makes no difference which artery is cannulated to directly measure the pulsatile pressure to obtain the average, or MAP or DBP, but to ensure accuracy, you always need to have the measuring pressure transducer zeroed to heart level. However, as the arterial blood vessels become narrower farther away anatomically from the aorta, the peak (systolic) pressure becomes augmented and

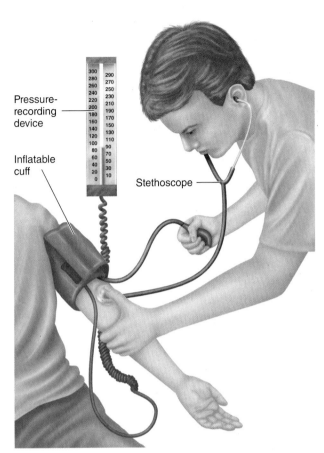

(a) Use of a sphygmomanometer in determining blood pressure

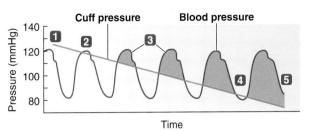

When blood pressure is 120/80:

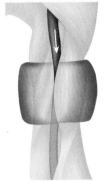

When cuff pressure is greater than 120 mm Hg and exceeds blood pressure throughout the cardiac cycle:

No blood flows through the vessel.

1 No sound is heard because no blood is flowing.

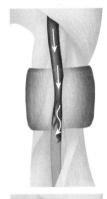

When cuff pressure is between 120 and 80 mm Hg:

Blood flow through the vessel is turbulent whenever blood pressure exceeds cuff pressure.

2 The first sound is heard at peak systolic pressure.

3 Intermittent sounds are produced by turbulent spurts of flow as blood pressure cyclically exceeds cuff pressure.

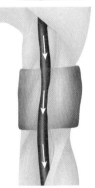

When cuff pressure is less than 80 mm Hg and is below blood pressure throughout the cardiac cycle:

Blood flows through the vessel in smooth, laminar fashion.

4 The last sound is heard at minimum diastolic pressure.

5 No sound is heard thereafter because of uninterrupted, smooth, laminar flow.

(b) Blood flow through the brachial artery in relation to cuff pressure and sounds

● **FIGURE 7.8 Auscultation.** (a) The pressure in the sphygmomanometer (inflatable cuff) can be varied to prevent or permit blood flow in the underlying brachial artery. Turbulent blood flow can be detected with a stethoscope, whereas smooth laminar flow and no flow are inaudible. (b) Red shaded areas in the graph are the times during which blood is flowing in the brachial artery. (From Sherwood, L. 2010. Figure 10.8 in *Human physiology.* 7th ed. Belmont. CA: Brooks/Cole-Cengage Learning.)

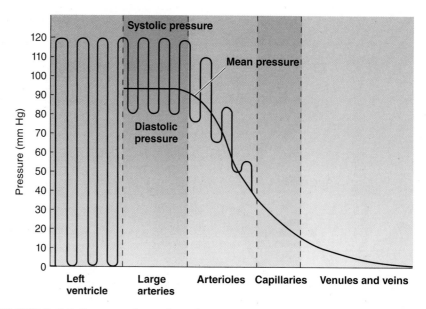

FIGURE 7.9 Pressures throughout the systemic circulation. Left ventricular pressure swings between a low pressure of 0 mm Hg during diastole to a high pressure of 120 mm Hg during systole. Arterial blood pressure, which fluctuates between a peak systolic pressure of 120 mm Hg and a low diastolic pressure of 80 mm Hg each cardiac cycle, is of the same magnitude throughout the large arteries. Because of the arterioles' high resistance, the pressure declines precipitously and the systolic-to-diastolic swings in pressure are converted to a nonpulsatile pressure when blood flows through the arterioles. The pressure continues to decline but at a slower rate as blood flows through the capillaries and venous system. (From Sherwood. L. 2010. Figure 10.9 in *Human physiology.* 7th ed. Belmont, CA: Brooks/Cole-Cengage Learning.)

does not reflect true systolic pressure. This augmentation of the pressure wave becomes more problematic with radial or brachial artery catheterization during exercise (see later in this chapter). Figure 7.9 summarizes the BPs that occur throughout the systemic circulation.

Clinically, direct catheterization of blood vessels is usually done in the resting state and poses little threat of movement complications; however, the systolic pressure wave augmentation from catheterization of a peripheral artery is always a factor to consider. In many exercise physiology laboratories around the world, arterial catheterizations of volunteer subjects have become routine procedures for skilled physicians.

The Cardiovascular System under Conditions of Exercise

Because we have briefly reviewed the cardiovascular system at rest, we are now ready to examine the system under conditions of exercise. There are two types of exercise: dynamic, or aerobic, and isometric (static), or resistance. Dynamic exercise involves rhythmic contractions that change muscle length and joint angles without generating large intramuscular forces; it primarily uses aerobic energy production and is sometimes called *aerobic exercise.* It includes activities such as running, bicycling, swimming, and so on. In contrast, isometric, or static, exercise primarily involves anaerobic energy production and also involves a sustained contraction that does not change muscle length and joint angles. Isometric exercise (static exercise) results in large increases in intramuscular force in direct relation to the absolute intensity of the contraction, or

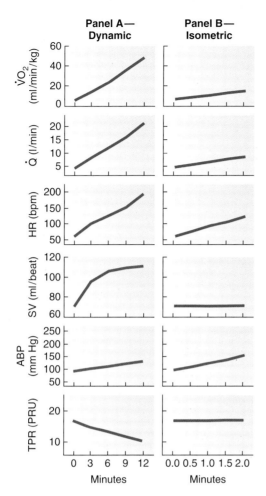

Panel A— Dynamic

Panel B— Isometric

$\dot{V}O_2$ (ml/min/kg)

$\dot{Q}$ (l/min)

HR (bpm)

SV (ml/beat)

ABP (mm Hg)

TPR (PRU)

Minutes

FIGURE 7.10 Cardiovascular responses to dynamic and isometric exercise. (From Mitchell, J. H., and P. B. Raven. 1994. Cardiovascular response and adaptation to exercise. Figure 17.2 in *Physical activity, fitness and health: International consensus statement* [pp. 286–298], edited by C. Bouchard, R. Shepard, and T. Stephens. Champaign. IL: Human Kinetics.)

the percentage of the individual's **maximal voluntary contraction** (% **MVC**). Figure 7.10 compares the average cardiovascular responses of a 30% MVC isometric exercise with that of maximal dynamic exercise.

When the isometric exercise involves some rhythmic dynamic contractions, it is termed *resistance exercise*. Therefore, an activity such as weight lifting is a form of resistance exercise; however, activities such as circuit weight training involve both aerobic and resistance exercises.

During progressive increases in dynamic exercise intensity, the circulatory response is directly related to the increase in exercise intensity until **maximal oxygen uptake ($\dot{V}O_2$ max)** is achieved. Similarly, the magnitude of the circulatory response

to isometric exercise is related to the intensity (% MVC) of the exercise and the amount of muscle mass being contracted (for example, arms vs. legs). However, during isometric exercise, the increase in $\dot{Q}$ is a result of the increases in HR only, whereas in dynamic exercise, $\dot{Q}$ increases as a result of increases in HR and SV. Another significant difference in the cardiovascular response to the two types of exercise is that in isometric exercise, the large increase in BP for a given **oxygen uptake ($\dot{V}O_2$)** is a result of an increase in $\dot{Q}$ into a vasoconstricted vasculature, whereas in dynamic exercise, the modest increase in arterial pressure is a balance between the increase in $\dot{Q}$ and the increases in total vascular conductance.

maximal voluntary contraction (MVC) The force generated by an individual's voluntary muscle contraction.

maximal oxygen uptake ($\dot{V}O_2$ max) The maximal rate of oxygen uptake ($\dot{V}O_2$) achieved during a progressive increase in work load exercise test.

oxygen uptake ($\dot{V}O_2$) The rate of oxygen uptake usually measured in liters/min.

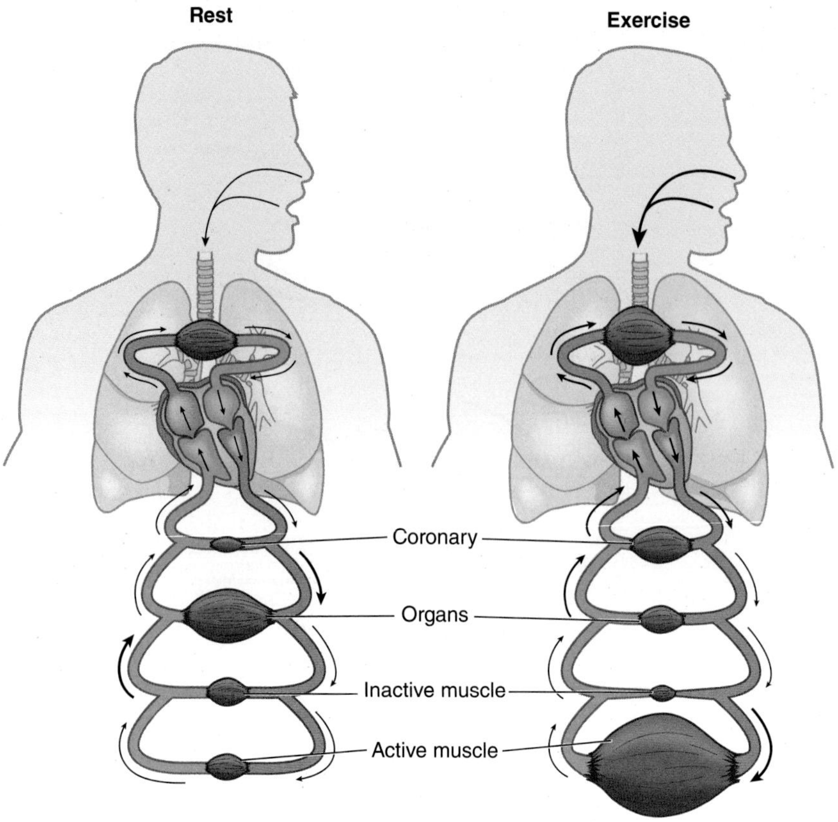

Rest

Exercise

Coronary

Organs

Inactive muscle

Active muscle

⊕ FIGURE 7.11 Schematic representation of the cardiovascular system at rest and during dynamic exercise. (Modified from J. T. Willerson and C. A. Sanders, editors. 1977. Figure 2, page 210 in *Clinical Cardiology*, Vol 3., *[The science and practice of clinical medicine]*, New York: Grune & Stratton (a subsidiary of Harcourt Brace Jovanovich).)

Dynamic Exercise Increases the Rate of Circulation and the Demands on the Body

During dynamic exercise, the rate of circulation increases up to a maximum of five to six times greater than at rest. A schematic representation of the cardiovascular system at rest and during dynamic exercise is presented in Figure 7.11. The increased speed of the circulation during exercise requires an increase in lung ventilation, rate of uptake of oxygen, pumping rate, and strength of heart contraction, and subsequently, flow of blood through the blood vessels, which results in increased oxygen being delivered to the exercising tissues. It is important to understand that any interruption or impairment of this process of oxygen delivery—caused by diseases of the lungs, heart, or blood vessels, and in some cases, rare genetic skeletal muscle diseases—will limit an individual's exercise

capacity. It is on this basis that the role of clinical exercise stress testing has evolved.

Without impairments of oxygen delivery and exercise performance imposed by disease, the function of the circulatory system can be improved up to an individual's genetic optimum by involvement in a program of regular endurance exercise training. The need to quantify the amount of training improvement that occurs and the need to determine the phenotype of genetically endowed performers (for example, the Kenyan middle- and long-distance runners) have pushed the practice of performance (or fitness) exercise testing to evolve (see Chapter 10).

Oxygen Uptake Increases during Dynamic Exercise

By comparing exercise with rest and by considering your own personal experiences, you can see that Q̇ (the quantity of blood pumped each minute by the heart, measured in L/min) increases during dynamic exercise. This occurs as HR (rate of beating, measured in beats/min) and SV (amount of blood pumped in each beat, measured in ml/beat) increase. This relationship is expressed mathematically as:

$$\dot{Q} \text{ (ml/min)} = \text{HR (beats/min)} \times \text{SV (ml/beat)} \quad [7.2]$$

Example calculation:

Given:

HR = 120 beats/min; SV = 100 ml/beat

Equation 7.2 becomes

$$120 \text{ beats/min} \times 100 \text{ ml/beat} = 12{,}000 \text{ ml/min} = 12 \text{ L/min}$$

The link between the rate of $\dot{V}O_2$ (in L/min; see also Chapter 10) and $\dot{Q}$ (L/min) is expressed mathematically as:

$$\dot{V}O_2 \text{ (L/min)} = \dot{Q} \text{ (L/min)} \times (a - v) O_2 \text{ difference (ml/L)} \quad [7.3]$$

This equation is known as the Fick equation, where a = the oxygen content of the arterial blood in ml/L, and v = the oxygen content of the venous blood in ml/L.

The term **(a − v) O₂ difference** is shorthand for the difference between the oxygen content of the arterial blood (measured in any artery) and the venous blood (measured in the pulmonary artery). This difference is an accurate, quantifiable representation of

the amount of oxygen extracted from the blood as it passes through the tissues.

Given:

$$\dot{V}O_2 = 500 \text{ ml/min} = 0.5 \text{ L/min};$$
$$\dot{Q} = 10 \text{ L/min}$$

Equation 7.3 becomes

$$0.5 \text{ L/min} / 10 \text{ L/min} = (a - v) O_2 \text{ difference} = 0.05 \text{ L/L} = 50 \text{ ml/L}$$

This means that for each liter of $\dot{Q}$, the tissues are extracting 50 ml oxygen.

(*Why is the oxygen content of the venous blood measured in the pulmonary artery?*)

From the relationships expressed in Equation 7.3, it can be deduced that $\dot{V}O_2$ max is a measure of the circulation's maximal capacity to deliver oxygen to the tissues. Therefore, Equation 7.3 can be rewritten to represent the maximal values as:

$$\dot{V}O_2 \text{ max} = \dot{Q} \text{ max} \times (a - v) O_2 \text{ diff max} \quad [7.4]$$

Calculate the following:

What is the $\dot{V}O_2$ max given a $\dot{Q}$ max of 20 L/min and (a − v) O₂ diff max of 180 ml/L?

HOTLINK *See the NASA website to learn more about the measurement of $\dot{V}O_2$ max:* http://ston.jsc.nasa.gov/collections/TRS/_techrep/TM-1998-104826.pdf.

(a − v) O₂ difference The amount of oxygen extracted by the tissues from one liter of blood.

inRETROSPECT

Measurement of Maximal Oxygen Uptake in Humans

A. V. Hill first conceived of the concept of maximal oxygen uptake ($\dot{V}O$ max) in humans in 1926 by predicting the amount of oxygen being used to achieve specific running speeds on a 400-meter cinder track. However, it was not until 1955 that Taylor, Buskirk, and Henschel established a valid and repeatable method of determining the $\dot{V}O_2$ max in humans in the laboratory by measuring ventilation and the expired gas concentrations during running exercise on a motor-driven treadmill. Then in 1958, Mitchell, Sproule, and Chapman made all of the necessary measurements of

the circulatory variables—HR, SV, and (a − v) O₂ difference (Equation 7.4) during treadmill exercise, using direct catheterization of the brachial artery and vein and dye dilution estimates of $\dot{Q}$, and measures of arterial and venous blood gases. Subsequent development of noninvasive foreign-gas rebreathing methods and fast-responding respiratory gas analyzers for accurately measuring $\dot{Q}$ have enabled the physician and nonphysician alike to routinely determine an individual's cardiovascular variables during submaximal and maximal exercise.

Normalization for Body Weight and Lean Body Mass

Because the amount of oxygen used by the body is related to the absolute amount of tissue using the oxygen for metabolism, both at rest and during exercise, exercise testing professionals and trainees use a method of normalizing the measurement of $\dot{V}O_2$ between subjects of different body weights (that is, ml O_2/kg of body weight) and different amounts of skeletal muscle (that is, ml O_2/kg of lean body mass or fat-free mass). Which normalization procedure used depends on what type of comparisons you are trying to make.

If you were to compare two individuals, both having a $\dot{V}O_2$ max of 5.0 L/min, you could conclude that they both have equal maximal circulatory capacities to deliver oxygen. However, Subject 1, a 25-year-old woman, weighs 70 kg, and Subject 2, a 25-year-old man, weighs 150 kg. Subject 1's $\dot{V}O_2$ max would be 5000 ml O_2/70 = 71.4 ml O_2/kg of her body weight; she is clearly an elite athlete. Subject 2's $\dot{V}O_2$ max would be 5000 ml O_2/150 = 33.3 ml O_2/kg of his body weight, which is below the average fitness level for 25-year-olds in the United States (normalized for body weight). Unfortunately, Subject 2's condition is fast becoming the norm for both men and women in the United States.

In the above example, we compared two individuals with different body weights; however, if we had also wanted to compare the differences related to sex, it would have been preferable to normalize the data to the individual's amount of lean body mass (muscle and bone tissue only; see Chapter 13). Such a comparison in the example above would only increase the differences between the female athlete and the sedentary unfit man.

Cardiac Output Is Progressively Increased during Progressive Increases in Intensity of Dynamic Exercise

It has become evident from the thousands of maximal dynamic exercise tests performed throughout the world that an invariant linear relationship exists between $\dot{Q}$ and $\dot{V}O_2$ from rest to maximal exercise (see Figure 7.12).

In healthy individuals, this relationship is expressed as approximating:

$$\dot{Q} \text{ (L/min)} = 5.5 \times \dot{V}O_2 \text{ (L/min)} + 5 \text{ (L/min)} \quad [7.5]$$

> Given a $\dot{V}O_2$ max of 5.5 L O_2, what is the individual's maximal $\dot{Q}$?

The approximations involve individual differences in the active skeletal muscle mass (metabolism) and hemoglobin concentrations (or the amount of oxygen being carried by the blood). The hemoglobin concentration of girls and premenopausal women is generally lower than that of boys and preclimacteric men, respectively, and explains most of the decreased $\dot{V}O_2$ max values observed between men and women, when normalized to lean body mass.

In rare cases, an individual (1/100,000) has a diagnosed muscle myopathy that, because of an enzyme deficiency, causes him or her to be unable to generate energy for ATP production. One such disease is McArdle disease, which is identified as an absence of the phosphorylase enzyme in the muscle, hence the metabolism of glycogen to glucose does not take place (for more details, see Chapter 4). At the beginning of exercise, the intracellular glucose

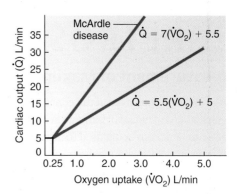

FIGURE 7.12 Schematic representation of the linear relationship between $\dot{V}O_2$ and $\dot{Q}$ during a progressive increase in dynamic exercise from rest to $\dot{V}O_2$ max in healthy normals and a McArdle disease patient. (© Cengage Learning 2013)

concentration is sufficient to support energy generation and ATP, but as the breakdown of glycogen is inhibited, the concentration of glucose in the cell decreases and becomes the limiting factor in the formation of ATP and results in excessive muscle pain and cessation of muscle contraction. However, while exercising, the muscles are sending neural signals to the brain (the exercise pressor reflex [EPR]) that identify a lack of energy to perform the exercise. These signals result in the cardiovascular center increasing the cardiac output ($\dot{Q}$) above that required to deliver the oxygen in healthy individuals, a condition known as a *hyperkinetic circulation* (see Figure 7.12).

Heart Rate and Stroke Volume

The increases in $\dot{Q}$ that occur during exercise in a normal healthy upright adult result from increases in HR and SV (see Figure 7.13).

In normally active healthy subjects at maximum exercise, there is usually a threefold increase in HR and a twofold increase in SV above resting values, resulting in a sixfold increase in $\dot{Q}$. In the highly trained endurance athlete, the increases in SV from rest to exercise do not exhibit a plateau and continue to have a progressive increase up to maximum and can result in an eightfold or greater increase in $\dot{Q}$. The reasons for this adaptation to endurance training are discussed in Chapter 8.

Heart Rate Increases during Dynamic Exercise

The relationship between HR and $\dot{V}O_2$ is linear and reproducible for each individual. The slope of the relationship between $\dot{V}O_2$ and HR is dependent on the individual's $\dot{V}O_2$ max and the individual's range of HR response (that is, HR rest to HR max; see Figure 7.14a).

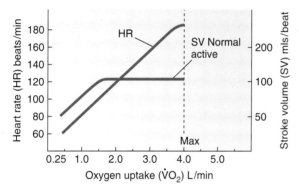

FIGURE 7.13 When normally active individuals progressively increase their exercise intensity from rest to $\dot{V}O_2$ max, their HR increases linearly and their SV increase plateaus at 40% $\dot{V}O_2$ max. (© Cengage Learning 2013)

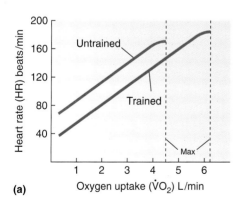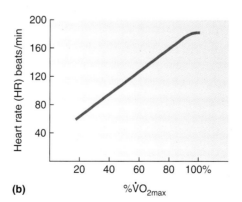

FIGURE 7.14 (a) Relationship between heart rate (HR) and oxygen uptake ($\dot{V}O_2$) up to maximal $\dot{V}O_2$ ($\dot{V}O_2$ max) for endurance exercise–trained and untrained individuals. (b) Relationship between HR and $\dot{V}O_2$ up to $\dot{V}O_2$ max for endurance exercise–trained and untrained individuals. (© Cengage Learning 2013)

These findings identify that for any given submaximal $\dot{V}O_2$, the HR of the trained individual will be lower than that of the untrained individual, but because the slope of the relationship between $\dot{Q}$ and $\dot{V}O_2$ is unchanged, regardless of training, the SV must be higher. However, the difference in the slope of the relationship is accounted for when the relationship between the HR responses to exercise (Y axis) are plotted against the increases in $\dot{V}O_2$ as relative to $\dot{V}O_2$ max, or % $\dot{V}O_2$ max (X axis) (see Figure 7.14b). Because the HR max of endurance-trained and untrained individuals of the same age are not different, it is best to design the endurance exercise training programs as a percentage of HR max. A more refined method of prescribing a training HR is to use the Karvonen formula, which accounts for the fitness difference in HR range (HR max − HR rest).

At birth, the population average for the average resting HR of the neonate is approximately 220 beats/min and is very near its maximal HR. During neonatal and infant development, the heart's intrinsic HR decreases and the ANS's control of the heart matures, resulting in a progressive reduction of the resting HR to the population's average resting HR of approximately 72 beats/min. As we age, our resting HR decreases and our maximal achievable HR is reduced because of a loss of pacemaker cells in the SA node, independent of the age-related loss of vagal control of the heart. The population average rate of this reduction is expressed as:

$$\text{HR max} = 220 - \text{age in years} \quad [7.6]$$

Notably, this relationship between age and maximal HR has been developed on a large population of average fit individuals and has a variance measure of 1 standard deviation equal to 10 beats/min. To encompass 98 percent of the adult population, individuals would be predicted to have a range of maximal HRs from 200 to 240 beats/min. However, a maximal HR of a mature young adult greater than 200 beats/min is rare, whereas HRs as high as 215 beats/min have been observed in teenagers.

If you rely on the age prediction formula of maximal HR to develop a training program for an individual health fitness or cardiac rehabilitation program, it may cause you to overpredict or underpredict the training stress. For example, a 60-year-old man wants you to devise a training program, and you decide to begin his training program at 60 percent HR max. Using the age prediction formula would require him to train at a HR of:

$$(220 - 60) \times 60\% = 160 \times 60/100$$
$$= 96 \text{ beats/min}$$

However, his measured maximal HR is 180 beats/min; therefore, for a 60 percent HR max training stimulus, he should be training at 108 beats/min. See Chapter 2 for further discussion about maximal HR and exercise training.

> Can you explain why it would be important to train individuals with different $\dot{V}O_2$ max values at the same % HR max than at the same absolute HRs?

Stroke Volume Increases during Dynamic Exercise

The heart functions to pump out what it receives from the systemic circulation, that is, the **venous return** or the amount of blood being delivered to the right side of the heart. Remember, the heart has two pumps—the right atrium and ventricle and the left atrium and ventricle—and the volume output of each pump is equal. SV is the amount of blood pumped by the heart in each beat and represents the difference between the heart's **end-diastolic volume (EDV)**—the volume of blood in the ventricles at the end of diastole—and its **end-systolic volume (ESV)**—the volume of blood in the ventricles at the end of systole (see Figure 7.15). This relationship can be expressed as:

$$\text{SV (ml/beat)} = \text{EDV (ml)} - \text{ESV (ml)} \quad [7.7]$$

venous return The amount of venous blood measured in liters returning to the heart in one minute.

end-diastolic volume (EDV) The volume of blood in the heart when the end of the heart muscle's relaxation is complete or when filling is complete.

end-systolic volume (ESV) The volume of blood in the heart when the heart muscle's contraction is maximal and emptying is complete.

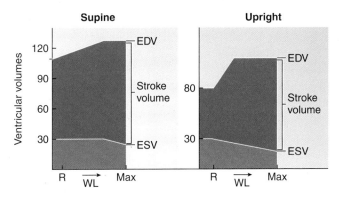

FIGURE 7.15 Left ventricular volumes for an untrained individual performing cycling exercise from rest to maximal exercise in the supine and upright positions. (Adapted from Poliner, L. R., G. J. Dehmer, S. E. Lewis, R. W. Parkey, C. G. Blomqvist, and J. T. Willerson. 1980. Left ventricular performance in normal subjects: A comparison of the responses to exercise in the upright and supine positions. *Circulation* 62:528–534.)

Example calculation:

Given: EDV = 200 ml

Equation 7.7 is 200 − 100 = SV = 100 ml/beat

$$ESV = 100 \text{ ml}$$

To estimate the heart's **ejection fraction**, divide the SV by the EDV related to it at the beginning of each beat. This measurement of ejection fraction is usually made in the left ventricle and provides a clinical estimate of the heart's clinical function, or health. See Table 7.1 for a listing of the normal ranges of cardiac volumes, ejection fraction, and heart rate measurements made at rest.

$$\text{Ejection fraction (\%)} = SV/EDV \times 100$$

or

$$(EDV − ESV) \times 100/EDV \qquad [7.8]$$

TABLE 7.1 Normative Volume Data for the Left Ventricle

Measure	Typical Value	Normal Range
end-diastolic volume (EDV)	120 ml	65–240 ml
end-systolic volume (ESV)	50 ml	16–143 ml
stroke volume (SV)	70 ml	55–100 ml
ejection fraction (E_f)	58%	55–70%
heart rate (HR)	72 bpm	
cardiac output ($\dot{Q}$)	4.9 L/minute	4.0–8.0 L/min

© Cengage Learning 2013

Example calculation:

Given: SV = 100 ml/beat; EDV = 200 ml

Ejection fraction = 100/200 = 50 percent

SV is directly related to **central blood volume (CBV)**. The posture in which the exercise is being performed affects the absolute value of the SV. In the supine position at rest, CBV, EDV, and SV are greater than in the upright position (see Figure 7.15).

During exercise in the supine position, such as in swimming the backstroke, increases in CBV, and, therefore, EDV and SV, result from the **muscle pump** (the action of the contracting skeletal muscles) increasing venous return. The measured EDV is regarded as the heart's **preload**.

During exercise in the upright position, such as walking, running, and upright bicycling, the muscle pump increases venous return and EDV to values equal to those of the resting supine position only for the normally active individual, even at maximal workloads (see Figure 7.15). When the $\dot{V}O_2$ of the workload performed in the supine position is the same as that performed in the upright position, the $\dot{Q}$ will be the same. Consequently, the HR of the supine workloads will be lower than the upright workloads.

(Why are heart rates different for supine and upright workloads?)

central blood volume (CBV) The volume of blood in the heart chambers, lungs, and central arterial blood vessels.

ejection fraction The amount of blood pumped each beat (stroke volume) divided by the end-diastolic volume, expressed as a percentage.

muscle pump The contracting skeletal muscles work in conjunction with competent venous valves to effectively drive blood back to heart.

preload The right atrial pressure for the right ventricle and the pulmonary wedge pressure for the left ventricle.

The data in Figure 7.15 provide insight into how the increasing SV associated with the increasing dynamic exercise workloads is ejected from the heart. The physiologists Frank and Starling studied this mechanism and determined that the increased venous return produced by the muscle pump increases EDV and, consequently, the filling pressure of the heart (preload). The increases in EDV and cardiac filling pressures increase the length of the cardiac muscle fibers, resulting in a greater intrafiber tension that results in a greater contraction force and a greater SV. This relationship is known as the **Frank–Starling mechanism**. The reductions in ESV and the increases in ejection fraction at the time when peak systolic pressure (afterload) is increasing are evidence of an increase in myocardial contractility.

From the data in Figure 7.15, you can see that the *increase in SV during supine* exercise is more reliant on the Frank–Starling mechanism until very near peak exercise. A combination of the Frank–Starling mechanism and increases in myocardial contractility is required to *increase SV during upright* exercise, especially when the increased venous return has achieved the supine EDV value. Involvement of myocardial contractility in generating the SV in the upright position occurs because of the need to generate a greater force of contraction to overcome the increasing aortic pressure, or MAP, in the upright compared with the constant MAP in the supine position. Consequently, the arterial pressure (afterload) indirectly affects the SV achieved.

> (*Why does the heart have to contract more strongly in the upright position?*)

In average fit individuals, when the supine EDV value is achieved during a progressive increase in the workload exercise test, the SV plateaus at approximately 40 percent $\dot{V}O_2$ max (see Figure 7.13). Therefore, further increases in $\dot{Q}$ are achieved only by increasing the HR. This SV plateau

is not present in highly trained endurance athletes. Currently, the reason for this difference between the trained and the untrained endurance athlete remains hotly debated. The two possible mechanisms, pericardial restraint and a balance between venous return and cardiac filling times, are discussed in Chapter 8.

HOTLINK *See the Cardiovascular Physiology Concepts website to learn more about ejection fraction:* **http://www.cvphysiology.com/Cardiac %20Function/CF012.htm**.

Venous Return Increases during Dynamic Exercise

Two additional mechanisms affect venous return at rest and during exercise: the muscle pump and the respiratory pump. They are generally regarded as auxiliary circulatory pumps.

Muscle Pump

The muscle pump requires the presence of competent, or working, venous valves. The large veins have one-way valves approximately 2 to 4 centimeters (cm) apart. These valves allow blood to move forward toward the heart but not backward into the capillaries. In addition, the venous valves counteract the effects of gravity in the upright position. During dynamic exercise, the combination of skeletal muscles contracting and the venous valve inhibiting retrograde flow away from the heart operates to provide a continuous pumping action of the blood toward the heart. Immediately after a muscle contraction (the first seconds of muscle relaxation), the veins exiting from the contracted muscle are empty, and the intravenous pressure approximates zero (see Figure 7.16). Because the venous valves prevent any backflow, the pressure gradient from the arterial (MAP, 90 mm Hg) to the venous side (venous pressure, 0) can be as high as 90 mm Hg. During exercise, the pressures in the legs can be as high as 200 mm Hg.

The importance of the venous valves in assisting the muscle contractions in returning blood to the heart is readily apparent in patients with a congenital absence

Frank–Starling mechanism As the length of the ventricular fibers are stretched, the contraction force of the fiber becomes greater.

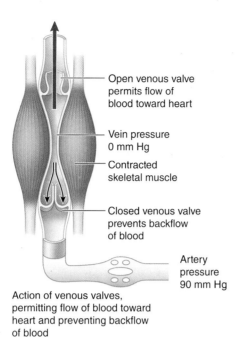

Open venous valve permits flow of blood toward heart

Vein pressure 0 mm Hg

Contracted skeletal muscle

Closed venous valve prevents backflow of blood

Artery pressure 90 mm Hg

Action of venous valves, permitting flow of blood toward heart and preventing backflow of blood

FIGURE 7.16 Function of venous valves. Venous valves permit the flow of blood toward the heart. (From Sherwood, L. 2010. Figure 10.32 in *Human physiology*, 7th ed. Belmont, CA: Brooks/Cole-Cengage Learning, and Rowell, L. B. 1993. Figure 1.14 in *Human cardiovascular control*. New York: Oxford University Press.)

of venous valves. The absence of the valves results in there being no mechanism to inhibit the backflow during the relaxation phase of the muscle after contraction of the muscle; hence EDV and Q̇ decrease instead of increasing.

As a consequence of the muscle pump mechanism, the greater the frequency and strength of the muscle contractions, the greater the venous return to the heart. When the upright posture is sustained for a long period and when the muscle contractions are at a minimum, the blood pools in the veins of the legs, resulting in an efflux of fluid from the veins into the tissues (edema) and marked declines in venous return, EDV, and cardiac filling pressure. This can result in **syncope**, or unconsciousness.

(Why does syncope occur during prolonged upright standing?)

The importance of the muscle pump to circulation is also apparent during long plane flights. After more than a 3- or 4-hour flight, in which muscle pump activity is reduced, you will notice puffiness, or tissue edema, in your legs. This can be a dangerous condition, as the flow through the venous system is very slow without the muscle pump, and clots known as **deep vein thromboses** will form. When these deep vein thromboses break loose, they can end up in the lungs as pulmonary emboli and in some instances, if not treated rapidly, can cause death. It is always advisable to exercise your legs on trips where you are in a seated position for long periods, such as in a car or plane.

In addition, the importance of the heart as the primary circulatory pump can be observed in patients who have a failing heart where the stroke volume and, therefore, the Q̇ are unable to generate an arterial pressure sufficient to drive the blood from the left side of the heart to the right side of the heart, causing the blood to pool in the leg veins. This occurs even though the muscle pump is functional. The muscle pump is weaker because of the poor delivery of oxygen to the active skeletal muscle, and the pooling of the blood in the leg veins results in tissue edema. This is why physicians press their fingers into the tissues surrounding the lower leg to judge the presence of edema.

deep vein thrombosis Usually a blood clot in the internal veins of the legs.

syncope Fainting.

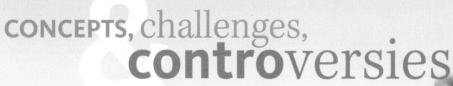

CONCEPTS, challenges, &controversies

Do Large Conduit Veins Actively Venoconstrict?

In the small peripheral veins, sympathetic activation of the alpha receptors produces venoconstriction and reduces the volume of blood in the smaller veins, resulting in an increased volume of blood being moved into the larger conduit veins returning to the heart. Controversy exists whether the larger conduit veins, such as the inferior vena cava, have alpha receptor-mediated venoconstriction. Currently, this may be one of the more important questions that needs to be answered.

respiratory pump Inspiration increases venous return, and expiration decreases venous return.

Respiratory Pump

The pumping action of the respiratory system is known as the **respiratory pump** and also increases venous return. Figure 7.17 illustrates the changes in intrapleural pressures during breathing, together with the flows measured in the inferior vena cava in the thorax and in the abdomen and the flows in the splanchnic circulation.

During the act of breathing, inspiration (breathing in) creates a negative pressure in the thorax and a positive pressure in the abdomen, which sucks and pushes blood, respectively, toward the right atria via the inferior vena cava. At the same time, the negative pressure in the thorax also draws the blood from the superior vena cava toward the right side of the heart. For

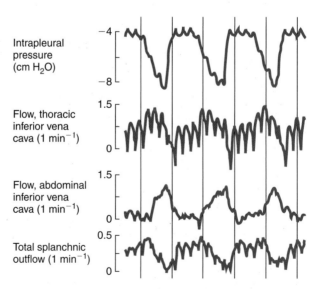

FIGURE 7.17 Respiratory muscle pump. Changes in intrapleural pressure and inferior vena caval blood flow in the thoracic and abdominal cavities and splanchnic bed during inspiration and expiration. (From Rowell, L. B. 1993. Figure 1.15 in *Human cardiovascular control*. New York: Oxford University Press, and Moreno, A. H., A. R. Burchell, R. Van der Woude, and J. H. Burke. 1967. Respiratory regulation of splanchnic and systemic venous return. *Am. J. Physiol.* 213:455–465.)

example, as we breathe out, the pressure in the thorax increases, thereby slowing the return of blood to the heart via the inferior and superior vena cava(e). However, a decrease in the abdominal pressure helps the flow out of the legs.

Because of the fluctuations in intrathoracic and intra-abdominal pressures, one would expect to observe large fluctuations in venous flow to the heart, resulting in large fluctuations in central venous and right atrial pressures. However, in healthy individuals, the liver serves as a buffer, or sump, to smooth out the pressure fluctuations and their effects on venous return.

During exercise, the venous return is increased in addition to the effects of the muscle pump because of the increase in breathing rate and the tidal volume of each breath.

The Arteriovenous Oxygen Difference Widens during Dynamic Exercise

The whole-body arteriovenous oxygen difference (the difference in content of oxygen in the systemic arterial and pulmonary arterial blood) widens from rest to maximal dynamic exercise (see Figure 7.18). As the intensity of exercise increases, a small amount of water is extracted from the blood for thermoregulation purposes (respiratory and sweating water loss), resulting in hemoconcentration and an increase in the oxygen-carrying capacity per unit volume of blood. However, the hemoconcentration does not alter arterial oxygen saturation or content.

One gram of hemoglobin binds 1.34 ml O_2. A healthy young adult male usually has 15 g hemoglobin per 100 ml blood, or 20 ml

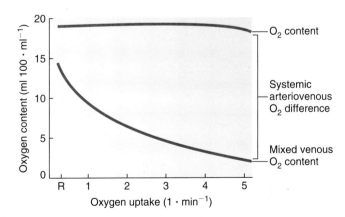

● **FIGURE 7.18** **Relationship between oxygen content (ml/100 ml blood) and oxygen uptake ($\dot{V}O_2$) during exercise to maximal oxygen uptake ($\dot{V}O_2$ max).** (From Rowell, L. B. 1993. Figure 5.15 in *Human cardiovascular control*. New York: Oxford University Press.)

O_2/100 ml blood. This value is usually referred to as 20 vol %; but to make it easier and to use the numeric values of the variables identified in Equation 7.3, you need to express it as 200 ml O_2/L arterial blood.

For example, in an individual with a resting $\dot{V}O_2$ of 250 ml O_2/min and a 5.0 L/min cardiac output ($\dot{Q}$), you can calculate, using Equation 7.3,

$$\dot{V}O_2 \text{ (L/min)} = \dot{Q} \text{ (L/min)} \times (a - v) \ O_2 \text{ difference (ml/L)}$$

$$250 \text{ ml/min} = 5 \text{ L/min} \times (a - v) \ O_2 \text{ difference (ml/L)}$$

$$(a - v) \ O_2 \text{ difference (ml/L)} = 250 \text{ ml/min} \div 5 \text{ L/min} = 50 \text{ ml/L}$$

The amount of oxygen extracted, or the $(a - v) \ O_2$ difference, is equal to 50 ml/L, which can be expressed as 5 vol %, or having a 5/20 = 1/4 = 25 percent extraction.

Explain why this means that the pulmonary artery blood (venous blood) would contain 15 vol % (150 ml O_2/L blood).

Usually a maximum of 85 percent of the available oxygen can be extracted from the blood at $\dot{V}O_2$ max, resulting in pulmonary artery blood containing approximately 3 vol %.

hemodynamics The study of the forces that move the blood within the cardiovascular system.

Practice calculation:
How much oxygen is being extracted by the tissues if the exercise requires a $\dot{V}O_2$ of 2.0 L/min and a $\dot{Q}$ of 16.0 L/min?

Principles of Hemodynamics Determine Blood Flow through the Systemic Blood Vessels during Dynamic Exercise

The interrelationship between the physical principles of pressure, flow, and resistance of blood flow is known as **hemodynamics**. The principles of hemodynamics are fundamental to how the blood flows within the vasculature of the circulatory system. Blood flows down a pressure gradient from the high pressure of the left side of the heart to the low pressure of the right side of the heart (see Figures 7.1, 7.11, and 7.19). Without a difference in pressure, there will be no flow.

In Figure 7.19, the left side of the heart is connected to the right side of the heart by a series of tubes. The flow of blood between the left side of the heart and the right side of the heart is directly proportional to the pressure difference between the left ventricle of the heart (P_1) and the right atrium of the heart (P_2). In other words, $P_1 - P_2 = \Delta P$. From Equation 7.1, that is, TPR = MAP/$\dot{Q}$, you can see that

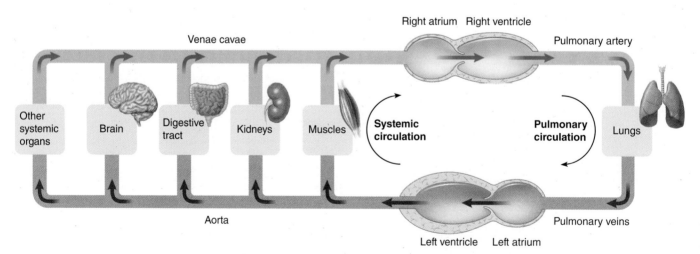

FIGURE 7.19 Dual pump action of the heart. Note the parallel pathways of blood flow through the systemic organs. (The relative volume of blood flowing through each organ is not drawn to scale.) (From Sherwood, L. 2010. Figure 9.2b in *Human physiology*, 7th ed. Belmont, CA: Brooks/Cole-Cengage Learning.)

resistance (R) of the blood vessel is related the pressure (P) in the vessel divided by the flow (Q̇) of blood passing through the vessel. Therefore, a sixfold increase in blood flow that is oftentimes required to perform exercise can be achieved two ways: (a) by a sixfold increase in arterial pressure, or (b) by a sixfold decrease in resistance.

Fortunately, increases in blood flow in animals are achieved by decreasing R, or the TPR, of the circulation in a greater proportion than by increasing the P or MAP. *(If a sixfold increase in arterial pressure was the only means of increasing blood flow, then in humans arterial pressures that exceed 500 to 600 mmHg would be required.)*

It is important to measure BP throughout maximal and submaximal exercise testing because a decrease in systolic arterial pressure, whether sudden or gradual, indicates a failing heart and reduced SV. A practical guide for exercise test monitoring is to realize that the systolic pressure reflects SV and diastolic pressure reflects vascular tone.

Resistance Arteries, or Arterioles, Provide Resistance to Blood Flow and Modify Blood Pressure

The major challenge to the circulatory system during dynamic or isometric exercise is to balance the regulation of arterial BP with the vascular regulation required to deliver adequate blood flow to the exercising muscles for oxygen delivery (see Figure 7.20).

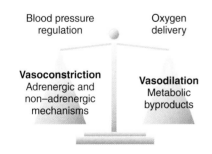

FIGURE 7.20 Regulation of blood flow and blood pressure during exercise. (Adapted from Buckwalter, J. B., and P. S. Clifford. 2001. The paradox of sympathetic vasoconstriction in exercising skeletal muscle. *Exerc. Sports Sci. Rev.* 29:159–163.)

The resistance to blood flow is affected by a number of physical properties of the blood vessels and the blood. Resistance is directly proportional to the length of the vessel and to the **viscosity** (thickness or density) of the blood, and is inversely proportional to the fourth power of the **radius**:

$$\text{Resistance} = \frac{\text{Length} \times \text{Viscosity}}{\text{Radius}^4} \quad [7.9]$$

Equation 7.9 indicates that:

i. If the length of the vessel is increased twofold, then the resistance is increased twofold.

ii. If the viscosity of the blood is increased twofold, then the resistance is increased twofold.

iii. If the radius of the vessel is decreased by half, then the resistance is increased 16-fold (that is, $2^4 = 16$).

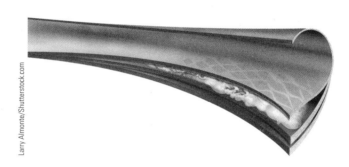

Larry Almonte/Shutterstock.com

Viscosity

Blood viscosity is made of two principal components: cells and plasma. The cells of the blood are the red blood cells (RBCs), white blood cells, and platelets. The plasma of the blood is the watery portion, which contains ions, proteins, metabolites, and endocrines. The proportion of blood made up by the cells is known as the hematocrit and generally ranges from 42 to 45 percent for a healthy, non-smoking, young male individual and 39 to 41 percent for a healthy, nonsmoking, young female individual. The cells in the blood are made up of approximately 90 percent RBCs and a 10 percent balance of white cells and platelets. An increase in the number of RBCs will increase the viscosity of the blood.

resistance (R) Calculated from the pressure difference from one end of a blood vessel to the other end divided by the blood flow in the blood vessel.

viscosity A measure of how sticky a fluid (blood) is.

radius Half the diameter of a circle (for example, half the diameter of a blood vessel).

aorta The large artery exiting the left
ventricle.

During dynamic exercise, hemocon-centration—that is, fluid shifting from the blood into the interstitium and loss of fluid through sweating and respiration—causes a loss of plasma and results in an increase in hematocrit and blood viscosity. Blood is much more viscous (sticky) than water. The higher the viscosity, the greater is the resistance to flow in the blood vessel; as shown in Equation 7.9, the smaller the blood vessel, the greater is the resistance to flow.

After maturation, blood vessel length and blood viscosity are relatively stable throughout life; therefore, the primary mechanism for the regulation of flow is the body's ability to change the diameter of the blood vessels, especially in the smaller resistance vessels. It is this ability to regulate the blood vessel's diameter (vasoconstriction or vasodilatation) that results in the redistribution of the Q̇ from the organs and inactive muscles to the active muscles during exercise. The anatomical difference between the diameters of the large conduit vessels and the smaller resistance vessels, that is, arterioles, is essential to generate the necessary pressure decrease from the high-pressure left side of the heart to the low-pressure right side of the heart in the circulation (see Figure 7.9).

Blood Vessels

The arterial blood vessels branch off of the main artery, the **aorta**, and form a vascular tree of blood vessels that decrease in diameter that perform specialized functions in regulating blood flow and pressure, and delivering oxygen to the tissues. The venous blood vessels collect the blood exiting from the capillaries and progressively increase their diameter until they enter the large collecting veins the superior and inferior vena cavae, also forming a vascular tree. Table 7.2 provides the structural and functional features of the arteries, arterioles, capillaries, and veins. All blood vessels have an inner lining of endothelial cells (known as the endothelium).

Arteries

Arteries have large diameters, offer little resistance to the blood flow coming from the heart, and are the main conduit vessels for the blood to deliver the oxygen to

● **TABLE** 7.2 **Features of Blood Vessels**

Feature	Aorta	Large Arterial Branches	Arterioles	Capillaries	Large Veins	Venae Cavae
Number	One	Several hundred	Half a million	Ten billion	Several hundred	Two
Wall Thickness	2 mm (2,000 μm)	1 mm (1,000 μm)	20 μm	1 μm	0.5 mm (500 μm)	1.5 mm (1,500 μm)
Internal Radius	1.25 cm (12,500 μm)	0.2 cm (2,000 μm)	30 μm	3.5 μm	0.5 cm (5,000 μm)	3 cm (30,000 μm)
Total Cross-Sectional Area	4.5 cm²	20 cm²	400 cm²	6,000 cm²	40 cm²	18 cm²
Special Features	Thick, highly elastic, walls; large radii		Highly muscular, well-innervated walls; small radii	Thin walled; large total cross-sectional area	Thin walled; highly distensible; large radii	
Functions	Passageway from the heart to the tissues; serve as a pressure reservoir		Primary resistance vessels; determine the distribution of cardiac output	Site of exchange; determine the distribution of extracellular fluid between the plasma and interstitial fluid	Passageway to the heart from the tissues; serve as a blood reservoir	

From Sherwood, L. 2004. Table 10.1 in *Human physiology,* 5th ed. Belmont, CA: Brooks/Cole-Cengage Learning.

tissues and organs of the body. The vessel wall of the artery is constructed in layers of tissue endothelium, smooth muscle cells, and collagen and elastin fibers (see Figure 7.21).

The collagen provides strength and the elastin enables the vessel to buffer the fluctuating increases and decreases in its velocity of the blood flow and enables the pulsatile pressure wave exiting the heart to be transduced, such that as it reaches the resistance arteries, or arterioles, and capillaries, the velocity of the blood flow is continuous and not pulsatile (see Figure 7.22).

During progressive increases in intensity of dynamic exercise, the pulsatile pressures of the fluctuations in blood flow velocity exiting the heart increase markedly, and yet because of the physical properties

of the blood vessel wall, the system is able to buffer the pressure waves before it reaches the resistance arteries (see Figure 7.22).

Resistance Arteries or Arterioles

Muscles with an abundance of red fibers and capillaries (slow-twitch oxidative fibers) have a higher blood flow than the muscles with more white fibers (fast-twitch low-oxidative fibers). During exercise, the major challenge to the neural regulatory system is to maintain control of BP whereas at the same time allowing increases in blood flow to the active skeletal muscles (see Figure 7.20). This is especially important in very heavy exercise, where it has been found that predictions from maximal blood flow observed in the

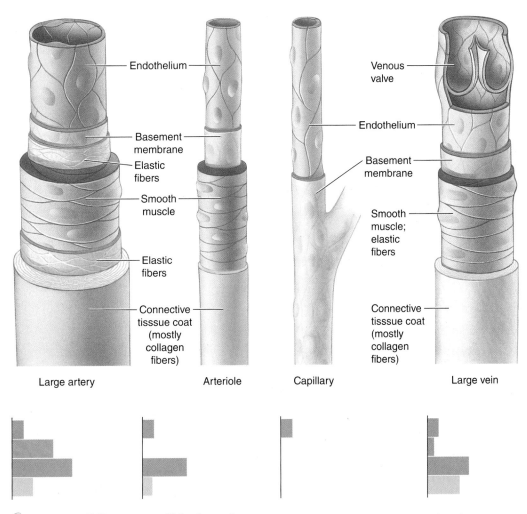

Large artery   Arteriole   Capillary   Large vein

● **F I G U R E 7.21 Features of blood vessels.** (From Sherwood, L. 2010. Figure 7.21 in *Human physiology*, 7th ed. Belmont, CA: Brooks/Cole-Cengage Learning.)

maximally vasodilated blood vessels of the quadriceps muscle, when used as a basis for the calculation of blood flow required for whole-body exercise, would far exceed maximal $\dot{Q}$ and result in a decrease in BP. The arterioles provide the primary regulation of blood flow into and within the skeletal muscle and organs of the body.

Because the transition from rest to exercise involves a change in BP and $\dot{Q}$, the baseline value of the calculated variable changes; therefore, it is necessary to normalize the changes in flow to a given change in BP, that is, **conductance (C)**, or blood flow per unit of arterial pressure, which can be calculated by rearranging Equation 7.1:

$$1/\text{Resistance} = \text{Conductance} = \dot{Q}/\text{MAP} \tag{7.10}$$

With this relationship, we can compare two different blood flows in relation to their BP and obtain an accurate picture of whether vasoconstriction or vasodilatation has occurred without the presence of a mathematical artifact because of differences in pressure (see Figure 7.22).

The reason for us to normalize the resistance response as a change in flow per unit of arterial pressure is that, although conductance is mathematically the reciprocal of resistance, that is, $(C) = 1/R$, the relationship is not linear but curvilinear (see Figure 7.23).

In Figure 7.23, for the same given change in conductance, that is, 0.02 on the X axis for C_1 and C_2, the change in resistance on the Y axis is 40 for R_1 and 2 for R_2 or a 20-fold difference in resistance changes. This mathematical difference could lead you to conclude a large degree of vasoconstriction had occurred between R_1 and R_2, yet the change in conductance or blood flow per unit of pressure for C_1 and C_2 is the same, indicating that no active change in vascular tone occurred. This becomes important when comparing blood flows between rest and exercise and between two or more exercise intensities, and is especially relevant when comparing blood flow changes in the brain that have a high degree of **blood vessel autoregulation** related to **myogenic tone** associated with increases and decreases in arterial pressure.

conductance (C) A measurement of a blood vessel's ability to convey blood.

blood vessel autoregulation The ability of the blood vessel to adjust its diameter to its initial diameter in response to stretch (vasodilatation) or contraction (vasoconstriction).

myogenic tone The intrinsic muscle tone of the blood vessels.

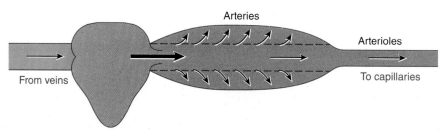

(a) Heart contracting and emptying

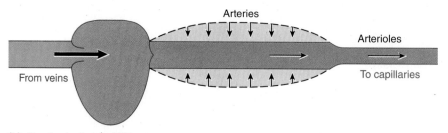

(b) Heart relaxing and filling

FIGURE 7.22 Arteries as a pressure reservoir. Because of their elasticity, arteries act as a pressure reservoir. (a) The elastic arteries distend during cardiac systole as more blood is ejected into them than drains off into the narrow, high-resistance arterioles downstream. (b) The elastic recoil of arteries during cardiac diastole continues driving the blood forward when the heart is not pumping. (From Sherwood, L. 2010. Figure 10.6 in *Human physiology*, 7th ed. Belmont, CA: Brooks/Cole-Cengage Learning.)

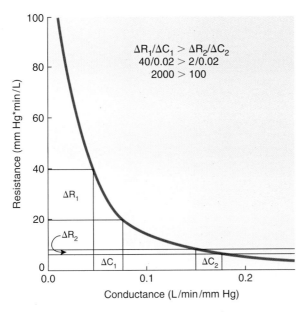

$$\Delta R_1 / \Delta C_1 > \Delta R_2 / \Delta C_2$$
$$40/0.02 > 2/0.02$$
$$2000 > 100$$

FIGURE 7.23 **Resistance versus conductance.** (Adapted from Figure 1 on page H 633 from O'Leary. D. 1991. Figure 1 in Regional vascular resistance vs. conductance: Which index for baroreflex responses? *Am. J. Physiol.* 260:H632–H637.)

Neural Control and Local Control

Both neural reflexes and local metabolic factors have important roles to play in balancing the blood flow and BP required. In general, the neural control is primary in regulating pressure, and the local factors are primary in regulating muscle blood flow (see Figures 7.6 and 7.20); therefore, it is the balance between the mechanisms of BP and blood flow modulation that provides the optimum regulation of both physiologic variables.

Neural control of the vasculature is provided by activation of the sympathetic nervous system, which during dynamic exercise increases as the intensity of exercise increases and results in intensity-related increases in norepinephrine-induced alpha-1 receptor–mediated contraction of the smooth muscles in the wall of the blood vessel, that is, vasoconstriction. In addition, during high sympathetic activity, vasoconstriction is enhanced by production of angiotensin II binding to the angiotensin I receptor and endothelin binding to the endothelin receptors of the vessel's smooth muscle cells.

In Figure 7.6, the increase in local metabolic activity results in vasodilatation caused by reductions in tissue PO_2, breakdown of ATP-producing adenosine, increased shear stress on the endothelium-releasing NO, and an endothelium-derived vasodilating factor caused by increases in blood flow. Much of the vasodilation is a result of the metabolic factors causing hyperpolarization of the **potassium ATP (K_{ATP})** channels of the smooth muscle cells, resulting in K^+ ion efflux and inhibition of the Ca^{2+} ion influx into the cell via the calcium channel.

Functional Sympatholysis

The increase in vascular conductance within the exercising muscles is restrained by sympathetic activity, but the amount of restraint is itself inhibited by the metabolites produced in direct relation to the intensity of exercise (that is, functional sympatholysis; see Figure 7.24). Much of this inhibition of vasoconstriction can be partially reversed by using a K_{ATP} channel blocker (glyburide) commonly prescribed for treatment of type 2 diabetes.

In contrast, in the nonexercising tissues and organs, the sympathetic vasoconstriction is not modulated by locally produced metabolites and the degree of vasoconstriction is directly related to the exercise-induced increase in sympathetic activity;

potassium ATP (K_{ATP}) A cell membrane channel that allows passage of potassium ions into and out of the cell.

that is, the greater the exercise intensity, the greater the effect of the increased sympathetic activity on the nonexercising skeletal muscle or organ blood flow (see Figure 7.24).

It is this local metabolic effect that provides the differential distribution of the effects of the exercise-induced increases in sympathetic activity that directs the increased $\dot{Q}$ to the active skeletal muscles.

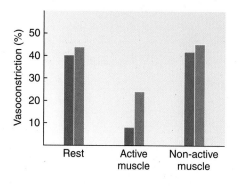

FIGURE 7.24 The (%) amount of vasoconstriction produced by 40 mmHg stimulation of the carotid baroreceptors in active and nonactive muscle vasculature: with (blue) and without (purple) oral ingestion of glyburide (K_{ATP} channel blockade). Exercise produced 75% reduction in vasoconstriction. Glyburide restored 40% (65% of the vasoconstriction) during exercise. Remember not all channels were blocked. (Adapted from Keller, D. M., S. Ogoh, S. Greene, A. Olivencia-Yurvati, and P. B. Raven. 2004. Inhibition of K_{ATP} channel activity augments baroreflex-mediated vasoconstriction in exercising human skeletal muscle. *J. Physiol.* 561:273–282.)

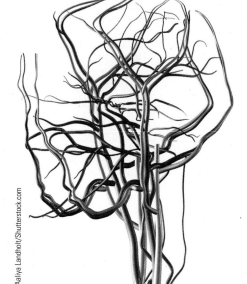

Aaliya Landholt/Shutterstock.com

Cerebral Circulation

Besides delivering oxygen to the active tissues by increasing $\dot{Q}$ and redistributing the flow away from inactive tissue and organs, another major role of the cardiovascular system is to ensure **cerebral circulation** (adequate blood flow or oxygen to the brain) during a variety of stressors. Standing upright in itself creates a stress, and when exercise is an additional stressor, regulation of blood flow becomes paramount. For example, when standing upright quickly from a squat position, you may experience light-headedness, or even fainting, because of a precipitous drop in BP, resulting in a lack of blood flow delivering oxygen to the brain. This feeling of light-headedness is a symptom of presyncope (pre-fainting). If you actually faint (lose consciousness), it is called *syncope*.

In many ways, the brain is similar to the skeletal muscle in its need for oxygen.

During exercise, the neural activity of the brain increases in relation to the mental and physical complexity of the exercise, and requires oxygen to be delivered in direct relation to the complexity and intensity of the exercise. Unless the heart begins to fail and reduces its delivery of oxygen to the brain, it is unlikely that you will experience symptoms of presyncope or syncope during exercise. However, during recovery from dynamic exercise, the muscle pump is voluntarily stopped or is reduced dependent on the type of recovery, and the respiratory pump effect diminishes as breathing rate and depth decrease. Subsequently, a postexercise hypotension (decrease in BP) may occur, resulting in a reduction in brain blood flow and possibly syncope. To accommodate the increased need for oxygen, exercise triggers a general vasodilatation of the cerebral blood vessels (the amount of vasodilatation

cerebral circulation The network of blood vessels that circulates blood throughout the brain.

is related to the intensity of the exercise and the thermal stress of the workload and the environment). The mechanism for this increase in blood flow has recently been reported to be an effect of the increase in Q̇ providing more flow to the brain and a cholinergic-NO vasodilator mechanism.

More insidious are the chronic outcomes of disturbances in brain blood flow associated with diseases associated with increases in sympathetic activity, such as hypertension, type 2 diabetes, obstructive sleep apnea, and congestive heart failure, and their resultant neurologic diseases, such as Alzheimer disease and senile dementia. Many forms of dementia are being identified as an end stage of type 2 diabetes, a hypersympathetic disease, which, if left untrea ted, results in vascular function abnormalities. These abnormalities can result in an earlier age-related onset of dementia. Such catastrophic diseases are a basis to strongly support prescribing exercise as a preventive health modality throughout life.

Cerebral Autoregulation Maintains a Constant Blood Flow over a Wide Range of Arterial Pressures

Arterial gas tensions of carbon dioxide (Pa_{CO_2}) and the ANS have major influences on the regulation of brain (cerebral) blood flow. However, steady-state cerebral blood flow (CBF) is primarily regulated by a mechanism called **cerebral autoregulation (CA)**, and because prior to the early 1980s, the measurement of CBF required steady-state conditions, it was termed static cerebral autoregulation (sCA). It has been demonstrated that at rest and during exercise, as Q̇ increases or decreases, the blood flow to the brain increases or decreases, respectively. The CA regulates CBF at a relatively constant change of flow (7 percent increase in CBF per 10-mm Hg increase in MAP) over a wide range of MAPs (60–150 mm Hg). This ability to regulate the flow by altering cerebral vascular resistance over such a wide range of pressures is unique to the brain. Outside of the 60- to 150-mm Hg

range of MAP, the CBF decreases and increases in direct relation to the changes in pressure. However, it has been found that in individuals with hypertension, a disease associated with increases in sympathetic activity, the pressure of the upper limit of sCA is extended to values greater than 200 mmHg (see Figure 7.25).

All blood vessels of the body have an intrinsic myogenic stretch-contraction property, which is the major mechanistic component of sCA. However, the sCA's greater capacity to autoregulate the brain's blood flow over the wide range of arterial pressures compared with that of the heart, kidney, and other organ beds, gives the cerebral circulation its uniqueness (see Figure 7.25). This unique property is probably related to its microcirculatory network and areas of distinct regional circulations that respond to different areas of the brain's metabolic activity. This network of regional circulations allows one area to vasodilate in response to increased metabolic activity and other areas to constrict as a means of buffering the effects of increases in the global perfusion pressure related to the exercise increases in Q̇ and the changes in intracranial pressure.

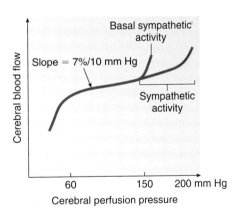

● FIGURE 7.25 Relationship between cerebral perfusion pressure (arterial blood pressure) and cerebral blood flow with and without increases in sympathetic activity.
(Adapted from D. D. Heistad and H. A. Kontos. Figure 11, page 165. Chapter 5, "Cerebral Circulation" in *Handbook of physiology Section 2, The Cardiovascular System*, Edited by J. T. Sheperd. F. M. Abboud and Stephen F. Geiger, Bethesda, MD: Publ. American Physiol. Soc.; Lucas S. J., Y. C. Tzeng, S. D. Galvin, K. N. Thomas, S. Ogoh, and P. N. Ainslie. 2010. Influence of changes in blood pressure on cerebral perfusion and oxygenation. *Hypertension* 55:698–705; and Panerai, R. B. 1998. Assessment of cerebral pressure autoregulation in humans—a review of measurement methods. *Physiol. Meas.* 19:305–338.)

cerebral autoregulation (CA) A primary means of regulating brain blood flow using blood vessel autoregulation over a wide range of blood pressures (60 mm Hg to 150 mm Hg).

Dynamic Cerebral Autoregulation

The development of **ultrasound technology** (the use of ultrasonic waves to image internal body structures) has enabled rapid noninvasive measurements of many internal organ systems and blood vessels. In particular, the development of transcranial Doppler (TCD) ultrasound and its clinical utility were demonstrated in the early 1980s, and measures of middle cerebral artery blood velocity in humans beat-to-beat at rest and during exercise were made possible. Recently, the use of advanced mathematical frequency analysis techniques on these beat-to-beat measures of cerebral blood velocity and BP has enabled investigators to define **dynamic cerebral autoregulation (dCA)**, that is, the beat-to-beat change in cerebral blood velocity per unit change in MAP. Initially, the use of TCD ultrasound was questioned because the diameter of the middle cerebral artery could not be measured at the same time as the measurement of velocity, so the investigator was unable to provide a value for flow. Subsequently, magnetic resonance imaging (MRI) demonstrated that the diameter of the middle cerebral artery was unchanged during a sympathetic stimulus. Therefore, it is generally accepted that the TCD measurements of cerebral blood velocity in the middle cerebral artery provide a valid index of CBF.

Other technologies of measuring blood flow within the brain using imaging techniques and radioactive materials are available but provide only small snapshots of the response and require that the head be immobile during the imaging. However, the imaging techniques do provide valuable clinical diagnostic information.

> **HOTLINK** *See the U.S. Department of Health & Human Services website for more information about physical activity recommendations to improve or maintain mental health:* http://www.health.gov/PAGuidelines/committeereport.aspx *(p. G8-1).*

Changes in Arterial Carbon Dioxide Increases and Decreases Brain Blood Flow

normocapnia An arterial carbon dioxide partial pressure of 40 mmHg.

hypercapnia An arterial carbon dioxide partial pressure of greater than 40 mmHg.

hypocapnia An arterial carbon dioxide partial pressure of less than 40 mmHg.

At rest, Pa_{CO_2} approximates 40 mm Hg (**normocapnia**) and is in equilibrium with the alveolar gas tension, whereas pulmonary artery or mixed venous carbon dioxide gas tension (Pv_{CO_2}) approximates 45 mm Hg. Brain blood flow is highly sensitive to changes in Pa_{CO_2} but is insensitive to changes in Pv_{CO_2}. An increase in Pa_{CO_2}, or **hypercapnia**, causes vasodilatation, whereas a decrease in Pa_{CO_2}, or **hypocapnia**, causes vasoconstriction in the arterial blood vessels of the brain. Thus, the hypercapnic changes increase brain blood flow, and hypocapnic changes decrease brain blood flow. The amount of brain blood flow, which is established by $\dot{Q}$, is regulated by sCA and Pa_{CO_2}. Furthermore, hypercapnia and hypocapnia increase and decrease dCA, respectively (see Figure 7.26).

During mild-to-moderate dynamic exercise, the CBF increases before the onset of respiratory compensation for metabolic acidosis (discussed in Chapters 9 and 10), whereas Pa_{CO_2} increases slightly toward hypercapnic tensions (40–50 mm Hg). However, during heavy to exhaustive exercise, Pa_{CO_2} decreases back to near resting values (40 mm Hg). This return to baseline values occurs because the hyperventilation (respiratory compensation) induced by the

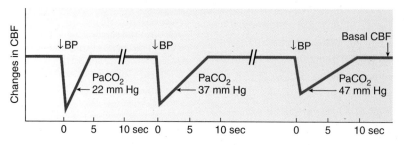

FIGURE 7.26 **Change in cerebral blood velocity (CBV) in response to a 25-mm Hg decline in blood pressure with increases and decreases in PaCO_2.** (Adapted from Aaslid, R., K. F. Lindegaard, W. Sorteberg, and H. Nornes. 1989. Figure 2 in Cerebral autoregulation dynamics in humans. *Stroke* 20:45–52.)

heavy exercise is a result of the acid-base buffering that occurs to counteract the exercise-induced metabolic acidosis. The slope of the relationship between Pa_{CO_2} and brain blood flow is significantly less than that observed at rest and suggests that the metabolites produced by the exercise reduces the effectiveness of CA (see Figure 7.27). Fortunately, both sCA and dCA are extended by the exercise-induced increases in sympathetic activity, thereby protecting the brain from hyperperfusion during the pulsatile increases in SBP that exceed the autoregulatory limits of sCA, that is, more than 150 mmHg (see Figure 7.25).

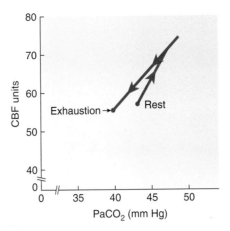

FIGURE 7.27 **Schematic representation of changes in Pa_{CO_2} cerebral blood volume at rest and during a 70 percent $\dot{V}O_2$ max cycle ride to exhaustion.** (Adapted from Ogoh, S., M. K. Dalsgaard, C. C. Yoshiga, E. A. Dawson, D. M. Keller, P. B. Raven, and N. H. Secher. 2005. Figure 2 in Dynamic cerebral autoregulation during exhaustive exercise in humans. *Am. J. Physiol. Heart. Circ. Physiol.* 288:H1461–H1467.)

The Autonomic Nervous System Affects Brain Blood Flow

Cerebral blood vessels are innervated by adrenergic sympathetic and cholinergic parasympathetic nerve fibers interfaced with their respective receptors. Their receptor densities are heterogeneously distributed throughout the blood vessels of the brain. Yet, the thought remains that the autonomic neural control of cerebral vessels was minimal, especially via the **arterial baroreflexes**. However, more current information indicates that the sympathoexcitation associated with dynamic or static exercise and baroreceptor activation does, indeed, affect brain blood flow regulation by increasing cerebral vascular tone (vasoconstriction).

arterial baroreflexes These include pressure-sensitive receptors in the carotid sinus and aortic arch, which signal the central nervous system that the blood pressure is too low or too high.

Isometric, Static, and Resistance Exercise

In a given muscle, a 100 percent maximal isometric voluntary contraction will activate the maximum number of muscle fibers, and will result in the highest intramuscular pressure and cause a complete cessation of blood flow through the muscle. With decreasing percentages of MVC, proportional to a decreasing number of fibers contracting, a proportional reduction in the obstruction to blood flow will occur. The length of time a submaximal % MVC can be maintained is inversely proportional to the % MVC (the greater the % MVC, the shorter the contraction time). The critical value of % MVC, below which long-lasting contractions can be held, range from 10 to 25 percent, and the physiologic reasons for this variance are probably related to muscle fiber type in the makeup of the muscle and the fixed position of the exercising muscle (see Chapter 3).

Less Oxygen Is Used to Generate Energy for Isometric Exercise Than Dynamic Exercise Requiring the Same Force

A comparison of the cardiovascular responses with progressive increases in dynamic exercise workloads and with a 3-minute 30 percent MVC isometric contraction is presented in Figure 7.10. The

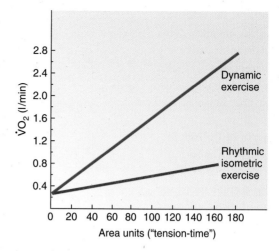

FIGURE 7.28 Oxygen uptake in relation to arbitrary units of tension-time. Upper curve: bicycling; lower curve: rhythmic static exercise. Data represent two subjects. (Adapted from Assmussen, E. 1981. Similarities and dissimilarities between static and dynamic exercise. Figure 1, page I-4 in *Static (isometric) exercise: Cardiovascular responses and neural control mechanisms* [American Heart Association monograph 76], edited by J. H. Mitchell, C. G. Blomqvist, A. R. Lind, B. Saltin, and J. T. Shepherd. Dallas, TX: American Heart Association; Proceedings of the 2nd Harry S. Moss International Symposium, Dallas, Texas, October 8–10, 1979. *Circ. Res.* 48(6 pt 2), I1–I188, 1981.)

primary difference between the two forms of exercise is that during dynamic exercise, the muscle shortens with contraction and lengthens during the relaxation, resulting in the muscle performing physical work. Whereas in contrast with dynamic exercise, the length of the muscle remains constant during isometric exercise and, therefore, by definition, no physical work is being performed, even though force is being produced that requires energy to be generated aerobically and anaerobically. The energy being transformed in either dynamic or isometric contractions can be summarized in the following equation:

$$E = A + kW \qquad [7.11]$$

where E corresponds to total energy transformed by the contraction, A is the energy connected to the production of the force, and W is the energy appearing as external work. During isometric contractions, W = 0.

(Why does W = 0 during isometric contractions?)

If we compare isometric and dynamic exercise at the same production of force (that is, A is the same for both isometric and dynamic exercise), the amount of oxygen used to generate the energy will be less for isometric exercise compared with the dynamic exercise requiring the same force (see Figure 7.28).

Cardiovascular Responses to Isometric Exercise Are Greatly Different Than Dynamic Exercise

The cardiovascular responses to light workload isometric exercise are only qualitatively different from the responses to heavy workload isometric exercise (see Figure 7.28). However, the cardiovascular responses are quantitatively different for dynamic exercise when performing equivalent light and heavy exercise workloads.

During isometric exercise, increases in intramuscular pressure restrict blood flow to the exercising muscle. This restriction to flow reduces the delivery of oxygen to the exercising muscle. Subsequently, more anaerobic energy production is required to maintain the heavy work of contraction, leading to an accumulation of metabolites.

(Why do the metabolites accumulate?)

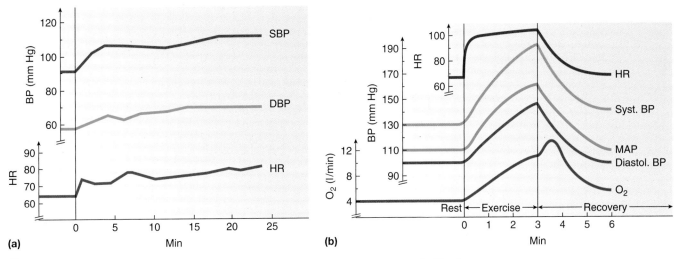

FIGURE 7.29 (a) Circulatory functions during light isometric exercise. DBP, diastolic blood pressure; HR, heart rate; SBP, systolic blood pressure. (b) Circulatory data from heavy isometric exercise. (a: Adapted from Assmussen, E. 1981. Similarities and dissimilarities between static and dynamic exercise. Figure 4. Page I-5 in *Static (isometric) exercise: Cardiovascular responses and neural control mechanisms* [American Heart Association monograph 76], edited by J. H. Mitchell, C. G. Blomqvist, A. R. Lind, B. Saltin, and J. T. Shepherd. Dallas, TX: American Heart Association; and Static (isometric) exercise. Cardiovascular responses and neural control mechanisms. Proceedings of the 2nd Harry S. Moss International Symposium, Dallas, Texas, October 8–10, 1979. *Circ. Res.* 48(6 pt 2), I1–I188, 1981; Fig 29b: adapted from Assmussen, E. 1981. Similarities and dissimilarities between static and dynamic exercise. Figure 6. Page I-7 in *Static (isometric) exercise: Cardiovascular responses and neural control mechanisms* [American Heart Association monograph 76], edited by J. H. Mitchell, C. G. Blomqvist, A. R. Lind, B. Saltin, and J. T. Shepherd. Dallas, TX: Proceedings of the 2nd Harry S. Moss International Symposium, Dallas, Texas, October 8–10, 1979. *Circ. Res.* 48(6 pt 2), I1–I188, 1981.)

This process occurs within the muscle and is proportional to the strength of the isometric contraction. The accumulation of metabolites activates chemical sensors within the muscle that tell the cardiovascular control center, by afferent neural networks connected to the cardiovascular system in the brain, that not enough oxygen is being delivered to the muscle. This message triggers a central stimulation of the cardiovascular system to try to increase the blood flow to the exercising muscle. This is why the increased cardiovascular responses identified in Figure 7.29 are larger than expected for the amount of oxygen required to perform the muscle contraction.

During an isometric muscle contraction, there is no increase in muscle pump activity and no increase in venous return. The neural signals from the muscle to the cardiovascular center result in a central sympathetic activation that increases the Q̇ by stimulating the HR without a change in SV. However, the increased sympathetic activity increases the total systemic vascular resistance to flow by causing vasoconstriction in the peripheral blood vessels. These responses result in a magnified BP response far in excess to the given exercise workload, if performed dynamically.

Indeed, during a maximum effort military press, arterial pressures, directly measured using a catheter placed in the aorta, exceeded a diastolic arterial pressure of 350 mm Hg and systolic pressures of 480 mm Hg for a calculated MAP of 393 mm Hg (see Figure 7.30a, page 246).

The increases in Q̇ do not increase blood flow to the active muscle because of the intramuscular restriction resulting from the isometric contraction. Instead, the increased flow is redirected to the nonworking muscles and the skin (the face and skin of an exercising person often become flushed). Remember, the amount of muscle mass used and the intensity of the exercise both correlate directly with the cardiovascular response.

At the beginning of the isometric contraction, the BP and brain blood flow are sharply increased, followed by a reduction in both over the time of the contraction.

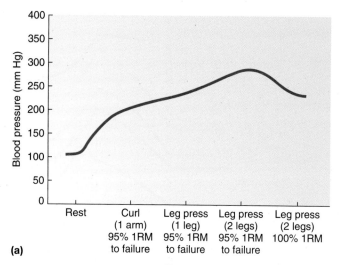

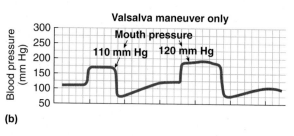

(a)

(b)

🔵 **FIGURE 7.30** **Blood pressure response to weight lifting.** (a) Peak systolic and diastolic blood pressures reached during various exercises. (b) Blood pressure responses in a single subject performing two maximal Valsalva maneuvers against a column of Hg while seated at rest. (a: Adapted from McDougall, J. D., D. Tuxen, D. G. Sale, J. R. Moroz, and J. R. Sutton. 1985. Figure 4 in Arterial blood pressure response to heavy resistance exercise. *J. Appl. Physiol.* 58:785–790; b: adapted from McDougall, J. D., D. Tuxen, D. G. Sale, J. R. Moroz, and J. R. Sutton. 1985. Figure 5 in Arterial blood pressure response to heavy resistance exercise. *J. Appl. Physiol.* 58:785–790.)

However, neither brain blood flow nor arterial BP is returned to normal while the contraction is being held. The BP and brain blood flow return to resting values rapidly after the contraction is released. If the isometric contraction is performed while holding the breath, the brain blood flow and BP responses are accentuated. This effect may prove to be dangerous for people with weak cerebral blood vessels (see Figure 7.30a). For more detailed information about the cardiovascular responses to static (isometric) exercise see selected reading reference, Mitchell et al, 1981.

Neural Control of the Circulation during Exercise

Exercise is now considered the *sine qua non* ("that which cannot be left out") in many investigations of neural integrated control mechanisms and in diagnostic evaluation of cardiovascular function (see Figure 7.31).

Central Command Controls the Cardiovascular Responses

At the onset of exercise, activation of **central command (CC)** involves a feed-forward set of neural signals emanating from the motor cortex that in parallel activate cardiovascular control centers in the brainstem (see Figure 7.31). This activation rapidly withdraws parasympathetic control of the heart, increasing HR, and increases sympathetic outflow to the heart and vasculature, increasing HR and regulating the sympathetic outflow to alter the vasomotor function of the blood vessels to ultimately regulate BP.

The amount of CC activation is directly proportional to the amount of motor activity required to perform the work. Therefore, in a progressive increase in workload exercise test, the CC activity increases in direct proportion to the increases in workload, resulting in progressive increases in

central command (CC) A feed-forward mechanism that controls the cardiovascular system.

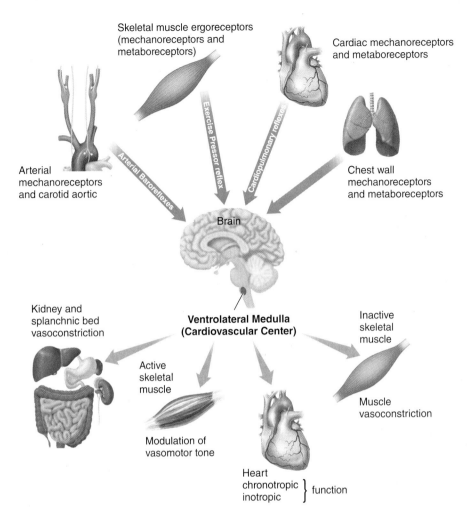

Skeletal muscle ergoreceptors
(mechanoreceptors and
metaboreceptors)

Cardiac mechanoreceptors
and metaboreceptors

Arterial
mechanoreceptors
and carotid aortic

Exercise Pressor reflex

Cardiopulmonary reflex

Arterial Baroreflexes

Chest wall
mechanoreceptors
and metaboreceptors

Brain

Kidney and
splanchnic bed
vasoconstriction

**Ventrolateral Medulla
(Cardiovascular Center)**

Inactive
skeletal
muscle

Active
skeletal
muscle

Muscle
vasoconstriction

Modulation of
vasomotor tone

Heart
chronotropic
inotropic } function

⊙ **FIGURE 7.31** **Schematic of the interaction of the neural regulation of the cardiovascular system during exercise.** (Adapted from Bouchard, C., R. J. Shepherd, and T. Stephens. 1994. Figure 17.3 in *Cardiovascular adaptation to physical activity in physical activity, fitness and health: International Proceedings and Consensus Statement.* Champaign, IL: Human Kinetics.)

HR and BP. In a unique set of experiments using a combination of hypnotic suggestion and brain mapping techniques during exercise and imagined exercise, the individual's own perception of effort has been shown to modulate the feed-forward neural signals of CC in providing the requisite cardiovascular response to exercise.

Activation of the Exercise Pressor Reflex Increases Heart Rate and Blood Pressure

Neural signals arising from the exercising muscle activate brainstem cardiovascular control centers resulting in an increase in

BP; this is called the **exercise pressor reflex (EPR)** (see Figure 7.31).

During exercise, stimulation of group III afferent nerves, which are within the skeletal muscle and sensitive to stretch or pressure (mechanical), and group IV afferent nerves, which are also within the skeletal muscle but sensitive to chemicals (metabolites), results in BP and HR increases via sympathetic activation and parasympathetic withdrawal, respectively. Similar to CC, progressive increases in workload will result in progressive increases in activation of the EPR, resulting in directly related increases in HR and sympathetic activity, causing increases in BP.

Recent work is beginning to identify the underlying intramuscular substrates

exercise pressor reflex (EPR) A feedback mechanism from the skeletal muscle to the brain to maintain oxygen delivery.

of stimulation, molecular signaling pathways of signal transduction from chemical to neural activity, and the neural networks and central nervous system's neural anatomy involved in EPR activation. These investigations are important for the exercise physiologist because the effects of the activated EPR are accentuated in heart disease patients; therefore, the planning of cardiac rehabilitation programs needs to account for an increased BP response to the exercise.

Arterial Baroreflexes Are Reset in Relation to the Intensity of Dynamic Exercise

The arterial baroreceptors have afferent nerves arising from the aortic arch and the carotid sinus (located at the bifurcation of the carotid artery) and going to the brain to interact within the cardiovascular center (see Figures 7.31 and 7.32) to reflexly regulate BP from one beat to the next by continually adjusting $\dot{Q}$ (via changes in HR) and vascular resistance (via changes in sympathetic activity). The operating point (OP), or pressure, around which these reflex adjustments occur is the MAP. During rest, when the MAP is increased, the HR ($\dot{Q}$) decreases and the vasculature vasodilates (via sympathetic withdrawal), which results in a decline in BP. When the MAP decreases, the opposite responses for the HR and vasculature occur and result in an increase in BP (see Figures 7.32 and 7.33).

However, because the HR and BP increase during exercise, it was thought for many years that the arterial baroreflex regulation of BP was either switched off or ignored. Since 1980, both animal and human experiments have shown that the arterial baroreflexes are reset in direct relation to the work intensity of dynamic exercise and operate around the prevailing arterial pressure, OP (see Figure 7.34), by modulating the appropriate reflex responses identified in Figure 7.33.

It has been identified that because of vagal withdrawal, the OP of the HR reflex is relocated to a point of lesser gain (sensitivity) on the reflex function curves in direct relation to the exercise intensity. Simultaneously, the responding and operating ranges of the curve are also reduced. In contrast, the BP reflex function curve resets without a change in its OP and operating or responding ranges. However, the centering point (the point of maximal gain [Gmax], or maximal sensitivity) of either of the function curves is unchanged.

Recent evidence has identified that the OP of the function curve during rest or exercise, by comparing exercise in the upright and supine positions, is a result of the inputs coming from CC, EPR, and CBV.

Activation of CC, EPR, or a combination of both is necessary for the arterial baroreflexes to be reset. For example, when exercise was simulated using electrical stimulation (a condition of no CC), along with the afferent pathway arising from the activated muscle blocked by epidural anesthesia (a condition of no EPR), or absent because of spinal injury, the BP did not increase, indicating that the arterial baroreflexes had not reset.

In summary, the overall consensus of how the arterial baroreflexes are reset is that the feed-forward mechanism of CC is primary, and the feedback mechanism of the EPR is a modulator of the resetting together with input from CBV. CC operates via withdrawal of parasympathetic control of the heart (increasing HR) and increased sympathetic activity to the heart and vasculature, whereas the EPR activates the sympathetic control of the vasculature. However, the specific central nervous system's neural circuits involved in arterial baroreflex resetting remain to be identified.

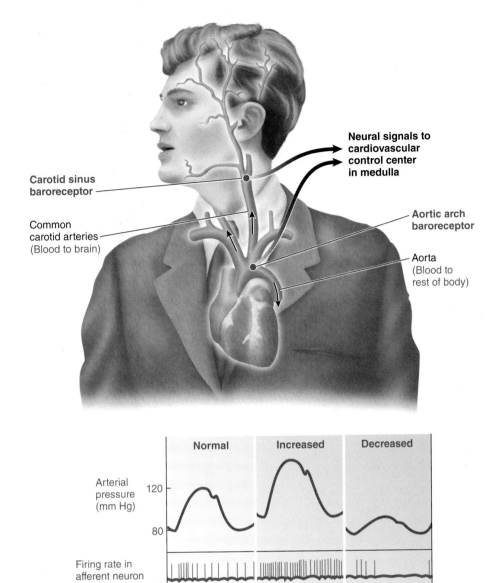

Normal Increased Decreased

Arterial pressure (mm Hg)

120

80

Firing rate in afferent neuron arising from carotid sinus baroreceptor

Time

Carotid sinus baroreceptor

Common carotid arteries (Blood to brain)

Neural signals to cardiovascular control center in medulla

Aortic arch baroreceptor

Aorta (Blood to rest of body)

● **FIGURE 7.32 Arterial baroreceptors.** (a) Location of the arterial baroreceptors. The arterial baroreceptors are strategically located to monitor the mean arterial blood pressure in the arteries that supply blood to the brain (carotid sinus baroreceptor) and to the rest of the body (aortic arch baroreceptor). (b) Firing rate in the afferent neuron from the carotid sinus baroreceptor in relation to the magnitude of mean arterial pressure. (a: From Sherwood, L. 2010. Figure 10.35 in *Human physiology.* 7th ed. Belmont, CA: Brooks/Cole-Cengage Learning; b: Sherwood, L. 2010. Figure 10.36 in *Human physiology.* 7th ed. Belmont, CA: Brooks/Cole-Cengage Learning.)

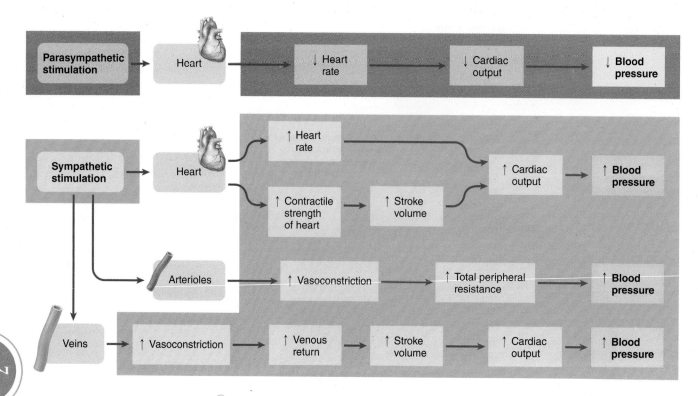

FIGURE 7.33 Summary of the effects of the parasympathetic and sympathetic nervous systems on factors that influence mean arterial blood pressure. (From Sherwood, L. 2010. Figure 10.37 in *Human physiology*, 7th ed. Belmont, CA: Brooks/Cole-Cengage Learning.)

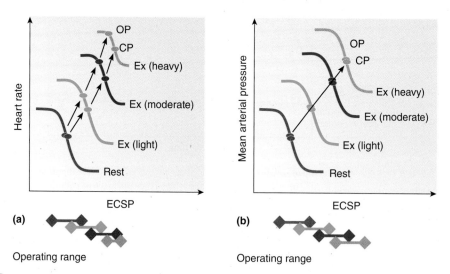

FIGURE 7.34 Arterial baroreflex control of heart rate and blood pressure resetting that occurs in direct relation to increasing exercise intensity. CP, centering point; OP, operating point. (Modified from Raven, P. B., P. J. Fadel, and S. Ogoh. 2006. Arterial baroreflex resetting during exercise: A current perspective. *Exp. Physiol.* 91(1):37–49.)

Autonomic Neural Controls Regulate the Cardiovascular Response to Exercise

It is important to note that all three neural mechanisms described earlier are part of the ANS and are involved in regulating the cardiovascular responses to exercise. The main goals of this regulatory system are to:

1. Increase Q̇ to deliver oxygen to the working muscles

2. Redistribute the increase in Q̇ to the working muscles and brain

3. Regulate arterial BP to provide adequate perfusion pressures in relation to oxygen demand without damaging the brain (see figure 7.35)

The regulation of arterial BP is paramount in protecting the brain from the large pulsatile increases in BP that occur with the large increases in Q̇ that are required in moderate to near-maximal dynamic or resistance exercise. At the onset of exercise, the CC activity sets the required BP in direct relation to the workload. This requires immediate resetting of the arterial baroreflexes to enable the HR to increase via parasympathetic withdrawal and begin to redirect the increased Q̇ to the exercising muscle via sympathetic activation. At the same time, muscle contractions activate the mechanoreceptors in the muscle, which signal the cardiovascular center to distribute blood flow to the muscle via further sympathetic activation and vasoconstriction of the blood vessels linked to the

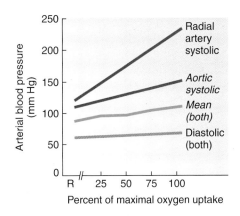

FIGURE 7.35 Increases in arterial blood pressure in relation to the percentage of maximal oxygen uptake ($\dot{V}O_2$ max) for radial and aortic pulse pressures. (Adapted from Rowell, L. B. 1993. Figure 5.11 in *Human cardiovascular control*. New York: Oxford University Press.)

organs and the nonactive skeletal muscles. The expected sympathetic vasoconstriction is partially inhibited by mechanisms of **functional sympatholysis**, to allow the increased blood flow to be delivered to the active muscle, even though the blood vessels of the active muscle are receiving the same increase in sympathetic activity as the inactive muscle (see Figure 7.6).

However, baroreflex control of BP is maintained via its control of sympathetic nerve activity to the blood vessels of both the active and inactive tissues. Because the active tissue has a higher volume of blood flowing through the vessels, the smaller vasoconstriction has a much larger effect in maintaining the arterial BP because it redistributes more blood centrally than the much greater vasoconstriction observed in the inactive tissue.

functional sympatholysis The inhibition of the effect of increased sympathetic activity at the blood vessel wall.

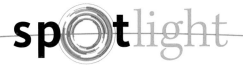

An Expert on the Autonomic Neural Control of the Circulation: Jere H. Mitchell, M.D.

Dr. Jere H. Mitchell (b. 1928), Professor of Cardiology at the University of Texas (UT), Southwestern Medical Center in Dallas, Texas, is recognized as a leader in the development of the scientific area known as the "Neural Control of the Circulation during Exercise."

After graduating from UT Southwestern's Medical School with his M.D. degree in 1954, Mitchell embarked on a career of clinical investigation, and by the time he completed his cardiology fellowship and a National Institutes of Health postdoctoral fellowship, he was recognized as a major investigator in the field of exercise physiology. In 1958, he was the first investigator to define the cardiovascular responses to a maximal oxygen uptake ($\dot{V}O$ max) test, and thereby provide a concise cardiovascular physiologic meaning of $\dot{V}O_2$ max. This work was published in *Journal of Clinical Investigation* in 1958.

His initial work was followed by 10 years of investigation into the central hemodynamic response to dynamic exercise and exercise training in healthy subjects and patients with cardiac disease. However, during this time, Dr. Mitchell was intrigued by the apparent relationship between muscle activity and the control of cardiovascular function. This interest led him to begin preliminary investigations of the interaction between the active skeletal muscle and cardiovascular function, and in 1963, he authored an article in *American Journal of Physiology* relating muscular activity and cardiovascular function. These initial works resulted in him proposing an integrative model of human exercise in a *Scientific American* article in 1965.

Mitchell was the driving force behind the landmark detraining study performed at UT Southwestern Medical Center in Dallas in collaboration with Dr. Bengt Saltin. This study of a group of people confined to complete bed rest for a period of 21 days documented the severe deconditioning of bed rest

and resulted in a change in the postsurgical treatments of patients, in that rather than ordering complete bed rest, doctors began requiring the patient to begin ambulation as soon as possible.

In 1972, Mitchell and McCloskey published their seminal findings on the exercise pressor reflex in *Journal of Physiology* (London). This work clearly identified that physiologic information relating the exercise state of the muscle (tension or metabolites) was sensed within the muscle and transmitted to the central nervous system via type III and IV nonmyelinated afferent neural fibers. Within 4 months of the publication of this initial article documenting the role of the type III and IV muscle afferents in the EPR, Mitchell, using human subjects, presented evidence for the role of CC and its interaction with the EPR in the cardiovascular response to exercise. Using unique experimental models, such as the decerebrate and spinal anesthetized cat and rat, the chronically instrumented awake and operant conditioned cat, and curarized and spinal anesthetized humans, he has defined the neuroanatomic pathways and physiologic function of the pathways involved in the neural control of the circulation.

in*Practice*

Examples of the Cardiovascular System and Exercise

The following sections provide some practical examples of how cardiovascular system adjustments to exercise are related to your area of interest.

Health/Fitness: Participation in regular exercise causes heart rate (HR) and systolic blood pressure (SBP) to be reduced at submaximal workloads after training (minimum of 6–8 weeks). For example, if you tested a client at 5 miles/hour on a treadmill when that client was deconditioned and tested that client again 6 to 8 weeks after cardiovascular conditioning at 5 miles/hour, you would observe marked reductions in the HR and SBP response. These adaptations in HR and SBP have been classically cited in exercise physiology research literature by scientists to document the effects of cardiovascular conditioning. The reductions in HR and SBP are commonly used as justification that the cardiovascular system becomes "more efficient" after aerobic conditioning.

Medicine: Participation in regular exercise causes the cardiovascular system to adapt, integrate, and change the cardiovascular responses to increased metabolic demands. The three neural systems—central command, the exercise pressor reflex, and the arterial baroreflexes—are part of the autonomic nervous system (ANS) and adapt specifically to the challenges of exercise, just as the skeletal muscles adapt.

Athletic Performance: Participation in regular high-intensity exercise significantly lowers the resting HRs of athletes compared with sedentary individuals. Endurance athletes have the lowest resting HRs, as low as 28 to 30 beats/min in marathoners (Clarence DeMar) and cyclists (Lance Armstrong). Resistance-trained athletes also have lower resting HRs than sedentary individuals, but usually are more in the range of 55 to 60 beats/min. This is probably due to the greater adaptations of the ANS control with aerobic (or cardiovascular) training compared with resistance (weight) training.

Rehabilitation: You have already learned in Chapter 2 that patients who participate in regular exercise via a cardiac rehabilitation program can acquire physiologic benefits from peripheral (skeletal muscles) and central (cardiac output) adaptations. Cardiac rehabilitation patients can also increase their strength safely and effectively by lifting weights (performing resistance exercise), but they need to be advised and reminded not to hold their breath. The cardiovascular blood pressure response to isometric exercise in healthy individuals is much higher than that for dynamic exercise; for cardiac patients, it would become clinically dangerous unless they perform low-intensity, high-repetition lifts without holding their breath.

 # Chapter Summary

- Clinically, the within normal limits (WNL) values for resting heart rate (HR) range between 50 and 80 beats/min. The systemic circulation consists of the blood flowing from the left ventricle to the right atrium, whereas the pulmonary circulation consists of blood flowing from the right ventricle to the left atrium.
- Mean arterial pressure (MAP) = cardiac output ($\dot{Q}$) × resistance.
- There are two types of exercise: dynamic, or aerobic; and resistance, a mixture of isometric (static) and dynamic.
- During dynamic exercise, the rate of circulation increases in an intensity-related manner up to a maximum of five to six times greater than at rest.
- During isometric contractions of greater than 30 percent maximal voluntary contraction (MVC), energy production occurs primarily by anaerobic processes and results in degrees of ischemia within the muscle directly related to % MVC, which activates the sympathetic nervous system and increases the blood pressure (BP) out of proportion to the oxygen uptake ($\dot{V}O_2$).
- $\dot{Q}$ = heart rate (HR) × stroke volume (SV).
- $\dot{V}O_2 = \dot{Q} \times (a - v) O_2$ difference.
- Venous return during dynamic exercise is assisted by the muscle and respiratory pumps. Blood flow in a vessel is influenced by the length of the vessel, the viscosity of the blood, and the radius of the vessel.
- Vasoconstriction and vasodilatation alter the radius vessel only and are the primary mechanisms of blood flow regulation.
- Blood flow in the brain is regulated by cerebral autoregulation (CA), but it is also influenced by $PaCO_2$ and the autonomic nervous system.
- The onset of exercise activation of central command (CC) involves a feed-forward set of neural signals emanating from the motor cortex and activating cardiovascular control centers in the brainstem, which rapidly withdraws parasympathetic control of the heart (increase in HR) and increases sympathetic outflow to the heart and vasculature (regulates BP).
- Currently, the overall consensus of how the arterial baroreflexes are reset is that the feed-forward mechanism of CC is primary and the feedback exercise pressor reflex mechanism is a modulator of the resetting.
- The main goals of this regulatory system are to increase $\dot{Q}$ to deliver oxygen to the working muscles, redistribute the $\dot{Q}$ to the working muscles, and regulate arterial BP.

 # Exercise Physiology Reality

CENGAGE brain To reinforce the exercise physiology concepts presented above, complete the laboratory exercises for Chapter 7. To access labs and other course materials for this text, please visit www.cengagebrain.com. See the preface on page xiii for details. Once you complete the exercises, have your instructor evaluate your prescriptions. Remember to use your lab experience to help guide you toward future success in exercise physiology.

Exercise Physiology Web Links

Access the following websites for further study of topics covered in this chapter:

- Find updates and quick links to sites related to the cardiovascular system and exercise physiology at our website. To access the course materials and companion resources for this text, please visit www.cengagebrain.com. See the preface on page xiii for details.

- Search for further information about research and the cardiovascular system and exercise at the American Physiological Society (APS) website: www.the-aps.org.

- Search for information about the cardiovascular system and exercise at the American College of Sports Medicine website: www.acsm.org.

- Search for more information about cardiovascular disease and the economic costs associated with this problem at the American Heart Association website: www.americanheart.org.

- Search for more information about research and the cardiovascular system and exercise at the Federation of American Societies for Experimental Biology website: www.faseb.org.

Study Questions

Review the Warm-Up Pre-Test questions you were asked to answer before reading Chapter 7. Test yourself once more to determine what you know now that you have completed the chapter.

The questions that follow will help you review this chapter. You will find the answers in the discussions on the pages provided.

1. Define the equation: $MAP/\dot{Q} = TPR$. *p. 220*

2. How is the maximal heart rate determined? *pp. 227–228*

3. Oxygen consumption has a central component and a peripheral component. Explain. *pp. 212–213*

4. What system enables the blood flow to be distributed to the exercising muscles? *pp. 236–238, 246–252*

5. Explain the relationship between stroke volume and ejection fraction. *p. 229*

6. Explain what happens to blood pressure as a result of an 85 percent MVC static exercise. *pp. 243–246*

7. What controversy exists regarding the brain's cerebral circulation during exercise? *pp. 240–243*

8. Briefly explain the theory of central command. *p. 246*

9. Explain the exercise pressor reflex. *pp. 247–248*

10. Explain how the cardiovascular response to exercise is regulated by autonomic neural controls. *pp. 246–251*

Selected References

Astrand, P. O., and K. Rodahl. 1986. *Textbook of work physiology: Physiological basis of exercise,* 3rd ed. New York: McGraw-Hill.

MacDougall, J. R., D. Tuxen, D. G. Sale, J. R. Moroz, and J. R. Sutton. 1985. Arterial blood pressure response to heavy resistance exercise. *J. Appl. Physiol.* 58:785–790.

Mitchell, J. H., B. J. Sproule, and C. B. Chapman. 1957. The physiological meaning of the maximal oxygen intake test. *J. Clin. Invest.* 37:538–547.

Mitchell, J. H., C. G. Blomqvist, A. R. Lind, B. Saltin, and J. T. Shepherd, editors. 1981. Static (isometric) exercise: Cardiovascular responses and neural control mechanisms

[American Heart Association monograph]. *Circ. Res.* 48(6 pt 2):1–188.

Mitchell, J. H., W. L. Haskell, and P. B. Raven. 1994. Classification of sports. *Med. Sci. Sports Exerc.* 86(Suppl. 2):S242–S245.

Raven, P. B., P. J. Fadel, and S. Ogoh. 2006. Arterial baroreflex resetting during exercise: A current perspective. *Exp. Physiol.* 91(1):37–49.

Raven, P. B., J. T. Potts, X. Shi, and J. A. Pawelczyk. 1999. Baroreceptor mediated reflex regulation of blood pressure during exercise. In *Exercise and circulation in health and disease* (pp. 3–24), edited by B. Saltin, R. Boushel, N. H. Secher, and J. H. Mitchell. Champaign, IL: Human Kinetics.

Rowell, L., editor. 1986. *Human circulation: Regulation during physical stress.* New York: Oxford University Press.

Secher, N. H., T. Seifert, and J. J. Van Lieshout. 2008. Cerebral blood flow and metabolism during exercise: Implications for fatigue. *J. Appl. Physiol.* 104:306–314.

Sherwood, Lauralee. 2010. Chapter 13, "The Respiratory System," pages 461–509, and Chapter 15, "Fluid and Acid-Base Balance," pages 557–587 in *Human physiology: From cells to systems,* 7th ed. Belmont, CA: Brooks/Cole-Cengage Learning.

Taylor, H. L., E. Buskirk, and A. Henschel. 1955. Maximal oxygen intake as an objective measure of cardiorespiratory performance. *J. Appl. Physiol.* 8:73–80.

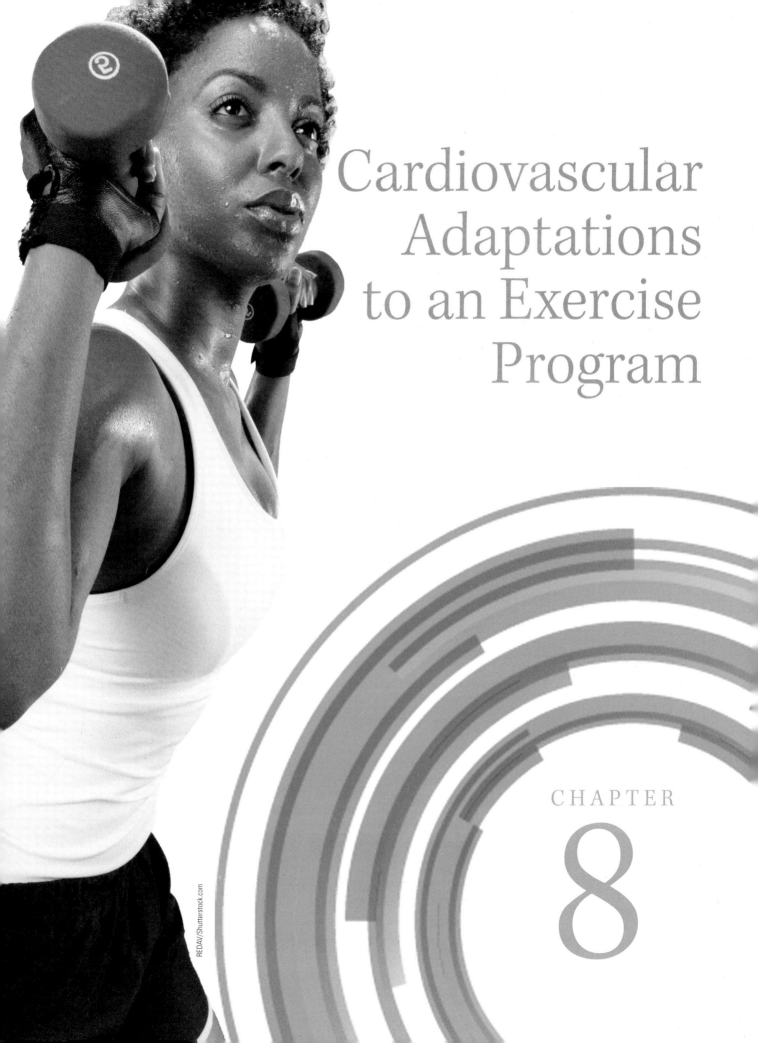

Cardiovascular Adaptations to an Exercise Program

CHAPTER

8

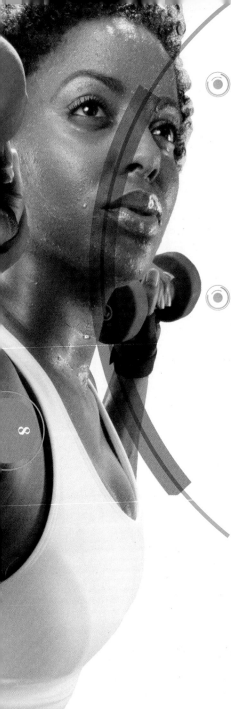

Warm-Up

CENGAGE **brain**

What do you already know about cardiovascular adaptations to endurance and resistance exercise training programs?

- Use the following Pre-Test or the online evaluation tools for Chapter 8 to determine how much you already know. To access the course materials and companion resources for this text, please visit **www.cengagebrain.com**. See the preface on page xiii for details.

- Need more review? Let the online assessments, animations, and tutorials for Chapter 8 help prepare you for class.

Pre-Test

1. What is the primary physiologic measure of circulatory capacity that distinguishes individuals with differing amounts of aerobic fitness?

2. What additional primary factor besides age, sex, body composition, and training program is an important factor for developing an individual's maximal oxygen uptake?

3. Endurance exercise training can result in a _____ percent increase in cardiac output.

4. Endurance exercise training results in a _____ in resting heart rate.

5. A significant increase in _____ _____ is the primary reason for the increase in cardiac output with aerobic endurance training.

6. Cardiac contractility is a measure of the strength of a cardiac contraction, and chronic endurance exercise training results in no change or minor _____ in cardiac contractility.

7. After 3 months of endurance exercise training, the number of capillaries per muscle fiber area _____.

8. Static exercise training results in _____ hypertrophy of the heart.

9. There is no change in blood pressure at rest after an endurance exercise training program because the vasculature has remodeled and there is a(n) _____ in total vascular compliance.

10. Endurance exercise training _____ the resting blood pressure of patients with hypertension.

1. maximal oxygen uptake ($\dot{V}O_2$ max); 2. genetics; 3. 100 percent; 4. decrease; 5. stroke volume; 6. increases; 7. increases; 8. concentric; 9. increase; 10. decreases

What You Will Learn in This Chapter

- How regular engagement in endurance (dynamic) exercise training increases maximal oxygen uptake ($\dot{V}O_2$ max)

- How regular engagement in endurance (dynamic) exercise training can change cardiac output

- How regular engagement in endurance (dynamic) exercise training can remodel the heart and the peripheral vasculature

- How isometric, or resistance, exercise training causes specific cardiovascular adaptations

QUICKSTART!

When you engage in regular endurance (dynamic) exercise training, how does your cardiovascular system adapt? How can you do more work with less fatigue? How long does it take to see positive cardiovascular adaptations with training? Do you think people who have had a previous heart attack benefit from engaging in a regular program of endurance (dynamic) exercise training? Answer yes or no, and explain your answer.

Introduction to Cardiovascular Adaptations to an Exercise Program

When a program of endurance exercise training is performed regularly, that is, three to four times per week, and the amount of training load is gradually increased over a period of weeks and months, the cardiovascular system adapts proportionally to meet the increased demand for oxygen delivery. When the adaptation of the individual's cardiovascular system reaches its genetic optimum for the delivery of oxygen to the working muscles, further training stress may not result in additional increases in cardiovascular function. It will, however, continue to stress the metabolic machinery (noted in Chapter 3) to increase its optimal use of the oxygen delivered and the tissue's capacity to use metabolically produced lactate from the type IIa and IIb fibers as an energy source for muscle and heart contraction (lactate shuttle; see Chapters 3 and 9) and brain metabolism (see Figure 8.1).

After the exercise physiologist/scientists demonstrated their ability to validly measure an individual's maximal oxygen uptake ($\dot{V}O_2$ max), it was surprising to many that the individual with the largest $\dot{V}O_2$ max value, measured in absolute (L O_2/min) or relative to body weight (ml O_2/Kg/min), did not always win the middle- to long-distance events. Indeed, the $\dot{V}O_2$ max values of Olympic champions of endurance events range from 72 to 94 ml O_2/kg/min and suggest that developing other factors, such as metabolic efficiency and economy of movement and/or skill in producing the necessary muscular power, are integral parts of a training program. In addition, as mentioned in Chapter 3, the training program must develop physiologic and psychological tolerance for withstanding the physical and psychological challenges of muscular fatigue to be an elite performer.

HOTLINK *See Chapter 3 for more information about muscular fatigue.*

This chapter provides an overview of the current knowledge regarding the adaptations of the cardiovascular system when undergoing an endurance exercise training program. In addition, whenever information is available regarding elite endurance athletes and cardiovascular-impaired patients, comparisons are drawn to emphasize the physiologic limits of both training and detraining. The cardiovascular adaptations to resistance exercise training (weight training) and the adaptations of the neural control of the cardiovascular system also are addressed. However, specific adaptations of the cerebral circulation to both dynamic and resistance exercise training have not been investigated to date. This chapter is organized in the same manner as Chapter 7, and each variable of the cardiovascular system is addressed in the same order.

inRETROSPECT

Bill Bowerman: Track Coach and NIKE, Inc. Cofounder

Bill Bowerman was born in Portland, Oregon, in 1913. He attended the University of Oregon, where he played football and majored in journalism. After graduation, Bowerman became a high school teacher and football coach, and then he joined the U.S. Army during World War II. After the war, he went back to high school coaching and got the opportunity to become the head track coach at the University of Oregon in 1948.

Coach Bowerman became one of the all-time most successful distance running coaches in the world. When he first started at the University of Oregon, interval training was very popular because numerous Olympian greats like Paavo Nurmi, "the flying Finn," used high-intensity training and pacing for success in distances from 1,500 meters to the marathon. However, coach Bowerman learned quickly that too much interval training (>2–3 days/week) without the proper amount of rest (what we call *periodization* now; see Chapter 2) increased the incidence of illness and injury in his runners. Bowerman learned to coach great runners like Steve Prefontaine and many others by having them finish workouts

feeling good and excited versus exhausted. Bowerman's teams at the University of Oregon won four NCAA national track titles with numerous individual titles, and 33 of his athletes became Olympians.

During his coaching career at the University of Oregon (1948–1973), coach Bowerman constantly experimented with running shoes, trying to make products that were light, provided support, and fit his runners properly. As a result, one of his former runners Phil Knight (now CEO of NIKE, Inc.) formed a partnership to distribute athletic footwear called Blue Ribbon Sports, which later became NIKE, Inc.

It is generally accepted that after coach Bowerman returned from a visit with Arthur Lydiard in New Zealand (1963), he introduced the concept of "jogging" as a fitness routine to the people of Oregon. Coach Bowerman used his journalist skills to write numerous articles and books (*Jogging*, written with cardiologist W. E. Harris in 1966, sold more than a million copies) about jogging for fitness, which subsequently sparked the "jogging craze" at that time in the United States.

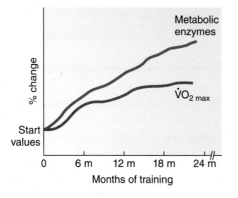

FIGURE 8.1 Endurance training adaptations. Schematic representation of the changes in maximal oxygen uptake ($\dot{V}O_2$ max) in relation to the changes that occur in the skeletal muscle's metabolic enzymes over a prolonged (≥2 years) period of endurance exercise training using the overload principles discussed in Chapters 2 and 3. (© Cengage Learning 2013)

Dynamic, or Endurance, Exercise Training

As noted in Chapter 2, endurance exercise training requires a regular and repetitive (once or twice a day) program of exercise incorporating rhythmic contractions of large muscle groups (running, swimming, bicycling, cross-country skiing, rowing, or walking) based on the training principles of progressive increases over time in frequency, duration, and intensity (see Chapters 2 and 3). If you are planning to be competitive, then the fourth principle of specificity also needs to be a part of your training program.

Increases in Oxygen Uptake above Rest Are Necessary to Perform Dynamic (or Aerobic) Exercise

The primary physiologic measure of circulatory capacity that distinguishes individuals with differing amounts of aerobic fitness is their $\dot{V}O_2$ max normalized to body weight (Figure 8.2).

There is a large range of values of $\dot{V}O_2$ max in healthy young adults; these are reflective of an individual's daily physical activities, dietary habits, cardiovascular health, and genetic makeup. In patients with severe cardiopulmonary disease, values less than 20 ml O_2/kg/min are often measured (see Table 8.1 for $\dot{V}O_2$ peak values for the classification of patients with heart failure), whereas in the elite endurance athletes (for example, cross-country

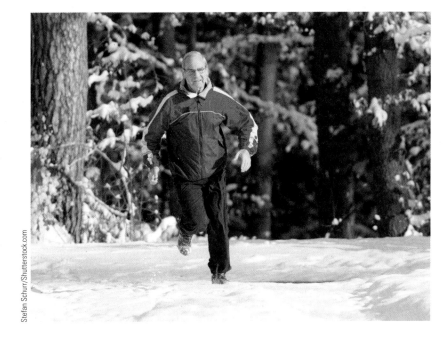

Stefan Schurr/Shutterstock.com

skiers), values that exceed 85 to 90 ml O_2/kg/min (see Figure 8.2) are not unusual.

In 1964, the New York chapter of the American Heart Association published a classification of the severity of heart failure in patients with heart disease linked to the symptom limitations identified during clinical exercise testing. In 2001, the American College of Cardiology modified the symptom classification; both are summarized in Table 8.1 and are linked to the measurement of $\dot{V}O_2$ peak.

In addition to the genetic component of training-induced increases in $\dot{V}O_2$ max, a number of other factors affect the amount of change in $\dot{V}O_2$ max following an exercise training program. These include:

1. The individual's $\dot{V}O_2$ max at the start of training

2. Age of the individual in training

3. Muscle mass involved

4. Frequency, intensity, and duration of training

5. Specificity

These factors are further discussed in the following subsections and are summarized in Figure 8.3.

KEY

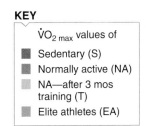

$\dot{V}O_2$ max values of

■ Sedentary (S)
■ Normally active (NA)
■ NA—after 3 mos training (T)
■ Elite athletes (EA)

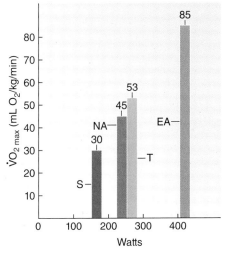

⬤ **FIGURE 8.2 Group differences in $\dot{V}O_2$ max values.** Differences in maximal oxygen uptake ($\dot{V}O_2$ max) between sedentary (S), normally active (NA), normally active that exercise trained for 3 months (T), and elite athletes (EA). (Modified from Rowell, L. B. 1993. Figure 5.1 in *Human cardiovascular control.* New York: Oxford University Press.)

CONCEPTS, challenges, & controversies

Genes or Exercise Training: What Contributes Most to Maximal Oxygen Uptake?

A controversy has arisen as to which provides the greatest proportional contribution to an individual's maximal oxygen uptake ($\dot{V}O_2$ max): the individual's genetic heritage or the amount (years × training load) of endurance training performed. Based on some earlier comparisons between fraternal and identical twins in which the identical twins had very similar $\dot{V}O_2$ max values, whereas fraternal twins had distinctly different $\dot{V}O_2$ max values, it was proposed that some 93 percent of $\dot{V}O_2$ max was a result of genetic endowment. However, after reviewing data obtained from long-term (>2 years) endurance training programs and reporting 44 percent improvement in $\dot{V}O_2$ max, the proportional contribution of genes versus training environment approaches a 50:50 split. Suffice it to say, "If you don't use it, you will lose it" regardless of your genetic optimum.

Another point of debate concerns the validity of the concept of the individual genetic component of adaptation to endurance training. The concept has significant scientific logic based on the many physiologic functions that have genetically based components. However, the technical difficulties of establishing appropriate controls for performing a definitive study are great enough that the answers have yet to be determined conclusively. The data of the **Heritage Study**, in which the genetic factors involved in establishing training adaptability were investigated using identical twins, do indeed indicate a strong role for a genetic component to one's adaptation to endurance exercise training.

HOTLINK *See the Pennington Biomedical Research Center website for more information about the Heritage Study:* **www.pbrc.edu/heritage/index.html**.

Heritage Study Funded by the National Heart, Lung, and Blood Institute of NIH since 1992. Its main goal is to study the role of the genotype in the cardiovascular and metabolic responses to exercise training of healthy subjects and to identify the genotype's role in influencing the exercise training effect on cardiovascular and diabetes risk factors.

TABLE 8.1 New York Heart Association (1964) and American College of Cardiology/American Heart Association (2001) Functional Classification of Patients with Heart Disease

New York Heart Association Functional Classification of Patients with Heart Disease (1964)	
Classification	**Criteria**
Class I	Patients with heart disease who have no symptoms of any kind; ordinary physical activity does not cause fatigue, palpitation, dyspnea, or anginal pain
Class II	Patients who are comfortable at rest but have symptoms with ordinary physical activity
Class III	Patients who are comfortable at rest but have symptoms with less than ordinary effort
Class IV	Patients who have symptoms at rest
American College of Cardiology–American Heart Association Classification of Chronic Heart Failure (2001)	
Stage	**Description**
A: High risk for developing heart failure	Hypertension, diabetes mellitus, CAD, family history of cardiomyopathy
B: Asymptomatic heart failure	Previous MI, LV dysfunction, valvular heart disease
C: Symptomatic heart failure	Structural heart disease, dyspnea and fatigue, impaired exercise tolerance
D: Refractory end-stage heart failure	Marked symptoms at rest despite maximal medical therapy

CAD, coronary artery disease; LV, left ventricular; MI, myocardial infarction.
(American Heart Association (1964) and American College of Cardiology (2001))

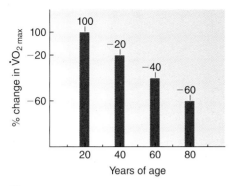

● FIGURE 8.3 Age-related reductions training increases in $\dot{V}O_2$ max. A generally accepted age-related decrease in the amount of increase in maximal oxygen uptake ($\dot{V}O_2$ max) achieved after a given period of exercise training. (© Cengage Learning 2013)

Beginning Maximal Oxygen Uptake

The greater the individual's $\dot{V}O_2$ max at the start of training, the smaller the increase in $\dot{V}O_2$ max that occurs after a given amount of training (see Figure 8.3).

Beginning Age

The effect of an adult's age at the beginning of training affects the amount of improvement one can expect to see; that is, the older the individual, the less is the increase in $\dot{V}O_2$ max after training (see Figure 8.3). However, in evaluating the data in Figure 8.3, it is important to note that the intensity of the training relative to the maximum heart rate (MHR; that is, $60\% \times [MHR - RHR] + RHR$, where RHR is resting heart rate) will be less; therefore, the total amount of total work and cardiac work performed by the older subjects in a given amount of time (3, 6, 9, or 12 months) will be far less than that of the younger subjects. This caveat will result in there being much less increase in the older individual's $\dot{V}O_2$ max regardless of an aging effect.

> Why will the training program based on the percentage of MHR result in there being less of a training stimulus to increase $\dot{V}O_2$ max? And how would you go about attempting to equalize the training stimulus?

In contrast, when endurance or strength training is performed during the pubescent years, the perception is that larger increases occur in $\dot{V}O_2$ max or strength, respectively, than for the same training program performed in the postpubescent period of development. Furthermore, it has been suggested that the effects of detraining are less for those who trained during the pubescent period. However, carefully controlled investigations of these controversial proposals have not been performed.

Beginning Muscle Mass

The absolute increase in $\dot{V}O_2$ max after training is directly related to the amount of muscle mass used during the training program. For example, the increase in $\dot{V}O_2$ max following a training program using one-legged knee extension exercise (such as one-legged kicking on a specially designed ergometer or one-legged cross-country skiing or cycling) will be less than if two-legged exercise was used during the training program. This will be more important for the one- or two-legged amputee, because the engineering design and specialized materials for the construction of prostheses has reached a point where the amputee can be as competitive as a nonhandicapped athlete. It was just prior to the 2008 Olympics that the International Olympic Committee ruled that a double-amputee equipped with prostheses will be unable to compete in the sprint competitions.

Frequency, Intensity, and Duration

Recall from Chapter 2 that the adaptive responses to endurance training are dependent on:

1. Frequency
2. Intensity
3. Duration

Increases in cardiovascular adaptation will continue to occur until the individual's genetic optimum is reached (see Figure 8.1).

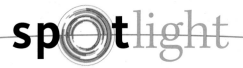

An Expert on Endurance Exercise Training for Middle-Distance: Arthur Lydiard

Arthur Lydiard was born in Eden Park, New Zealand. He grew up to become one of the foremost middle-distance (800 meters to marathon) running coaches in the world. Although Lydiard dropped out of school at age 16 to work in a shoe factory, he became self-educated about applied exercise physiology principles and developed scientifically based training methods that are still modeled today by competitive athletes and coaches. He was able to learn about endurance training by using himself as a model and ran up to 250 miles in 1 week to test his endurance and adaptation abilities.

Lydiard became interested in developing new methods of training after a fellow older rugby club member took him out on a 5-mile run and embarrassed him. Although Lydiard was not known as a fast runner, he began training regularly 7 days a week, for up to 12 miles a day, and eventually became a New Zealand marathon champion twice (1953 and 1955), with a best time of 2:39.05. By conducting training experiments on himself and others who joined him in training, Lydiard discovered how to combine long, slow distance training, interval training, Fartlek (speed play) training, and effective strategies for peaking for competition.

Lydiard informally coached several New Zealand marathon runners who won the national marathon title 11 times between 1958 and 1970. In 1960, he helped coach Murray Halberg and Peter Snell to win Olympic gold medals in the 5,000 and 800 meters, respectively. In the 1964 Olympics, under Lydiard's leadership, Snell stunned the world by winning gold again in the 800-meter final and followed it up with another gold medal in the 1,500 meters.

Following his coaching successes with individual athletes, Lydiard began sharing his methods with coaches throughout the world who were willing to listen. Although many often shunned his training methods, Arthur Lydiard continued to influence successful runners and coaches until his death at the age of 87. Often called the father of the "jogging" craze in the United States (because of his relationship with Bill Bowerman, the successful University of Oregon track coach), he was able to successfully develop and integrate the present-day concepts of neuromuscular responses and adaptations related to exercise.

Specificity

Another factor involved in adaptation for performance is that of the specificity of training (see Chapter 2). The simple fact is that even though you can train an elite endurance swimmer to have a large $\dot{V}O_2$ max by using running as the mode of training, her swimming performance will be well below that of other elite swimmers trained with swimming.

A wide range of individual values of $\dot{V}O_2$ max and a large range of endurance performance exists within the general population. When the measures of $\dot{V}O_2$ max and endurance performance, assessed by a 1.5-mile run or the distance traveled in 12 minutes, are correlated, the correlation coefficient is strong (0.9), suggesting that a measure of $\dot{V}O_2$ max predicts endurance performance (Figure 8.4; see Chapter 10).

However, if one were to compare individual world-class or elite middle-distance runners and marathoners, it would *not* always be the one with the highest $\dot{V}O_2$ max who would win a competitive race. This fact identifies that performance in endurance events is not all about $\dot{V}O_2$ max but can and does include a multitude of factors, such as the specificity of training, the capacity of the metabolic machinery supporting muscle contraction, muscle fiber type and plasticity, neuroendocrine regulation, psychological traits, and the degree of acclimatization to environmental challenges.

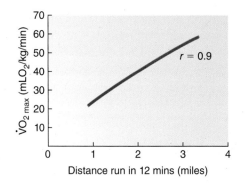

● **FIGURE 8.4** **The relationship between distances run in 12 minutes and maximal oxygen uptake ($\dot{V}O_2$ max).** (Modified from Cooper, K. H. 1968. A means of assessing maximal oxygen intake. Correlation between field and treadmill testing. *JAMA* 203:201–204.)

Examples of the Benefits of $\dot{V}O_2$ Max versus Endurance Training

Two Olympic gold medal athletes who made use of these adaptations were Peter Snell of New Zealand and Frank Shorter of the United States. Peter Snell won gold medals for the 800-meter race in the 1960 Rome Olympics and the 800- and 1500-meter races in the 1964 Tokyo Olympics; he also broke the world record for time for the 1-mile race in 1962 (3:54.4) and again in 1964 (3:54.1).

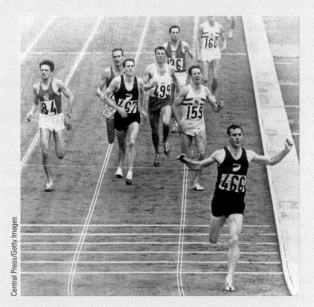

Peter Snell winning the 1,500-meter gold medal in the Tokyo Olympics.

The current world record for the mile run is 3:43.13, run by Hicham El Guerrouj of Morocco in 1999. Whether better training methods or the new style tartan track surfaces and high-technology running shoes provided the 11-second difference between 1964 and 1999 is only speculation. However, Snell's treadmill-measured $\dot{V}O_2$ max was a mere 72 ml O_2/kg/min, or 5.6 L O_2/min, a value that when compared with other elite athletes at the time was rather average. How, then, was he able to achieve such exceptional middle-distance performances?

Snell trained under the tutelage of Arthur Lydiard, an internationally renowned New Zealand middle- and long-distance track coach, who was a proponent of long, slow distance training runs interspersed with "speed play" (Fartlek) training up and down the sand dunes of New Zealand's North Island coastal shores. It was Snell's belief that even though he had achieved his optimum cardiovascular performance earlier in 1962, it was his training regimen that enabled the adaptation of the metabolic machinery of the muscle to continue to adapt, and thereby enable the muscles to use the delivered oxygen more efficiently, resulting in his ability to generate such superior athletic performances.

Frank Shorter from the United States won an Olympic gold medal for the marathon in record time at the 1972 Munich Olympic Games and also had a measured $\dot{V}O_2$ max of 72 ml O_2/kg/min (the same as Snell's).

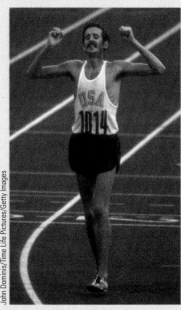

Shorter winning the 1972 Munich Olympic Games gold medal in the marathon.

Shorter was also a practitioner of the long, slow distance training runs interspersed with speed play (Fartlek) training. It is important to understand that long, slow distance training to the elite athlete is not as you and I know slowly to be. Many of these training runs were for a distance of 20 or more miles run at a 5- to 6-min/mile pace. The current world record time for the 26-mile marathon requires the runner to run each mile in 4 minutes 44 seconds.

However, similar to Snell, Shorter achieved his genetic optimum for cardiovascular adaptation but continued to train his skeletal muscle's metabolic machinery to more efficiently use the oxygen delivered and the metabolic lactate produced. Indeed, when tested on a treadmill running at 90 percent $\dot{V}O_2$ max, his blood lactate value was well below the lactate threshold (see Chapters 2, 4, 7, 9, and 10).

Many elite competitors in Snell's and Shorter's races had higher $\dot{V}O_2$ max values, yet the competitors were unable to defeat them in the races they all had specifically trained for.

Endurance Exercise Training Results in Rapid Central Circulatory Adaptations

In Equation 7.3 (see Chapter 7), we identified the relationships between HR, stroke volume (SV; that is, cardiac output), and arteriovenous oxygen difference at $\dot{V}O_2$ max.

Figure 8.5 presents a cross-sectional comparison of these variables for a patient with heart disease with a $\dot{V}O_2$ max of 1.5 L/min, an average fit sedentary individual with a $\dot{V}O_2$ max of 3.0 L/min, and an elite endurance-trained athlete with a $\dot{V}O_2$ max of 5.6 L/min.

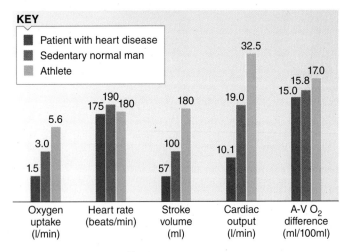

FIGURE 8.5 Maximal cardiovascular and oxygen uptake values. Maximal oxygen uptake ($\dot{V}O_2$ max) values and related central circulation variable of a male patient with heart disease, a sedentary healthy normal man, and an endurance athlete. (From Blomqvist, G. 1974. Exercise physiology related to diagnosis of coronary artery disease. In *Coronary heart disease: Prevention, detection, rehabilitation with emphasis on exercise testing* [pp. 2–1 to 2–26], edited by S. M. Fox III. Denver, CO: Department of Professional Education, International Medical Corporation.)

From these data it is readily apparent that the difference in maximal SV between the three individuals results in the differences in maximal cardiac output and $\dot{V}O_2$ max. Indeed, the effect of an individual's left heart pump function on the achievable maximal SV at MHRs is generally accepted as the limiting factor to an individual's maximal cardiac output, and hence his/her $\dot{V}O_2$ max.

The slight differences in maximal arteriovenous oxygen difference are significant between each of the individuals, but they are not large enough to account for the large differences in $\dot{V}O_2$ max.

> Explain physiologically the cause of the differences in arteriovenous oxygen at $\dot{V}O_2$ max.

Endurance Exercise Training Programs Result in Increases in Maximal Cardiac Output

Endurance exercise training can result in a near doubling of an elite athlete's maximal cardiac output without changing the resting or submaximal cardiac outputs. Furthermore, the invariant linear relationship between cardiac output and $\dot{V}O_2$ (described in Chapter 7) is unchanged by endurance exercise training (see Figure 8.6).

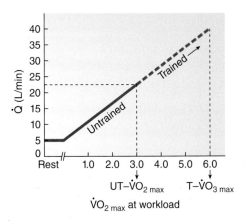

FIGURE 8.6 The relationship between oxygen uptake ($\dot{V}O_2$) and cardiac output ($\dot{Q}$) in untrained (UT) and endurance exercise–trained (T) individuals.
(© Cengage Learning 2013)

How endurance exercise training changes cardiac structure and function and its response to exercise are discussed later in this chapter. Training that consists of resistance exercise, or weight lifting, does not result in an increase in the maximal cardiac output.

Endurance Exercise Training Programs Result in Decreases in Resting and Submaximal Heart Rates

Endurance exercise training results in a decrease ranging from 10 to 40 beats/min in RHRs and submaximal workload HRs but only minor differences at MHR (see Figure 8.7a).

These differences in RHRs and submaximal HRs between endurance-trained and untrained individuals are due to an increase in the degree of vagal control on the cells of the sinoatrial (SA) node and their intrinsic firing rate. An increased vagal control reduces the SA node cell's firing rate and decreases the HR, and a decrease in vagal control increases the SA node cell's firing rate and increases the HR. However, if we plot the HR response to exercise in relation to the individual's percentage of $\dot{V}O_2$ max (%$\dot{V}O_2$ max), the difference between the trained and untrained individuals disappears (see Figure 8.7b).

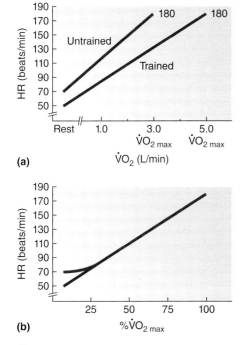

(a)

(b)

● FIGURE 8.7 Relationship between HR and $\dot{V}O_2$. (a) Relationship between heart rate (HR) and oxygen uptake ($\dot{V}O_2$) from rest to maximal $\dot{V}O_2$ ($\dot{V}O_2$ max) of endurance exercise–trained and untrained subjects. (b) Relationship between HR and %$\dot{V}O_2$ max from rest to 100 percent $\dot{V}O_2$ max of exercise-trained and untrained subjects. (© Cengage Learning 2013)

> Explain why when you relate the absolute HRs to absolute $\dot{V}O_2$, the HRs of the trained individuals are lower than the untrained individuals at submaximal workloads, but are not different when related to the %$\dot{V}O_2$ max.

Despite a multitude of investigations into the effects of endurance exercise training on MHR, it remains unclear whether MHR is reduced, unchanged, or, in some cases, increased. In general, the trend is for endurance exercise training to decrease the MHR.

Endurance Exercise Training Affects the Neural Control of Heart Rate

The neural control of HR involves the following factors:

1. Intrinsic rhythm of the SA node cells, or the **intrinsic heart rate (IHR)**

2. Parasympathetic (vagal) influence on the IHR

3. Sympathetic influence on the IHR

At rest in healthy individuals, the vagal activity has a proportionally greater influence on HR than the sympathetic activity. At the beginning of dynamic exercise, the HR increases primarily because of vagal withdrawal and a gradual increase in sympathetic activity. As the intensity of the exercise gets progressively higher, the balance between the vagal influence and the sympathetic influence on HR is reversed and the sympathetic activity becomes predominate. In contrast with the findings of earlier investigations, the vagus has a small but significant influence on HR and arterial baroreflex-mediated HR responses during high-intensity exercise and even at

intrinsic heart rate (IHR) The heart rate that is measured when the sympathetic and parasympathetic neural influence is fully blocked by metoprolol (β-1 selective receptor) and atropine (muscarinic receptor), respectively.

maximum exercise. Immediately on cessation of exercise, the vagus becomes fully re-engaged and is the primary mechanism in the slowing of the HR during recovery (see Figure 8.8).

In healthy sedentary individuals with RHRs ranging from 60 to 80 beats/min, the rate and depth of breathing are involuntarily controlled, and the time between successive PQRST waves is relatively stable. However, close inspection of the time between successive P waves identifies a slight shortening of the P – P time interval during inspiration and a slight lengthening of the P – P time interval during expiration. These changes in time intervals between successive electrocardiographic (ECG) waves, when analyzed as a change in frequency in a specific time period, is defined as the **heart rate variability** and provides an assessment of the integration between the neural control of the respiratory and circulatory systems (see Figure 8.9).

The rate and depth of breathing and the rate of the heart's beating are controlled by the respiratory center and the cardiovascular center, respectively, located within the medulla oblongata. However, in addition to these central mechanisms, the lungs and the respiratory muscles provide feedback information regarding the depth of breathing to the respiratory center, which, in turn, modulates the cardiovascular center's output influencing the HR. A third neural input comes into play during inspiration and expiration, and is known as the **Bainbridge reflex**. During inspiration, the amount of blood returning to the heart (venous return) increases and stretches the right atrium's mechanoreceptor cells, causing them to stimulate the afferent (C-fibers) connected to the mechanoreceptors to send signals to the medulla, which, in turn, decreases the vagal outflow from the nucleus ambiguus to the heart (that is, withdraws the vagal outflow) and increases the SA node firing (that is, increases the HR).

Describe the reflex pathway during expiration and explain how it affects the HR. In formulating your answer, use the previous text and Figure 8.9.

HOTLINK *See Chapter 7 for more information about the ECG definitions of the P, QRS complex, and T waves.*

Bainbridge reflex An increase in heart rate due to an increase in right atrial pressure caused by an increase in venous return. Sometimes called the *atrial reflex.*

heart rate variability A physiological phenomenon where the time interval between consecutive heart beats or R-R intervals varies.

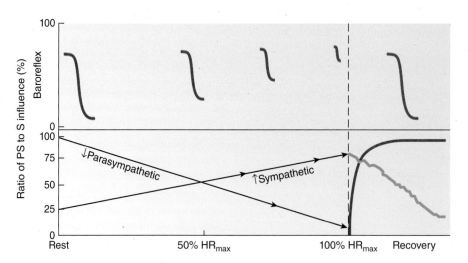

FIGURE 8.8 Balance between parasympathetic and sympathetic neural activity on heart rate (HR) and the arterial baroreflex control of the HR during progressive increases in exercise intensity and recovery. See text for explanation of Figure 8.8. (© Cengage Learning 2013)

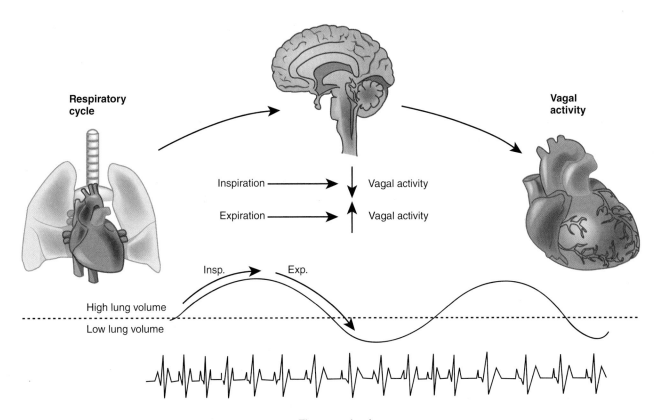

Insp. — **Exp.**

High lung volume
Low lung volume

Three mechanisms:

1. **Resp. & CV center**

2. **Afferents from lung**

3. **Bainbridge reflex**

FIGURE 8.9 Changes in vagal activity during inspiration and expiration that result in changes in heart rate. See text for explanation of Figure 8.9. (© Cengage Learning 2013)

Respiratory Sinus Arrhythmia

Elite athletes have RHRs between 30 and 40 beats/min. In the well-trained endurance athlete with the exceptionally low HRs, the propagation of the electrical depolarization originates from the SA node, indicating a maintained sinus rhythm. The maintenance of a sinus rhythm is related to the training-induced increased influence of parasympathetic control of the heart and is generally referred to as an increase in vagal tone. This training-induced increase in vagal tone results in the decreased RHRs and submaximal HRs, and the appearance of **respiratory sinus arrhythmia (RSA)** (see Figure 8.9).

Most, if not all, well-trained endurance athletes exhibit RSA, and the degree of RSA is associated with the amount of vagal (parasympathetic) control of the HR. Athletes with RHRs less than 60 beats/min usually exhibit RSA, and those with HRs of 30 to 40 beats/min always have pronounced RSA. The presence of RSA can be visually determined from an ECG record and is quantified over time by measuring the standard deviation around the average (mean) HR. In addition, bioengineering techniques of measuring the HR variability in the frequency domain identify from measures of **power spectral density** that the high-frequency variability

respiratory sinus arrhythmia (RSA)
A naturally occurring variation in heart rate that occurs during respiration.

power spectral density Describes how the power of a signal or time series is distributed with respect to frequency is used to analyze heart rate variability and breathing variability by transforming (using a mathematical process termed **Fast Fourier Transform analysis**) the time domain to the frequency domain.

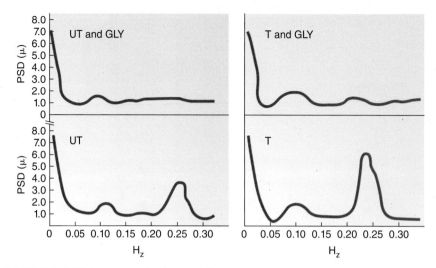

FIGURE 8.10 Heart rate (HR) variability power spectral density of an endurance exercise-trained (T) subject and an untrained (UT) subject breathing at a frequency of 15 breaths/min (that is, 0.25 Hz) without and with blockade of the parasympathetic nerve action at the muscarinic receptors on the heart using glycopyrrolate (GLY).

(© Cengage Learning 2013)

occurs in synchrony with the respiration (Figure 8.10).

Note the greater prominence of the power spectral density at 0.25 Hz (a breathing frequency of 15 breaths/min) of the trained subject compared with the untrained subject. In addition, the synchrony between respiratory variability and HR variability is disrupted, and the variation in HR over time of both the trained and untrained subjects is removed when a selective vagal blockade (atropine or glycopyrrolate) is used.

Adaptations of Stroke Volume to a Program of Endurance Exercise Training

The supine or upright resting and maximal SV can double as a result of endurance exercise training and is the primary reason for the increase in maximal cardiac output. An average fit sedentary individual's SV plateaus at a relative workload of 40 percent $\dot{V}O_2$ max, and it is maintained relatively constant up to 100 percent $\dot{V}O_2$ max. However, in the highly trained endurance athlete, SV continues to increase up to 100 percent $\dot{V}O_2$ max (see Figure 8.11).

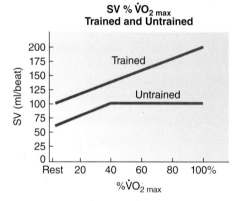

FIGURE 8.11 Drawing of the changes in stroke volume (SV) with increases in dynamic exercise workloads related to the individual's maximal oxygen uptake ($\dot{V}O_2$ max), that is, %$\dot{V}O_2$ max.

(© Cengage Learning 2013)

The physiologic explanation for the plateau in SV at 40 percent $\dot{V}O_2$ max in the healthy average fit individual and the absence of the plateau in the endurance exercise-trained athlete remains in question. However, the following two scenarios provide a simple explanation for the differences between the trained and untrained subjects without providing clear indications of the structural and molecular biologic mechanisms involved in the training adaptations:

1. The appearance of the plateau of SV at 40 percent $\dot{V}O_2$ max in the sedentary healthy individuals appears to be related to a balance between cardiac filling time (a factor of the R-R interval) and volume and the rate of venous return (a factor of the muscle and respiratory pumps; see Chapter 7) and its effect on the cardiac filling volume; that is, as the pulse interval decreases (increasing HR), more volume must be entering the heart at a faster rate just to maintain the ejection volume of each beat constant.

2. In contrast, the continuously increasing SV up to $\dot{V}O_2$ max in the endurance exercise-trained athlete suggests that the venous return volume entering the heart for each decrease in R-R interval (that is, increase in HR) is greater and enables a greater ejection fraction volume to be achieved for each beat via the Frank–Starling mechanism and increases in myocardial contractility in direct relation to the progressively increasing $\dot{V}O_2$ required for the increasing workloads.

For these changes to occur, the following adaptive responses to the endurance exercise training are required:

1. Pericardial restraint and remodeling of the pericardium

2. Cardiac remodeling and hypertrophy

3. Possible increases in cardiac contractility

4. Vascular remodeling and growth

5. Blood volume expansion

Pericardial Restraint

The concept that the heart's SV can be limited by pericardial restraint emanates from the **cardiac tamponade patient**, in whom as the fluid volume between the pericardium and the myocardium increases, the volume of the heart gets restrained from completely filling; consequently, the reduction in the resting cardiac output of the tamponade patient results from a reduction in SV.

The presence of pericardial restraint on the SV of an exercising human was first demonstrated in a patient with an implanted pacemaker requiring an open pericardium. The patient's HR was set using the pacemaker at 100 beats/min during rest and while performing progressive workload cycling up to 2 L O_2/min (see Figure 8.12).

Because the HR was fixed at a rate of 100 beats/min during exercise, the increases in cardiac output must have been a result of increases in SV related to the unrestrained increase in end-diastolic volume (remember, the pericardium is slit open). However, it should also be noted that as the workload increased, the end-systolic volume decreased, resulting in an increased ejection fraction indicating an increase in myocardial contractility. This response is slightly different from that identified previously in healthy subjects with their pericardium intact (see Figure 7.15).

In addition, in an experiment using exercising dogs, before and after pericardiectomy, significant increases in SV were observed at workloads much greater than the workload at which the plateau in SV was observed with the pericardium intact (that is, load 1; see Figure 8.13).

As foxhounds have untrained $\dot{V}O_2$ max values of 90 ml O_2/kg plus and had evidence of pericardial restraint only near maximal exercise, and the fact that the patient with a slit pericardium did not exhibit a plateau in SV with increasing workload exercise, it appears that pericardial restraint will only be a factor at near-maximal exercise. Because pericardial restraint of an endurance exercise-trained individual is not observed (see Figure 8.11), even at maximal exercise, some form of cellular remodeling of the pericardium must occur in response to the endurance exercise training.

cardiac tamponade patient A patient with a life-threatening situation in which there is such a large amount of blood or other fluid inside the pericardial sac around the heart that it interferes with the performance of the heart.

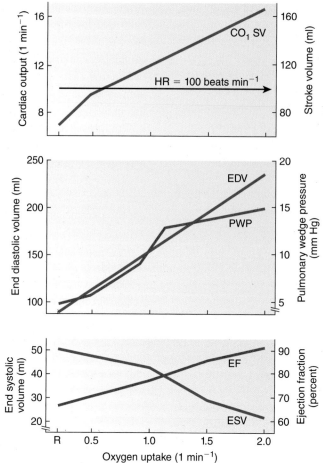

FIGURE 8.12 The heart function of a patient with a pacemaker implant and a split pericardium response to upright cycling during progressive increases in workload. (From Rowell, L. B. 1993. Figure 5-9 in *Human cardiovascular control*. New York: Oxford University Press.)

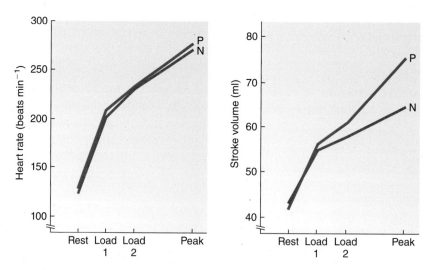

FIGURE 8.13 The heart function of a foxhound's response to progressive increases in workload exercise before and after pericardiectomy. (From Rowell. L. B. 1993. Figure 5-10 in *Human cardiovascular control*. New York: Oxford University Press.)

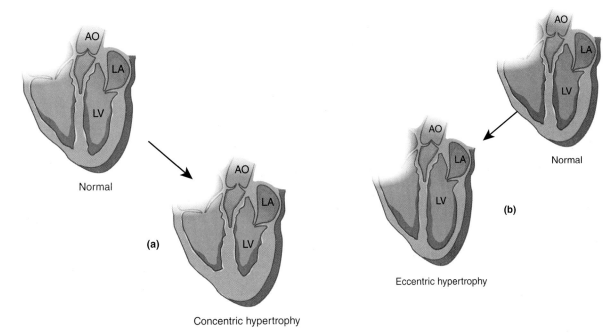

Normal

Concentric hypertrophy

(a)

Normal

Eccentric hypertrophy

(b)

FIGURE 8.14 Changes in heart structure. (a) Schematic representation of the differences in wall thickness between a normal healthy heart and a concentric hypertrophied heart during the first 3 months of endurance exercise training or after a resistance exercise training program. (b) Schematic representation of the differences in left ventricular (LV) chamber volume between a normal healthy heart and an eccentric hypertrophied heart after 6 to 9 months or more of endurance exercise training. (© Cengage Learning 2013)

Cardiac Remodeling and Hypertrophy and Blood Volume

The cardiac hypertrophy that results from the training program is directly related to the intensity and duration of the exercise training program and the changes in fitness or $\dot{V}O_2$ max. During a typical overload principle training program, the heart initially adapts to the increased preload of the larger central blood volume during exercise by increasing its left ventricular (LV) mass (concentric hypertrophy; see Figure 8.14a), resulting in an increase in the heart's LV wall thickness. As the training continues and blood volumes increase, the ventricular chambers of the heart increase their volumes without reducing the thickness of the chamber walls. This adaptation is called *eccentric hypertrophy* (see Figure 8.14b).

For example, in a 1-year endurance exercise training program performed by investigators at the Institute for Exercise and Environmental Medicine (University of Texas Southwestern/Presbyterian Hospital in Dallas), magnetic resonance images of the subjects' hearts were made every 3 months to determine the progression of the changes in heart mass and chamber

diameters. After the initial 3 months of training, the adaptation of the left ventricle was an increase in mass, that is, concentric hypertrophy. After 6 months, the increases in LV mass stopped (see Figure 8.15).

However, with continued training over a 6- to 12-month period, the LV chamber diameters increased because of the sustained training-induced increases in blood volume and the intermittent training increases in wall stress related to the increased cardiac filling volumes. These training-induced increases resulted in the often reported eccentric hypertrophy of endurance exercise-trained athletes (see Figure 8.16).

In contrast, the right ventricle establishes eccentric hypertrophy during the first few months of training. In addition, the

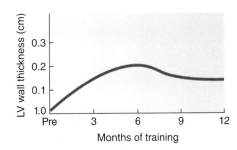

FIGURE 8.15 Changes in wall thickness. The increases in left ventricular wall thickness in 3-month intervals over 1 year of endurance exercise training. No significant changes after 3 months. (Unpublished data provided by B. J. Levine, M.D., Director of the Institute of Exercise and Environmental Medicine in Dallas, TX.)

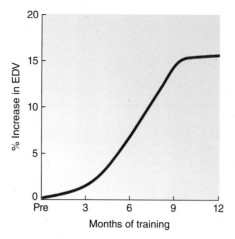

compliance (C) The change in volume (ΔV) over the change in pressure (ΔP).

FIGURE 8.16 Changes in end diastolic volume. The increases in left ventricular end-diastolic volumes [EDVs] in 3-month intervals over 1 year of endurance exercise training. Significant increases from 3 to 9 months. (Unpublished data provided by B. J. Levine M.D., Director of the Institute of Exercise and Environmental Medicine in Dallas, TX.)

pulmonary capillary wedge pressure (PCWP) An indirect measurement of the left atrial pressure obtained by wedging a catheter into a small pulmonary artery tightly enough to block flow from behind and in order to sample the pressure beyond. This measurement is used as a measure of the filling pressure of the left ventricle.

Example Calculation of Ventricular Compliance

A fundamental concept you need to grasp to understand how heart, lungs, and blood vessels function is the measurement of **compliance (C)**. Simply stated, compliance is the amount of change in volume (ΔV) that occurs for a given change in pressure (ΔP), or

$$C = \Delta V / \Delta P \qquad [8.1]$$

When the PCWP of the sedentary subjects decreases from 15 to 5 mm Hg during LBNP, the SV decreases from 85 to 60 ml and the C = 25/10 = 2.5 ml/mm Hg. When the PCWP of the athlete decreases from 15 to 5 mm Hg during LBNP, the SV decreases from 130 to 85 ml and the C = 45/10 = 4.5 ml/mm Hg. These calculations indicate that the athletes' LV compliance is nearly twice as compliant as the sedentary subjects (see Figure 8.17).

During the LBNP, the endurance-trained subjects had greater reductions in SVs (that is, end-diastolic volume data used in the sample calculation above) for a given reduction in the heart's filling pressure. The endurance-trained athletes' left ventricles were more compliant after the 12-month training period, as well as in the cross-sectional comparison with their aged-matched sedentary counterparts.

left atrial and right ventricular dimensions of athletes exhibiting the LV eccentric hypertrophy of the endurance-trained athlete are increased.

Before and after the exercise training program, these same investigators measured the changes in SVs and **pulmonary capillary wedge pressures (PCWPs)** during a simulated orthostatic challenge using lower body negative pressure (LBNP) to assess LV compliance in cross-sectional and longitudinal investigations (see Figure 8.17).

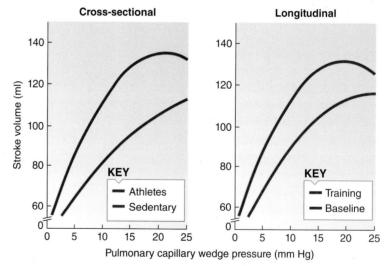

FIGURE 8.17 Training-induced changes in LV compliance. Levine's data documenting the changes in left ventricular compliance [SV × PCWP] after 1 year of endurance exercise training. (Levine's cross-sectional data: Levine B. D., L. D. Lane, J. C. Buckey, D. B. Friedman, and C. G. Blomqvist. 1991. Left ventricular pressure-volume and Frank–Starling relations in endurance athletes. Implications for orthostatic tolerance and exercise performance. *Circulation* 84:1016–1023. Lines drawn without standard error bars.)

These findings provide a physiologic explanation as to "why well-trained endurance athletes often have syncopal episodes (fainting) when standing up from a supine, bent knee or sitting position." A simple muscle tensing maneuver, such as crossing the legs and squeezing the buttock muscles, has been found to counteract the presyncopal symptoms.

In earlier times when ECGs were the only noninvasive means of assessing LV mass, the QRS complex in standard leads of the endurance athlete exceeded 15 mm (reflecting a large ventricular muscle mass) because of the earlier described training-induced physiologic hypertrophy. These adaptations are similar to volume overload conditions that exist in such pathologic states as aortic or mitral valve regurgitation and also result in eccentric hypertrophy (see Figure 8.14b). At the same time, the presence of the training-induced very slow HR, together with the cardiac hypertrophy of the athletes, resulted in a mistaken identification of the **"athlete's heart"** being classified as a pathologic hypertrophy.

However, the eccentric hypertrophy of the endurance-trained athlete is accompanied by slight outward increases in ventricular wall thickness. Hence the current understanding is that the structural and functional changes observed after a period of endurance exercise training are a healthy adaptation. In contrast, the eccentric hypertrophy of the pathologic volume stress associated with valvular regurgitation, or volume overload caused by congestive heart failure, result in ventricular wall thinning without changes in ventricular muscle mass.

The current use of M-mode echocardiographic evaluations, magnetic resonance imaging, or both enables reproducible and more accurate measures of wall thickness, diameters, and mass, and provides the physiologic basis for a more accurate diagnosis of the "athlete's heart."

HOTLINK *Use your favorite search engine for sites such as* **http://www.aha.org/** *to find more information on "athlete's heart."*

The increased SVs that occur with endurance exercise training are associated with training-induced increases in blood volume and plasma volume. However, the increase in ventricular diameter has been related to the increase in central blood volume associated with the training-induced increase in total blood volume. This concept remains controversial because the blood volume expansion has not been sufficiently documented to occur at the same time that changes in wall thickness and chamber size have been shown to occur.

The amount of tension generated in the heart wall is described by **Laplace's law**:

$$Twall = (P \times r) \qquad [8.2]$$

where Twall is wall tension, P is the ventricular chamber pressure, and r is radius of the heart chamber.

From Laplace's law (Equation 8.2), the increase in ventricular pressure during each heartbeat caused by the larger central blood volumes and venous return will increase the wall stress, or tension (T), which, in turn, stimulates signaling of cardiac muscle fiber growth. The resultant increase in fiber diameter increases the thickness of the ventricular walls, which enables the increase in wall stress to be reduced back to normal because the tension is distributed over a larger cross-sectional area of the chamber wall:

$$Twall/A \qquad [8.3]$$

where Twall is the tension in the wall, and A is the cross-sectional area of the wall.

It is proposed that the increased central blood volume results in increases in volume and pressure within the chambers of the heart causing chamber dilatation (physiologic hypertrophy) and a reduction in pressure. This volume overload chamber dilatation is present in many valvular disorders and in the patient with congestive heart failure. Why the training-induced dilatation of heart chambers of the endurance-trained individual occurs without wall thinning as compared with wall thinning associated with the heart failure-induced chamber enlargement (pathologic hypertrophy) is unknown. Molecular biologists are attempting to discern the cellular mechanisms involved in the two types of hypertrophy.

Laplace's law States that there is an inverse relationship between the inside surface tension of a sphere and its radius. In the cardiovascular system a small heart chamber or blood vessel exhibits a greater inward force than a large heart chamber or blood vessel. Also called the *Law of Laplace*.

"athlete's heart" Describes the enlarged ventricular chambers that result from endurance training without a change in ventricular wall thickness (eccentric hypertrophy) and a decrease in resting and submaximal heart rates.

Another important functional outcome of the training-induced cardiac remodeling is the increase in chamber compliance, especially ventricular compliance. The increase in ventricular compliance together with the training-induced bradycardia and central blood volume results in the heart filling over a longer diastolic time and being able to receive a larger volume of venous return for a given change in ventricular pressure. The larger blood volume within the ventricles at the end of diastole will result in a greater stretch of the cardiac muscle fibers and via the Frank–Starling mechanism a greater SV (see Figure 8.15; see also the explanation of the Frank–Starling mechanism in Chapter 7.)

This increased stretch of the cardiac muscle fibers is probably the molecular biologic signal for growth of the dormant satellite cells present within the cardiac striated muscle. From cross-sectional comparisons, the largest increase in wall thickness and chamber diameters has been noted in professional road cyclists and rowers. The anatomic changes that occur within heart cells are identified as cardiac remodeling. The benefit of these anatomic changes in endurance-trained athletes is related to the heart's ability to increase its SV during dynamic exercise, thereby allowing for a greater maximal cardiac output while maintaining a constant wall tension. The result of the increase in maximal cardiac output is that it provides a greater capacity to deliver oxygen, that is, $\dot{V}O_2$ max (see Figure 8.18).

Cardiac Contractility

Cardiac contractility is a measure of the strength, or vigor, of a cardiac contraction when the **preload, or cardiac filling pressure (end-diastolic fiber length)**, HR and **afterload, or arterial pressure**, are constant. This is a difficult measure to make in isolation from changes in the length–tension (Frank–Starling) or interval strength (HR) effects. It is generally accepted that myocardial contractility increases during progressive increases in exercise workload (see Figure 7.15); however,

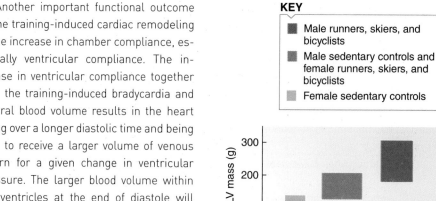

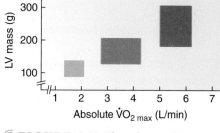

KEY

■ Male runners, skiers, and bicyclists
■ Male sedentary controls and female runners, skiers, and bicyclists
■ Female sedentary controls

● FIGURE 8.18 The relationship between absolute maximal oxygen uptake ($\dot{V}O_2$ max; L/min) and left ventricular (LV) mass (in grams) of male and female endurance athletes and sedentary individuals. (Based on data on LV mass and $\dot{V}O_2$ max presented by Mitchell, J. H., and P. B. Raven. 1994. Cardiovascular adaptation to physical activity. Chapter 17 in *Physical activity fitness and health: International proceedings and consensus statement* [pp. 296], edited by C. Bouchard, R. J. Shephard, and T. Stephens. Champaign, IL: Human Kinetics.)

attempts to measure changes in contractility at rest or during exercise after a period of endurance exercise training have suggested no change or changes so small that current measurement methods are unable to detect them.

Vascular Remodeling and Growth

Despite the increased blood volume at rest and the increases in maximal cardiac output and SV that occur after an endurance exercise training program, arterial blood pressure in healthy individuals at rest and during submaximal and maximal exercise remains unchanged; indeed, at maximal exercise, it is sometimes lower. These findings suggest that the microcirculatory volume within the trained skeletal muscle must have increased as a result of substantial vascular remodeling of conduit arteries and arterioles, and angiogenic growth of new capillaries (see Figure 8.19).

These changes result in increased vascular compliance and total vascular conductance (see Figure 8.20). In addition, there is direct relationship between $\dot{V}O_2$

preload, or cardiac filling pressure (end-diastolic fiber length) The initial stretching of the cardiac myocytes prior to contraction. Preload, therefore, is related to the sarcomere length. Because sarcomere length cannot be determined in the intact heart, other indices of preload are used such as ventricular end-diastolic volume or pressure.

afterload, or arterial pressure Generally thought of as the "load" that the heart ejects blood against. In simple terms, the afterload is closely related to the mean aortic pressure.

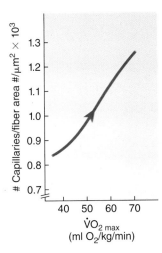

FIGURE 8.19 Relationship between maximal oxygen uptake ($\dot{V}O_2$ max; ml O_2/kg/min) and the number of capillaries per fiber area (number/$\mu m^2 \times 10^3$). (Based on Rowell, L. B. 1993. Figure 7-19 in *Human cardiovascular control.* New York: Oxford University Press.)

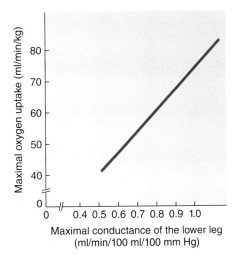

FIGURE 8.21 Relationship between maximal oxygen uptake ($\dot{V}O_2$ max) and maximal leg vascular conductance. (Based on data from Snell, P. G., W. H. Martin, J. C. Buckey, and C. G. Blomqvist. 1987. Maximal vascular leg conductance in trained and untrained men. *J. Appl. Physiol.* 62:606–610.)

max and an individual's reactive hyperemic leg blood flow response to suprasystolic leg cuff occlusion during heel-raising exercise. This finding suggests that the higher an individual's $\dot{V}O_2$ max that occurs as a result of endurance exercise training, the greater his/her capacity to vasodilate the blood vessels (see Figure 8.21). Therefore, as the maximal cardiac output increases in response to endurance exercise training, the muscle's maximal capacity to receive blood flow increases as a result of the increases in the vessel's compliance and vasodilatation capacity (see Figure 8.22).

Notably, if the vasculature supplying the active skeletal muscle during whole-body exercise were to be maximally dilated, the muscle's capacity of receiving the blood flow would exceed the heart's ability to increase its cardiac output, even if one were sedentary and the vascular adaptations to endurance exercise training would make the situation worse. Indeed, as described in Chapter 7, the balance between active

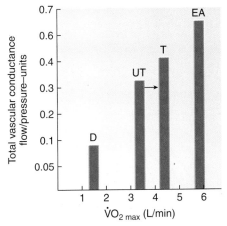

FIGURE 8.20 Relationship between maximal oxygen uptake ($\dot{V}O_2$ max; L/min) and total vascular conductance. (Based on Rowell, L. B. 1993. Figure 5-12 in *Human cardiovascular control.* New York: Oxford University Press.)

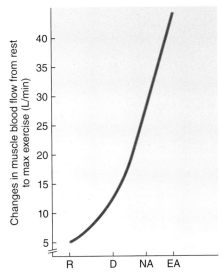

FIGURE 8.22 Changes in maximal leg blood flow from rest to maximal dynamic exercise of detrained (D), normally active (NA), and elite endurance athletes (EEA). (Redrawn from data presented in Rowell, L. B. 1993. Figure 7-7 in *Human cardiovascular control.* New York: Oxford University Press.)

sympathetic vasoconstriction and functional sympatholysis of the blood vessels is essential to maintain control of arterial blood pressure.

> Explain the balance between functional sympatholysis and sympathetic vasoconstriction of the active muscle's vasculature.

Arteriovenous Oxygen Difference

You have learned that an endurance exercise training program increases the number of capillaries per muscle fiber area, and that the capillary density of active skeletal muscle is directly related to $\dot{V}O_2$ max. In conjunction with these vascular changes, endurance exercise training increases hemoglobin (the oxygen-carrying protein; see Chapter 9) content of the red blood cell and the myoglobin (oxygen-carrying) protein in the skeletal muscle. In addition, oxidative enzymes of the trained skeletal muscle are increased, which, together with the training adaptations of the vasculature and the heart, result in a greater capacity to deliver, extract, and utilize oxygen within the active skeletal muscle. The increased capacity to extract oxygen should be reflected in a greater $(a - v)O_2$ difference maximum; but when compared as a percentage change, the total body extraction of oxygen from the blood is relatively unchanged from pretraining to post-training. The main difference in extraction is observed in the trained skeletal muscle bed. Although some investigators suggest that the increase in the maximal extraction of oxygen from the blood, or the $(a - v)O_2$ difference maximum, can increase $\dot{V}O_2$ max after an endurance exercise training program by as much as 50 percent, a more generally accepted increase suggests that it is less than 20 percent (see Figure 8.23).

Cardiac Work

In addition to the increased vagal control of the heart following an endurance exercise training program, other changes occur that reduce the submaximal HR and sympathetic activity at any given oxygen uptake. Thus, there is an increased efficiency of the heart's function. This increased efficiency of heart function is identified by a reduction in the **double product**, or the HR multiplied by systolic blood pressure (**HR × SBP**), at submaximal workloads. The double product is directly related to **myocardial oxygen consumption**, or the work of the heart, in generating the cardiac output (see Figure 8.24).

double product (HR × SBP) The mathematical product of heart rate times the systolic blood pressure; an index of the workload of the heart.

myocardial oxygen consumption The amount of oxygen consumed by the heart in a given unit of time (1 minute); is directly related to the double product.

KEY
- Oxidative enzymes
- Capillary density
- Oxygen uptake
- Cardiac output
- A–$\dot{V}O_2$ diff

⬤ **FIGURE 8.23** Average percentage changes in a normally active individual's oxygen-carrying and delivery capacity after years of endurance exercise training.
(© Cengage Learning 2013)

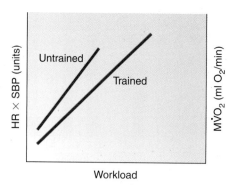

⬤ **FIGURE 8.24** Differences in the cardiac work of the heart before and after endurance exercise training. (© Cengage Learning 2013)

Resistance Exercise Training

In contrast with dynamic exercise training, resistance exercise training results in only one major change in cardiovascular function, that is, marked concentric hypertrophy of the heart.

(What is concentric cardiac hypertrophy?)

Resistance exercise training, or weight training, causes an increase in lean body mass as a result of muscle fiber hypertrophy and hyperplasia (5–20 percent) via dormant satellite (stem) cell activation (see Chapter 3).

Both cardiac and skeletal muscle are classified as striated muscle, and in the early 1980s, a major controversy arose with respect to whether the weight training-induced hypertrophy of skeletal muscle was only a result of an increase in muscle fiber diameter (a dogma held for more than 100 years) or whether an increase in the number of fibers was a part of the skeletal muscle hypertrophy (see Figure 8.25; see also Chapter 3 for a detailed discussion of this controversy).

The proposal whether a similar mechanism of cardiac stem cell activation occurs has stimulated a major controversy. Resistance exercise training primarily uses anaerobic metabolism to provide the energy for the muscle to contract; hence there is relatively little change in $\dot{V}O_2$ max. If $\dot{V}O_2$ max does increase, it is probably more related to a dynamic component of the exercise training program, such as that involved in circuit weight training. In addition, RHRs, blood pressure, and total blood volume are unchanged. Because of the increase in maximal voluntary contraction (MVC) of the trained muscle or groups of muscles, when the response to resistance exercise is expressed as a percentage of

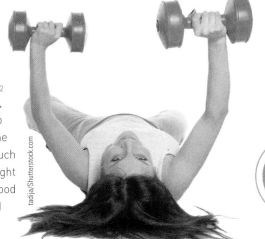

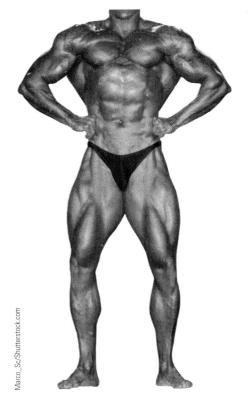

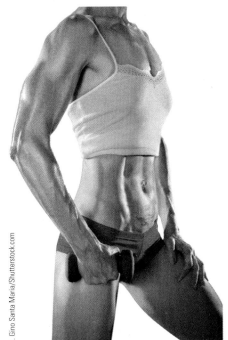

● **FIGURE** 8.25

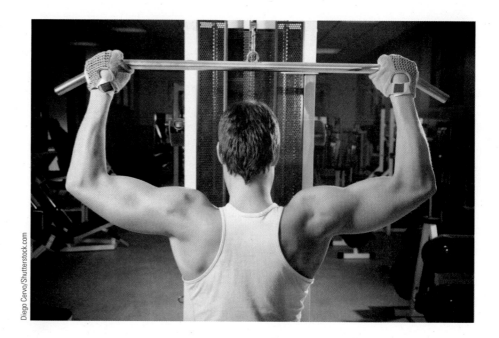

Diego Cervo/Shutterstock.com

MVC (%MVC), the resistance exercise training program does not change the HR and blood pressure responses to the exercise. However, the absolute HR and blood pressure responses are lower for a given MVC.

This reduction in absolute cardiovascular stress provides a rationale for including weight training in a preventative health program throughout life. As we get older and lose strength because of disuse atrophy, the simple MVC challenges (for example, a stuck jelly jar lid) become more difficult and the pressor response becomes magnified and increases the risk for stroke. Perhaps a regimen of weight training throughout life provides the heart a reserve to overcome the acute pressure overload on the left ventricle imposed by the daily resistance exercise challenges.

As noted previously, the cardiovascular response to resistance exercise is an exaggerated exercise pressor response elicited by the muscle ischemia invoked by the muscle contraction (see Chapter 7). The increased pressor response causes a pressure overload on the heart. This pressure overload is similar to that which accompanies systemic hypertension and aortic stenosis. Subsequently, the resistance exercise-trained athlete usually has concentric cardiac hypertrophy of the left ventricle, a disproportional thickening of the intraventricular septum and posterior

walls without LV chamber enlargement. When the increase in heart mass is normalized for body weight or body surface area, the weight-trained athletes are no different than normal sedentary individuals but have much less cardiac hypertrophy than an endurance-trained athlete (see Figure 8.26).

The use of anabolic steroids increases the wall thicknesses of the resistance-trained athlete and can cause a pathologic restriction on the aortic outflow tract, a high risk for sudden cardiac arrest.

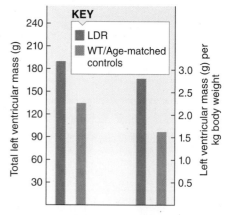

● **FIGURE 8.26 Differences in left ventricular mass between endurance- and weight-trained athletes and age-matched control subjects.** (Based on Longhurst, J. C., A. R. Kelly, W. J. Gonyea, and J. H. Mitchell. 1980. Echocardiographic left ventricular masses in distance runners and weight lifters. *J. Appl. Physiol.* 48:154–162.)

Whether resistance exercise training produces similar changes to the vasculature as observed with endurance exercise training has not been identified. However, because static exercise has significant beneficial effects on bone health and muscle strength, and also may develop protection against untimely pressure overloads on the heart and the brain, it is recommended that a preventative health program include both dynamic and static exercise training.

Neural Control of the Circulation

Chapter 7 explained that the fundamental mechanisms associated with the neural control of the circulation were central command, the exercise pressor reflex, and the arterial and cardiopulmonary baroreflexes (see Figure 7.31). The main goals of these regulatory mechanisms are:

1. To increase cardiac output and delivery of oxygen to the working muscles by redistributing the cardiac output to the working muscles

2. To regulate arterial blood pressure

The effects of a regular endurance exercise training program on the neural control of the circulation are manifested in the effective responses described earlier for the HR and the vasculature. However, when the responses are normalized from pretraining to post-training by relating the responses to the $\%\dot{V}O_2$ max before and after training to account for the increases in $\dot{V}O_2$ max, the differences disappear (see Figure 8.7).

It has been known since the 1970s that, for a given workload performed before a program of endurance exercise training, the amount of circulating norepinephrine spilled over into the circulation (a marker of autonomic nervous system activation) would be higher than when the same workload was performed after a training program (see Figure 8.27a). However, by relating the norepinephrine concentration to the change in $\%\dot{V}O_2$ max, the differences were eliminated (see Figure 8.27b).

Physiologic Adaptations to a Program of Endurance Exercise Training Often Cause Incidences of Presyncope

Because of the training-induced increases in central blood volume and the resting SV, the aortic arterial baroreflex and the

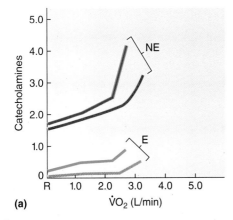
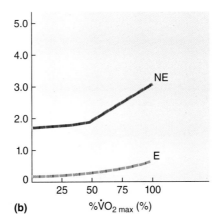

FIGURE 8.27 Changes in plasma catecholamine (norepinephrine [NE] and epinephrine [E]) concentrations during dynamic exercise before (a) and after (b) a 7-week intensive endurance exercise training program. (Based on Hartley, L. H., J. W. Mason, R. P. Hogan, L. G. Jones, T. A. Kotchen, E. H. Mougey, F. E. Wherry, L. L. Pennington, and P. T. Ricketts. 1972. Multiple hormonal responses to graded exercise in relation to physical training. *J. Appl. Physiol.* 33:602–606.)

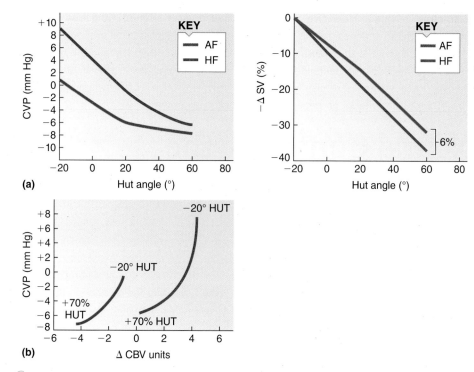

FIGURE 8.28 Changes in CVP, SV, and CBV during tilt. (a) Cross-sectional comparison decreases in the central venous pressure and stroke volumes of average fit (AF) and endurance exercise-trained high fit (HF) individuals during 70-degree head-up tilt (HUT). (b) Cross-sectional comparison changes in central venous pressure in relation to decreases in central blood volume of AF and endurance exercise-trained HF individuals during 70-degree HUT. (a: Based on Ogoh, S., S. Volianitis, P. Nissen, D. W. Wray, N. H. Secher, and P. B. Raven. 2003. Carotid baroreflex responsiveness to head-up tilt-induced central hypovolaemia: Effect of aerobic fitness. *J. Physiol.* 551[Pt 2]:601–608.)

cardiopulmonary baroreflex appear to be less responsive to orthostatic challenges. These reductions in baroreflex sensitivity, together with the cardiac remodeling, increases in cardiac compliance, and consequent greater declines in SV during orthostasis, result in the elite endurance athletes being more prone to orthostatic hypotension and syncope (see Figure 8.28).

Central Nervous System Adaptation

The loci of the dynamic exercise training-induced adaptations within the central nervous system have not been identified. From animal studies, it appears that the central neural outflow of efferent sympathetic neural activity is reduced (down-regulated)

in response to the repetitive bouts of exercise associated with a treadmill running training program. These findings strongly suggest that the training program not only adapts the muscles of the heart and skeleton, but the neural networks of the brain as well. Indeed, once the heart and skeletal muscle have reached their genetic optimum, the superior performances of the elite athletes may lie in the degree of neural adaptation in the central nervous system, enabling the individual's ability to psychophysically monitor their physiologic stress in relation to their maximal performance. These types of adaptations may well explain why the superior well-trained athlete does not confirm the existence of a "wall" when performing in endurance events.

Cardiovascular Deconditioning

Because of the successful introduction of antibiotics and childhood vaccinations against infections and infectious diseases,

together with the antiviral medications and vaccines, and the public health policies of providing healthy drinking water and sanitation, the life expectancy of the Western industrialized nations has grown to an age exceeding 80 years. Indeed, in the United States today, there are more than 1 million people older than 100 years and 32 million older than 65 years. This growth in the aged population has led to the general conception that as we age we lose physical fitness and cardiovascular health. However, since the introduction of jogging as a healthy lifestyle activity in the 1960s, the question whether aging per se is the reason for the loss of cardiovascular fitness or whether it is the increasingly greater percentage of time spent in a sedentary lifestyle that is the cause needs to be answered.

In what has become recognized as a classic investigation in 1966, a group of investigators at the University of Texas Southwestern Medical Center asked five (two active and three sedentary) men to undergo complete bed rest for a period of 21 days; the study became known as the **Dallas bed-rest study**. The active subjects lost significantly more $\dot{V}O_2$ max than the sedentary subjects. The group rate of loss of $\dot{V}O_2$ max was later calculated to be 250 ml O_2/kg/min/year, or 26 percent. After the 21 days of bed rest, each of the subjects underwent a supervised endurance exercise training program for 60 days (5 days/ week). The sedentary subjects restored their $\dot{V}O_2$ max to their initial values in 10 to

11 days, and at the end of the 60-day training period exceeded their initial pre-bed rest $\dot{V}O_2$ max value by 40 percent. In contrast, the two active subjects required the full 60 days of endurance exercise training to return to their pre-bed rest $\dot{V}O_2$ max values (see Figure 8.29).

> Explain the difference between the training responses of the sedentary compared with the active subjects.

Results of the Dallas Bed-Rest Study Resulted in Major Changes in Clinical Practice and Developments in Microgravity Deconditioning Investigations

The three major outcomes of the classical Dallas bed-rest study are:

1. Recovery from surgery required early ambulation instead of the usually prescribed complete bed rest.

2. The initial concept developed in the late 1950s of an active cardiac rehabilitation program after "a heart attack" was confirmed.

3. It was recognized that bed-rest deconditioning was similar to the deconditioning associated with the microgravity exposure of spaceflight. Therefore, many bed-rest facilities were built to investigate short- and long-term deconditioning of microgravity.

HOTLINK *Use your favorite search engine to investigate the negative physiologic effects of bed rest using the keywords "NASA bed-rest studies."*

Sedentary Living

After the completion of the Dallas bed-rest study, the same subjects underwent follow-up $\dot{V}O_2$ max testing 30 and 40 years later. The results documented that the

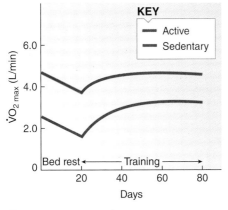

● FIGURE 8.29 $\dot{V}O_2$ max response to bed rest and training. Changes in maximal oxygen uptake ($\dot{V}O_2$ max) with 21 days of bed rest and 60 days of exercise training response to exercise after bed rest and after training. (Based on Saltin, B., G. Blomqvist, J. H. Mitchell, R. L. Johnson Jr., K. Wildenthal, and C. B. Chapman. 1968. Response to exercise after bed rest and after training. *Circulation* 38[5 Suppl]:VII1–VII78.)

Dallas bed-rest study A historical classic study conducted at the University of Texas Southwestern Medical Center in Dallas under the direction of Jere H. Mitchell. M.D. and Bengt Saltin, M.D./Ph.D.

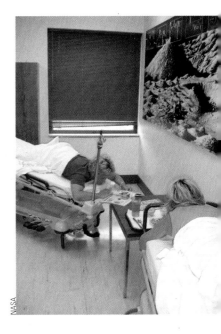

NASA

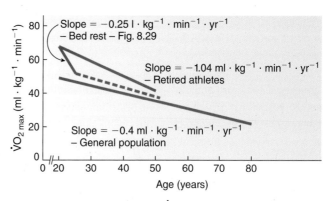

FIGURE 8.30 Age-related decreases in $\dot{V}O_2$ max. Decreases in maximal oxygen uptake ($\dot{V}O_2$ max) with increasing age, bed rest, and deconditioning. (Redrawn from Raven, P. B., and J. H. Mitchell. 1980. The effect of aging on the cardiovascular response dynamic and static exercise. Figure 2 in *The Aging Heart* [Vol. 12], edited by M. L. Weisfeldt. New York: Raven Press.)

subject's $\dot{V}O_2$ max declined 27 percent and was equivalent to the 26 percent decline caused by the 21 days of bed rest. However, between the ages of 50 to 60 years, the annual decline of $\dot{V}O_2$ max was four times greater (55 ml/min/year) than that which had occurred between the ages of 20 and 50 years (12 ml/min/year).

In comparison with the rate of loss of 1.04 ml O_2/kg/min/year $\dot{V}O_2$ max of the well-trained endurance athletes aged 20 to 35 years who became sedentary between the ages of 40 and 60 years, the bed rest had a 250 times greater deconditioning effect (see Figure 8.30).

In general, the data of many cross-sectional studies across an age range of 20 to 80 years indicate that age-related deconditioning in the general population occurs at an average rate of 0.45 ml O_2/kg/min/year. However, in a well-designed longitudinal training study performed in San Diego between 1970 and 1990, 15 volunteer men, who had an average age of 35 years at the beginning of the study, were recruited. Each of the recruited subjects' training programs was supervised 4 to 5 times/week, and the adherence to the training regimen was near 90 percent for all of the training days. Between years 25 and 33 of the training program, 4 of the original 15 subjects died. In contrast with the 0.45-ml O_2/kg/min/year decline in $\dot{V}O_2$ max that has been reported for the general population; the regular exercise training reduced the age-related yearly loss by 33 percent to 0.30 ml O_2/kg/min/year (see Figure 8.31).

Lifestyle

The physiologic changes, especially the cardiovascular changes, associated with the Dallas bed-rest deconditioning study were the opposite of the changes observed after an endurance exercise training program. Whether the time spent in training on a daily basis provides an economy of effort in maintaining one's health is for the individual to decide; however, both the Dallas and the San Diego studies emphasize the need to maintain an active lifestyle to optimize one's life expectancy. After completion of the 21 days of complete bed rest in the Dallas study, the subjects were intensively aerobically trained using a program of walk, jog, and run for a period of 60 days. The two subjects who were active before bed rest were only able to train their $\dot{V}O_2$ max back to their pre–bed-rest $\dot{V}O_2$ max. In contrast, the three subjects who were sedentary before the bed rest

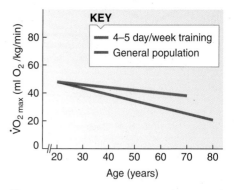

FIGURE 8.31 Age-related decreases in $\dot{V}O_2$ max with training. Changes in maximal oxygen uptake ($\dot{V}O_2$ max) over 20 years of regular exercise training compared with the general population's age-related rate of loss of $\dot{V}O_2$ max. (© Cengage Learning 2013)

were able to increase their $\dot{V}O_2$ max some 33 percent greater than their pre–bed-rest value.

There are two obvious situations in which the rapid and serious deleterious effects of bed rest become manifest:

1. A prolonged bed-rest recovery from traumas and injuries that require surgery

2. The tendency for the elderly confined to nursing homes to retire to bed or the armchair. In extended-care populations, some 63 percent become bedridden for the rest of their lives within 1 year of entering the home.

in*Practice*

Examples of Cardiovascular Adaptations to an Exercise Program

This section provides some practical examples, from a variety of professional areas with regards to the cardiovascular system and variables related to exercise.

Health/Fitness: Heart rate (HR) monitoring at rest and during exercise is a practical, non-invasive method that practitioners and participants in exercise can use for a variety of reasons, such as measuring the intensity of exercise, exercise testing, monitoring recovery from exercise, evaluating training improvements, preventing injuries, and optimizing rehabilitation. Many brands and types of heart rate monitors are available commercially. Although HR monitoring has become popular, many advocates of HR monitoring forget that there can be as much as 20 to 25% error in estimating the energy cost of exercise via HR monitoring. Day-to-day HR variation, overtraining, the type of exercise (static versus dynamic), cardiovascular drift (heart rate increases over time with continued exercise, 20–40 minutes), hydration status, temperature, and altitude all can significantly influence the HR and energy–cost relationship.

Medicine: You have learned previously about cardiac remodeling like left ventricular hypertrophy (LVH), but sometimes physiological changes in the heart like the development of hypertrophic cardiomyopathy (HCM) can become life threatening. HCM is a heritable disease that affects males significantly more than females and is the leading cause of sudden cardiac death (SCD) in young athletes (< age 30). The HCM heart has gross thickening (concentric) of the left ventricle walls with no dilation/decrease in LV chamber size, which can essentially reduce blood flow to the coronary arteries and the heart. There are few symptoms associated with the early development of HCM, and the problem is often missed, even with quality pre-participation sport participation exams (unless expensive echocardiography is used to determine heart dimensions). However, knowing if a person has a family history of HCM (death of a family member in their 40s or 50s) or has had syncope (fainting) during exercise (not necessarily after) can be helpful in screening for those at risk for SCD.

Athletic Performance: Participation in regular high-intensity exercise has been shown to produce LVH and LV dilation in endurance and strength athletes (the athletic heart) that is associated with eccentric or concentric hypertrophy changes. These physiologic changes to exercise are considered normal, and they have been shown to be reversible once training is stopped (detraining). Exercise causes the release of growth factors and neurotransmitters that stimulate receptors to mediate positive changes in LV mass and LV dilation.

Rehabilitation: Beta-blocker drugs are commonly prescribed for patients with hypertension and coronary artery disease (CAD), in addition to exercise training. Because beta-blockers lower resting and exercise heart rates and blood pressures, some professionals in the 1980s questioned whether patients could achieve a significant training effect while taking either selective medications (preferred because they primarily block only heart beta$_1$ receptors) or non-selective medications (block heart and beta$_2$ receptors of the lung and periphery). Researchers have since reported that patients with CAD who are treated with beta-blockers of any type can expect significant benefits with exercise training, and when possible, beta$_1$-selective blockers should be prescribed for those with uncomplicated hypertension versus non-selective beta-blockers for those who are exercising. See Gordon, N.F., Duncan, J.J., 1991. *Medicine and Science in Sports and Exercise*, 2(6): 668–676.

Chapter Summary

- When a training program of exercise is prescribed following the principles of intensity, frequency, duration, and specificity, the individual can achieve his or her genetic optimum maximal oxygen uptake ($\dot{V}O_2$ max).

- Although the relationship between maximum endurance performance and $\dot{V}O_2$ max is strong in a population with a wide range of $\dot{V}O_2$ max, the measurement of $\dot{V}O_2$ max is not absolutely predictive of elite endurance performance.

- The physiologic changes associated with a regularly performed program of exercise are increases in $\dot{V}O_2$ max, maximum cardiac output, stroke volume (SV) at rest and at max, total vascular conductance at rest and at maximum, and arteriovenous oxygen difference at maximum.

- Exercise training increases total blood volume and plasma volume. The maximal heart rate (MHR) is either unchanged or slightly decreased.

- Resting heart rates (RHRs) and submaximal HRs at a given workload after exercise training are reduced because of an increase in vagal tone.

- The cardiac remodeling and hypertrophy, and the angiogenic vascular and compliance changes are a result of molecular biologic mechanisms of remodeling.

- During progressive increases in dynamic exercise workloads, the SV of the average fit plateaus at 40 percent $\dot{V}O_2$ max, whereas the well-trained endurance athlete does not have evidence of a plateau in SV until near maximum cardiac output. The fitness-related differences in the SV may be related to pericardial restraint and cardiac filling time and ejection volume.

- All the changes associated with a regular program of exercise are reversed with detraining and even further with bed-rest deconditioning.

- The benefits of improved cardiovascular function associated with exercise training programs together with other ancillary health benefits have resulted in the development of prescribed cardiac rehabilitation programs.

- Static exercise training produces only a little improvement in cardiovascular function, and the concentric cardiac hypertrophy, although large, is in proportion to the increase in lean body mass.

Exercise Physiology Reality

CENGAGEbrain   To reinforce the exercise physiology concepts presented above, complete the laboratory exercises for Chapter 8. To access labs and other course materials for this text, please visit www.cengagebrain.com. See the preface on page xiii for details. Once you completed the exercises, have your instructor evaluate your work. Remember to use your lab experience to help guide you toward future success in exercise physiology.

Exercise Physiology Web Links

Access the following websites for further study of topics covered in this chapter:

- Find updates and quick links to cardiovascular adaptations to exercise at our website. To access the course materials and companion resources for this text, please visit www.cengagebrain.com. See the preface on page xiii for details.

- Search for further information about research and the cardiovascular system at the American Physiological Society website: http://www.the-aps.org.

- Search for information about cardiovascular physiology training and the American College of Sports Medicine at: http://www.acsm.org.

- Search for more information about cardiovascular physiology training at the U.S. National Heart, Lung, and Blood Institute information site: http://www.nhlbi.nih.gov/.
- Search for more information about cardiovascular physiology training at the American Heart Association website: http://www.americanheart.org.
- Search for more information about research and cardiovascular physiology training at the Federation of American Societies for Experimental Biology website: http://www.faseb.org.
- Search YouTube for video clips that provide examples of cardiovascular physiology training: http://youtube.com.

Study Questions

Review the Warm-Up Pre-Test questions you were asked to answer before reading Chapter 8. Test yourself once more to determine what you know now that you have completed the chapter.

The questions that follow will help you review this chapter. You will find the answers in the discussions on the pages provided.

1. How much influence does genetics have on a client's $\dot{V}O_2$ max? *p. 262*
2. How does the "specificity of training" principle apply to endurance performance? *p. 264*
3. What happens to MHR after intensive exercise training? Why? *p. 267*
4. What does pericardial remodeling refer to? *p. 271*
5. What is the difference between normal and abnormal cardiac hypertrophy? *pp. 273–276*
6. What happens to the arteriovenous oxygen difference after a 3-month endurance exercise training program? *p. 278*
7. How can $\dot{V}O_2$ max increase via static training? *p. 279*
8. What does the use of anabolic steroids do to the heart? *p. 280*
9. Why are elite endurance athletes more prone to hypotension and syncope? *p. 282*
10. What happens to one of your clients who undergoes cardiovascular deconditioning? *pp. 282–284*

Selected References

Astrand, P. O., and K. Rodahl. 1986. *Textbook of work physiology: Physiological basis of exercise,* 3rd ed. New York: McGraw-Hill.

Blomqvist, C. G., and B. Saltin. 1983. Cardiovascular adaptations to physical training. *Ann. Rev. Physiol.* 45:169–190.

Levine, B. D., D. L. Lane, J. C. Buckey, D. B. Friedman, and C. G. Blomqvist. 1991. Left ventricular pressure-volume and Frank–Starling relations in endurance athletes: Implications for orthostatic tolerance and exercise performance. *Circulation* 84:1016–1023.

Mitchell, J. H., and P. B. Raven. 1994. Cardiovascular adaptation to physical activity. Chapter 17 in *Physical activity fitness and health: International proceedings and consensus statement* (pp. 286–301), edited by C. Bouchard, R. J. Shephard, and T. Stephens. Champaign, IL: Human Kinetics.

Raven, P. B., and J. H. Mitchell. 1980. The effect of aging on the cardiovascular response dynamic and static exercise. In *The aging heart* (Vol. 12, pp. 1–323), edited by M. L. Weisfeldt. New York: Raven Press.

Rowell, L. B. 1974. Human cardiovascular adjustments to exercise and thermal stress. *Physiol. Rev.* 54:75–159.

Rowell, L. B. 1993. *Human cardiovascular control.* New York: Oxford University Press.

Saltin, B. 1969. Physiological effects of physical conditioning. *Med. Sci. Sports* 1:50–56.

Saltin, B. 1986. Physiological adaptation to physical conditioning. *Acta. Med. Scand. Suppl.* 711:11–24.

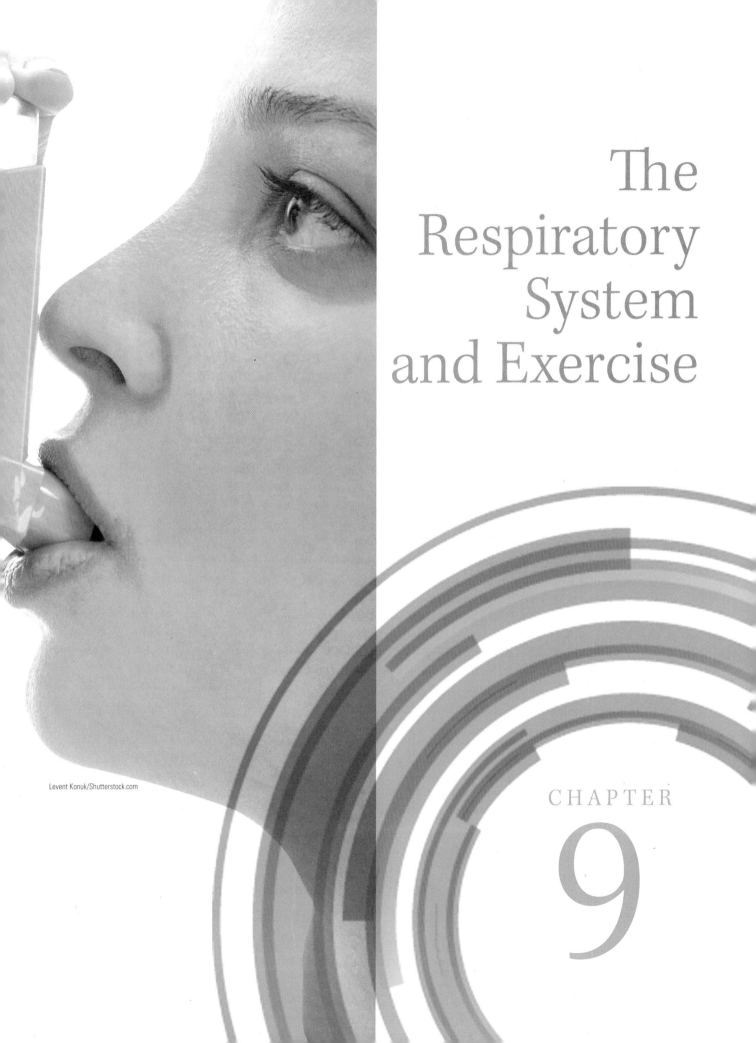

The Respiratory System and Exercise

CHAPTER

9

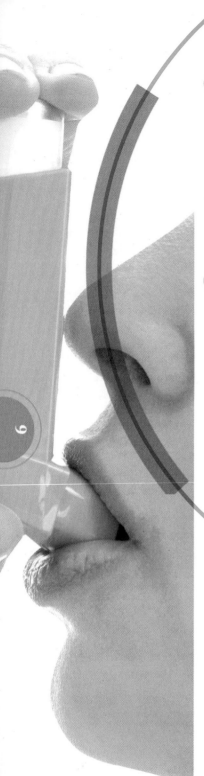

What do you already know about the respiratory system?

- Use the following Pre-Test or the online evaluation tools for Chapter 9 to determine how much you already know. To access the course materials and companion resources for this text, please visit **www.cengagebrain.com**. See the preface on page xiii for details.

- Need more review? Let the online assessments, animations, and tutorials for Chapter 9 help prepare you for class.

Pre-Test

1. Air is normally moved into and out of the lungs through a process called _____.

2. Intra-alveolar, intrapleural, and _____ pressures are major determinants for ventilation.

3. The _____ nerve innervates the diaphragm.

4. Intrapleural pressure is less than intra-alveolar pressure during _____.

5. Total lung capacity is equal to vital capacity and _____ _____.

6. The differences between alveolar air and atmospheric air are that alveolar air is humidified and has a _____ PO_2 than atmospheric air.

7. The PO_2 gradient between alveolar air and pulmonary capillaries favors diffusion of O_2 from _____ into pulmonary capillaries.

8. Hypoxia is the condition of having insufficient O_2 at the cellular level and can be caused by anemia, inadequate hemoglobin saturation and low arterial PO_2, and decreased _____ delivery.

9. The two main central stimuli for ventilation are _____ and _____.

10. Ventilation can be altered by swallowing, pain, sneezing, and _____ independent of gas exchange.

1. ventilation; 2. atmospheric; 3. phrenic; 4. inspiration; 5. residual volume; 6. lower; 7. alveoli; 8. oxygen; 9. $PaCO_2$; pH; 10. coughing

What You Will Learn in This Chapter

- How the respiratory system functions in response to the challenges of endurance exercise

- How oxygen is transferred from the lungs to the tissues during endurance exercise

- How the respiratory system functions in acid–base regulation during endurance exercise

- How regular engagement in endurance exercise (training) influences the respiratory system

QUICKSTART!

What happens to your breathing when you engage in exercise? Do you know anyone who suffers from asthma when he exercises? If so, what causes his asthma? What recommendations can you provide to help control his asthma, particularly so he can continue to engage in regular exercise?

Introduction to the Respiratory System and Exercise

This chapter has the following goals:

1. To review the fundamental anatomy and physiology of the respiratory system

2. To explain how oxygen is extracted from the air and carbon dioxide is exhaled from the blood

3. To show how oxygen and carbon dioxide are transported in the blood

4. To detail how acid–base balance is regulated during exercise

Specifically, this chapter focuses on how the range of workloads, or intensity, of the endurance exercise from light to moderate to heavy to very heavy exhaustive exercise (or work) alters the response of the **respiratory system** to maintain oxygen saturation of the blood and at the same time maintain acid–base balance.

respiratory system Designed to obtain oxygen from the ambient air for use by the body's cells and to utilize and eliminate the carbon dioxide produced.

Pulmonary Ventilation

Pulmonary ventilation is defined as the movement of air into and out of the lungs during the act of breathing. Breathing in, or *inspiration*, is active and requires contraction of the muscles of the chest wall and the diaphragm (see Figure 9.1).

At rest, the diaphragm is the main respiratory muscle; however, during forced inspiration, the intercostal (chest wall) muscles also become involved. By contracting these muscles, the diaphragm is pushed down into the abdominal cavity, lifting up the chest wall away from the spine, creating a negative pressure within the thorax and the lung compared with the air pressure outside the body, and thereby causing air to flow into the lungs. In contrast, the act of breathing out, or *exhalation*, occurs when the diaphragm and chest wall muscles relax; however, during forced exhalation, the intercostal (chest wall) muscles also become involved. The relaxation of the expiratory muscles squeezes the air in the lungs and creates a greater pressure in the lungs compared with the air pressure outside of the lungs, thereby causing the air to flow out of the lungs (see Figure 9.1, page 294).

During the inspiration of one breath, the work of the respiratory muscles is directly related to the resistance to the air flowing into the lungs through the large conducting airways. The air flowing through the large conducting airways accounts for 80 percent of the resistance. The lung tissue that makes up the bulk of the respiratory airways and surface of the lungs, where gas exchange occurs, is pliable and soft. In this area of the lungs, the resistance is low and accounts for the remaining 20 percent of the lungs' total airway resistance (Figure 9.2, page 295).

> Why do we need to create a negative pressure in the lung compared with the ambient pressure during inspiration?

At any given ventilation, the resistance to the airflow is directly related to the pressure difference at the two ends of the airway:

$$\text{Resistance} = \frac{P_1 - P_2}{\text{Airflow}} \qquad [9.1]$$

This equation is the same as presented for resistance to blood flow in Chapter 7

pulmonary ventilation The movement of air into and out of the lungs during the act of breathing.

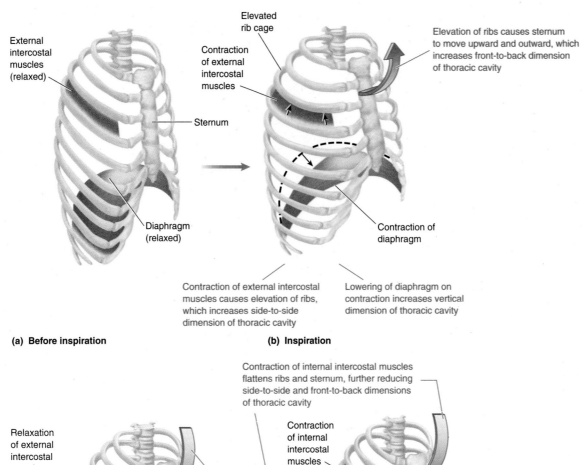

External intercostal muscles (relaxed)

Sternum

Diaphragm (relaxed)

(a) Before inspiration

Elevated rib cage

Contraction of external intercostal muscles

Elevation of ribs causes sternum to move upward and outward, which increases front-to-back dimension of thoracic cavity

Contraction of diaphragm

Contraction of external intercostal muscles causes elevation of ribs, which increases side-to-side dimension of thoracic cavity

Lowering of diaphragm on contraction increases vertical dimension of thoracic cavity

(b) Inspiration

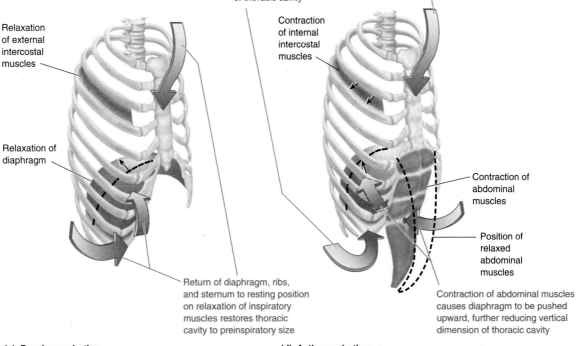

Relaxation of external intercostal muscles

Relaxation of diaphragm

Return of diaphragm, ribs, and sternum to resting position on relaxation of inspiratory muscles restores thoracic cavity to preinspiratory size

(c) Passive expiration

Contraction of internal intercostal muscles flattens ribs and sternum, further reducing side-to-side and front-to-back dimensions of thoracic cavity

Contraction of internal intercostal muscles

Contraction of abdominal muscles

Position of relaxed abdominal muscles

Contraction of abdominal muscles causes diaphragm to be pushed upward, further reducing vertical dimension of thoracic cavity

(d) Active expiration

⊙ **FIGURE 9.1 Respiratory muscle activity during inspiration and expiration.** (a) Before inspiration, all respiratory muscles are relaxed. (b) During inspiration, the diaphragm descends on contraction, increasing the vertical dimension of the thoracic cavity. Contraction of the external intercostals muscles elevates the ribs and subsequently the sternum to enlarge the thoracic cavity from front to back and from side to side. (c) During *quiet passive expiration*, the diaphragm relaxes, reducing the volume of the thoracic cavity from its peak inspiratory size. As the external intercostal muscles relax, the elevated rib cage falls because of the force of gravity. This also reduces the volume of the thoracic cavity. (d) During *active expiration*, contraction of the abdominal muscles increases the intra-abdominal pressure, exerting an upward force on the diaphragm. This reduces the vertical dimension of the thoracic cavity further than it is reduced during quiet passive expiration. Contraction of the internal intercostal muscles decreases the front-to-back and side-to-side dimensions by flattening the ribs and sternum. (From Sherwood, L. 2010. Figures 13.12a and 13.12b in *Human physiology*, 7th ed. Belmont, CA: Brooks/Cole-Cengage Learning.)

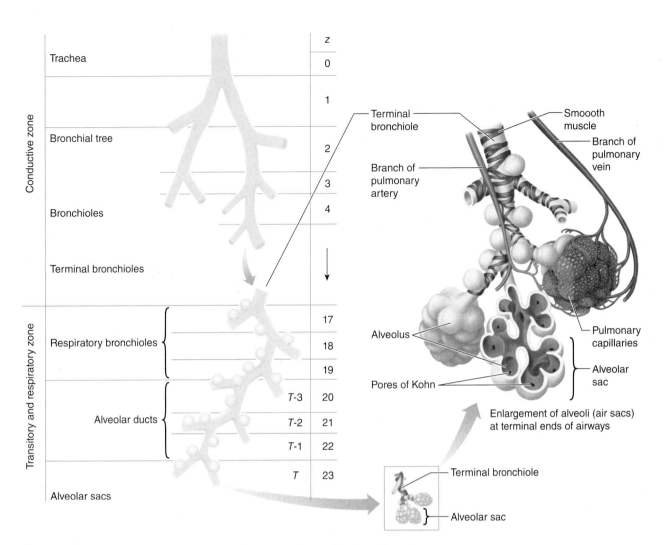

FIGURE 9.2 Schematic relationships between the conductive and respiratory zones and the anatomic components of the lung. (Composite of Sherwood, L. 2010. Figure 13.12, Chapter 13, "The Respiratory System" in *Human physiology*, 7th ed. Belmont, CA: Brooks/Cole-Cengage Learning, and Weibel, E. R. 1963. Figure 5.2 in *Morphometry of the human lung*. Berlin: Springer-Verlag OHG.)

and is another variation of the equation of **Ohm's law**. As noted in Chapter 7, the greatest effect on resistance to flow is the diameter of the tube the fluid is flowing through. Recall the following equation:

$$\text{Resistance} = \frac{\text{length} \times \text{viscosity}}{\text{radius}^4} \quad [9.2]$$

This relationship identifies that a two-fold reduction in the radius of the airway will increase the resistance to airflow some 16-fold, regardless of whether the air is flowing into or out of the lung.

Work of Breathing

During each breath there is a relationship between the pressure across the lung and the volume of air in the lung. Remember from basic physics that force × distance = work.

The *force* generated by the lung is reflected by the change in pressure, and the *distance* is the change in volume that occurs in relation to the pressure change. Therefore, the *work of breathing* can be calculated from the following:

Work of breathing (W) =
    change in pressure (ΔP) ×
        change in volume (ΔV)

The lung works by contracting and relaxing the muscles of the chest wall to move the chest wall and the lungs to overcome the resistance to the airflow into and out of the lung, and at the same time overcome

Ohm's law The relationship between the voltage (V), current (I) and resistance (R), and is usually written V = IR.

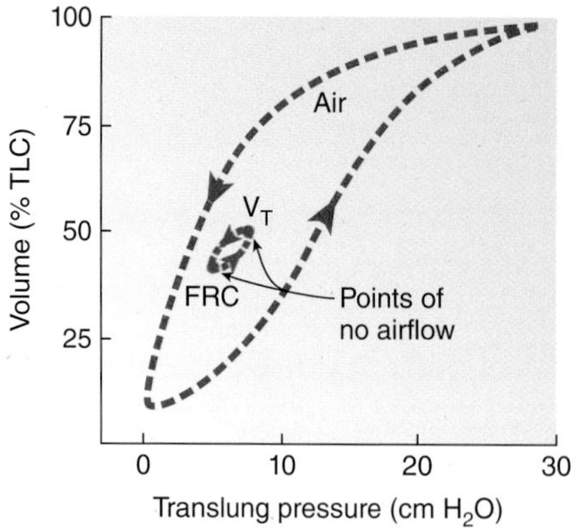

maximal expired (e) ventilation (Ve max) The maximal volume of air moved for 1 minute (L/min) when maximal exercise is being performed.

FIGURE 9.3 Inflation–deflation pressure–volume curve. The direction of inspiration and exhalation is shown by the arrows. The difference between the inflation and deflation pressure–volume curves is due to the variation in surface tension with changes in lung volume. Note the slope of the line joining points of no airflow. This slope is less steep than the slope from the deflation pressure–volume curve at the same lung volume. (From Koeppen, B. M., and B. A. Stanton. 2008. Figure 21-15 in *Berne & Levy Physiology*, 6th ed. New York: Elsevier.)

ventilation volume The volume (ml) of air that is moved into or out of the lung per unit time, usually recorded in 1 minute (L/min).

tidal volume (V_T) The volume of air that is moved into or out of the lung in each breath (ml/breath).

the elastic recoil of the lung tissue (see Figure 9.3).

During exercise, the **ventilation volume** of each breath increases and the number of breaths per minute increases, which results in increasing the work of the lung and the respiratory muscles in direct relation to the work intensity. These increases in breath volume and rate of breathing are needed to increase the delivery of oxygen to the working muscles. However, the lung regulates its breathing frequency to a minimum rate that is the most economical in terms of energy expended for the mechanical work required to ventilate the lung at a given work intensity. Therefore, the breathing frequency decreases and the **tidal volume (V_T)** increases when the mechanical work of the lung is increased for a given intensity of exercise (such as for firefighters or mine rescuers working with respiratory protection equipment). Later in this chapter, the mechanical properties of the lung and its effects on exercise performance are discussed.

HOTLINK *Visit the course materials for Chapter 9 for more details on the mechanics of ventilation.*

Minute Ventilation Is the Amount (Volume) of Air Breathed into and out of the Lungs in 1 Minute

The range in **maximal expired (e) ventilation (Ve max)** depends on the workload achieved, and the size and age of the individual. During maximal exercise, the minute ventilation can range from 125 to 200 L/min (Figure 9.4a). In general, the thorax (chest) of males is larger than females, resulting in males having larger V_T per breath than females during rest and exercise. The relationship between thoracic volume and V_T—that is, the larger the thoracic volume, the larger the V_T during rest and exercise—also explains many sex differences in breathing rates and ventilation volumes during rest and exercise (see Table 9.1, page 298).

A positive correlation exists between pulmonary ventilation volume and the oxygen uptake ($\dot{V}O_2$) measured during a progressive increase in the workload exercise test (see Figure 9.4b, page 297). However, because of respiratory control mechanisms associated

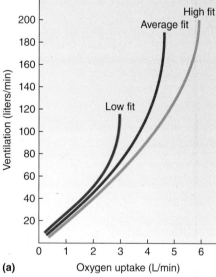

(a)

FIGURE 9.4 Relationship of ventilation to oxygen uptake during exercise. (a) Ventilation response to progressive increases in exercise intensity of low, average, and high fit men. (Modified from Astrand, P.-O., and Rodaahl. 1986. Figure 5.9 in *Textbook of Work Physiology: Physiological Basis of Exercise*, 3rd ed. New York: McGraw-Hill Book Co. Original data from Saltin, B., and P.-O Astrand. 1967. Maximal oxygen uptake in athletes. *J. Appl. Physiol.* 23:353–358.)

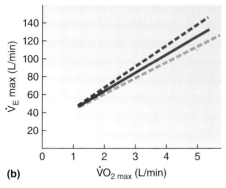

(b)

FIGURE 9.4 (b) **Relationship between maximal pulmonary ventilation and maximal oxygen uptake during running treadmill exercise.** (Modified from Astrand, P. O., and Rodaahl. 1986. Figure 5.10 in *Textbook of Work Physiology: Physiological Basis of Exercise,* 3rd ed. New York: McGraw-Hill Book Co. Original data from Saltin, B., and P. O. Astrand. 1967. Maximal oxygen uptake in athletes. *J. Appl. Physiol.* 23:353–358.)

with the regulation of the acid–base status of the blood, the minute ventilation increases exponentially above a threshold workload, or $\dot{V}O_2$, at which there is an extra stimulus from the central and peripheral chemoreceptors that are sensitive to arterial carbon dioxide (CO_2) and hydrogen ion concentration (pH) to increase ventilation (see Figure 9.4a). This threshold workload is generally defined as the **ventilation threshold**. In addition, because of its measured association with an increase in blood lactate concentrations, it is sometimes referred to as the *lactate threshold*. This threshold is termed the *anaerobic threshold* in some older texts, and coaches and other professionals have used it to convey the concept that the ventilation is increased by an anaerobic stimulus.

ventilation threshold The exponential increases in ventilation above a threshold workload, or $\dot{V}O_2$, during a progressive increase in workload exercise test.

inRETROSPECT

The Onset of the Lactate Threshold

The lactate threshold was initially identified by the appearance of lactate in the venous blood by Margaria, Edwards, and Dill in 1932 at the Harvard Fatigue Laboratory. They exercised subjects on a treadmill that was driven by a motor and gear system that was scavenged from a Boston city tram that had two speeds, 3.5 and 7.0 miles/hour. The investigators drew venous blood samples during the progressive increase in exercise intensity achieved by increasing the slope (or grade) of the treadmill.

Much later in 1983, Wasserman and Whipp observed in some cases the presence of the ventilation threshold as being at the same workload as the lactate threshold by using sophisticated noninvasive breath-by-breath respiratory gas analysis techniques and venous blood sampling during progressive increases in bicycle exercise workloads. These same investigators linked the appearance of lactate in the blood as being an indication of anaerobic conditions within the exercising muscle, as pyruvate conversion to lactate is an anaerobic process, and coined the term *anaerobic threshold* to indicate the threshold. It was the use of the term *anaerobic threshold* that resulted in an ensuing controversy.

However, more recent information using radioactive labeled carbohydrate has clearly identified that the appearance of lactate in the venous blood is not an indication of an onset of anaerobic conditions in the muscle, but rather one of an imbalance between lactate production and lactate clearance within the muscle. Indeed, the glycolytic pathway for the anaerobic processes of producing energy from the metabolism of glucose and glycogen that produces lactate and pyruvate is operating continuously regardless of one's activity. However, when the intensity of the exercise for adenosine triphosphate (ATP) production exceeds the Krebs cycle's rate of ATP production, the excess pyruvate generated by glycolysis is stopped from entering the Krebs cycle and converted to lactate by lactate dehydrogenase, a chemical process that occurs without oxygen and is termed *anaerobic* (see Chapter 4). Furthermore, it has been demonstrated that during exercise, the white fast glycolytic fibers of the exercising muscle produce lactate, and this lactate is "shuttled" within the muscle to the slow oxidative fibers to be used as a substrate for aerobic energy production. In addition, the lactate released into the venous blood is recirculated (shuttled) and taken up by the exercising muscles, the beating heart, and the metabolically active brain, where it is also used as a substrate for aerobic energy production. Furthermore, during exercise, lactate is the major gluconeogenic precursor for hepatic gluconeogenesis.

		Men						Women			
Ht (cm)	Age (yrs)	VC	FRC	RV	TLC	Ht (cm)	Age (yrs)	VC	FRC	RV	TLC
155	20	3.97	2.72	1.13	5.10	145	20	2.81	1.96	1.00	3.81
	30	3.65	2.72	1.30	4.95		30	2.63	1.96	1.08	3.71
	40	3.35	2.72	1.45	4.80		40	2.45	1.96	1.16	3.61
	50	3.04	2.72	1.61	4.65		50	2.27	1.96	1.24	3.51
	60	2.73	2.72	1.77	4.50		60	2.09	1.96	1.32	3.41
	70	2.42	2.72	1.91	4.35		70	1.91	1.96	1.40	3.31
160	20	4.30	2.98	1.27	5.57	150	20	3.08	2.20	1.05	4.13
	30	4.00	2.98	1.42	5.12		30	2.89	2.20	1.14	4.03
	40	3.70	2.98	1.57	5.27		40	2.71	2.20	1.22	3.93
	50	3.40	2.98	1.72	5.12		50	2.53	2.20	1.30	3.83
	60	3.10	2.98	1.87	4.97		60	2.35	2.20	1.38	3.73
	70	2.80	2.98	2.02	4.82		70	2.17	2.20	1.46	3.63
165	20	4.62	3.23	1.42	6.04	155	20	3.34	2.43	1.19	4.53
	30	4.32	3.23	1.57	5.89		30	3.15	2.43	1.28	4.43
	40	4.02	3.23	1.72	5.74		40	2.97	2.43	1.36	4.33
	50	3.72	3.23	1.87	5.59		50	2.79	2.43	1.44	4.23
	60	3.42	3.23	2.02	5.44		60	2.61	2.43	1.52	4.13
	70	3.12	3.23	2.17	5.29		70	2.43	2.43	1.60	4.03
170	20	4.94	3.48	1.57	6.51	160	20	3.60	2.67	1.32	4.92
	30	4.64	3.48	1.72	6.36		30	3.41	2.67	1.41	4.82
	40	4.35	3.48	1.86	6.21		40	3.22	2.67	1.50	4.72
	50	4.05	3.48	2.01	6.06		50	3.05	2.67	1.57	4.62
	60	3.74	3.48	2.17	5.91		60	2.87	2.67	1.65	4.52
	70	3.44	3.48	2.32	5.76		70	2.69	2.67	1.73	4.42
175	20	5.26	3.74	1.73	6.98	165	20	3.88	2.90	1.44	5.32
	30	4.96	3.74	1.87	6.83		30	3.68	2.90	1.54	5.22
	40	4.66	3.74	2.02	6.68		40	3.50	2.90	1.62	5.12
	50	4.36	3.74	2.17	6.53		50	3.32	2.90	1.70	5.02
	60	4.06	3.74	2.32	6.38		60	3.14	2.90	1.78	4.92
	70	3.76	3.74	2.47	6.23		70	2.96	2.90	1.86	4.82
180	20	5.58	3.99	1.87	7.45	170	20	4.13	3.14	1.58	5.71
	30	5.28	3.99	2.02	7.30		30	3.94	3.14	1.67	5.61
	40	4.98	3.99	2.17	7.15		40	3.76	3.14	1.75	5.51
	50	4.68	3.99	2.32	7.00		50	3.58	3.14	1.83	5.41
	60	4.38	3.99	2.47	6.85		60	3.40	3.14	1.91	5.31
	70	4.08	3.99	2.62	6.70		70	3.22	3.14	1.99	5.21
185	20	5.90	4.25	2.02	7.92	175	20	4.38	3.37	1.80	6.18
	30	5.60	4.25	2.17	7.77		30	4.20	3.37	1.90	6.10
	40	5.30	4.25	2.32	7.62		40	4.02	3.37	2.00	6.02
	50	5.00	4.25	2.47	7.47		50	3.84	3.37	2.10	5.94
	60	4.70	4.25	2.62	7.32		60	3.66	3.37	2.20	5.86
	70	4.40	4.25	2.77	7.17		70	3.38	3.37	2.40	5.78

From Bates, D. V., P. T. Macklem, and R. V. Christie. 1971. Tables 2-7 and Table 2-8 in *Respiratory function in disease*, 2nd ed. Philadelphia: W.B. Saunders Co.

Effects of Endurance Exercise Training on the Ventilation Threshold

Generally, in an average fit individual, the ventilation threshold occurs at approximately 60 percent maximal oxygen uptake ($\dot{V}O_2$ max) during a dynamic progressive workload exercise test. Elite endurance-trained athletes have ventilation thresholds measured at 85 to 90 percent $\dot{V}O_2$ max (see Figure 9.4a). For example, the higher and the faster the dynamic exercise workload you can perform without having lactate appear in the blood, the greater the capacity to use your aerobic machinery to generate

ATP. However, the type of endurance training you perform, such as interval versus long, slow-distance training, also affects the way the muscle's energy generation mechanisms adapt and use lactate as a substrate. Generally, the increase in ventilation threshold is a marker of the training effect of endurance exercise on the exercising muscle's increase in its internal lactate shuttle capacity and mitochondrial energy-generating mechanisms. For example, endurance runners who primarily train using the long, slow-distance method of training (remember, for the more elite runner, "slow" means a sub-5- to -6-minute mile time for 20 miles or more) usually have ventilation thresholds at 80 to 90 percent $\dot{V}O_2$ max, whereas the middle-distance runners who use "speed-play" and "interval training" methods usually have ventilation thresholds around 70 percent $\dot{V}O_2$ max and usually have much higher maximal lactate concentrations. This physiologic response to endurance exercise training is common to all types of endurance exercise besides running, for example, bicycling, rowing, cross-country skiing, and swimming. One important caveat for using the ventilation threshold as a marker of the endurance training effect is that glycogen stores need to be optimum for the individual, because glycogen depletion results in the ventilatory threshold occurring at a lower workload than the lactate threshold. In addition, during cycling, the higher the pedal frequency is, the lower is the workload at which the lactate threshold occurs. One practical way of recognizing when you have passed the ventilatory threshold while out jogging or training with a friend is when you cannot carry a conversation without grunting or gasping out the words.

HOTLINK *See the following website of Edward F. Coyle, Ph.D., for more information about exercise endurance training on factors like ventilation threshold:* http://www.edb.utexas.edu/coyle/.

Dyspnea Index

In general, a healthy individual's maximal exercise ventilation volume ($\dot{V}_e$ max in L/min) approximates 70 percent of the individual's clinically measured maximal voluntary ventilation in 15 seconds (MVV.15;

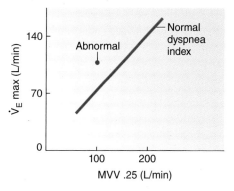

FIGURE 9.5 Dyspnea index. Relationship between the maximal voluntary ventilation in 25 seconds (MVV.25) pulmonary function test and maximal exercise ventilation — dyspnea index — MVV.25/V_E max × 100. Normal = 70%. (© Cengage Learning 2013)

expressed as L/min). This ratio has been termed the **dyspnea index**, an index of the feeling of breathlessness.

When this ratio is exceeded, it is oftentimes a sign of cardiorespiratory disease or psychobiologic stress resulting from anxiety or panic. For example, an individual with a $\dot{V}_e$ max of 125 L/min and an MVV.15 of 162.5 L/min has a dyspnea index of 70 percent and is identified as normal and healthy. However, another person with a $\dot{V}_e$ max of 144 L/min and a MVV.15 of 180 L/min has a dyspnea index of 80 percent and is probably excessively ventilating at maximal exercise. In endurance-trained athletes, such as marathon runners and cross-country skiers, this generalization may not hold because some have reached a dyspnea index value of 80 to 85 percent (similar to the exercise intensity at the appearance of the ventilatory or lactate threshold) but without the feeling of breathlessness (Figure 9.5).

Gas Laws

Gas volumes are affected by two ideal gas laws, Boyle's law and Charles's law. Because not all clinical lung function and exercise testing are performed at the same ambient pressures or temperatures, standard practice is to normalize the pulmonary volume measures to normal body temperature (37°C) and the ambient barometric pressure saturated with water vapor, or **body temperature** (in degrees Kelvin) **pressure saturated (BTPS)**. However,

dyspnea index The ratio of the ventilation volume at maximal workload ($\dot{V}_e$ max in L/min) to their clinically measured maximal voluntary ventilation in 15 seconds (MVV.15; expressed as L/min).

body temperature pressure saturated (BTPS) A correction factor used to standardize (equilibrate) the measured ventilation volumes to the body's temperature of 37°C to the absolute temperature of 273° K and the barometric pressure plus the 47 mm Hg water vapor pressure at 37°C.

when measuring $\dot{V}O_2$, the partial pressures of water vapor do not affect the diffusion gradient for O_2 or CO_2, resulting in the calculated volume for $\dot{V}O_2$ or CO_2 being normalized to **standard temperature** (in degrees Kelvin) **pressure dry** (with correction for water vapor) **(STPD)**.

For healthy adults who are not excessively overweight, that is, individuals with body mass indices less than 25, normalization of pulmonary volumes across age and sex can be accomplished by dividing by an individual's height. Clinical pulmonary function measured capacities of the lungs, that is, vital capacity (VC) and total lung capacity, are directly related to height cubed (ht^3). During resting breathing, there is always an end-expiratory pause, where the elastic recoil forces of the lungs equal the chest wall expansion forces. This end-expiratory pause is used as a point from which all lung volume measurements are made.

Tidal Volume and Breathing Frequency Increase during Exercise

The volume of air brought into or out of the lungs in one breath is known as the V_T, and the number of breaths per minute is the breathing, or respiratory frequency (f). Therefore, the amount of ventilation volume ($\dot{V}$) respired in 1 minute can be expressed by the following equation:

$$\dot{V} = V_T \times f \qquad [9.3]$$

Young healthy adult men have resting ventilation volumes ($\dot{V}e$) ranging from 6.0 to 8.0 L/min and respiratory frequencies (f) ranging from 12 to 15 breaths/min.

(Calculate the range of resting V_T you would expect to see in young healthy adult men.)

Respiratory frequencies (f) at maximal exercise range from 40 to 50 breaths/min and result in V_T ranging from 3.0 to 4.0 L (Figure 9.6).

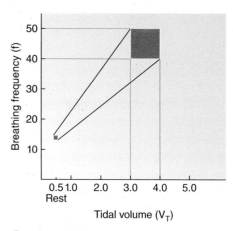

FIGURE 9.6 Range of tidal volumes and breathing frequencies from rest to maximal exercise. (© Cengage Learning 2013)

When comparing rest and exercise ventilation volumes ($V_T \times f$), it is obvious that the increased ventilation volume of maximal exercise is achieved by increasing the breathing frequency three to four times and the V_T by six to seven times. Because V_T is the volume of the breath expelled each breath, the V_T of the lungs is similar to the heart's stroke volume, and respiratory frequency (f) is similar to the heart's rate, or beats/minute (see Chapter 7). Lung capacities are associated with an individual's height, and the VC (measured in liters) is directly and linearly related to an individual's $\dot{V}O_2$ max (measured in L/min; Figure 9.7). An individual's maximal V_T (measured in liters) achieved during maximal exercise is also related to their VC (measured in liters; Figure 9.8).

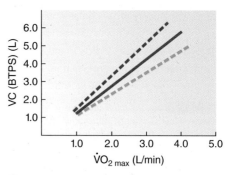

FIGURE 9.7 Relationship between maximal oxygen uptake and vital capacity. (Modified from Astrand, P.-O., and Rodaahl. Figure 5.12a in *Textbook of Work Physiology: Physiological Basis of Exercise*, 3rd ed. New York: McGraw-Hill Book Co.,1986. Original source from Astrand, P-O. 1952. *Experimental studies of physical work capacity in relation to sex and age.* Copenhagen: Munksgaard.)

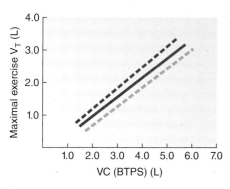

FIGURE 9.8 Relationship between vital capacity and tidal volumes at maximal exercise. (Modified from Astrand, P.-O., and Rodaahl. 1986. Figure 5.8 in *Textbook of Work Physiology: Physiological Basis of Exercise*, 3rd ed. New York: McGraw-Hill Book Co. Original source from Astrand, P.-O. 1952. *Experimental studies of physical work capacity in relation to sex and age*. Copenhagen: Munksgaard.)

Because these relationships are clearly related to anatomic dimensions of the thorax and the height of the individual, it should be obvious that when comparing individuals of different heights and weights, you should normalize the data. For example, in a comparison of pulmonary function values of elite athletes with average fit individuals normalized to their height, the athletes had larger VCs per centimeter height than the larger average fit individuals, who had larger absolute (L) VCs. Furthermore, because the relationship between breathing frequency and V_T operates to achieve the lowest work of breathing, or **energy cost**, the breathing rate at any given ventilation volume results in an optimal V_T, which at maximum exercise averages 55 percent of VC. This breathing rate is involuntarily and spontaneously controlled for each individual. How the regulation and optimization of V_T and respiratory frequency (f) occurs is a research area of great interest.

Remember, we have been discussing the effects of breathing one breath in and one breath out; however, we always discuss pulmonary ventilation over a period usually for 1 minute. When the V_T are added together for the number of breaths that occur in 1 minute, a ventilation volume per minute (L/min) is obtained. As we breathe faster and deeper during exercise, all the changes identified for one breath

accumulate over the minute to increase the alveolar ventilation of the lungs and, therefore, increase the $\dot{V}O_2$ and $\dot{V}CO_2$ exhalation. In stressful conditions (such as firefighting), individuals who are prone to anxiety attacks will increase, and continue to increase, their breathing frequency out of proportion to the oxygen demand. This is defined as a hyperventilation response and, in many instances, results in "blowing off" CO_2. This "blowing off" of CO_2 is defined as **hyperventilation**, and in individuals susceptible to severe "panic attacks," this can result in unconsciousness. In actual firefighting, it is not uncommon that even the most experienced firefighters hyperventilate and, in some instances, respond by removing their respiratory protection while fighting fires in enclosed spaces, resulting in death. Similar situations have been found to occur in scuba and deep-sea diving.

Practical Challenges in Everyday Jobs Requiring Physical Work and Endurance Exercise Training

The primary property of air pollution that exacerbates injury to the lung is the concentration of particulates in the air you are breathing. As the intensity of work (exercise) increases, the breathing frequency and the volume of each breath increases, and during an air pollution episode, this results in an increased dose/breath of the pollutants reaching the respiratory lung tissue, that is, the area of the lung where gas exchange occurs. Therefore, it is not wise to exercise train during an air pollution alert or in the vicinity of a lot of airborne particulates. A few examples of activities in which the respiratory airways can be damaged are smoking, firefighting, dust particles in the air, and industrial work such as mining, cement making, sand blasting, and working with asbestos. Many of these industrial exposures without adequate respiratory protection result in specific cancers; however, the initial effects of the damage are very difficult to detect by routine pulmonary function testing, and it is not until you experience

hyperventilation An excess ventilation that causes a reduction in the arterial carbon dioxide tension, or $PaCO_2$.

energy cost Calculated in calories from the amount of oxygen used to perform the work.

symptoms of breathlessness and the start of chronic obstructive pulmonary disease (COPD), a condition when the damage is irreversible, that you realize you may have a disease. The Occupational Safety and Health Administration mandates respiratory protection programs for all industrial work sites where particulate exposure is part of the job.

> Can you name any routine jobs you do around the house or garden that will increase your exposure to particulate pollution?

HOTLINK See the Occupational Safety and Health Administration website (**http://osha.gov/**) for more information about respiratory protection.

Alveolar Ventilation Is the Inspiration and Expiration of Air into and out of the Alveoli

The lungs are divided into two main sections: the conducting zone and the respiratory zone. The section that is made up of the dividing airways of the trachea, bronchial tree, bronchioles, and terminal bronchioles is known as the *conducting zone* (see Figure 9.2, page 295). These tubes conduct the air from the mouth and nose to the depths of the lung where gas exchange occurs. Within the conducting airways, no gas exchange in and out of the body occurs; this makes up the anatomic **dead space** volume of the lung (V_D). The section made up of the deeper airways of the lung continues to divide into smaller and smaller tubes, known as the respiratory bronchioles, which then terminate at the alveolar sacs. This section of the lung is known as the *respiratory zone* (see Figure 9.2).

In the respiratory zone airways and alveoli, respiration, or gas exchange between the air and blood, occurs. Because the conducting airways transfer the air only from the mouth to the respiratory zone, part of

each V_T does not reach the gas exchange areas of the lung and, therefore, does not take part in gas exchange and is identified as the *anatomic V_D*, and the air that moves into and out of the lung in this area is referred to as *dead space ventilation* (Figure 9.9). The **alveolar volume** (V_A) is the area of the lung where gas exchange between the air and blood occurs and is often referred to as the **alveolar ventilation** volume or the effective V_T.

If the alveoli of the lung were spread out on a two-dimensional surface, the adult lung surface area would match the size of a doubles tennis court. The ease and rapidity of diffusion of gases across the alveolar membrane is directly related to the surface area of the alveoli. Diseases that affect the surface area of the alveoli, such as **emphysema**, cause an impairment of gas exchange, resulting in a reduction of $\dot{V}O_2$ and retention of CO_2.

During an expiration of one breath, the air of the V_D is expired first and has the same mixture of gases (20.9 percent O_2, 0.03 percent CO_2, and 79.07 N_2) as the inspired air. During the same expired breath and after the expiration of the V_D, the air contained in the alveolar gas follows (see Figure 9.9, page 303). Because of the gas exchange that occurs at the alveoli that results from alveolar ventilation, the alveolar gases have a higher percentage of CO_2 and a lower percentage of O_2. The volume relationships of the lung can be summarized by the following equation:

$$V_T = V_A + V_D \qquad [9.4]$$

Example calculation

At rest, if $V_T = 500$ ml and $V_D = 150$ ml, the remaining fresh air that reaches the alveoli, or V_A, is 350 ml.

Because this new fresh air reaching the alveoli is diluted by approximately 3,500 ml air remaining in the lung at the end of expiration, which is known as the *functional residual capacity*, the breath-to-breath variations in gas concentrations in the alveoli, and in the blood passing through the lung, are relatively small.

---

alveolar volume The area of the lung where gas exchange between the air and blood occurs and is often referred to as the alveolar ventilation volume or the effective V_T.

alveolar ventilation The effective tidal volume (V_T).

emphysema An obstructive disease of the lung where the alveolar membrane is destroyed.

dead space Space made up of the airways and alveoli of the lung where no gas exchange occurs. In healthy lungs this usually the conducting airways only.

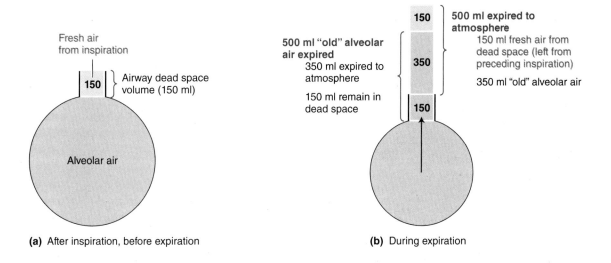

(a) After inspiration, before expiration

(b) During expiration

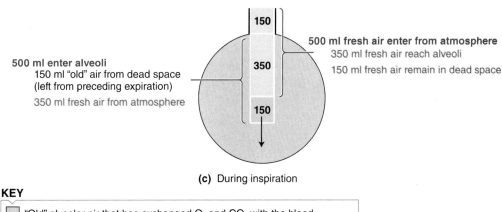

(c) During inspiration

KEY

| | "Old" alveolar air that has exchanged O_2 and CO_2 with the blood |
| | Fresh atmospheric air that has not exchanged O_2 and CO_2 with the blood |

FIGURE 9.9 Effect of dead air space volume on exchange of tidal volume between the atmosphere and the alveoli. (From Sherwood, L. 2010. Figures 13.22a, 13.22b, and 13.22c in Chapter 13, "The Respiratory System" in *Human physiology*, 7th ed. Belmont, CA: Brooks/Cole-Cengage Learning.)

A number of situations occur in which some of the fresh air reaching the alveoli are not perfused (**perfusion** is the blood within the circulatory system that circulates through or over the tissues), or are poorly perfused, by the blood carried in the lung's network of capillaries. These alveoli will not be able to exchange alveolar gas with the blood and are identified as an additional dead space. Calculations can be made to identify this additional V_D. When this additional V_D is added to the anatomic dead space volume (aV_A), a measure of the *physiologic dead space* (pV_D) is obtained. At rest and even during heavy exercise, when lung perfusion is maximized, the physiologic dead space always exceeds the anatomical dead space because of the presence of small anatomic and physiologic shunts or mismatches between diffusion and perfusion.

Dead Space Ventilation

During voluntary breathing at rest, healthy individuals are rarely aware of their breathing; however, in patients with lung disease who have increases in dead space ventilation, the patients become very aware of their breathing.

perfusion The passage of a fluid (blood) through a vessel or tissue.

Why does a patient
with COPD have
an increase in
dead space?

is breathed to achieve 1.0 L $\dot{V}O_2$. After the ventilation threshold has been reached, VE will increase exponentially to 30 to 35 L/L O_2 during maximal exercise (Figures 9.4a and 9.10a).

Snorkeling is another example of an activity requiring an increase in dead space ventilation. The snorkeling tube is an extension of the V_D. Therefore, total ventilation has to be increased, and the work of breathing increases to obtain the same amount of oxygen. If the length of the snorkeling tube were increased to enable the swimmer to snorkel at a depth of 3 feet (1/2 atmosphere), the external pressure on the chest wall would equal the largest external pressure the inspiratory muscles can overcome.

Ventilation Equivalent for Oxygen

By dividing the expired ventilation volume ($\dot{V}_E$) by the volume of oxygen consumed ($\dot{V}O_2$), we obtain a ratio ($\dot{V}_E/\dot{V}O_2$) that identifies the efficiency of the ventilation to provide 1 L oxygen for the body's metabolism. This relationship is known as the **ventilation equivalent for oxygen ($\dot{V}EO_2$)**.

$$VEO_2 = \dot{V}_E/\dot{V}O_2 \qquad [9.5]$$

At rest and up to moderately heavy exercise, the VE is 20 to 25; that is, 20 to 25 L air

Ventilation Equivalent for Carbon Dioxide

Similar to $\dot{V}_E/\dot{V}O_2$, the **ventilation equivalent for carbon dioxide ($\dot{V}_E/\dot{V}CO_2$)** is defined as the ventilation volume (L/min) related to the exhaled CO_2 (L/min), and is expressed as follows:

$$VECO_2 = \dot{V}_E/\dot{V}CO_2 \qquad [9.6]$$

The $\dot{V}EO_2$ and $\dot{V}ECO_2$ (see Figure 9.10b) relationships when related to workload or $\dot{V}O_2$ provide an accurate detection of the onset of the ventilation threshold. In Chapter 10, you will learn how to use $\dot{V}EO_2$ and $\dot{V}ECO_2$ ratios to identify changes related to the body's control of ventilation.

Gas Exchange within the Lung

You have learned how the lung operates to draw air into the lung and provide breath-by-breath ventilation of the alveoli both at rest and during exercise, we can now move on to the details of gas exchange. When new fresh air reaches the alveoli, there is an exchange of oxygen from the alveolar

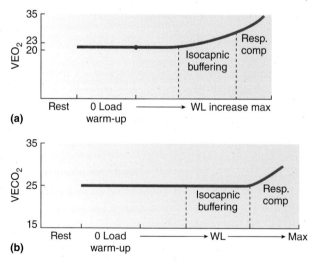

FIGURE 9.10 Schematic representation of the changes in the ventilatory equivalent for oxygen ($\dot{V}EO_2$) that occurs between rest and maximal exercise. (Modified from Wasserman, K., J. E. Hansen, D. Y. Sue, and B. J. Whipp. 1987. Figure 2.10 in *Principles of exercise testing and interpretation*. Philadelphia: Lea & Febiger.)

air to the blood and CO_2 from the blood to the air.

The physical mechanism by which gases move is known as **diffusion**. Diffusion occurs from high to low gas pressures (or tensions), and the difference between the high and low pressures is known as the diffusion gradient. Gases flow down a gradient, or from a high gas pressure to a low gas pressure. This gradient is represented by the following equation:

$$\text{Diffusion gradient} = P_1 - P_2 \quad [9.7]$$

where P_1 is the higher pressure and P_2 is the lower pressure.

For example, at rest, the pressure of oxygen in the alveolar gas (PA) after inspiration is 100 mm Hg (P_1), and the pressure of oxygen in the venous blood returning to the lung is 40 mm Hg (P_2). Using Equation 9.7, $P_1 - P_2 = 100$ mm Hg $- 40$ mm Hg, we calculate that the diffusion gradient is 60 mm Hg, which results in the oxygen leaving the alveolar air and entering the blood. The exchange of oxygen at the lung to the blood is the point at which venous blood becomes arterialized. This exchange of gases occurs as a result of a set of physical laws discovered by a number of historically renowned scientists, whose names are attached to the specific laws they discovered.

Dalton's Law of Partial Pressures

Dalton's law of partial pressures states that the total pressure of a mixture of gases is equal to the sum of the pressure that each gas independently exerts. Air contains 20.9 percent O_2; 0.03 percent CO_2; 0.94 percent inert gases (helium and argon); and 78.13 percent N_2. At sea level, ambient air pressure is 760 mm Hg and nitrogen (N_2) is physiologically inert. Physiologically inert means that the volume of N_2 inspired is equal to the volume of N_2 expired when the body is in nitrogen balance. Therefore, many respiratory calculations use measures of inspired and expired N_2 as markers for correcting differences between the inspired and expired volumes of air related to the **respiratory exchange ratio (RER)**. The RER is the ratio of the amount of CO_2 expired to the amount of O_2 used in the metabolic processes, that is, $\dot{V}CO_2/\dot{V}O_2$.

For example, when the metabolism uses a mixture of fats and carbohydrates as substrates for the production of energy, the RER approximates 0.8 and identifies that the volume of CO_2 produced is 80 percent the volume of O_2 used. Because N_2 is physiologically inert, the volume of N_2 inspired will be less than the volume of N_2 expired, and the ratio between inspired and expired N_2 percentages is used to correct the ventilation volumes.

To calculate the partial pressure of each gas within the gas mixture, you need to multiply the percentage of the specific gas in the mixture by the ambient pressure, which at sea level is 760 mm Hg. Therefore, the partial pressure (P) of each gas in the inspired air at the mouth is:

$PO_2 = 20.9$ percent $\times$ 760 mm Hg
   $= 159$ mm Hg

$PCO_2 = 0.03$ percent $\times$ 760 mm Hg
   $= 0.023$ mm Hg (usually accepted as zero)

$P\text{inert} = 0.94$ percent $\times$ 760 mm Hg
   $= 7$ mm Hg

$PN_2 = 78.13$ percent $\times$ 760 mm Hg
   $= 594$ mm Hg

Total $= 760$ mm Hg

As shown, the majority of the total pressure of the inspired ambient air is made up of oxygen and nitrogen. The partial pressure of water vapor within the lung at 37°C (98.6°F body temperature) is 47 mm Hg; therefore, the PO_2 at the alveoli is: 20.9 percent $\times$ (760 mm Hg $- 47$ mm Hg) $= 149$ mm Hg, if no CO_2 is present. However, the alveolar partial pressure of carbon dioxide (P_ACO_2) at rest approximates 45 mm Hg, resulting in the alveolar partial pressure of oxygen (P_AO_2) being (149 $- 45$) mm Hg, or 104 mm Hg.

(Explain this result using Dalton's law of partial pressures.)

diffusion The net movement of solutes and gases across a semi-permeable membrane from a high concentration/pressure to a low concentration/pressure. The high to low difference in concentrations/pressure is known as the diffusion gradient.

Dalton's law Dalton's law of partial pressures states that the total pressure of a mixture of gases is equal to the sum of the pressure that each gas independently exerts.

respiratory exchange ratio (RER) The ratio of the amount of CO_2 expired to the amount of O_2 used in the metabolic processes, that is, $\dot{V}CO_2/\dot{V}O_2$.

Fick's law Fick's law of diffusion of
gases states that the rate (velocity) at
which a gas (V gas) is transferred across
a tissue membrane is proportional to
the tissue membrane's surface area (A),
the diffusion coefficient (D) of the gas,
and the difference between the partial
pressures of the gas on each side of
the tissue membrane ($P_1 - P_2$), and is
inversely proportional to the thickness
(T) of the tissue membrane.

Fick's Law of Diffusion of Gases

Fick's law of diffusion of gases states that
the rate (velocity) at which a gas ($\dot{V}$ gas) is
transferred across a tissue membrane is
proportional to the tissue membrane's surface area (A), the diffusion coefficient (D) of
the gas, and the difference between the
partial pressures of the gas on each side of
the tissue membrane ($P_1 - P_2$), and is inversely proportional to the thickness (T) of
the tissue membrane. These relationships
are expressed in the following equation:

$$\dot{V} \text{ gas} = A/T \times D \times (P_1 - P_2) \quad [9.8]$$

The human lung is designed to optimize the
transfer of oxygen from the air to the blood
in that the surface area of the alveoli for gas
exchange is large. For the gas to enter the
bloodstream, the gas must diffuse across the
alveolar cell, the capillary endothelial cell,
and interstitial space that form the respiratory membrane. The respiratory membrane
is very thin (approximately 1/3 micrometer),
and the diffusion gradient ($P_1 - P_2$) from the
alveolus to the blood is very large (60 mm Hg).
The easy transfer of oxygen from the alveolar
air to the blood is essential during maximal
exercise, where the speed of the circulation
of the blood through the lung can be six to
eight times faster than at rest.

Henry's Law of Solubility of Gases

Henry's law of solubility of gases states
that at equilibrium, the amount of oxygen
dissolved in the blood is directly proportional to the partial pressure of oxygen
in the alveolar air. In other words, oxygen
from the alveolar air will continue to dis-
solve in the blood circulating around the
alveoli until the PO_2 of the blood equals the
PO_2 of the alveoli at any given temperature.

Notably, this law explains only the oxygen dissolved in the blood and not the
amount of oxygen combined with the **hemoglobin (Hb)**. However, it is the difference
in P_AO_2 and the PO_2 of the dissolved oxygen
in the arterial blood (PaO_2) that makes up
the diffusion gradient ($P_AO_2 - PaO_2$) for the
transfer of oxygen. Another way of looking
at it is to understand that once the combination of oxygen to Hb occurs, the oxygen

Henry's law Henry's law of solubility
of gases states that at equilibrium, the
amount of a gas dissolved in a fluid is
directly proportional to the partial pressure of the gas in the air.

hemoglobin (Hb) The large iron-
bearing protein molecule contained
in the red blood cells, which primarily
combines with oxygen in the lungs to
carry it to the body's tissues via circulation.

has no effective partial pressure, or the Hb
molecule is acting as a sponge soaking up
the oxygen and not allowing it to contribute to the partial pressure of the oxygen
in the blood. It is important to realize that
this sponge effect of Hb is reversible and is
linked to the PO_2.

Similarly, the transfer of CO_2 from the
mixed venous blood to the alveolar air follows the same principles of gas exchange
and solubility outlined for oxygen, with the
exception that the diffusion gradient for CO_2
is much less (approximately 5–10 mm Hg).
However, other physical characteristics
of CO_2 aid in the transfer of CO_2 from the
blood to the alveolar air.

These same three laws of gas exchange
that are a part of the respiration of oxygen
and CO_2 at the lung are also guiding principles for the exchange of oxygen from the
blood to the tissues of the body and of CO_2
from the tissues of the body to the blood.
Figure 9.11 on page 307 summarizes these
exchanges.

Lung Blood Flow Enables the Exchange of Gases

The right atrium receives blood from both
the inferior and superior vena cava. As the
blood goes from the right atrium to the
right ventricle across the tricuspid valve,
a mixing of the two sources of blood from
the systemic circulation occurs and results
in mixed venous blood. This mixed venous
blood is pumped via the right ventricle into
the pulmonary artery (the only example of
an artery carrying venous blood) into the
pulmonary circulation to enable gas exchange to occur. When the mixed venous
blood picks up the oxygen in exchange for
the CO_2, the blood is arterialized, and it is
carried from the pulmonary circulation to
the left atrium via the pulmonary vein (an
example of arterialized blood being carried
within a vein).

At rest, the right and left ventricles
pump the same amount of blood, approximately 5.0 L/min, through the pulmonary
and systemic circulations, respectively.
As the cardiac output increases in response to increasing exercise workloads,

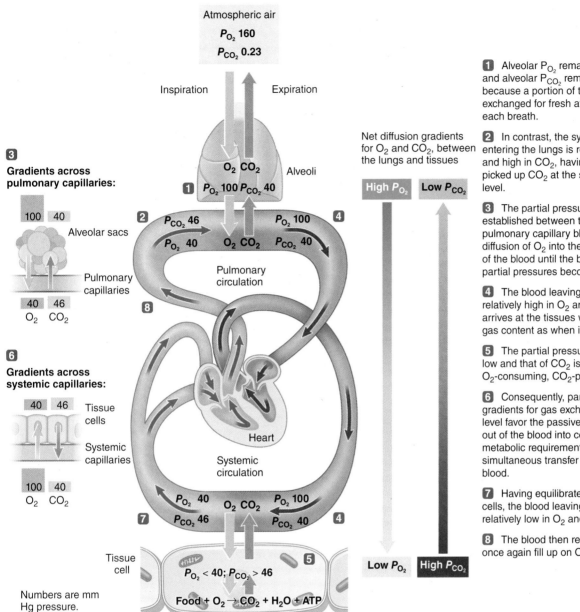

Atmospheric air

P_{O_2} 160

P_{CO_2} 0.23

Inspiration　Expiration

3

Gradients across pulmonary capillaries:

| 100 | 40 |

Alveolar sacs

Pulmonary capillaries

| 40 | 46 |
| O_2 | CO_2 |

6

Gradients across systemic capillaries:

| 40 | 46 | Tissue cells
| 100 | 40 |
| O_2 | CO_2 |

Systemic capillaries

Numbers are mm Hg pressure.

O_2　CO_2　Alveoli

1 P_{O_2} 100 P_{CO_2} 40

2 P_{CO_2} 46　　　P_{O_2} 100 **4**

P_{O_2} 40　O_2 CO_2　P_{CO_2} 40

Pulmonary circulation

8

Heart

Systemic circulation

P_{O_2} 40　O_2 CO_2　P_{O_2} 100

7 P_{CO_2} 46　　　P_{CO_2} 40 **4**

Tissue cell

P_{O_2} < 40; P_{CO_2} > 46　**5**

Food + O_2 → CO_2 + H_2O + ATP

Net diffusion gradients for O_2 and CO_2, between the lungs and tissues

High P_{O_2}　**Low P_{CO_2}**

Low P_{O_2}　**High P_{CO_2}**

1 Alveolar P_{O_2} remains relatively high and alveolar P_{CO_2} remains relatively low because a portion of the alveolar air is exchanged for fresh atmospheric air with each breath.

2 In contrast, the systemic venous blood entering the lungs is relatively low in O_2 and high in CO_2, having given up O_2 and picked up CO_2 at the systemic capillary level.

3 The partial pressure gradients established between the alveolar air and pulmonary capillary blood induce passive diffusion of O_2 into the blood and CO_2 out of the blood until the blood and alveolar partial pressures become equal.

4 The blood leaving the lungs is thus relatively high in O_2 and low in CO_2. It arrives at the tissues with the same blood-gas content as when it left the lungs.

5 The partial pressure of O_2 is relatively low and that of CO_2 is relatively high in the O_2-consuming, CO_2-producing tissue cells.

6 Consequently, partial pressure gradients for gas exchange at the tissue level favor the passive movement of O_2 out of the blood into cells to support their metabolic requirements and also favor the simultaneous transfer of CO_2 into the blood.

7 Having equilibrated with the tissue cells, the blood leaving the tissues is relatively low in O_2 and high in CO_2.

8 The blood then returns to the lungs to once again fill up on O_2 and dump off CO_2.

FIGURE 9.11 Exchange of oxygen and carbon dioxide at the lungs and tissues. (From Sherwood, L. 2010. Figure 13.26 in Chapter 13, "The Respiratory System" in *Human physiology*, 7th ed. Belmont, CA: Brooks/Cole-Cengage Learning.)

the pulmonary blood flow increases to the exact same cardiac output provided to the systemic circulation by the left ventricles (values >20–25 L/min). This increase in pulmonary blood flow is accomplished by the recruitment of unused capillaries that exist within the lung at rest. The increase in the number of open capillaries enables the increase in blood flow without causing large increases in pulmonary artery blood pressure and also results in an increase in the lung's blood volume. The increase

in lung blood volume together with the increase in flow provides the lung a greater volume of blood per unit time, which enables the exchange of gases to occur rapidly enough to limit the amount of oxygen desaturation in the arterialized blood exiting the lung via the pulmonary vein.

However, this is not always true for the highly trained endurance athlete and individuals with diffusion diseases, such as cystic fibrosis, bronchitis, and congestive heart failure.

Ventilation and Perfusion Must Match

Air is brought into the lungs, and the lungs provide a constant source of new oxygen to exchange with the CO_2 carried in the blood. For an optimum exchange of gases to occur, the ventilated alveoli must be matched with the blood flow surrounding the alveoli, or perfusion of the alveoli (Figure 9.12).

This matching is identified by the ratio of ventilation ($\dot{V}$) to perfusion, or cardiac output ($\dot{Q}$), or the $\dot{V}/\dot{Q}$ ratio. The perfect $\dot{V}/\dot{Q}$ ratio would be 1.0. In many airway diseases, such as the group of diseases known as COPD, a mismatch exists between ventilation being too low for the normal perfusion of the alveoli in that region, which results in no or too little oxygen being added to the blood and a retention of the CO_2 in the blood; this results in the $\dot{V}/\dot{Q}$ ratio being less than 1.0. In conditions where regions of the lung are underperfused, such as in congestive heart failure or blocked lung capillaries, the $\dot{V}/\dot{Q}$ ratio is greater than 1.0.

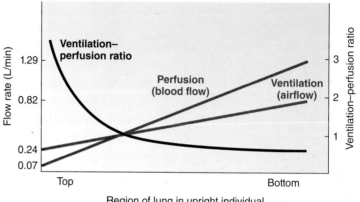

(a) Regional ventilation and perfusion rates and ventilation–perfusion ratios in the lungs

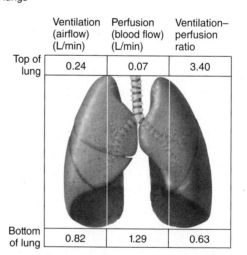

	Ventilation (airflow) (L/min)	Perfusion (blood flow) (L/min)	Ventilation–perfusion ratio
Top of lung	0.24	0.07	3.40
Bottom of lung	0.82	1.29	0.63

(b) Ventilation and perfusion rates and ventilation–perfusion ratios at top and bottom of lungs

FIGURE 9.12 Differences in ventilation–perfusion ratios throughout the lung because of gravitational effects when standing upright. (a) Regional ventilation and perfusion rates and ventilation–perfusion ratios in the lungs. (b) Ventilation and perfusion rates and ventilation–perfusion ratios at top and bottom of lungs. (From Sherwood, L. 2010. Figures 13.24a and 13.24b in Chapter 13, "The Respiratory System" in *Human physiology*, 7th ed. Belmont, CA: Brooks/Cole-Cengage Learning.)

TABLE 9.2 Pressure Relationships in Lung Zones

Zone 1	Apex of lung	PA > Pa > Pv
Zone 2	Middle of lung	Pa > PA > Pv
Zone 3	Base of lung	Pa > Pv > PA

© Cengage Learning 2013

In an upright healthy individual with normal lung function and circulation, the V̇/Q̇ ratio is different in different regions (zones) of the lung (see Figure 9.12b; Table 9.2). The zones of the lung are dependent on the relationship between the pressure in the pulmonary artery (the vessel [Pa] coming from the right side of the heart and going to the lung), the pressure in the pulmonary vein (the vessel [Pv] coming from the lung and going to the left side of the heart), and the pressure in the alveoli (PA).

Because of the effect of gravity and the base of the lung being below the heart and the apex of the lung being above the heart, the volume of blood perfusing the lung is greatest at the base and least at the apex of the lung. However, even though ventilation is greater at the base of the lung than at the apex, the V̇/Q̇ ratio at the base

of the lung (zone 3) is less than 1.0, which is indicative of an area of overperfusion or underventilation. In contrast, the V̇/Q̇ ratio at the apex of the lung (zone 1) is greater than 1.0, which is indicative of an area of underperfusion or overventilation (see Figure 9.12).

For example, ventilation at the apex of the lung (zone 1) is 0.3 L/min, and the blood flow is 0.15 L/min, which means the V̇/Q̇ ratio is 2. However, ventilation at the base of the lung (zone 3) is 0.9 L/min, and the blood flow is 1.4 L/min, which means the V̇/Q̇ ratio is 0.64.

During light-to-moderate exercise, the matching of blood flow to ventilation increases in all zones of the lung, resulting in an overall lung V̇/Q̇ ratio approximating 1.0. However, in very heavy dynamic exercise performed by highly trained endurance athletes, the capillary recruitment, and hence pulmonary blood volume, reaches a maximum before the achievement of maximal flow (cardiac output) through the lung. The faster the blood flows through the fixed volume of the lung, the shorter the transit time (through the lung), and the less time the blood has to load oxygen to the blood (Figure 9.13).

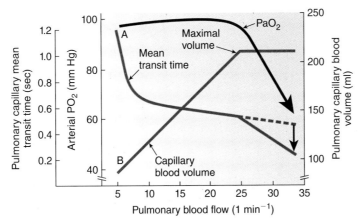

FIGURE 9.13 Theoretical explanation of arterial hypoxemia during severe exercise in endurance athletes. Line A shows computed mean transit times for red cells through pulmonary capillaries with increasing pulmonary blood flow. Line B shows estimated average pulmonary capillary blood volume with increasing blood flow. As long as capillary blood volume increases with pulmonary blood flow, mean transit time is sufficient to permit alveolar–capillary oxygen equilibration. In some athletes, flow increases beyond the point at which capillary volume can increase (shown here at 25 L/min), causing mean transit time to decline suddenly (smaller arrow). Heavy line at top (labeled PaO₂) shows the decline in arterial partial pressure of oxygen (PaO₂) that accompanies the sudden decline in mean transit time. In this scheme, hypoxemia is caused by a diffusion limitation caused by very brief mean transit times. (From Rowell, L. B. 1993. Figure 9.11 in *Human cardiovascular control.* New York: Oxford University Press.)

This decrease in transit time can, in some individual athletes, result in oxygen desaturation of the arterial blood. Figure 9.14 illustrates the effect of the elite athletes and their high maximal cardiac outputs on arterial desaturation.

It was previously thought that mismatch between speed of the pulmonary blood flow of the elite athlete performing high-intensity exercise and the rate of diffusion of oxygen across the respiratory membrane was the primary cause for the **oxyhemoglobin desaturation**, or **exercise-induced arterial hypoxemia (EIAH)**. However, recently, other reasons in addition to the perfusion/diffusion mismatch have been identified that appear to be related to thoracic volume and endurance exercise training.

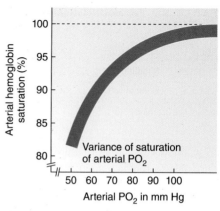

● FIGURE 9.14 Average values for decreases in arterial hemoglobin saturation during heavy intensity exercise. (From Rowell, L. B. 1993. Figure 9.11 in *Human cardiovascular control*. New York: Oxford University Press, adapted from Dempsey, J. A., P. G. Hanson, and K. S. Henderson. 1984. Exercise-induced arterial hypoxemia in healthy human subjects at sea level. *J. Physiol.* 355:161–175.)

oxyhemoglobin desaturation When the hemoglobin is not 100% saturated with oxygen.

exercise-induced arterial hypoxemia (EIAH) When the hemoglobin is not completely saturated with oxygen after passing through the lung during exercise.

Endurance Exercise Training

It is generally accepted that endurance exercise and weight training have little effect on lung tissue in terms of growth or regeneration. This means that, unlike the cardiovascular system, once you lose it, it is gone forever (smokers beware). However, recent work identifies that specific growth factors may play a role in lung tissue regeneration.

Another generally accepted truism before the 1980s was that the lung could never limit exercise performance in a healthy individual. However, this truism has been rejected because it had been demonstrated in endurance exercise-trained men that the skeletal muscle's demand for oxygen could exceed the lung's capacity to take up oxygen, thereby resulting in arterial oxygen desaturation, or exercise-induced arterial hypoxemia (EIAH), and limited exercise performance (Figure 9.15).

Subsequently, EIAH has been demonstrated in young adult women, endurance-trained elderly athletes, and high-intensity endurance athletic events, such as time trials. However, it appears that the mismatch between perfusion and diffusion produced by high pulmonary blood flows of the endurance-trained athlete is not the

only reason for the arterial desaturation. Other reasons include:

1a. Using measurements of breath-by-breath tidal flow–volume loops during exercise, researchers have found that individuals with a lung architecture that restricts the flow–volume envelope of each breath achieving the required pulmonary ventilation results in a flow restriction during inspiration and expiration, and interferes with gas exchange producing EIAH and increases the work of breathing.

1b. In some individuals, the presence of subclinical hyperactive airways results in mild airway constriction and a reduction of the flow–volume envelope. The mild airway constriction impairs gas exchange, resulting in EIAH, and also increases the work of breathing, which if the exercise is prolonged will result in respiratory muscle fatigue. The initial treatment for the hyperactive airway athlete was to use low doses of bronchodilators; however, one of the unexpected

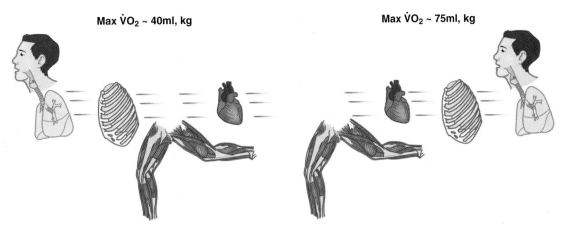

Max $\dot{V}O_2$ ~ 40ml, kg   Max $\dot{V}O_2$ ~ 75ml, kg

FIGURE 9.15 High maximal oxygen uptake ($\dot{V}O_2$ max) increases *demand* on the lung and respiratory muscle with little or no change in their *capacity*. (Adapted from Dempsey, J. A. 1986. J. B. Wolffe memorial lecture. Is the lung built for exercise? *Med. Sci. Sports Exerc.* 18(2):143–155.)

consequences of the more effective drugs was their enhancement of the individual's performance, which was not associated with pulmonary vessel reactivity. As a result, these drugs were banned by the World Anti-Doping Agency (WADA).

2. Some individuals have small intra-cardiac or intrapulmonary shunts (where venous blood bypasses the alveoli and, therefore, the arterial blood is not fully saturated with oxygen), which cause a widening of the alveolar–arterial oxygen pressure difference resulting in EIAH (see earlier section Ventilation and Perfusion Must Match). Even these small and probably insignificant shunts for everyday living activities may prove to limit elite performance. Research into identifying the presence of these small shunts during heavy-intensity exercise continues but is proving technically challenging.

3. Fatigue of the respiratory muscles may cause limitations in perfor-mance. Generally, the diaphragm (the primary respiratory muscle) has a high oxidative capacity with multiple blood vessels that are resistant to va-soconstriction, and it rarely fatigues during exercise. However, during pro-longed exercise at 80 to 85 percent

$\dot{V}O_2$ max, the work of breathing be-comes so strenuous that the dia-phragm has been shown to fatigue and limit exercise performance. An-other compounding factor involved in the increased cost of breathing dur-ing exercise is that the respiratory muscle's demand for oxygen can ex-ceed its delivery of oxygen, thereby activating the exercise pressor reflex (see Chapter 7) and producing a va-soconstriction in the exercising mus-cles. In effect, this is a situation where the work of the lungs to in-crease the $\dot{V}O_2$ required for the chest wall muscles to perform the exercise is stealing blood and oxygen from the exercising muscles (Figure 9.16).

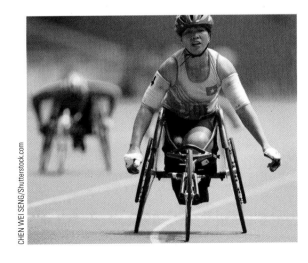

CHEN WEI SENG/Shutterstock.com

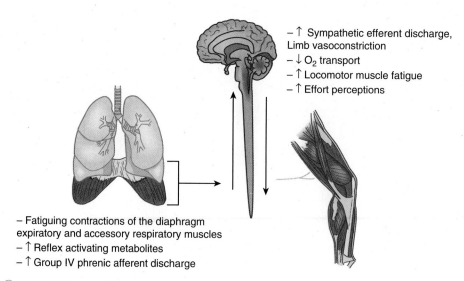

- ↑ Sympathetic efferent discharge, Limb vasoconstriction
- ↓ O_2 transport
- ↑ Locomotor muscle fatigue
- ↑ Effort perceptions

- Fatiguing contractions of the diaphragm expiratory and accessory respiratory muscles
- ↑ Reflex activating metabolites
- ↑ Group IV phrenic afferent discharge

FIGURE 9.16 The respiratory muscle metaboreflex. (Modified from Dempsey, J. A., A. W. Sheel, C. M. St. Croix, and B. J. Morgan. 2002. Respiratory influences on sympathetic vasomotor outflow in humans. *Respir. Physiol. Neurobiol.* 130:3–20, 2002, and Romer, L. M., and M. I. Polkey. 2008. Exercise-induced respiratory muscle fatigue: Implications for performance. *J. Appl. Physiol.* 104(3):879–888.)

Whether training of the respiratory muscles by inspiring and expiring against a resistance will enable the athletic individual to overcome respiratory muscle fatigue is a subject of intense investigation. Respiratory muscle endurance training is proving beneficial for exercise performance by healthy individuals and in patients with restrictive or obstructive pulmonary diseases during activities of daily living.

HOTLINK *Conduct an Internet search using your favorite search engine on clinical case studies on exercise testing and respiration, such as research papers found on PubMed (**http://www.ncbi.nlm.nih.gov/pubmed/**).*

Transport of Oxygen from the Lungs to the Tissues

Now that we understand how oxygen is brought into the body from the ambient air and exchanged with CO_2 from the blood at the alveoli of the lung, we need to trace how both gases are transported in the blood and exchanged at the tissues.

Dalton's law of partial pressures and Charles's law of dissolved gases in fluids relate the air pressure of the gas to its partial pressure of the gas in a fluid. At sea level, only a small amount of oxygen is dissolved in the blood (0.3 ml O_2/100 ml blood), but it is important to understand that it is the amount of gas dissolved in the fluid that provides its partial pressure.

Fortunately, humans have developed a large protein molecule (Hb) that combines with oxygen. Because of this combination, no active partial pressure is attributable to the oxygen when it is combined with Hb. In other words, the Hb acts as a sponge that soaks up oxygen until all of its carrying sites (the sites containing iron, or heme groups) are completely combined with oxygen. Indeed, 99 percent of oxygen transported by the blood is chemically bound to Hb.

Hb is carried in the red blood cell (RBC), or **erythrocyte**. Each molecule of Hb has four binding sites for oxygen, and therefore carries four molecules of oxygen when fully saturated. The combination of oxygen with Hb is called *oxyhemoglobin*. The Hb that gives up its oxygen is known as *deoxyhemoglobin*.

A healthy man has an Hb concentration of 15 g/100 ml blood. A healthy woman has an Hb concentration of 13 g/100 ml blood. Hb combines 1.34 ml oxygen/g Hb. The amount of oxygen actually bound to Hb is called the *oxygen content*. For a healthy man, the oxygen content is $15 \times 1.34 = 20.1$ ml/100 ml blood.

The oxygen-carrying capacity of the blood is the sum of the amount of oxygen dissolved (0.3 ml O_2/100 ml blood) and the oxygen content bound to the Hb of the blood. For a healthy man, the oxygen-carrying capacity is $20.1 + 0.3 = 20.4$ ml O_2/100 ml blood.

(What is the oxygen-carrying capacity for a healthy woman?)

The percentage of Hb saturated by oxygen is calculated by:

Percentage oxyhemoglobin saturation = O_2 content/O_2 carrying-capacity   [9.9]

For example, percent oxyhemoglobin saturation = $20.1/20.4 \times 100 = 99$ percent.

Sports Anemia

Many endurance athletes who use high-mileage running training programs often adhere to diets that are low in iron and vitamin B_{12}. In addition, the continuous pounding of the feet on hard surfaces for long distances during each training session has been found to break down the RBCs in the capillary vessels of the feet. These dietary practices and the high volume of endurance training can result in a condition of sports anemia from the breakdown of RBCs and insufficient iron uptake from the diet. Because of the differences in total Hb in women compared with men, this appears to be more prevalent in women.

Calculate the oxygen-carrying capacity of a young woman with an Hb concentration of 6 g/100 ml blood.

(What would be her exercise capacity: normal, low, or high?)

HOTLINK *Search PubMed (http://www.ncbi.nlm.nih.gov/pubmed/) for research articles on sports anemia.*

In many Third World countries, severe anemia caused by poor nutrition or parasitic infestation, such as hookworm anemia, results in a reduced number of RBCs, a reduced amount of hemoglobin in the RBC, or a combination of both. The presence of anemia in many of these populations reduces the working productivity of the nation.

When the arterial blood circulates through the capillaries of the tissues of the organs and skeletal muscles, the pressure of oxygen dissolved in the arterialized capillary blood is greater than in the tissues. This difference in pressure provides a diffusion gradient from the blood to the tissues, resulting in a transfer of oxygen from the blood to the tissues down the diffusion gradient. Remember, it is the difference in pressure of O_2 in the blood and in the tissues that enables the unloading of the O_2. It is not the amount of O_2 being carried by the Hb. Note that we use the terms *loading* and *unloading* of oxygen to describe the flow of oxygen to and from the blood, respectively.

The actual transfer of oxygen from the blood to the mitochondria of the cells within the skeletal muscle tissue is aided by **myoglobin (Mb)**, a smaller protein molecule similar to the Hb molecule in the blood, but stored within the striated and smooth muscle tissues of the heart, skeletal muscle, and blood vessels. The physical association of oxygen onto and dissociation from the Hb molecule, respectively, is based on a complex, yet predictable, kinetic relationship between the stereochemistry of the oxyhemoglobin molecule and tissue oxygen pressure, generally known as the *oxyhemoglobin dissociation curve*.

erythrocyte A red blood cell (RBC).

myoglobin (Mb) The large iron-bearing protein molecule contained in the muscle.

The Oxyhemoglobin Dissociation Curve Describes the Loading and Unloading of Oxygen

The Hb molecule has stereochemical properties, which provides it a unique ability to load and unload oxygen in relation to the partial pressures of O_2 in the air and tissues. Figure 9.17, the **oxyhemoglobin (O_2–Hb) dissociation curve**, describes the relationship between PO_2 and the percentage of the Hb that is saturated with O_2.

Note its sigmoid shape and how it is flat at the top and bottom of the curve and steep and linear in the middle of the curve. This shape represents the unique kinetics of the binding of four molecules of oxygen to one molecule of Hb. The first molecule of O_2 is slowly combined with the Hb molecule (first flat portion of the curve), after which the

Hb molecule rotates to allow the next two molecules of O_2 to combine very rapidly (the steep linear portion of the curve). The kinetics of the combination of the fourth O_2 molecule to the Hb molecule is slow and results in the final flat portion of the curve. During the unloading of O_2 from the Hb molecule, the reverse of the loading process occurs.

For example, at the lung's capillary blood–alveolar air interface during rest, the P_AO_2 at sea level is calculated as follows:

$$PiO_2 = (760 - 47) \text{ mm Hg} \times 20.9 \text{ percent}$$
$$= 149 \text{ mm Hg} \qquad [9.10]$$

$$P_AO_2 = 149 \text{ mm Hg} - 45 \text{ mm Hg}$$
$$= 104 \text{ mm Hg}$$

where PiO_2 is partial pressure of inspired oxygen, 760 mm Hg is sea level barometric pressure, 47 mm Hg is the lung's water vapor pressure at 37°C (body temperature), and 45 mm Hg is the P_ACO_2.

oxyhemoglobin (O_2–Hb) dissociation curve Describes the relationship between the pressure of O_2 and the percentage of the Hb that is saturated with O_2.

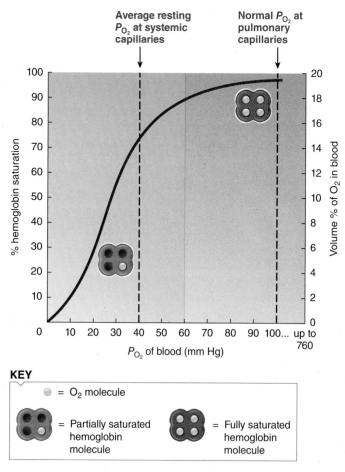

KEY

- ● = O_2 molecule
- = Partially saturated hemoglobin molecule
- = Fully saturated hemoglobin molecule

● **FIGURE 9.17 Oxygen–hemoglobin (O_2–Hb) dissociation (saturation) curve.** (From Sherwood, L. 2010. Figure 13.28 in Chapter 13, "The Respiratory System" in *Human physiology,* 7th ed. Belmont, CA: Brooks/Cole-Cengage Learning.)

However, because the new inspired O_2 is mixed and diluted with the larger volume of old air in the functional residual capacity, the actual P_AO_2 approximates 100 to 105 mm Hg. The mixed venous blood arriving at the lung's capillary–alveolar air interface has approximately 40 mm Hg PO_2 (or is 75–80 percent saturated; see Figure 9.17). Therefore, as the blood passes through the lung, the 60 to 65 mm Hg diffusion gradient enables the oxygen to enter the blood, which then combines with the Hb in the RBC until the Hb is nearly fully saturated, or arterialized, and the PaO_2 of the blood is nearly equivalent to the P_AO_2.

At rest, the metabolic rate of the tissues is low, using some 250 to 300 ml O_2/min. With a 5.0 L/min cardiac output, from Chapter 7 you should be able to calculate the whole-body oxygen extraction, or the arteriovenous oxygen difference (a − v O_2 difference), to be 50 to 60 ml/L blood.

> For practice, calculate what the (a − v)O_2 difference is during exercise with a cardiac output of 10.0 L/min and $\dot{V}O_2$ of 1.0 L/min.

As the intensity of exercise increases from mild to moderate to heavy and on up to exhaustion, the skeletal muscle tissue PO_2 (PtO_2) gets progressively lower and can attain PtO_2 values less than 18 mm Hg. During this type of exercise, the cardiac output increases to values in excess of 25 to 30 L/min, causing the transit time of the blood through the muscle to be brief and requiring a rapid unloading of the oxygen from the blood to the tissues. The beauty of the Hb molecule is its ability to release the O_2 rapidly in response to the decreases in PtO_2; that is, the steep linear portion of the curve is a reflection of the increasing difference between PaO_2 and PtO_2 (see Figure 9.17). In addition, other properties of the Hb molecule related to metabolism assist in this rapid unloading of oxygen.

At sea level, barometric P_AO_2 of 100 mm Hg result in 99 percent saturation of Hb. However, it is important for you to understand the difference between a partial pressure of oxygen (PO_2), percentage saturation of Hb, oxygen content, and oxygen-carrying capacity, especially if you want to understand exercise physiology at altitude and underwater.

At sea level, you can increase the PO_2 threefold by pressurizing a scuba tank to 3 atmospheres (2,280 mm Hg × 0.21 = 479 mm Hg) or having a person breathe room air in a hyperbaric chamber pressurized to 3 atmospheres. From the oxyhemoglobin dissociation curve, you can deduce that despite the large increase in PiO_2 (160 to 479 mm Hg), and therefore alveolar partial pressure of oxygen (P_AO_2), you will only add a further 1 percent of saturation to the Hb.

In contrast, because of Henry's law, the amount of O_2 dissolved in the blood will increase threefold from 0.3 to 0.9 ml O_2/100 ml. This can be increased even further if you breathe 100 percent O_2 at 3 atmospheres, resulting in a PiO_2 of 2,280 mm Hg, which raises the dissolved oxygen to 4.3 ml/100 ml blood and increases the oxygen-carrying capacity to 24.4 ml O_2/100 ml blood. This small increase in the volume of dissolved oxygen probably seems inconsequential, but it has been shown to be an extremely potent way of attacking

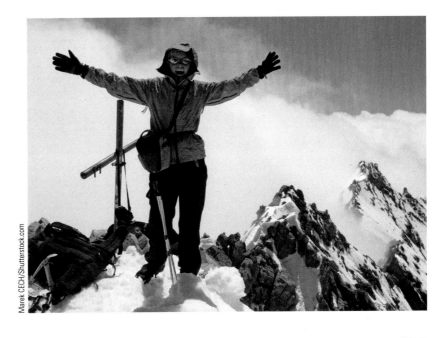

Marek CECH/Shutterstock.com

blood pH The measure of hydrogen ion (H^+) concentration in the blood.

Bohr effect Occurs when excess H^+ and or CO_2 bind with the Hb molecule and reduces the Hb molecule's affinity for oxygen.

2,3-diphosphoglycerate (DPG) Produced during metabolism within the RBC. As the DPG concentration increases, the O_2–Hb shifts to the right enabling an unloading of oxygen from the RBC at a higher PO_2.

gangrenous tissue, if blood flow to the area is available. This clinical example shows that it is not the quantity of oxygen that is physiologically active but the PO_2.

Given that aerobic metabolism is the human's fundamental mechanism of generating the energy for motor activity, it is easy to assume that adding oxygen to the inspired air would improve physical performance. However, the increase in performance occurs only when the ambient PO_2 is low, that is, at altitude.

It is important to realize that breathing 100 percent O_2 for long periods at sea level can be highly toxic, and in the early days of deep sea and scuba diving, the breathing of 100 percent O_2 under increased atmospheric pressure proved fatal in many instances.

Blood pH, Blood Temperature, and 2,3-Diphosphoglycerate Concentration Affects the Binding of Oxygen

The binding of O_2 to Hb at any given PO_2 is affected by blood pH, the temperature of the blood, and the amount of **2,3-diphosphoglycerate** (DPG; Figure 9.18).

Blood pH

As the acidity of the blood increases, **blood pH** decreases from its normal value of 7.4 at rest. In heavy exercise, it can reach values of 7.2. The change of 0.2 appears to be a minor decline, but remember, it is measured on a logarithmic scale. The increase in blood acidity weakens the bond between Hb and oxygen, and causes the oxygen to dissociate from the Hb at a higher PO_2, which results in a rightward shift in the O_2–Hb dissociation curve (see Figure 9.18). In contrast, if the pH increases, as it does at altitude (pH 7.6), the blood becomes more alkaline. The higher the pH, or more alkaline the blood becomes, the stronger the binding between O_2 and Hb, which results in O_2 dissociating from Hb at a lower PO_2 and a leftward shift in the O_2–Hb dissociation curve (see Figure 9.18).

The influence of acid, or pH, on the O_2–Hb dissociation curve is known as the **Bohr effect**. Generally, the Bohr effect is used to describe the rightward shift in the O_2–Hb dissociation curve. The rightward shift in the O_2–Hb dissociation curve is beneficial during heavy exercise because it unloads the oxygen at a higher PaO_2 in the acid conditions that exist within the exercising

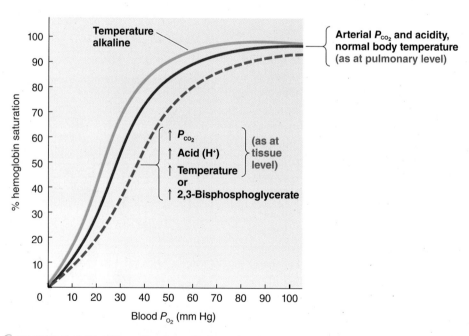

FIGURE 9.18 Effect of increased PCO_2 H^+, temperature, and 2,3-bisphosphoglycolerate on the oxygen–hemoglobin (O_2–Hb) curve. (From Sherwood, L. 2010. Figure 13.30 in Chapter 13, "The Respiratory System" in *Human physiology.* 7th ed. Belmont, CA: Brooks/Cole-Cengage Learning.)

skeletal muscle. Proteins can act as buffers in acidic solutions by binding with hydrogen ions (H^+), or protons. Therefore, the Hb molecule is an important protein available in the blood for buffering the large number of protons produced during exercise.

HOTLINK *Visit the course materials for Chapter 9 for more information on blood pH.*

Blood Temperature

Similar to the Bohr effect, an increase in the temperature of the blood causes a loosening of the O_2–Hb bond, resulting in a rightward shift in the O_2–Hb dissociation curve. In contrast, a decrease in the blood temperature results in a strengthening of the O_2–Hb bond, resulting in a leftward shift in the O_2–Hb dissociation curve (see Figure 9.18).

The muscle contractions of dynamic exercise have been found to be approximately 25 to 27 percent efficient, which indicates that a large amount of the metabolic energy generated to perform the exercise is wasted and is converted to heat within the muscle. This heat is transferred to the blood as it passes through the exercising muscle. Therefore, as the blood circulates through the exercising muscle, an increase in blood temperature facilitates O_2–Hb dissociation and O_2 unloading to the tissues. In the lung, the conditions are reversed because the ventilation of the lung is cooling the blood. Therefore, conditions for stronger binding of O_2 to Hb (leftward shift in the O_2–Hb dissociation curve) are present, resulting in a facilitation of the loading of oxygen to the blood.

2,3-Diphosphoglycerate (2,3 DPG)

The mature RBC lacks a nucleus and mitochondria, and relies solely on anaerobic glycolysis for its energy needs. A by-product of glycolysis is 2,3 DPG. An increase in the RBC's content of 2,3 DPG has been found to shift the O_2–Hb curve to the right. However, at sea level, acute exercise has little effect on the amount of 2,3 DPG, hence the Bohr effect and the increase in muscle temperature during exercise have a more

prominent role in the unloading of O_2 from the blood to the exercising muscles. Endurance exercise training at sea level, and more so using a paradigm of high-altitude living and low-altitude training (known as *Hi-Lo training*), results in an increased concentration of DPG within the RBC. The effect of a Hi-Lo training program on 2,3 DPG concentration in the RBC has proved to be beneficial to endurance performance.

Myoglobin (Mb) Provides Oxygen at the Beginning of Exercise

The final link in the transport of O_2 from air to the exercising muscle requires the unloading of the oxygen from Hb in the blood within the exercising muscle and its transfer to the respiratory chain of the mitochondria of the muscle cell. This transfer is aided by another oxygen-binding protein: Mb. Mb is similar in structure to Hb but is one fourth its weight. Mb has a greater affinity for oxygen (some 240 times greater); therefore, the O_2–Mb dissociation curve is much steeper (hyperbolic) than the O_2–Hb dissociation curve (Figure 9.19).

The O_2–Mb curve has an extreme leftward shift compared with the O_2–Hb curve. The practical outcome of the shape of the curve, because of its greater affinity for O_2, is that it binds O_2 at a PO_2 less than 20 mm Hg and unloads O_2 at a PO_2 as low as 1.0 mm Hg. This enables the delivery of O_2 to the mitochondria during heavy exercise where a PO_2 of 1 to 2 mm Hg has been recorded in the skeletal muscle.

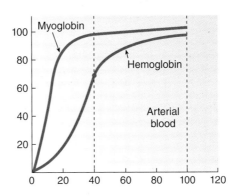

FIGURE 9.19 Comparison of the dissociation curve for myoglobin and hemoglobin. (© Cengage Learning 2013)

Mb is present in large amounts in slow-twitch skeletal muscle fibers (type I or red) and cardiac muscle fibers (muscles with high aerobic capacity). Intermediate (type I and II) muscle fibers have less concentration of Mb than type I fibers. White muscle, or fast-twitch muscle fiber (type II), has only minor amounts of Mb (see Chapter 3 for a review of muscle fiber types).

It is thought that Mb acts as an O_2 depot and has an important role in providing O_2 to the mitochondria at the beginning of exercise. At the transition from rest to exercise, there is a time lag between the onset of the muscle contraction and the increase in O_2 delivery to the muscle. The O_2 depot of the O_2–Mb molecule can be a source for the immediate delivery of O_2 and, in effect, acts as a facilitator of the transition from rest to an increase in O_2 delivery to the tissues and the time it takes for the cardiorespiratory system to deliver the O_2 to the tissues.

To what degree the O_2–Mb stores reduce the O_2 deficit at the beginning of exercise is unknown. The amount of O_2 required as part of the increased $\dot{V}O_2$ after exercise as a payback of the O_2 disassociated from O_2–Mb is also unknown. Notably, the muscles of highly trained endurance athletes have large quantities of red fiber, possibly because of three adaptations of the slow oxidative type I fibers to endurance exercise training:

1. Increase in mitochondrial number and their complexity, resulting in an increased iron content in the electron transport chain (primary)

2. Increase in number of capillaries, which during section or biopsy have residual blood within the capillaries

3. Increase in Mb content (however, not all investigators agree)

All three of these adaptations appear to be linked to the endurance-trained athlete's O_2 onset kinetics being faster than an average fit individual and also appears to play a role in the lactate shuttle between white and red fibers.

blood doping To transfuse whole blood or synthetic blood into a competitor to increase their oxygen-carrying capacity.

EPO Erythropoietin is the hormone released from the kidney in response to low PO_2 in the blood that stimulates RBC production in the bone marrow.

CONCEPTS, challenges, & controversies

Altitude Training or Hypoxic Training for Endurance Performance?

In preparing for the Mexico City Olympic Games in 1968, many athletes trained at altitudes of 8,000 feet or more to hopefully increase their red blood cell (RBC) volume (polycythemia). This was based on the concept that the ambient hypoxia-induced stimulation of erythropoietin (EPO) increases in red cell production while the athletes trained for their specific endurance event. Unfortunately, for many low-altitude–adapted athletes, they soon found out that they were unable to train at the same intensity and for same duration at altitude that they were accustomed to at the lower altitudes. Most of these athletes actually detrained and performed way below expectations in their Olympic events. However, the altitude stimulus of EPO production and the resultant increase in RBCs was not forgotten.

Clinically, it has been known for years that a means of increasing RBC volume into a hemorrhaged or anemic patient was to transfuse whole blood. This led to the idea of acutely increasing an athlete's RBC volume by the process of **"blood doping"** or the use of synthetic **"EPO"** infusions. Both of these procedures have been empirically found to decrease

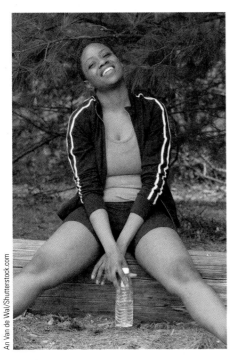

performance times and experimentally to increase $\dot{V}O_2$ max, which for many endurance athletes competing for a gold medal is worth the risk for death.

In blood doping involving a matched donor (homologous transfusion), the risk for infection and blood type incompatibility that may lead to shock and death is much greater than a transfusion of blood that is obtained from the recipient themselves (autologous transfusion). Initially, when EPO infusions became a method of choice in increasing RBC volumes for the athlete, the relationship between infused dose and the increase in RBC volume was unknown. Therefore, the use of EPO was suspected in a number of cases of unexpected deaths of endurance event competitors because of an increase in hematocrit and an exponential increase in blood viscosity, causing stroke or myocardial infarction. It should be recognized that these methods of enhancing performance are unethical and are banned by the World Anti-Doping Agency (WADA) and the national governing bodies of the individual sports and athletics.

In the late 1990s, the concept was advanced that if athletes lived at a relatively high altitude (approximately 16 to 18 hours/day) but trained (approximately 6 to 8 hours/day) at a low altitude (sometimes referred to as Hi-Lo altitude training), they would benefit from the natural hypoxic-stimulated EPO production, resulting in increased RBC volume. These changes have been demonstrated to increase $\dot{V}O_2$ max and decrease performance time. Indeed, when a group of athletes lived at 8,250 feet (2,500 meters) and trained at 4,125 feet (1,250 meters) for 4 weeks with dietary iron supplementation, they significantly increased their $\dot{V}O_2$ max (5 percent) and RBC volume (8 percent), and decreased their 5,000-meter time 1.5 percent. These findings, coupled with the knowledge that at one time it was a common practice for the Nordic Ski teams of Scandinavia to use "nitrogen houses" (a house that is plumbed to vary the altitude inside the house by introducing nitrogen into the circulating air of the house) during preparation for competition, has resulted in a defined industry that manufactures individual and/or group nitrogen tents. This has resulted in a major debate with WADA as to whether this provides economically advantaged countries or athletic teams an unfair advantage. This concern has curtailed the practice for using engineered Hi-Lo training atmospheres; however, there is no move to stop the practice using natural environmental changes in altitude.

Transport of Carbon Dioxide from the Tissues to the Lungs

The end products of aerobic and anaerobic metabolism within the cell are water, CO_2, energy, and lactate. At rest, the PCO_2 of the tissues ($PtCO_2$) is 46 mm Hg. The PCO_2 of the blood arriving at the respiratory arterioles ($PaCO_2$) in the tissues is 40 mm Hg, resulting in a diffusion gradient from the tissues to the blood of 6 mm Hg. (Remember,

carbonic acid (H_2CO_3) The combination of H^+ (ion) or acid with the bicarbonate (ion) or base.

bicarbonate ion (HCO_3^-) The base (salt) of carbonic acid.

gas flows down a tissue gradient from high pressure to low pressure, that is, from 46 to 40 mm Hg for CO_2).

The CO_2 is transported from the tissues to the alveoli in the blood in three ways:

1. 70 percent as **bicarbonate ion (HCO_3^-)**

2. 20 percent as carbaminohemoglobin (that is, bound to the Hb)

3. 10 percent dissolved in plasma

These three forms of CO_2 transportation are shown in Figure 9.20.

Some of the CO_2 dissolves in the plasma (10 percent) and another 20 percent combines with the Hb to form carbaminohemoglobin. However, the major (70 percent) transport mechanism for carrying CO_2 in

the blood is the HCO_3^-. The increase in PCO_2 in the venous blood because of diffusion from the tissues causes HCO_3^- to combine with water to form **carbonic acid (H_2CO_3)**. This combination, or reaction, is catalyzed by carbonic anhydrase within the RBC. H_2CO_3 is a weak acid and easily disassociates into a hydrogen ion and a bicarbonate ion. The hydrogen ion binds to the Hb (reduced Hb), and the bicarbonate ion diffuses out of the RBC. The bicarbonate ion is negatively charged and results in an electrochemical imbalance across the cell membrane. A chloride ion enters the RBC in a 1:1 exchange with the bicarbonate ion to keep the cell membrane electrochemically balanced, or neutral. This shift in ions is known as the *chloride shift*.

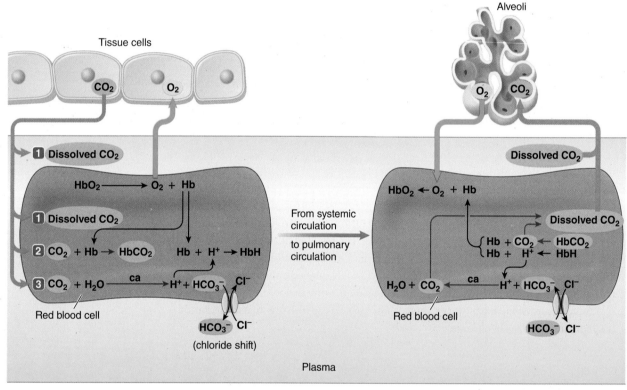

ca = Carbonic anhydrase

FIGURE 9.20 Carbon dioxide (CO_2) transport in the blood. CO_2 picked up at the tissue level is transported in the blood to the lungs in three ways: (1) physically dissolved, (2) bound to hemoglobin (Hb), and (3) as bicarbonate ion (HCO_3). Hb is present only in the red blood cells, as is carbonic anhydrase, the enzyme that catalyzes the production of HCO_3^-. The H^+ generated during the production of HCO_3^- also binds to Hb. Bicarbonate moves by facilitated diffusion down its concentration gradient out of the red blood cell into the plasma, and chloride (Cl^-) moves by means of the same passive carrier into the red blood cell down the electrical gradient created by the outward diffusion of HCO_3^-. The reactions that occur at the tissue level are reversed at the pulmonary level, where CO_2 diffuses out of the blood to enter the alveoli. (From Sherwood, L. 2010. Figure 13.31 in *Human physiology*, 7th ed. Belmont, CA: Brooks/Cole-Cengage Learning.)

When the blood reaches the alveoli of the lung, a reverse chloride shift occurs, in that a bicarbonate ion enters the RBC in exchange for the chloride ion, which then combines with a hydrogen ion and is released from the reduced Hb. When oxygen is loaded onto Hb, it releases hydrogen ions bound to the Hb and they combine with CO_2 to form H_2CO_3, which then disassociates into water and CO_2, and then diffuses from the RBC to the plasma. The CO_2 dissolved in the plasma diffuses across the respiratory membrane into the alveoli. The carbaminohemoglobin in the RBC releases its CO_2 as oxygen combines with Hb, and it also diffuses across the respiratory membrane into the alveoli (see Figure 9.20).

(What anatomic structures make up the respiratory membrane?)

Acid–Base Balance

Recall from your introductory chemistry and human physiology classes that the body's normal pH is 7.4, a value higher than the neutral pH value of 7.0. However, when pH values are higher than 7.4 in the body, or when the hydrogen ions decrease, the body is said to be more alkalotic. In contrast, when the hydrogen ions increase and the pH decreases to less than 7.4, the body is said to be more acidic. The lowest pH value of blood consistent with life is 6.8, and in very heavy exercise, pH values have been reported to be as low as 7.0. However, intramuscular pH values have been reported as low as 6.4 in heavy exhaustive exercise.

Exercise in hypoxic (low PO_2) environments, such as mountaineering, downhill and cross-country skiing at altitude, can result in blood pH values of 7.8 (alkalosis), because the peripheral chemoreceptors sense the low PO_2 and via central nervous system mechanisms increase the ventilation in excess of the ventilation for the $\dot{V}O_2$ required for the exercise at sea level, resulting in an increase in the rate and depth of breathing, that is, hyperventilation. Hyperventilation is by definition "blows of CO_2" at the lung, and this mechanism reduces the amount of acid in the blood, defined as alkalosis:

$$H^+ + HCO_3^- \rightleftharpoons H_2CO_3 \rightleftharpoons CO_2 + H_2O$$
[9.11]

If our physiologic mechanisms fail to maintain **acid–base balance**, the consequence may be fatal. For example, many of the deaths that have occurred during sporting events, which were unexplained by underlying genetic or pathologic conditions, were most likely a result of acid–base disturbances that resulted in cardiac arrhythmia and sudden death.

By far, the most common form of acid production occurs via the process of metabolism. Even at rest, the body's metabolic processes produce acids. Consequently, depending on the intensity of the exercise, the rate of acid production is proportionally increased with increasing intensity. Therefore, the body needs to have a rapid way of protecting itself and neutralizing the acids. Three main **metabolic acids** are produced:

1. *Volatile acids:* The most important volatile metabolic acid produced is CO_2. Although not truly an acid, it is the end product of the oxidation of carbohydrates, fats, and proteins, which in the presence of **carbonic anhydrase** reacts with water to produce H_2CO_3. Subsequently, the H_2CO_3 breaks down to hydrogen and bicarbonate ions.

   As you have learned previously, CO_2 is carried by the blood back to the lung and expired from the lung in exchange for the uptake of oxygen.

acid–base balance The balance between the hydrogen ion (acid) and the bicarbonate ion (base) in the blood.

metabolic acids The most abundant metabolic acid is CO_2 and although not a true acid, it is the end result of the breakdown of carbonic acid; by reason of its exchange at the lung, CO_2 is a primary regulator of the acid–base status during exercise.

carbonic anhydrase The enzyme catalyst for the rapid breakdown of carbonic acid to CO_2 and H_2O.

Indeed, it is this process of CO_2 elimination at the lung that provides the body with the rapid responding system to balance the production of acids resulting from metabolism.

2. *Fixed acids:* Both sulfuric and phosphoric acid are fixed acids and are products of the metabolism of some amino acids and phospholipids and nucleic acids, respectively. The production of fixed acids is linked more with dietary metabolism than to the metabolic production of energy for exercise. The hydrogen ions produced by the metabolic production of fixed acids are excreted by the kidney as ammonium ions (NH_4) and sodium biphosphate (NaH_2PO_4).

   The importance of this process during exercise is relatively minor during athletic events of short duration. However, in events like the Comrades Marathon (90 km) in South Africa and the Tour de France bicycle race (3,200 km over 3 weeks), the kidney's ability to clear the fixed acids becomes important. Indeed, if the concentration of ammonia is allowed to build because of a reduction in kidney function, neurologic brain function can be impaired.

3. *Organic acids:* The primary organic acid resulting from the metabolism of carbohydrate and fat is lactic acid. At rest, the production of lactic acid is slow enough to allow its resultant CO_2 to be expired at the lung without challenging the regulation of the body's pH. However, during heavy exercise above the ventilation (lactate) threshold, the production of lactic acid challenges the body's pH regulatory capacity.

   If the intensity and duration of exercise results in the production of lactic acid being greater than the body's ability to use (lactate within the muscle, heart, and brain) or eliminate it in a 1:1 ratio, then the tissue and blood lactate concentrations will increase. The decrease in

intramuscular pH impairs exercise performance in three ways because of the increases in hydrogen ion concentration:

1. It interferes with the enzymatic ability of the energy-producing machinery of the muscle cell to produce ATP.

2. It hinders the contractile process of the skeletal muscle by competing with calcium for the binding sites on the troponin molecule.

3. It inhibits SR calcium release.

In acute bouts of high-intensity exercise (100- to 400-meter sprints), there is an accumulation of inorganic phosphates and hydrogen ions within the fibers that impair contractile protein function, resulting in reduced force output. This reduction in force output comes on suddenly and is commonly referred to as "jelly legs."

The initial process by which the body combats excess hydrogen ion production is its **buffering capacity**. A buffer resists changes in pH by removing excess hydrogen ions and by adding hydrogen ions when they are reduced. The first buffering

buffering capacity The capacity of a buffer to resist changes in pH by removing excess hydrogen ions and by adding hydrogen ions when they are reduced.

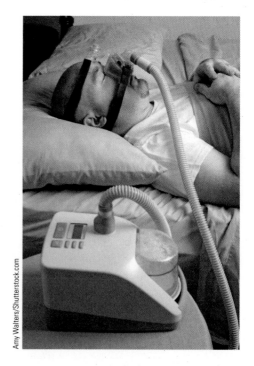

Amy Walters/Shutterstock.com

process occurs in the cell as both proteins and phosphates can reversibly bind excess hydrogen ions. For example, intracellular phosphocreatine buffers hydrogen ions at the beginning of exercise during the anaerobic processes of the oxygen deficit. In addition, both the weak phosphoric acids and bicarbonate ions are available in the skeletal muscle to act as buffers.

However, the primary buffering capacity for the excess lactic acid produced in exercise is found in the blood. The blood has three major buffering systems:

1. Proteins
2. Hb
3. Bicarbonate

Similar to the intracellular proteins of the muscle, the extracellular proteins, or plasma proteins, of the blood contain weak acids, which act as buffers when required. However, the small quantities of blood proteins that are present do not make them very useful, especially in heavy exercise when the hydrogen ion production is very large.

In contrast, Hb within RBCs is especially important because it has six times the buffering capacity of the plasma proteins. Furthermore, as Hb becomes deoxygenated in the capillaries, its ability to bind hydrogen ions is enhanced at the time when hydrogen ions are formed in the blood from the breakdown of H_2CO_3 after CO_2 enters the blood from the tissues. When the deoxygenated Hb becomes oxygenated in the lung, the bound CO_2 is released and diffuses from the blood into the alveoli and becomes part of the gas exchange process described earlier.

However, because of its rapidity of action, the bicarbonate buffer system is by far the most important buffer system in the body, especially during exercise. The CO_2 produced in the tissue cells diffuses into the blood, and because of its solubility, is dissolved in the plasma and the cytoplasm of the RBC. The CO_2 in the plasma and the RBC combines with water to form H_2CO_3, which then disassociates to form hydrogen ions and bicarbonate ions (see Equation 9.11 and Figure 9.20).

The bicarbonate ion in the RBC exchanges with the chloride ion from the plasma, as per the chloride shift, and combines with the leftover sodium ions to form sodium bicarbonate ($NaHCO_3$). The sodium bicarbonate of the plasma then interacts with the lactic acid that has exited from the muscle into the blood because of an imbalance between lactate production and clearance (see Figure 9.20):

$$Na + HCO_3^- + H^+ + La \rightleftharpoons$$
$$NaLa + H_2CO_3 \rightleftharpoons H_2O + CO_2 \quad [9.12]$$

At the lung, the resultant CO_2 is expired as a part of the gas exchange mechanism described previously, which is in direct relation to the metabolic demand of the exercise.

In summary, the body uses three strategies for defending against acidosis: It buffers immediately, respires from the lung during each breath, and excretes the excess acids via the kidney over the long term.

Control of Ventilation

We noted earlier that at rest and low-intensity exercise, inspiration, which involves the contraction of the diaphragm and costal (or chest wall) muscles, is an active process, whereas expiration is a passive relaxation of the same respiratory muscles. Control of these respiratory muscles occurs via the motor nerves of the spinal cord, the activity of which are under the control of the respiratory control center located in the medulla oblongata. Within the respiratory center, two groups of neurons, the ventral respiratory group and the dorsal respiratory group, fire in a rhythmic

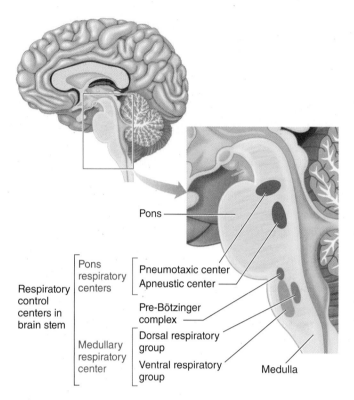

Pons

Respiratory control centers in brain stem
- Pons respiratory centers
  - Pneumotaxic center
  - Apneustic center
- Medullary respiratory center
  - Pre-Bötzinger complex
  - Dorsal respiratory group
  - Ventral respiratory group

Medulla

FIGURE 9.21 **Respiratory control centers in the brainstem.** (From Sherwood, L. 2010. Figure 13.33 in Chapter 13, "The Respiratory System" in *Human physiology*, 7th ed. Belmont, CA: Brooks/Cole-Cengage Learning.)

central chemoreceptors Located in the medulla oblongata and separate from the respiratory centers, sense changes in hydrogen ion concentration caused by changes in CO_2 within the brain's extracellular fluid (ECF).

pattern and make up the respiratory rhythmicity center. It is this rhythmicity center that provides the timing of the rhythm of breathing in and out (Figure 9.21).

Two other areas anatomically located within the pons in the brainstem, the apneustic area and the pneumotaxic area, interface with the rhythmicity center and control the time of inspiration and the depth of each breath, respectively (see Figure 9.21).

External neural input (central command and/or the exercise pressor reflex) ($PaCO_2$, H^+ ions, PaO_2, and potassium ions) to the respiratory control center also modify ventilation of the lung to affect changes in acid–base status in response to the demands of exercise and altitude in delivering oxygen to the tissues. The external humoral receptors of the body are known as the chemoreceptors, and they react to chemical stimuli sensed within the tissues and fluids of the body. Depending on their location within or outside of the brain, they

are identified as central or peripheral chemoreceptors, respectively.

HOTLINK *See Chapter 7 for more information on central command and the pressor reflex.*

Central Chemoreceptors Provide Humoral Control of Ventilation

The anatomic location of the **central chemoreceptors** is located within the medulla oblongata but is distinctly separated from the respiratory center. Increases in cerebrospinal fluid concentrations of hydrogen ions and PCO_2 cause increases in ventilation, whereas decreases in hydrogen ion concentration and PCO_2 decrease ventilation. Indeed, the central chemoreceptors are more sensitive to changes in PCO_2 and H^+ than are the peripheral chemoreceptors and are generally regarded as the primary source of humoral control of ventilation.

ịnRETROSPECT

History of Neural Control of Ventilation during Exercise

In 1855, Christian Bohr became Professor of Physiology at the University of Copenhagen and director of a laboratory investigating respiration, digestion, and metabolism. He developed a lifelong interest in the transport of oxygen and carbon dioxide in the blood while he was working with Carl Ludwig in Germany. He was the first investigator to identify the effects of carbon dioxide on the oxyhemoglobin–dissociation curve (that is, the Bohr effect).

(*What is the Bohr effect on the oxyhemoglobin–dissociation curve?*)

Without the Bohr effect, the unloading of oxygen from Hb in the exercising muscle would be impaired. Christian Bohr was the father of Niels Bohr, the Danish Nobel Prize-winning nuclear physicist. However, Christian Bohr's fame in the physiology world was enhanced by his graduate students who later in their careers accomplished more. One of his students was August Krogh (1874–1949), the 1920 Nobel Prize winner for identifying oxygen diffusion at the lung and tissue and capillary recruitment in both the lung and muscle during exercise. Another student was Karl Albert Hasselbalch, who defined the "Hendersen–Hasselbalch equation," standardizing the measurement of pH of the blood and defining acidosis. In addition, Hendersen was the founder and first director of the Famous Harvard Fatigue Laboratory,

which in the 1930s became recognized as the leading Exercise and Work Physiology research program in the United States.

One of Hasselbach's students, Johannes Lindhard, M.D. (1870–1947), joined the University of Copenhagen in 1909 and was invited by Krogh to collaborate in investigating the many "human integrative physiology" questions raised by isometric and dynamic exercise. This collaboration is recognized as the birth of "exercise physiology," specifically, the neural control of the circulation and respiration. Based on identifying the brief latency in the time of the increase in the ventilation and the increase in the absorption of oxygen at the beginning of exercise, Krogh and Lindhard postulated a neural mechanism (*cortical irradiation* first suggested in 1895) as being responsible for the increases. This concept of a neural mechanism of parallel cortical neural irradiation to the muscles and the heart and respiratory control centers was based on the work of Johansson in 1895, who demonstrated that the increases in pulse rate and ventilation occurred only during voluntary contractions and not with passive movement, or electrical stimulation, of a rabbit's leg muscles. Indeed, the concept of "**central command**" in being the initiator of the increase in ventilation at the beginning of exercise and increasing the ventilation in parallel to increases in exercise intensity was confirmed in human experiments in 1972.

Peripheral Chemoreceptors Provide Control of Ventilation

The **peripheral chemoreceptors** located in the aortic arch are termed the *aortic bodies*, and those located in the bifurcation of the common carotid artery are termed the *carotid bodies*. The aortic bodies and the carotid bodies are anatomically located in similar structures as the aortic and carotid baroreceptors, respectively. Both the aortic and carotid bodies respond to increases in $PaCO_2$, arterial H^+, and potassium ion concentrations by increasing ventilation, whereas a reduction in PaO_2 to less than

75 to 80 mm Hg (identified as a hypoxic threshold) also stimulates increases in ventilation (Figures 9.22 and 9.23, page 326). It is not unusual after vascular procedures involving bilateral carotid artery resection to remove atherosclerotic plaques in the area of the carotid bifurcations, to have a partial loss of control of ventilation and blood pressure.

Neural Control of Ventilation during Exercise

It is generally recognized that the neural control of ventilation developed at about the same time as that already described

peripheral chemoreceptors The aortic and carotid bodies located in the aortic arch and the bifurcation of the carotid artery and respond to increases in $PaCO_2$, arterial H^+, and potassium ion concentrations by increasing ventilation. A reduction in PaO_2 to less than 75 to 80 mm Hg (identified as a hypoxic threshold) also stimulates the peripheral chemoreceptors and increase ventilation.

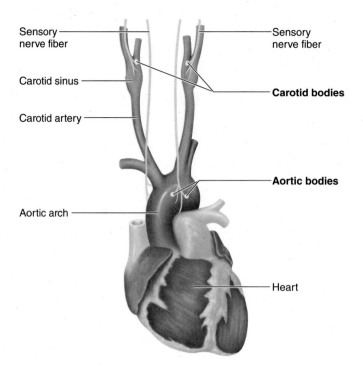

● **FIGURE 9.22 Location of the peripheral chemoreceptors.** The carotid bodies are located in the carotid sinus, and the aortic bodies are located in the aortic arch. (From Sherwood, L. 2010. Figure 13.34 in Chapter 13, "The Respiratory System" in *Human physiology*, 7th ed. Belmont, CA: Brooks/Cole-Cengage Learning.)

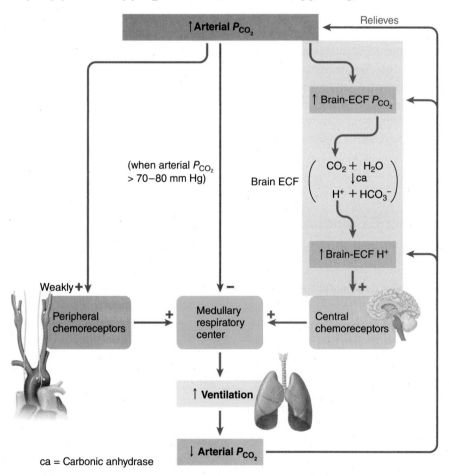

● **FIGURE 9.23 Effect of increased arterial partial pressure of oxygen (PCO₂) on ventilation.** (From Sherwood, L. 2010. Figure 13.35 in Chapter 13, "The Respiratory System" in *Human physiology*, 7th ed. Belmont, CA: Brooks/Cole-Cengage Learning.)

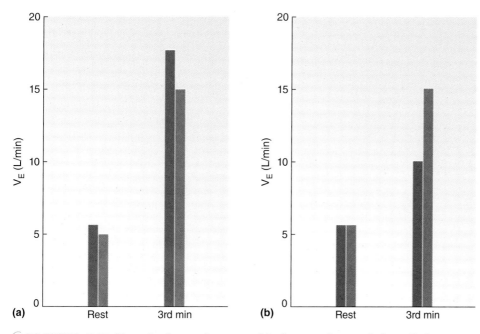

● FIGURE 9.24 The role of central command in the neural control of ventilation.
(a) Ventilation response from rest to 20 percent maximum voluntary contraction (MVC) without (blue bars) and with (purple bars) agonist tendon vibration induced decrease in central command (CC). Note that the 3-L/min reduction in exercise ventilation when CC was reduced (purple bars). (b) Ventilation response from rest to 35 percent MVC without (blue bars) and with antagonist tendon variation induced increase in CC. Note that the 5-L/min increase in exercise-induced ventilation when CC was increased (purple bars). (Modified from Goodwin, G. M., D. I. McCloskey, and J. H. Mitchell. 1972. Cardiovascular and respiratory responses to changes in central command during isometric exercise at constant muscle tension. *J. Physiol.* 226:173–190.)

for the cardiovascular system in Chapter 7. At this time, we provide a brief review of the specific developments and current thinking regarding the neural control of the ventilatory response to exercise. Experiments using the tendon vibration technique (described in Chapter 7) identified that when you performed muscle contractions (exercise) while central command was being assisted by agonist tendon vibration, the ventilation response to the exercise was less than if it was performed without assistance. When the muscle contraction (exercise) was performed against an inhibition of the contraction produced by antagonist tendon vibration, the ventilation response was increased (Figure 9.24).

Subsequently, in experiments using decerebrate animal preparations and stimulation of the mesencephalic locomotor region within the brain (a central nervous system nucleus that appears to be a relay on the pathway used by central command), walking was initiated, and at the same time, an increase in ventilation began. In humans, central command was manipulated by using hypnotic suggestion of an increase in bicycle workloads, whereas the actual work remained the same (100 W) as that without hypnotic suggestion. During the suggested increase in workload, ventilation was increased (see Figure 9.25, page 328).

These animal and human experiments confirm the role of central command in the parallel activation of motor activity and ventilation. However, what is not known is whether central command affects the sensitivity of the central or peripheral chemoreceptors to CO_2 in a similar way that it affects resetting of the arterial baroreflexes (see Chapter 7).

Using "in vivo" animal experiments and selective anesthesia of afferent nerves emanating from electrically contracting skeletal muscles, investigators found that neural signals arising from the activated skeletal muscle interface with the respiratory control center in the medulla oblongata and cause a reflex increase in ventilation (Figure 9.26, page 328).

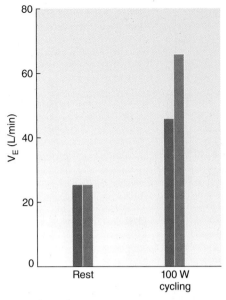

FIGURE 9.25 Hypnotic suggestion and exercise ventilation. Ventilation response from rest to 100-W steady-state cycling exercise without (open bars) and with (hatched bars) hypnotic suggestion of increased effort. (Modified from Morgan, W.P., P. B. Raven, B. L. Drinkwater and S. M. Horvath. 1973. Figure 2 in "Perceptual and metabolic responsivity to standard bicycle ergometry following various hypnotic suggestions" *Int. J. Clin. Exp. Hypn.* 21:86–101.)

Recently, researchers found that by slowing the venous outflow from the legs using leg cuffs inflated to 90 mm Hg, and thereby increasing intramuscular lactate concentrations in the femoral veins (an index of increased metabolic acidosis in the exercising leg) during cycling exercise, the signal for the exponential increase in ventilation (ventilation threshold) occurs at a lower workload, or $\dot{V}O_2$ (Figure 9.27).

This finding indicates that a signal for increased ventilation can be an intramuscular neural signal to the respiratory center in the brain, which in the control condition coincidentally occurs at the same time that the intramuscular lactate is beginning to flow into the circulation from the skeletal muscles involved in performing the exercise and the chest wall muscles involved in pulmonary ventilation.

From the data from both animal and human studies presented in Figures 9.24, page 327, through 9.27, page 328, the schematic model in Figure 9.28, page 329, summarizes the neural control of the ventilation.

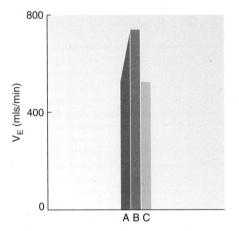

FIGURE 9.26 Exercise pressor reflex control of ventilation. Ventilatory response to 15-second isometric contraction of a cat's triceps surae muscle without ischemia (A), with ischemia (B), and with ischemia and afferent nerves cut (C). (Modified from McCloskey, D.L. and J. H. Mitchell. 1972. Figure 2 in Reflex cardiovascular and respiratory responses originating in exercising muscle. *J. Physiol.* 224:173–186.)

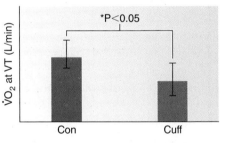

FIGURE 9.27 Activation of muscle chemoreceptors during exercise stimulates ventilation. Estimates of oxygen uptake ($\dot{V}O_2$) ventilatory threshold (VT) during progressive increases in workload cycling exercise without (con) and with (cuff) leg cuff occlusion at 90 mm Hg. (Modified from Smith, S. A., K. M. Gallagher, K. M. Norton, R. G. Querry, R. M. Welch-O'Connor, and P. B. Raven. 1999. Figure 6 in Ventilatory responses to dynamic exercise elicited by intramuscular pressure sensors. *Med. Sci. Sports and Exerc.* 31:277–286.)

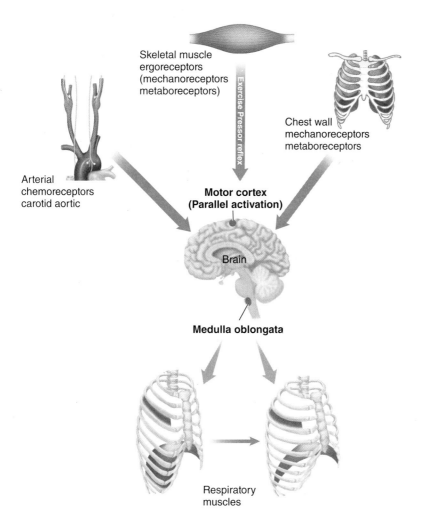

Arterial
chemoreceptors
carotid aortic

Skeletal muscle
ergoreceptors
(mechanoreceptors
metaboreceptors)

Exercise Pressor reflex

Chest wall
mechanoreceptors
metaboreceptors

Motor cortex
(Parallel activation)

Brain

Medulla oblongata

Respiratory
muscles

FIGURE 9.28 Schematic model of the neural control of pulmonary ventilation during exercise. (© Cengage Learning 2013)

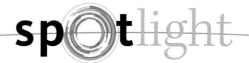

An Expert on the Respiratory System and Exercise: Karlman Wasserman, M.D., Ph.D.

Dr. Karlman Wasserman was born in Brooklyn, New York, in 1927. He earned a Bachelor of Arts in basic engineering and chemistry from Upsala College in 1948. He earned a Ph.D. in physiology from Tulane University in 1951 and also earned his M.D. degree in 1958. He completed postgraduate training at John Hopkins University (1958–1959) and at the Cardiovascular Research Institute at the University of California in San Francisco (1959–1961).

Wasserman was one of the pioneers who first used exercise testing to study the interaction of cardiovascular, ventilatory, and metabolic responses in humans. He has authored more than 270 journal articles, 8 books, 39 book chapters, and numerous scientific reviews in his professional career. He is

currently a professor emeritus at the UCLA School of Medicine where he first started as an associate professor in 1967. Wasserman also served as the Chief of the Division of Respiratory and Critical Care Physiology at the Medical Center in Torrance, California, from 1967 to 1997.

Wasserman is perhaps best known for describing the concept of measuring the "anaerobic threshold" by using ventilatory and cardiovascular responses to exercise testing. He describes how he became involved with his research interests that have lasted nearly 50 years in the following paragraphs.

After a year internship in medicine on the Osler Service at Johns Hopkins, Wasserman arrived in San Francisco as a special National Institutes of Health Fellow of Dr.

Julius H. Comroe, Jr., in July 1959. Dr. Comroe was Director of the new Cardiovascular Research Institute at the University of California, San Francisco. Dr. Comroe, Jr., called me into his office and posed the following question to me: "Can we develop a method to detect heart disease earlier, before it compromises the patient?" Why the question? Why ask me?

Personal Recollections

In November 1960, Dr. Comroe had just returned from the Annual Scientific Sessions of the American Heart Association. During the meeting, the fact that the incidences of coronary artery disease and heart failure were increasing at an alarming (epidemic) rate was widely discussed. I pointed out that the rate of buffering of the accumulating lactic acid might be observable in the exhaled gas and quantified, possibly breath by breath. Comroe then quickly stopped the discussion and told me, "Go do it." I thought that the problem would be resolved by the time I was due to take my new position at Stanford. However, I didn't appreciate at the time (1) that other investigators were skeptical that there was an anaerobic or lactate threshold, or 2) that the accumulating lactate was buffered by HCO_3.

Cardiopulmonary exercise testing is now a well-established diagnostic tool, used by multiple medical disciplines. It is invaluable in the grading of the severity of impairment of organ systems involved in the support of muscle respiration, a process essential for the production of energy for muscle contraction. Specifically, it is currently used to establish the cause of exercise intolerance resulting from the symptoms of exertional dyspnea, fatigue, or pain (differential diagnosis). Cardiologists use it to prioritize patients with heart failure for heart transplantation according to the severity of the physiologic impairment. It is also used to detect myocardial dyskinesis caused by myocardial ischemia during exercise. In addition, it is unsurpassed as a noninvasive tool to diagnose pulmonary vascular disorders causing ventilation/perfusion mismatching and the opening of right-to-left shunts during exercise, abnormalities that lead to exertional dyspnea.

Anesthesiologists responsible for bringing patients through surgery and providing postoperative care have used cardiopulmonary exercise testing to identify which patients are apt to have an unfavorable course after surgery and to be at greatest risk for not surviving the postoperative period. Both cardiologists and pulmonologists rely on it as a method to objectively document the effectiveness of treatments, including drugs, surgical procedures, and exercise training, in the correction of the dysfunctional physiology resulting in exercise intolerance.

This brief overview of how the field of cardiopulmonary exercise testing in health and disease came about illustrates how the process of discovery shaped later developments. It started with an observation (prevalence of heart disease was on the rise), followed by a question related to the observation (How can we detect heart disease in its early stages?). Observation and question are essential elements of discovery. This was followed by the integration of operationally factual information that could be extended by the investigator into a hypothesis that could be tested. As is true of most research, important side discoveries were made along the way toward solving the original question. Examples are the effect of phosphocreatine splitting on early exercise gas exchange kinetics, the timing and mechanism of potassium efflux from muscle at the start of exercise, the likely mechanism for Hb and plasma sodium concentration increase during exercise, the critical capillary PO_2, how the development of the exercise lactic acidosis affects O_2 transport to muscle, and how regulation of arterial H^+ affects ventilatory control during exercise.

in*Practice*

Examples of the Respiratory System and Exercise

The following section provides practical examples of how the respiratory system and exercise are related to your area of interest (review the future career table from Chapter 1).

Health/Fitness: Asthma is the most common reason students miss physical education classes or athletes have to modify their practice time for sport. **Asthma** is a disease that causes the air passages in the lungs to swell or narrow (bronchospasm), making it harder for athletes to breathe. Signs and symptoms of asthma include:

- Coughing
- Wheezing (a hoarse whistling sound heard during exhalation)
- Shortness of breathe
- Chest tightness

Strenuous exercise acts as a common trigger for bronchospasm in athletes. Other common triggers for asthmatic attacks are:

- Poor medical management
- Air pollution (mold, pollen, tobacco, dust mites)
- Emotions (like laughing or crying)
- Allergies
- Exposure to cold air

Medicine: Cystic fibrosis (CF) is a congenital metabolic disorder that causes an inability to clear the lungs of secretions (mucus). The thick mucus in patients with CF also limits their ability to release digestive enzymes, which results in malnutrition, poor weight gain, and poor growth. CF patients also lose large amounts of salt in their sweat. CF occurs in about 1 in 3,500 births. Patients with CF usually take many medications to control their disease; however, regular participation in exercise helps patients with CF clear their lungs of mucus, stimulates coughing, improves heart and lung function, and can improve the psychological outlook for most patients with CF. Patients with CF should be encouraged to maintain their hydration when engaging in exercise, and to monitor their caloric expenditure and intake balance.

In the case of obstructive lung disease, the airflow out of the lung is obstructed because of airway narrowing (asthma), plugging of the small airways (bronchitis, inflammation of the lung tissue resulting in mucus production), or no elastic recoil of the lung tissue (emphysema) and, therefore, requires the act of expiration to become active, resulting in increased work in breathing. Unfortunately, the act of contracting the expiratory muscles can cause the airways to collapse, especially in advanced disease cases, which can further obstruct airflow out of the lung.

In the case of restrictive lung disease, the airflow into the lung is restricted because of chest wall abnormalities or fibrotic disease of the lung tissue (elastin fibers losing their elastic property). Remember, the act of inspiration is active, and the contraction of the inspiratory muscles requires energy to generate the forces of contraction to shorten the muscle. If the lung tissue is fibrotic, the amount of force required to contract the respiratory muscles to expand the chest wall increases and, therefore, the work of breathing increases.

The lung minimizes the work of breathing for each breath. When a resistance to breathing in or out (such as wearing a firefighter's respirator) is present, the V_T of the breath gets bigger and breathing is less frequent. In many of the chronic obstructive lung diseases (COPD), such as asthma, bronchitis, emphysema, or combinations of two or three of these, the work of breathing becomes so hard that patients become worried about where the next breath will come from. Therefore, the thought of having to increase their breathing just to walk becomes frightening.

HOTLINK *For more information about firefighters, mine rescue industrial respirators, and scuba, visit the National Institutes of Health website:* http://www.nih.gov/.

Athletic Performance: The one obstructive lung disease that the physical educator, coach, and recreational and competitive athlete needs to be aware of, because it may come on suddenly, is asthma. In susceptible individuals, "exercise" can induce the bronchoconstriction of asthma (known as *exercise-induced asthma*). The presence of pollutants and pesticides in the air can also result in an allergic asthma episode during athletic events where pesticides have been used. A large number (25–50 percent) of swim athletes may have chosen swimming as their event because the higher humidity of the inspired air is associated with a significant reduction in the number of episodes of exercise-induced asthma.

asthma A disease that produces spasmodic contractions of the bronchi, which results from direct irritation or reflex irritation of the bronchial mucosal membranes, especially in sensitized individuals.

Athletes who have asthma often do not admit or tell their coaches about their symptoms and blame them on being deconditioned or having a cold. Because athletes will deny their symptoms, coaches and athletic trainers need to be aware of the signs that suggest an athlete is experiencing asthmatic problems. These signs include:

- Frequent use of inhalers
- Sensitivity to cold air
- Repeated complaints of feeling winded or tiring easily
- Dizziness
- Stomachache
- Frequent colds or clearing of the throat
- Muscle cramps
- Poorer performance than their training would predict

Asthma should not eliminate athletes from participating in sport. However, coaches should help athletes learn to properly manage their asthma before small problems become major ones. Coaches should encourage their asthmatic athletes to do the following:

- Make sure they see their doctor and get a checkup (often by a specialist like an allergist), and encourage them to be open and honest with their physician and make sure they let their physician know if their asthma gets worse.
- Make sure they always have their inhaler close by and have trainers carry backup inhalers when the team travels. As with all medications, do not let anyone use someone else's inhaler.

- Make sure they have a 15-minute minimum warm-up that includes balance or agility drills, walking, jogging, stretching, or submaximal short sprints.
- Make sure they stop exercising slowly and have at least a 10-minute cool-down after activity.
- Make sure that in cold weather they cover their mouths and noses with scarves or face masks to warm air before it reaches their airways; this will help prevent bronchospasm.
- Do not make fun of athletes with asthma because they have a potentially serious health problem that can become worse if they learn to ignore their basic symptoms. An athlete may need to stop practice/competition because of an asthmatic attack, and it should be treated as a safety precaution, not punishment for the athlete.

Rehabilitation: Many physical therapists and clinical athletic trainers find themselves working with patients who have chronic obstructive pulmonary disease (COPD), which is usually associated with chronic bronchitis, emphysema, and asthma, in addition to their most current physical ailment. To successfully treat these types of patients, therapists and trainers need to thoroughly understand pulmonary function testing and norms for healthy and compromised clients. They will also need to be able to determine and/or understand arterial blood gases and arterial oxygen saturation (SaO_2) in pulmonary patients and modify their traditional exercise training protocols as necessary.

Chapter Summary

- Pulmonary ventilation is defined as the movement of air into and out of the lungs during the act of breathing. Breathing in, or inspiration, is active and requires contraction of the muscles of the chest wall and the diaphragm.
- In many of the chronic obstructive lung diseases (COPD), such as asthma, bronchitis, emphysema, or combinations of two or three of these, the work of breathing can become so hard that the patient worries where the next breath will come from. Therefore, the thought of having to walk can become frightening.
- During maximal exercise, ventilation volumes can range from 125 to 200 L/min. Generally, in an average fit individual, the ventilation threshold occurs at approximately 60 percent $\dot{V}O_2$ max during a dynamic progressive workload exercise test.

- Dalton's law of partial pressures states that the total pressure of a mixture of gases is equal to the sum of the pressure that each gas independently exerts.
- Fick's law of diffusion of gases states that the rate (velocity) at which a gas (V gas) is transferred across a tissue membrane is proportional to the tissue membrane's surface area (A), the diffusion coefficient (D) of the gas, and the difference between the partial pressures of the gas on each side of the tissue membrane ($P_1 - P_2$), and is inversely proportional to the thickness (T) of the tissue membrane.
- Henry's law of solubility of gases states that at equilibrium, the amount of oxygen dissolved in the blood is directly proportional to the partial pressure of oxygen in the alveolar air.

- As the acidity of the blood increases, the pH of the blood decreases from its normal value of 7.4. In heavy exercise, pH values can reach 7.2. Similar to the Bohr effect, an increase in the temperature of the blood causes a loosening of the O_2–Hb bond, resulting in a rightward shift in the O_2–Hb dissociation curve.

- The effect of a Hi-Lo training program on DPG concentration in the red blood cell has proved beneficial to endurance performance. It is thought that Mb acts as an O_2 depot that plays an important role in providing O_2 to the mitochondria at the beginning of exercise.

- Carbon dioxide is transported in the blood in three ways: 70 percent as a bicarbonate ion (HCO_3^-), 20 percent as carbaminohemoglobin, and 10 percent dissolved in plasma. The initial process by which the body combats excess hydrogen ion production is its buffering capacity. A buffer resists changes in pH by removing excess hydrogen ions and by adding hydrogen ions when they are reduced.

- Ventilation is controlled via neural, hormonal, and chemoreceptor factors. It is generally accepted that endurance and weight exercise training have little effect on lung tissue in terms of growth or increase in function. This means that, unlike the cardiovascular system, once you lose it, it is gone forever.

Exercise Physiology Reality

CENGAGE brain   To reinforce the exercise physiology concepts presented above, complete the laboratory exercises for Chapter 9. To access labs and other course materials for this text, please visit www.cengagebrain.com. See the preface on page xiii for details. Once you complete the exercises, have your instructor evaluate your prescriptions. Remember to use your lab experience to help guide you toward future success in exercise physiology.

Exercise Physiology Web Links

Access the following websites for further study of topics covered in this chapter:

- Find updates and quick links to these and other exercise physiology–related sites at our website. To access the course materials and companion resources for this text, please visit www.cengagebrain.com. See the preface on page xiii for details.

- Search for further information about research and the respiratory system at the American Physiological Society (APS) website: http://www.the-aps.org.

- Search for information about respiratory physiology and the American College of Sports Medicine at: http://www.acsm.org.

- Search for more information about respiratory training at the U.S. Government National Heart, Lung, and Blood Institute website: http://www.nhlbi.nih.gov.

- Search for more information about research and respiratory physiology training at the Federation of American Societies for Experimental Biology website: http://www.faseb.org.

Study Questions

Review the Warm-Up Pre-Test questions you were asked to answer before reading Chapter 9. Test yourself once more to determine what you know now that you have completed the chapter.

The questions that follow will help you review this chapter. You will find the answers in the discussions on the pages provided.

1. Define the term *pulmonary ventilation,* and describe why ventilation volume and tidal volume are important factors in exercise. *pp. 291–295*

2. Why is having a higher ventilation threshold beneficial to an endurance athlete? *pp. 296–297*

3. Explain why Dalton's, Fick's, and Henry's laws are important in gas exchange within the lungs. *pp. 302–305*

4. Explain how oxygen is transported from the lungs to the tissues. *pp. 310–317*

5. Describe the oxyhemoglobin dissociation curve. *pp. 312–317*

6. Describe the Bohr effect. Why is it important? *pp. 314–317*

7. What are the three ways carbon dioxide is transported in the blood, and which way is the major transport mechanism? *pp. 317–319*

8. Explain why acid–base balance is important. *pp. 319–321*

9. Explain when the exercise pressor reflex is activated during exercise training and what occurs during this process? *pp. 321–327*

Selected References

Dempsey, J. A. 2006. Classical perspectives: Is the healthy respiratory system (always) built for exercise? *J. Physiol.* 576:339–340.

Dempsey, J. A., D. C. McKenzie, H. C. Haverkamp, and M. W. Eldridge. 2008. Update in the understanding of respiratory limitations to exercise performance in fit, active adults. *Chest* 134:613–622.

Eichner, R. 2007. Blood doping: Infusion, erythropoietin and artificial blood. *Sports Med.* 37:389–391.

Ekblom, B., G. Wilson, and P. O. Astrand. 1976. Central circulation during exercise after venesection and reinfusion of red blood cells. *J. Appl. Physiol.* 40:379–383.

Levine, B. J., and J. Stray-Gundersen. 1997. Living high-training low: Effect of moderate-altitude acclimatization with low-altitude training on performance *J. Appl. Physiol.* 83(1):102–112.

Saltin, B., and P-O Astrand. 1967. Maximal oxygen uptake in athletes. *J. Appl. Physiol.* 23:353–358.

Sherwood, L. 2010. Chapter 13, "The Respiratory System" in *Human physiology,* 7th ed. Belmont, CA: Brooks/Cole-Cengage Learning.

Sherwood, L. 2010. Chapter 15, "Fluid and Acid–Base Balance" in *Human physiology,* 7th ed. Belmont, CA: Brooks/Cole-Cengage Learning.

Van Hall, G. 2009. Blood lactate is an important energy source for the human brain. *J. Cereb. Blood Flow Metab.* 29:1121–1129.

Wasserman, K. 1984. The anaerobic threshold measurement to evaluate exercise performance. *Am. Rev. Respir. Dis.* 129:535–540.

Whipp, B. J. 1983. Ventilatory control during exercise in humans. *Annu. Rev. Physiol.* 45:393–413.

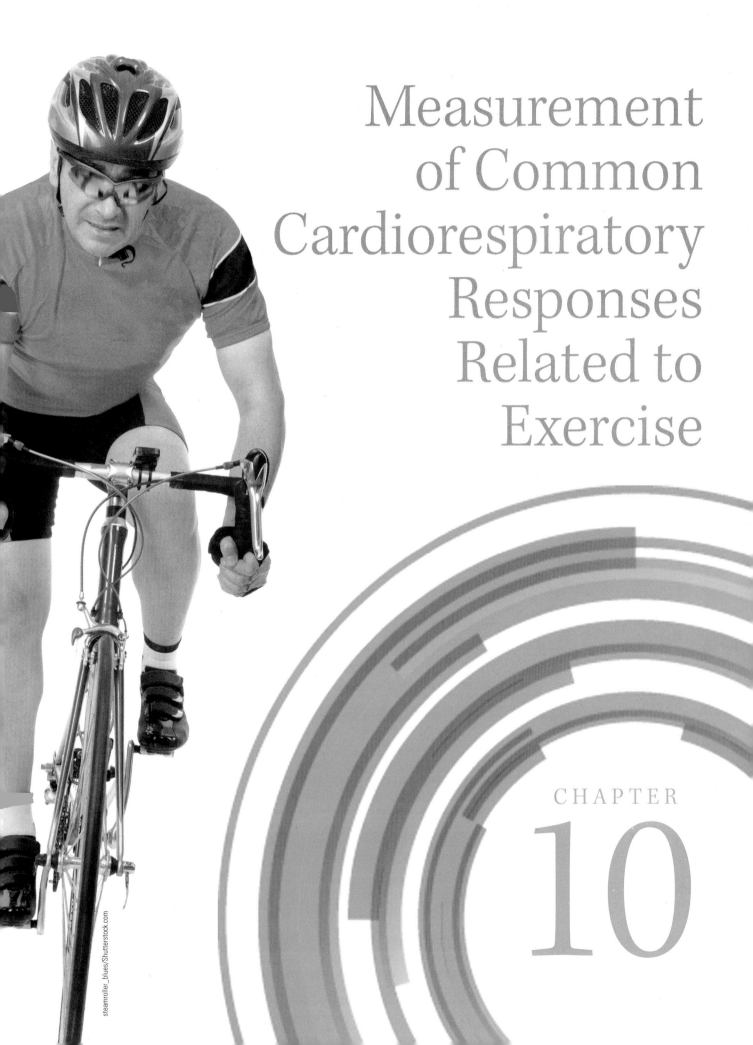

Measurement of Common Cardiorespiratory Responses Related to Exercise

CHAPTER

10

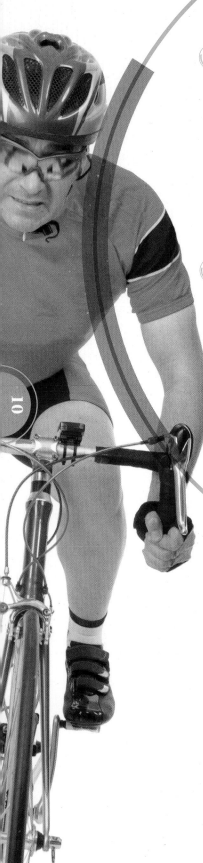

What do you already know about the measurement of common cardiorespiratory responses?

- Use the following Pre-Test or the online evaluation tools for Chapter 10 to determine how much you already know. To access the course materials and companion resources for this text, please visit www.cengagebrain.com. See the preface on page xiii for details.

- Need more review? Let the online assessments, animations, and tutorials for Chapter 10 help prepare you for class.

Pre-Test

1. A(n) _____ _____ test should last 10 seconds or less and be performed at maximal intensity.

2. A(n) _____ _____ test should last 10 seconds or longer and less than 2 to 3 minutes at high intensity.

3. The assessment of aerobic capacity ($\dot{V}O_2$ max) requires at least a minimum of _____ to _____ minutes.

4. _____ and _____ are the two most commonly used machines to measure aerobic capacity ($\dot{V}O_2$ max).

5. The appearance of lactate in the venous blood indicating a greater production of lactate than the clearance of lactate is called _____ _____.

6. If your exercise heart rate is between 130 and 150 beats/min, you are working at a(n) _____ to _____ intensity.

7. Exercise _____ _____ response to submaximal exercise testing is a physiologic variable usually measured to help predict maximal aerobic capacity ($\dot{V}O_2$ max).

8. A(n) _____ is used to predict a third variable using two scales with other known variables or values.

9. The point where an individual can maintain a specific submaximal workload for several minutes without fatigue in endurance events is called _____ _____.

10. The oxygen cost at a given speed or workload is defined as _____.

1. anaerobic power; 2. anaerobic capacity; 3. 10; 15; 4. Treadmill; cycle; 5. lactate threshold or ventilatory threshold; 6. moderate; vigorous; 7. heart rate; 8. nomogram; 9. critical power; 10. economy

What You Will Learn in This Chapter

- Important linkages between the discipline of exercise physiology and measurement

- Current concepts about performing and evaluating common anaerobic abilities related to exercise

- Current concepts about performing common cardiorespiratory response evaluations related to exercise

- Common measurements that provide important physiologic assessment data related to Health/Fitness, Medicine, Athletic Performance, and Rehabilitation

QUICKSTART!

Have you ever had to test your own anaerobic power ability, like running a 40-yard dash for time? How about testing your aerobic ability by running a mile-and-a-half for time? Why did your coach or physical education teacher have you perform tests like these? What did they reveal about your anaerobic and aerobic abilities?

Introduction to Measurement of Common Cardiorespiratory Responses Related to Exercise

Chapter 2 explained that developing effective exercise prescriptions depended on the art and science of exercise physiology. In this chapter, you will learn that the testing and interpretation of anaerobic and aerobic abilities depends on the linkages between the academic disciplines of exercise physiology and tests and measurement.

Figure 10.1 illustrates a variety of physiologic factors (variables) that can influence exercise abilities along a physical performance continuum. It is important for you to understand how the factors in Figure 10.1, as well as others, can affect the exercise performance of your clients' ability to achieve long-term functional health

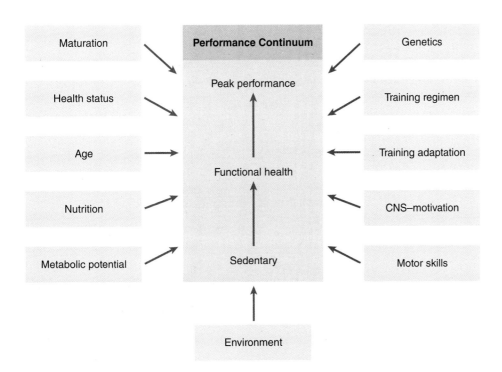

● **FIGURE 10.1 Physiologic factors that influence the exercise performance continuum.** (© Cengage Learning 2013)

(see Chapter 1), and their potential for peak performance, if so desired. Remember, the maintenance of a sedentary lifestyle is *not* consistent with long-term functional health.

The measurement of the factors illustrated in Figure 10.1 need to be considered for all client-related performance goals, and the assessment of each factor (at least at a basic level) can help you design more optimal exercise plans and exercise prescriptions based on the goals of your clients. Test selection should be based on the energy pathways stressed by the exercises and performance events (review the spectrum of energy demands in Chapter 2) that your clients choose to participate in. It is important for you to learn to select appropriate tests for performance evaluation that meet your specific desired needs of accuracy, practicality, ease of use, time, cost, and interpretation. In this chapter, you will learn about considerations for exercise test selection, examples of tests that measure anaerobic and aerobic performance, and practical considerations related to the practice of exercise testing.

Essential Exercise Testing Considerations

Effective anaerobic and aerobic assessments require valid, reliable, and objective measurements that include:

Test selection: Exercise physiology–related tests generally fall into the categories of **laboratory tests** (very controlled, usually focused on one client at a time, and performances are commonly directly measured) and **field tests** (conducted in more practical settings where multiple clients can often be tested at one time and performance times or distances are measured and related to estimated physiologic measures). Both types of tests can provide valuable exercise performance information but require some up-front thought on your behalf to enhance specific interpretation (see "Laboratory and Field Models to Evaluate Body Composition" section in Chapter 13 for a more detailed discussion). Testing should be done at regular intervals, depending on which physiologic factor you are measuring, because the dose responsiveness of the variable will vary (for example, 2–3 weeks to several months), to determine exercise program effectiveness.

Validity: Valid testing refers to the ability of the test selected to test what you want it to test. Tests that correlate highly to performance measures are preferred (look for a minimum correlation [r] of 0.80, with $r > 0.90$ being preferred).

Reliability: Reliable testing refers to the ability of a test to consistently categorize your client's performance abilities; tests that are consistent correlate highly to multiple measures over time (look for a minimum correlation [r] of 0.80, with $r > 0.90$ being preferred).

Objectivity: Objective refers to tests that have a defined scoring system, are administered by trained personnel, and where at least two trained testers score the same test and get similar scores.

The outcomes of this type of testing (including effective interpretations) can be used for the following exercise science applications:

- Placement—classify clients by abilities

- Diagnosis—classify weaknesses, strengths, and health problems

- Evaluation of achievement—can be used to evaluate improvement and provide feedback

- Prediction—can be used to predict future performance

laboratory tests Exercise physiology-related tests that are very controlled and focused on one client at a time. Physiologic variables are measured using invasive and non-invasive techniques, whereas exercise performances are directly measured.

field tests Exercise physiology-related tests that are conducted in more practical settings, where multiple clients can often be tested at one time and performance times or distances are measured and related to estimated physiologic measures.

validity The ability of a selected test to evaluate what you want it to test.

reliability The ability of a test to repeatedly measure performance abilities or physiologic variables and provide the same result.

objectivity Tests that have a defined scoring system, are administered by trained personnel, and where at least two trained testers score the same test and get similar scores.

- Program evaluation—used to determine the program effectiveness

- Motivation—can be used to provide incentives for improvement

- Education—can be used to teach clients to perform exercise more effectively

Some other considerations that can help make your performance testing more effective are:

- Make the tests as specific as possible and related to the mode of exercise to be enhanced

- Control the testing environment as much as possible

- Consider variations in client performance by age, sex, and seasonal issues

- Interpret the results in a timely manner and give applicable, practical feedback

Scoring: The results of tests can be scored using **normative values**, which are based on performance of a group of people, often using percentages (that is, 10th–90th percentile), or **criterion-referenced values**, based on an individual score, often expressed as pass/fail or the achievement of a health standard (that is, systolic blood pressure ≤140/90 mm Hg).

Test interpretation: The ability to explain exercise physiology testing results to your clients is essential, and yet oftentimes ignored or provided superficially. If you do not or cannot explain test results and provide your clients with effective messages to improve their exercise performance, you are probably better off not testing at all. Effective exercise testing requires meaningful and timely feedback to your clients, and requires you to think about why you are testing your client and whether the test(s) you have chosen will help them reach their exercise goals.

Regularly assessing the exercise performance of your clients will provide you with valuable information about the effectiveness of your exercise training programs. However, it is important to understand that even very sophisticated testing procedures with standardized results have limitations. Performance testing is one important tool you will need in your exercise science career, but testing should not be considered as a magic bullet to ultimately predict future exercise performance. For a more thorough review of measuring anaerobic abilities and cardiorespiratory responses to exercise testing, refer to the Selected References at the end of this chapter, specifically the *ASCM's Guidelines for Exercise Testing and Prescription* (2010), Maud and Foster (2006), McDougall et al. (1991), and Baumgartner et al. (2006).

(Why would you use a field test versus a laboratory test to determine the physiologic abilities of a client?)

normative values Based on the performance of a group of people and are often expressed as percentages (that is, within the 10th to 90th percentile).

criterion-referenced values Based on an individual score and are often expressed as pass/fail or the achievement of a health standard (that is, systolic blood pressure ≤140/90 mm Hg).

Overview of Testing for Anaerobic Power and Anaerobic Capacity

The concept of anaerobic (or nonoxidative) power was discussed in Chapter 2, and can be evaluated using tests that measure peak power in the laboratory or by field testing.

Anaerobic power tests as previously defined should last 10 seconds or less and are performed at maximum intensities. Table 10.1 contains examples of common

TABLE 10.1 Common Laboratory and Field Tests of Anaerobic Power

Laboratory Methods	Field Tests
Force plates	Vertical jump
Linear position transducers	Hand grip strength
Accelerometers	1 repetition maximum
Computerized isometric dynamometry	40-yard dash
Wingate bike testing	Margaria stair-climbing test

© Cengage Learning 2013

peak anaerobic power The maximum anaerobic power, whereas the predominant energy source is ATP/CP and the anaerobic breakdown of carbohydrate.

laboratory and field tests to determine the anaerobic power abilities of your clients. The procedures for administering the anaerobic power tests and the performance standards for each test listed in Table 10.1 can be found at various commercially available websites listed in Hot Links boxes in this chapter, as well as the Selected References at the end of the chapter.

HOTLINK *Search for more information about anaerobic exercise tests at the following commercial websites:* http://www.exrx.net, http://www.brianmac.co.uk, *or* http://www.topendsports.com.

One example of an anaerobic power laboratory type test would include using the Wingate anaerobic power cycle test for 30 seconds and using a measure of the first 5-second period that can be used as an index of peak power, which has been

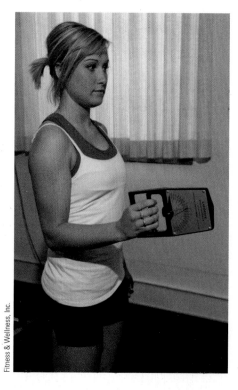

Fitness & Wellness, Inc.

described by Bar-Or (1987) and others. In this test, a Monark cycle ergometer is pedaled by a client at a resistance based on the client's sex, age, and fitness level (0.075 kg/kg body weight or less). After a general warm-up, a client rides as rapidly as possible in a seated position and the resistance is applied immediately and a timer is started. The cycle must be equipped with a photocell to count flywheel revolutions, and peak power can be calculated by using the following formula:

Peak anaerobic power (maximum anaerobic power recorded in watts) = (flywheel revolutions/min for the highest 5-second period × 1.615 meter) × (resistance [kg] × 9.8)   [10.1]

Normative values for absolute and relative (as per body weight/kg) Wingate peak anaerobic power values for physically active male and female individuals available for ages ranging from 18 to 28 years have been developed and can be found via the websites provided in the Exercise Physiology Web Links or the Selected References at the end of this chapter.

Example Using the Wingate Test

If you had a male client who was 20 years old and generated 545 watts of absolute power (or about 8.2 watts/kg body weight), he would be categorized as having average peak anaerobic power for his age and sex. You could use his Wingate power assessment data (see Figure 10.2 for an example of the patterns of power output for two clients during a Wingate cycle test) to plan an exercise training program to improve his peak anaerobic power to achieve his specific performance goals.

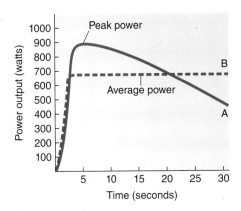

FIGURE 10.2 Examples of peak anaerobic power and mean anaerobic power (between subject A and subject B).
(© Cengage Learning 2013)

HOTLINK *Visit the following sites for more information about Wingate cycle testing:* http://www.brianmac.co.uk/want.htm *and* http://www.topendsports.com/testing/tests/wingate.htm.

An example of an anaerobic power field type test would include using the 1 Repetition (REP) Maximum (1 RM) test to determine how much your client can lift (for example, a bench press) one time, or by using a 5 RM or 10 RM test to predict a 1 RM (recommended for novice clients, youth clients, and elderly clients). In this test, a client performs a light warm-up, lifting 5 to 10 repetitions at approximately 40 to 60 percent intensity followed by 1 minute of rest, and then lifting 3 to 5 repetitions at approximately 60 to 80 percent intensity. The client then attempts to lift a maximum amount one time. The 1 RM should be achieved within three to five attempts to prevent excessive fatigue. There are several prediction equations that you can use to predict 1 RM from 5 RM or 10 RM (see Exercise Physiology Web Links and Selected References at the end of this chapter for more information).

Another example of a simple field test to estimate peak anaerobic power is the static hand grip test. This test takes a minimum amount of time and assesses the isometric (static) strength of a client, which is positively associated (but not perfectly) to dynamic power and fitness like the 1 RM described previously. Although anaerobic power field tests are positively correlated with laboratory measures, they do not measure power output over time and

therefore produce greater errors in predicting performance. The test procedure for static hand grip strength and the associated fitness categories based on performance are provided in Figure 10.3.

The concept of anaerobic capacity (or mean anaerobic capacity) testing requires that your clients perform for 10 seconds or longer but less than 2 to 3 minutes at high intensities. Table 10.2 contains examples of common laboratory and field tests to determine the anaerobic capacity abilities of your clients. The procedures for administering the anaerobic capacity tests and the performance standards for each test are listed in Table 10.2 and can be found in Hot Link boxes and Selected References at the end of this chapter.

One example of an anaerobic capacity laboratory type test would include using

1. Adjust the width of the dynamometer* so the middle bones of your fingers rest on the distant end of the dynamometer grip.
2. Use your dominant hand for this test. Place your elbow at a 90° angle and about 2 inches away from the body.
3. Now grip as hard as you can for a few seconds. Do not move any other body part as you perform the test (do not flex or extend the elbow, do not move the elbow away or toward the body, and do not lean forward or backward during the test).
4. Record the dynamometer reading in pounds (if reading is in kilograms, multiply by 2.2046).
5. Three trials are allowed for this test. Use the highest reading for your final test score. Look up your percentile rank for this test in Table 7.1.
6. Based on your percentile rank, obtain the hand grip strength fitness category according to the following guidelines:

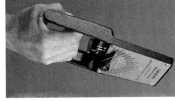

Percentile Rank	Fitness Category
≥90	Excellent
70–80	Good
50–60	Average
30–40	Fair
≤20	Poor

*A Lafayette model 78010 dynamometer is recommended for this test (Lafayette Instruments Co., Sagamore and North 9th Street, Lafayette, IN 47903).

FIGURE 10.3 Sample procedure for the hand grip strength test. As shown, subject is using a Lafayette model 78010 dynamometer from Lafayette Instruments, Sagamore and North 9th Street, Lafayette, IN 47903. (From Hoeger, W. W. K., and S. A. Hoeger. 2010. Figure 7.2 in *Lifetime physical fitness & wellness*, 11th ed. Belmont, CA: Brooks/Cole-Cengage Learning.)

TABLE 10.2 Common Laboratory and Field Tests of Anaerobic Capacity	
Laboratory Methods	**Field Tests**
Force plates	Continuous jumping tests
Linear position transducers	Multiple lifts to fatigue
Accelerometers	Multiple short sprint performance
Computerized isometric dynamometry	Sport-specific drills
Wingate bike testing	Sit to stand tests

© Cengage Learning 2013

mean anaerobic power The ability to maintain a high percentage of peak anaerobic power for several seconds.

fatigue index The ability to maintain a high percentage of peak anaerobic power for several seconds.

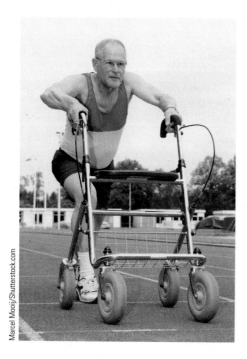

Marcel Mooij/Shutterstock.com

the Wingate Anaerobic Power Cycle test for 30 seconds again. However, to test for anaerobic capacity, the client would perform the Wingate Cycle test for 30 seconds, and **mean anaerobic power** (or capacity) could be calculated by using the following formula:

Mean anaerobic power (watts) = (flywheel revolutions/min for 30 seconds × 1.615) × (resistance [kg] × 9.8) [10.2]

A **fatigue index** can also be calculated for clients based on the differences between their peak anaerobic power and mean anaerobic power performances by using the following formula:

Fatigue index = (peak power − [lowest power/peak power]) × 100 [10.3]

As highlighted previously for anaerobic power, published normative values for physically active male and female individuals are available in the scientific literature. The power curve that represents mean aerobic power (over the full 30 seconds of testing), as was identified in Figure 10.2, can be used to compare individual performances and as benchmarks for training to enhance performance.

An example of an anaerobic capacity type field test (sometimes referred to as "gassers") would include performing a sport-specific test, such as sprinting across an American football field and back two times without stopping (about 200 yards). Norms could be developed for players over the course of a season to determine whether there are improvements in a player's anaerobic capacity. Remember, in sports like American football, for most positions, high levels of anaerobic power and anaerobic capacity are important for optimal performance.

Another example of a simple field test to estimate anaerobic capacity for older individuals is the sit to stand test. Several muscular endurance tests for seniors (age 60–90+) require clients to perform physical activities such as timed walks for several yards, but the sit to standing test determines how many times an individual can move from a sitting position in a chair to standing for 30 seconds. Sit to stand tests, or chair tests, for seniors have been found to correlate highly with walking speed, stair-climbing ability, and the risk for falling. If you have a 65-year-old female client who can stand 15 times in 30 seconds, she would have average muscular endurance (predictive anaerobic capacity). You could use her performance score to develop exercise programming to help her increase her strength and muscular endurance, and that should help reduce her risk for falls.

Have you ever taken an anaerobic performance test? Did you get feedback that helped you achieve your personal goals? If not, how can you make sure you give your clients effective feedback about their performances?

Practical Considerations for Anaerobic Exercise Testing

Unlike the measurement of oxygen uptake ($\dot{V}O_2$) for aerobic performance (see later for more details), there is no one single anaerobic measurement technique that has been recognized as the gold standard that over time has been consistently associated with anaerobic work. Anaerobic performance depends heavily on an individual's ability to recruit, rate code, and synchronize a large number of fast-twitch fibers rapidly. Limiting factors associated with anaerobic performance include the individual's genetic predisposition to the amount of fast-twitch fibers he or she possesses in a given muscle group. Other factors that affect anaerobic work performance are the individual's training state, age, and sex. Factors associated with motivation (central nervous system arousal) and the learning effects of comprehending how to optimally perform an anaerobic type of test can negatively affect anaerobic test performance, perhaps even more so than in aerobic exercise testing. Aerobic exercise testing consistently allows for more warm-up time and is linear in nature with regard to gradually increasing workloads as compared with anaerobic exercise testing.

Although exercise physiologists and other exercise scientists have traditionally used anaerobic field tests to assess anaerobic performance, many of these tests, such as the vertical jump, 40-yard dash, and some sport-specific assessments, do not correlate well (lower validity than is desired) with more accepted laboratory anaerobic measures. However, when multiple traditional field tests are given to clients (for example, at a football combine test—speed, agility, strength/power) and the results are evaluated collectively, they do provide better predictability of anaerobic performance than any single test. Thus, many of the anaerobic tests that exercise physiologists rely on are traditional and popular, even though many present measurement challenges that are often difficult to control and interpret.

HOTLINK *Search YouTube (http://www.youtube.com) for anaerobic tests. Rate your top 10 videos on how well the clips explain the details of the specific test based on what you have learned thus far.*

Overview of Testing Aerobic Power and Aerobic Capacity

Earlier chapters detailed the physiologic processes by which oxygen (O_2) was extracted from the air we breathe and delivered to the body's tissues. During exercise testing, and especially maximal exercise testing, the large increases in metabolic demand for the production of adenosine triphosphate (ATP) require large increases in O_2 delivery to the active skeletal muscles. At the same time, the increased production of carbon dioxide (CO_2) and hydrogen ions resulting from the anaerobic and aerobic metabolic processes require rapid buffering, transportation, and removal of CO_2 at the lungs to avoid acute tissue acidosis. Figure 10.4 provides a schematic representation of the close coupling of the cardiovascular and pulmonary systems' physiologic responses necessary to ensure adequate delivery of O_2 and removal of metabolic by-products to support the metabolic demand of the exercise.

Performance of maximal exercise during which **maximal oxygen uptake ($\dot{V}O_2$ max, or aerobic power)** is achieved provides a major challenge to the cardiorespiratory control systems.

maximal oxygen uptake ($\dot{V}O_2$ max) Measured using the general principle of progressively increasing workloads and measuring the increase in $\dot{V}O_2$ until a plateau of $\dot{V}O_2$ is achieved (that is, $\dot{V}O_2$ max) that increases no further despite a continued increase in workload.

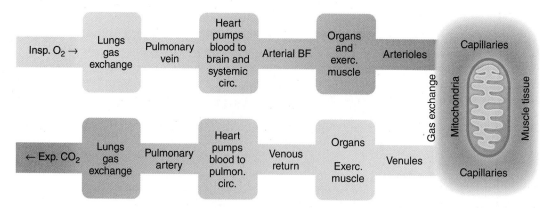

FIGURE 10.4 Schematic diagram tracing the transport of oxygen (O_2) from the inspired air from the lungs to the muscle tissue and the mitochondria, and its exchange with carbon dioxide (CO_2) and its transport back to the lungs for exchange with O_2 and exhalation. (Adapted from Wasserman, K., J. E. Hansen, D. K. Sue, and B. J. Whipp, editors. 1987. Figure 1-1 in *Principles of exercise testing and interpretation*. Philadelphia: Lea & Febiger.)

Measurement of Maximal Oxygen Uptake (or Aerobic Power)

There are a number of practical and physiologic considerations in determining an individual's $\dot{V}O_2$ max, which is measured using the general principle of progressively increasing workloads, and measuring the increase in $\dot{V}O_2$ until a plateau of $\dot{V}O_2$ is achieved (that is, $\dot{V}O_2$ max), a plateau that increases no further despite a continued increase in workload (see Figure 10.5).

The achievement of $\dot{V}O_2$ max is accompanied by large increases in venous blood lactate concentrations (10–20 mM), sampled 3 to 5 minutes into recovery, and a **respiratory exchange ratio (RER — $\dot{V}O_2/\dot{V}CO_2$)** greater than 1.1 at the time the subject is unable to continue.

> (What term would you use to describe a client's breathing when the RER is greater than 1.0?)

To determine the amount of O_2 the body uses at rest, submaximal and maximal exercise requires the measurement of the difference between the inspired and expired volumes of O_2 over a given amount of time while performing the exercise. In general, the measurement time is usually for 1 minute, that is, liters of oxygen per minute (L O_2/min). In the laboratory, the traditional method of measuring the amount of O_2 used required that we collect the volume of expired air in a Douglas bag (named after the inventor of the bags) at 1-minute intervals (see Figure 10.6).

The bag's volume of expired air, percentage of O_2, and percentage of CO_2 were analyzed and based on a number of valid assumptions involving the physical gas laws and the physiologic inert property of nitrogen at sea level; the metabolic use of O_2 and CO_2 production and the volumes of inspired and expired O_2 also were calculated. Thus, the difference between the inspired oxygen volume ($\dot{V}iO_2$) and the expired oxygen volume ($\dot{V}eO_2$) is the $\dot{V}O_2$ (measured in L/min).

Since the development of electronic devices for the rapid measurements of gas concentrations, volumes of air of each breath, and their electronic interface with personal computer systems, the tedium of measuring $\dot{V}O_2$ has been reduced markedly. However, a word of caution to you the practitioner is that if the appropriate calibrations of each monitoring machine are not performed before the testing, then the

respiratory exchange ratio (RER — $\dot{V}O_2/\dot{V}CO_2$) The ratio of expired carbon dioxide to the amount of oxygen uptake. Values over 1.00 indicate hyperventilation.

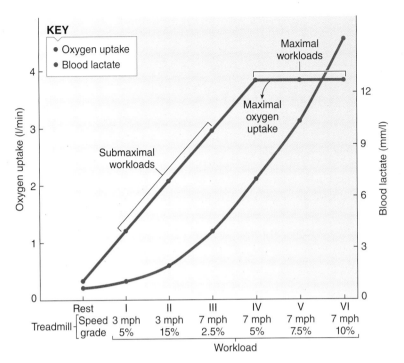

FIGURE 10.5 Determination of maximal oxygen uptake (in L/min) on a motor-driven treadmill. (From Mitchell, J. H., and C. G. Blomqvist. 1971. Maximal oxygen uptake. *N. Engl. J. Med.* 284:1018–1022.)

measurements you make may not be accurate. This point cannot be overemphasized, because many a test has had to be discarded because of mistakes calibrating the monitoring machine, the computer's data acquisition system, and the data output. Unfortunately, our reliance on computer outputs providing the correct information is only as good as the accuracy of data being acquired and calibrations of the monitors to provide that assurance.

HOTLINK *For a calculation of $\dot{V}O_2$ per minute, visit* **http://ston.jsc.nasa.gov/collections/TRS/ _techrep/TM-1998-104826.pdf**.

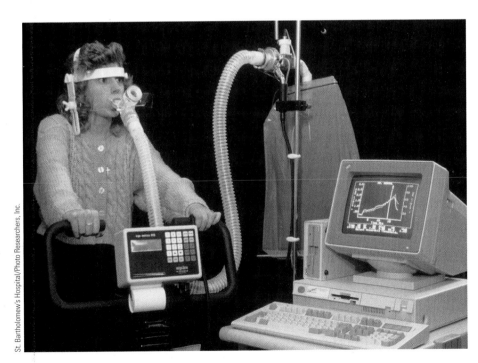

FIGURE 10.6 Maximal exercise testing using a Douglas bag method of gas collection.

CONCEPTS, challenges, & controversies

Is the Plateau of Oxygen Uptake a Reality?

Because many investigators were (and are) unable to generate a plateau of oxygen uptake ($\dot{V}O_2$) as the criterion for identifying an individual's maximal oxygen uptake ($\dot{V}O_2$ max) during progressive increase in workload maximal exercise testing, the concept of the existence of a plateau of $\dot{V}O_2$ as being an attainable measurement was challenged. An alternative hypothesis proposed the existence of a central nervous system "Governor" (restraint). This proposal suggested the existence of some unidentified cardiac afferents that warned the central nervous system of impending cardiac ischemia, which resulted in a centrally generated signal to cause the individual to stop exercising. However, a more recent study, performed at the Institute of Exercise and Environmental Medicine in Dallas, required 52 subjects to perform $\dot{V}O_2$ max and supramaximal $\dot{V}O_2$ tests at a work requirement 30 percent greater than that previously achieved during the incremental exercise test. These experiments used the Douglas bag gas collection protocols of the classic study of 1955 (see Figure 10.6). The incremental exercise and supramaximal exercise tests were performed on three separate occasions (separated by weeks) resulting in a total of 156 incremental exercise tests and 156 supramaximal exercise tests (see Figure 10.7).

The $\dot{V}O_2$ reached a maximum in the incremental exercise tests and was not different from the $\dot{V}O_2$ with the 30 percent supramaximal workload exercise test. Therefore, a measurement of $\dot{V}O_2$ max that exhibits a plateau during a progressive increase in workload exercise was concluded to be a valid index of the individual's maximal limit of their cardiorespiratory system's capacity to deliver O_2 to the tissues.

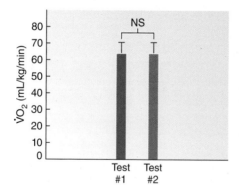

FIGURE 10.7 Comparison of a progressive increase in workload running maximal oxygen uptake ($\dot{V}O_2$ max) test (test 1) with a 30 percent greater workload running supramaximal test (test 2). (Adapted from Hawkins, M. N., P. B. Raven, P. G. Snell, J. Stray-Gundersen, and B. J. Levine. 2007. Maximal oxygen uptake as a parametric measure of cardiorespiratory capacity. *Med. Sci. Sports Exerc.* 39:103–107.)

inRETROSPECT

History of Validation: The Maximal Oxygen Uptake Exercise Test

In the classic study of 1955 in which the plateau of oxygen uptake ($\dot{V}O_2$) was demonstrated, 115 subjects performed 3 maximal exercise tests on a motor-driven treadmill over a 3- to 5-day period for each subject. The exercise test consisted of a 10- minute warm-up at submaximal workload (based on the subject's exercise history) followed by a 3-minute running exercise at 7 miles/hour on an uphill grade initially determined based on the subjects' predicted fitness from their exercise histories. Douglas bag gas collections for 1 minute were collected for each minute of the 3-minute test and analyzed for percentage of O_2 and CO_2 using the micro-Scholander manual gas volume technique and for bag volume using a Tissot gasometer. Each successive day the test was repeated at an increase in grade of 2.5 percent until the measured $\dot{V}O_2$ differed by less than 2.1 ml/kg/min. This difference in $\dot{V}O_2$ was calculated to be half to a third of that expected from the increase in grade. All but 7 subjects (of the 115 total subjects) achieved a plateau in $\dot{V}O_2$ on day 2 or 3 of testing. A change in grade was chosen above changing the running speed because many of the subjects were unable to run fast enough to be able to biomechanically achieve the speeds necessary to achieve a plateau in $\dot{V}O_2$.

Measurement of Aerobic Capacity

The assessment of aerobic capacity requires tests that last a minimum of 15 to 20 minutes in duration. Activities such as running a fast time for 3 miles, a 1-hour cycling time trial, or participating in a competitive triathlon require high aerobic capacities ($\geq$85 percent of $\dot{V}O_2$ max). Usually tests of aerobic capacity are activity specific and would most likely be performed as field tests in a time trial situation. An example of an aerobic capacity test for competitive distance runners (3–6 miles or 5–10 kilometers) is a 30-minute steady-state run, whereas a subject would try to maintain at least 85 percent of their **velocity at $\dot{V}O_2$ max (v$\dot{V}O_2$ max)**, which can be determined by various laboratory and field $\dot{V}O_2$ max testing procedures. Other assessments that are associated with aerobic capacity include tests to determine **exercise economy** (the $\dot{V}O_2$ cost at a given speed or workload) and tests to determine **critical power** (the point where a client can maintain a specific submaximal power output for several minutes without fatigue).

Exercise economy is often associated with exercise efficiency by coaches and exercise practitioners, which is a much more difficult factor to measure because efficiency includes the elasticity (stored energy-recoil) properties of muscles and biomechanical factors that cannot be obtained easily. The measurement of exercise economy (commonly done for running, cycling, and swimming) can be achieved by having a client perform a multiple-stage discontinuous exercise test to $\dot{V}O_2$ max, whereas the $\dot{V}O_2$ of the client can be measured at each stage of the test. Figure 10.8

velocity at $\dot{V}O_2$ max (v$\dot{V}O_2$ max) The performance speed of an athlete, such as running at which the running speed (v$\dot{V}O_2$ max) of $\dot{V}O_2$ max occurs.

exercise economy Energy required to perform the work divided by the actual energy cost measured performing the work; see efficiency.

critical power The work rate at which a person can maintain a constant submaximal power output for several minutes without fatigue.

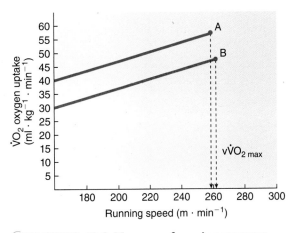

FIGURE 10.8 Measures of running economy of two runners, A and B. Runner B is running with greater economy because she is using less oxygen for a given running speed. (© Cengage Learning 2013)

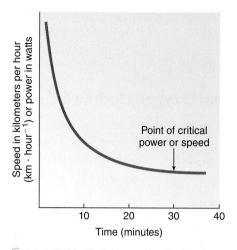

Speed in kilometers per hour
(km · hour⁻¹) or power in watts

Point of critical
power or speed

Time (minutes)

FIGURE 10.9 Example of critical power (speed) for a runner. (Modified from Maud, P., and C. Foster, editors. 2006. *Physiological assessment of human fitness,* 2nd ed. Champaign, IL: Human Kinetics.)

illustrates a running economy test example for two runners who have different $\dot{V}O_2$ max values and running economy curves but similar maximal performance times (velocity of $\dot{V}O_2$ max, or $v\dot{V}O_2$ max). By measuring exercise economy, you can develop and implement training strategies that can allow clients to recruit less muscle mass to perform at the same intensity, improve $\dot{V}O_2$ max, and exercise economy.

Critical power (or speed, for activities such as running, cycling, and swimming) can be evaluated in an exercise laboratory by having a client perform several exercise bouts to exhaustion over the course of several days. Figure 10.9 illustrates an example of the point of critical power (speed) for a runner who is able to maintain his running speed for several minutes (20–40 minutes) before fatigue. Critical power is a strong predictor of success in endurance sports and essentially predicts the percentage of $\dot{V}O_2$ max (that is, the $v\dot{V}O_2$ max for runners).

HOTLINK *Search the Internet for sport-specific references to learn more about the measurement (or estimation) of economy and critical power at sites such as* **http://jap.physiology.org/content/86/5/1527.long.**

Why would it be important to know the running economy and the critical power of an athletic client you are working with?

Practical Considerations for Aerobic Exercise Testing

There are a number of practical considerations for aerobic exercise testing (as there are for anaerobic exercise testing), including the duration of the test; the type of exercise performed by a client; assessment of peak performance; and other variables, such as age, sedentary lifestyle, and disease.

1. *Duration of test protocol:* In young healthy adult subjects, the time of the test should be greater than 2 minutes and no longer than 6 to 7 minutes (see Figure 10.10).

2. *Type of exercise:* To determine the true $\dot{V}O_2$ max of an active individual, remember to use a progressive exercise test that specifically uses the exercise the individual usually performs (see Chapter 2 for more about the specificity of exercise training). The exercise should be aerobic and require the use of large

Lisa F. Young/Shutterstock.com

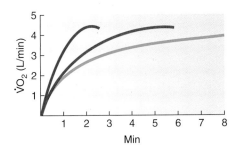

FIGURE 10.10 Maximal oxygen uptake ($\dot{V}O_2$ max test) duration is determined by the rate of increase in workload. (Modified from Åstrand, P-O., and K. Rodaahl. 1986. Figure 7.4 in *Textbook of work physiology: Physiological basis of exercise*, 3rd ed. New York: McGraw-Hill.)

muscle masses performing rhythmic dynamic exercise. For example, if you are testing a rower by having her run on a treadmill, the $\dot{V}O_2$ max you measure will be far less than her rowing $\dot{V}O_2$ max. Generally, a $\dot{V}O_2$ max of the U.S. population measured using a bicycle ergometer protocol is 6 to 10 percent lower than the walking or running treadmill measures of $\dot{V}O_2$ max, except in bicyclists. In populations who use a bicycle as their main form of transportation, such as in the Scandinavian countries, it is not unusual for the $\dot{V}O_2$ max measured on a bicycle to be equal to or higher than the treadmill $\dot{V}O_2$ max.

3. *Performance testing:* It is important for you to distinguish between performance testing and $\dot{V}O_2$ max testing. As defined in Chapters 7 and 8, $\dot{V}O_2$ max is a measure of the circulation's maximal capacity to deliver O_2, and when correlated with a performance test, such as an individual's time to run a specific distance, within the general population with a wide range of aerobic fitness, 80 percent of the time the $\dot{V}O_2$ max measure significantly predicts the performance time. Now, if you were to try and rank the performance of an elite middle-distance runner running a 1,500-meter race from the runner's $\dot{V}O_2$ max, your success rate would be well below 20 percent. In other

words, performance testing should be separated from $\dot{V}O_2$ max testing.

4. *Age, sedentary lifestyle, and disease:* If, as is usual for the general population of the United States, we live sedentary lifestyles, starting in the early teenage years or in the presence of a disease that can limit performance because of symptoms, a slower progression of increases in workload during the $\dot{V}O_2$ max testing needs to be used. Indeed, many of the clinical exercise treadmill testing protocols have been specifically developed to address these issues. In the interest of economy of time, many laboratories combine the incremental workload increase testing protocol to determine both the $\dot{V}O_2$ max and performance in sedentary and aging population studies.

In many cases, local fatigue of the exercising muscles probably causes the subject to stop exercising before a true plateau can be achieved. The value of $\dot{V}O_2$ that is measured at the time of cessation of the test without a verifiable plateau is usually referred to as $\dot{V}O_2$ peak. However, if the increase in absolute $\dot{V}O_2$ measured in the last minute of exercise is less than 50 ml/min and is accompanied by a RER greater than 1.1 and a 3- to 5-minute postexercise venous lactate concentration of 10 to 15 mM, it is generally accepted as being a measure of $\dot{V}O_2$ max.

If you were testing a contender for the next Tour de France cycling championship, what type of exercise test would you choose and what exercise protocol would you use? How could you find more information to confirm that you are making a good choice?

Incremental Load Exercise Testing

Regardless of the mode of exercise testing (that is, treadmill, bicycle ergometer, rowing ergometer), the principle of progressively increasing the workload (metabolic rate) at specific time intervals results in progressive increases in the breath-by-breath respiratory responses until a maximal effort is achieved or, as in some cases, the exercise needs to be stopped because of clinical symptoms (see Figure 10.11).

In Figure 10.11, the bicycle ergometer work rate was increased at 1-minute intervals after a warm-up period of 4 minutes of zero load pedaling. As the work rate increases, you will observe linear and rapid increases in $\dot{V}_eO_2$ and $\dot{V}_eCO_2$ and measured

⬤ **FIGURE 10.11 Schematic representation of the ventilatory responses to a progressive increase in workload exercise test.** As noted in Figure 9.10, the ventilation threshold (VT) is identified as the workload (WL), or oxygen uptake ($\dot{V}O_2$), at P^1, that is when the ventilatory equivalent for oxygen (VEO₂) increases and ventilatory equivalent for carbon dioxide (VECO₂) is maintained constant as a result of an increase in ventilation resulting in an increased exhalation of carbon dioxide (CO₂). (Adapted from Wasserman, K., J. E. Hansen, D. Y. Sue, and B. J. Whipp. 1987. Figure 2.10 in *Principles of exercise testing and interpretation*. Philadelphia: Lea & Febiger.)

expired ventilation volume ($\dot{V}e$). This continues until the **ventilation threshold**, or the appearance of lactate in the venous blood indicating a greater production of lactate than the clearance of lactate, is reached, at which time the $\dot{V}_eCO_2$ expired is greater than the $\dot{V}_eO_2$ because the CO_2 generated from the buffering reaction of the bicarbonate with the lactic acid is added to the metabolically produced CO_2. At this workload, the increase in $\dot{V}e$ is equivalent to the increase in $\dot{V}eCO_2$ (defined as isocapnic buffering) and results in a constant **ventilatory equivalent for CO₂** (that is, $VECO_2 = \dot{V}e/\dot{V}_eCO_2$). However, at this same ventilation threshold workload, the $\dot{V}e/\dot{V}_eO_2$ ratio, or ventilatory equivalent for O₂ (that is, VEO₂) is increased. If you remember that the chemoreceptor drive to ventilation is primarily a result of CO₂, then the workload at which the increase in the VEO₂ occurs without a change in VECO₂ is the workload at which the ventilation threshold begins (see Figure 10.11). These measures provide a sensitive, noninvasive method of identifying the ventilation threshold without having to actually measure arterial or venous lactate concentrations.

HOTLINK *See the Concepts, Challenges, & Controversies feature in Chapter 9 for more details about the measurement of the ventilation threshold.*

As the work rate is increased further, the $\dot{V}e$ increases more rapidly and results in arterial CO₂ (PaCO₂) and end-tidal CO₂ (PetCO₂) values decreasing (that is, hyperventilation) and identifies the work rate at which the respiratory compensation for the metabolic acidosis begins. In many of the breath-by-breath gas analyzers that have a rapid-response analyzer for CO₂, the decrease in PetCO₂ can be detected noninvasively, in healthy subjects with no lung function abnormalities, because PetCO₂ differs from PaCO₂ by as little as 1 mm Hg.

TABLE 10.3 Classification of Work Intensities

Level of Intensity	$\dot{V}O_2$	HR	Tvent	Duration
Mild	0.5 L/min	<90 beats/min	<<	Very prolonged Limited by boredom
Moderate	0.5–1.5 L/min	90–130 beats/min	<	Prolonged Substrate limited
Heavy	1.5–2.0 L/min	130–150 beats/min	>	Substrate and acidosis limited
Severe/Exhaustive	>2.0 L/min	>150 beats/min	>>	Limited by uncompensated acidosis

HR, heart rate; Tvent, ventilatory threshold; $\dot{V}O_2$, oxygen uptake.
Adapted from Åstrand, P-O., and K. Rodaahl. 1986. *Textbook of work physiology: Physiological basis of exercise,* 3rd ed. New York: McGraw-Hill.

Measures of Oxygen Uptake and Heart Rate Are Used to Identify Work Intensity of Specific Industrial and Home Household Tasks

The identification of the work rates associated with the ventilation threshold, together with the equivalent $\dot{V}O_2$ and heart rate (HR), has led to the development of a qualitative description of work intensities (see Table 10.3).

Clinical Maximal Exercise Testing

Many clinical symptom-limited maximal exercise tests have been developed from the progressive increase in workload maximal testing protocols used for healthy individuals. The name of the physician who first used and published the testing protocol has usually been associated with the test. Hence the Balke treadmill test (named after Bruno Balke), the Bruce treadmill test (named after Robert Bruce), and the Ellestad treadmill test (named after Marvin Ellestad) are all tests that have gained acceptance in the clinical arena of exercise testing. Even though many of the test protocols can be adapted to the bicycle ergometer, the treadmill test is the one most often used in the United States because bicycling is not an everyday activity of the U.S. population, and hence the subjects often cease cycling because of leg fatigue only. However, when ambulation is difficult for the patient, a new form of progressively stressing the cardiovascular system using increasing doses of cardiovascular-stimulating drugs has been developed.

Perhaps the most often used test is the Bruce maximal stress test. The test protocol and predicted metabolic outcomes (presented in metabolic equivalents [METS]) are provided in Table 10.4.

HOTLINK *Search the Internet to determine specific differences between the Balke, Bruce, and Ellestad treadmill test protocols. An example website to review is:* http://www.brianmac.co.uk.

TABLE 10.4 Bruce Treadmill Exercise Test Protocol

Characteristics	Stage				
	I	II	III	IV	V
Duration (minutes)	3	3	3	3	3
Speed (miles/hour)	1.7	2.5	3.4	4.2	5.0
Grade (percent)	10.0	12.0	14.0	16.0	18.0
METS*	4	6–7	8–9	15–16	21

*1 MET, a metabolic unit, is 3.5 ml O_2 uptake $\cdot$ kg^{-1} $\cdot$ min^{-1}.
Adapted from Bruce, R. A. 1971. Exercise testing of patients with coronary heart disease. Principles and normal standards for evaluation. *Ann. Clin. Res.* 3:323–332.

> *Why would you choose to use the Balke treadmill test protocol instead of the Bruce treadmill test protocol? To answer the question, you will need to go to the URL link.*

Metabolic Equivalents

Chapter 2 explained that intensity can be expressed in METS (1 MET = 3.5 ml O_2 kg/L/min = 1 Kcal), and workload intensities via the various methods of aerobic power and aerobic capacity can also be expressed in METS. The total workload completed during exercise testing can be measured or predicted in METS based on age and sex. For example, the average maximal working capacity for a 40-year-old man is 10 METs.

Ratings of Perceived Exertion

One's cardiorespiratory and metabolic responses to exercise provide psychobiologic cues that enables each individual to rate their perception of effort as a rating of perceived exertion (RPE), as described in Chapters 2 and 9 (see Table 10.5).

● TABLE 10.5 Rating of Perceived Exertion Scales

Original Rating Scale		Revised Rating Scale	
6		0	Nothing at all
7	Very, very light	0.5	Very, very light (just noticeable)
8		1	Very light
9	Very light	2	Light (weak)
10		3	Moderate
11	Fairly light	4	Somewhat hard
12		5	Heavy (strong)
13	Somewhat hard	6	
14		7	Very heavy
15	Hard	8	
16		9	
17	Very hard	10	Very, very heavy (almost max)
18		*	Maximal
19	Very, very hard		
20			

Borg, G. 1982. Psychological Bases of Physical Exertion. *Med. Sci. Sports Exerc.* 14:377–381.

The RPE provides a field assessment of the stress of the particular activity and is used to rate an individual's workload during cardiac rehabilitation, exercise training, exercise stress testing, and athletic performance. A large number of investigations have identified that an individual's RPE is influenced by personality structure, training status, physiologic responses, sex, and environmental conditions. These interactions have been identified to be especially important during stressful activities, such as diving using self-contained underwater breathing apparatus or firefighting using self-contained breathing apparatus.

An especially significant result from experiments into the manipulation of an individual's RPE using hypnosis, while performing constant load exercise, is that areas of the brain have been identified using brain mapping techniques that correlate with animal studies investigating the locus of central command. In addition, having the subject under hypnosis and having him imagine performing an isometric hand grip exercise has enabled investigators

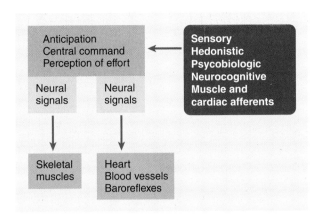

● **FIGURE 10.12 Schematic representation of the peripheral and central sensory inputs that modulate the central command's neural regulation of the skeletal muscular and cardiovascular systems during exercise.** (Adapted from Williamson, J. W. 2010. The relevance of central command for the neural cardiovascular control of exercise. *Exp. Physiol.* 95:1043–1048.)

to identify areas of the cortex involved in the cardiorespiratory responses to exercise independent of the individual actually performing any exercise. Previously, we have identified that central command (see Chapters 7 and 9) was thought to be the primary factor in activating and establishing the operating point of the cardiovascular and respiratory systems. However, the data from the experiments using hypnosis suggest that it may be relying on feedback from a perceptual center in the brain to fine-tune the degree of activation necessary (see Figure 10.12).

HOTLINK *See Chapters 7 and 9 to review the concepts surrounding central command.*

Oxygen Deficit

At the onset of exercise, the muscles immediately require energy to be released from the ATP stored in the muscle to enable muscle contraction. However, the increase in O_2 delivery and the $\dot{V}O_2$ lags behind the demand for the energy released from the ATP until a steady state in $\dot{V}O_2$ is achieved. During this period, the energy demand of the exercise is partially met by anaerobic processes and is defined as an **oxygen deficit**. In Figure 10.13a, the shaded portion identifies the oxygen deficit and is defined as the difference between the $\dot{V}O_2$ in the initial minutes of the exercise and the $\dot{V}O_2$ required to perform the exercise, which, in this case, is the steady-state $\dot{V}O_2$. In short bouts of intense exercise where steady state is never achieved (100-meter sprint), the oxygen deficit continues to increase (see Figure 10.13b). A large body of evidence indicates the anaerobic metabolic processes: first,

the ATP-CP (creatine phosphate) energy system is followed by the glycolytic energy system, resulting in lactate production to provide ATP to the working muscles during the oxygen deficit.

These anaerobic energy-producing mechanisms occur both at the beginning of exercise (see Figure 10.13a, page 352) and at the time when $\dot{V}O_2$ max is achieved yet the individual is continuing to exercise (see Figure 10.13b, page 352).

At steady state, the muscle's ATP requirements are met by aerobic metabolism. Most of the lactate produced within the muscle during the oxygen deficit is "shuttled" within the muscle between the fast glycolytic fibers to the oxidative fibers and oxidized. A minor portion is converted to glycogen or glucose. Hence the old idea that the lactate produced during the oxygen deficit was repaid postexercise as a part of an "oxygen debt" is not valid.

oxygen deficit The difference between the $\dot{V}O_2$ measured in the initial minutes of the exercise and the calculated $\dot{V}O_2$ required to perform the exercise.

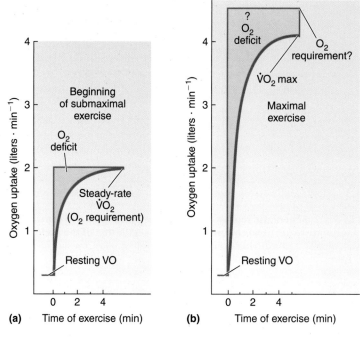

FIGURE 10.13 **(a) Oxygen deficit incurred at the beginning of steady-state submaximal exercise. (b) Oxygen deficit incurred at the end of a non–steady-state maximal oxygen uptake test.** (Adapted from Brooks. G. A., T. D. Fahey, and T. P. White. 1996. Figures 10-5a and 10-5b in *Exercise physiology: Human bioenergetics and its applications*, 2nd ed. Mountain View, CA: Mayfield Publishing Company.)

The oxygen deficit of an aerobically trained athlete at the beginning of exercise asked to perform a given amount of work at steady state is always less than an untrained sedentary individual or a weight-trained individual (see Figure 10.14). This finding suggests that the aerobic exercise trained athlete has more oxymyoglobin stores readily available to support the up-regulated aerobic energy production of ATP, and consequently reduces lactic acid production during the period of oxygen deficit.

HOTLINK *Access the following website for more information about procedures for exercise physiology laboratory measures:* http://ston.jsc.nasa.gov/collections/TRS/_techrep/TM-1998-104826.pdf.

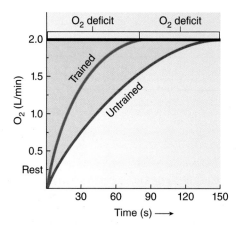

FIGURE 10.14 **Comparison of oxygen deficits of endurance-trained and untrained individuals performing 2.0 L/min steady-state dynamic exercise.** (© Cengage Learning 2013)

Excess Postexercise Oxygen Consumption

The idea that the excess O_2 consumed after exercise was the body's way of paying back a debt of O_2 associated with producing ATP anaerobically during exercise (that is, an O_2 debt) has been discounted since the radioisotope tracer studies were performed in the 1980s. However, these tracer studies only confirmed earlier work performed in 1936, which challenged the concept of the recovery O_2 being related to the amount of lactate produced during the exercise. A detailed analysis of the **excess postexercise oxygen consumption (EPOC)** identified that the $\dot{V}O_2$ does not return to resting values immediately, and that after mild exercise, the recovery $\dot{V}O_2$/time relationship fits a single exponential curve after mild exercise and a more complex double exponential after moderate-to-maximal exercise (see Figure 10.15). Unfortunately, use of the term O_2 debt remains in effect even though its physiologic definition is inaccurate.

A more cogent explanation of EPOC is the finding that excess O_2 consumption occurs when the **efficiency** between mitochondrial oxidation and phosphorylation of substrates (that is, ATP production)

decreases. This occurs during exercise for the following reasons:

1. Metabolic heat production increases within the active skeletal muscle during exercise and decreases the coupling efficiency between oxidation and phosphorylation.

2. Links between lipolysis, fatty acid metabolism, thyroid hormone, and catecholamines produced during exercise increase sodium and potassium membrane pump activity, requiring increases in mitochondrial oxidative phosphorylation and an increase in O_2 consumption.

3. During muscle contraction, calcium is released from the cell's sarcoplasmic reticulum and taken up by the mitochondria and, in turn, increases the mitochondrial O_2 consumption.

During EPOC, the excess O_2 consumption can be attributed to the body's gradual cooling and the return of cellular membrane sodium-potassium pump function and metabolism to resting, or homeostatic operation. In contrast with the O_2 debt theory of lactic acid oxidation being the main cause for the excess O_2 consumption, the EPOC facts identify that the excess O_2 consumption is required to restore homeostasis without the involvement of lactate. In fact, lactate metabolism during exercise and recovery from exercise involves the "lactate shuttle," which serves as a fuel and a gluconeogenic precursor.

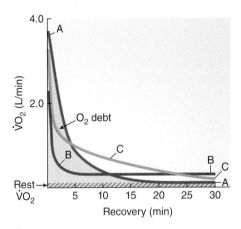

⦿ **FIGURE 10.15 The oxygen debt recovery curve (A) after a moderate-intensity steady-state exercise bout is composed of a fast single component curve (B) and a second slow component curve (C).** The striped area under curve A–the shaded area identifying resting oxygen uptake ($\dot{V}O_2$) = oxygen debt. (Adapted from Brooks, G. A., T. D. Fahey, and T. P. White. 1996. Figures 10-6a 10-6b, and 10-6c in *Exercise physiology: Human bioenergetics and its applications.* 2nd ed. Mountain View, CA: Mayfield Publishing Company.)

(What are the major differences between oxygen deficit and EPOC?)

Submaximal Exercise

At the advent of the Industrial Revolution, the individual's ability to repeatedly perform submaximal work for prolonged periods, without rest and at the highest work intensity possible day in and day out

without cumulative fatigue or injury, was of vital importance to worker productivity for all manner of industrial work. During the periods of World War I and II and the increase of overtime work, the problems of cumulative fatigue, muscle soreness, and injury became an issue of national importance. However, it was not until the Scandinavian countries required an assessment of the ratio of health costs to worker productivity in industries using production line work practices that a quantitative analysis was undertaken.

The Scandinavian investigations identified that an individual's $\dot{V}O_2$ max played an important part in his or her sustained productivity. Active healthy individuals can walk or run approximately 1 h at 50 percent $\dot{V}O_2$ max, keeping $\dot{V}O_2$, cardiac output ($\dot{Q}$), and HR constant, without an elevation in blood or muscle lactate. However, when asked to repeat the same duration and intensity of exercise after a 10-minute break in each hour for 8 hours, the resultant cumulative fatigue was such that the subjects could not repeat a similar work protocol the following day. Indeed, a number of studies evaluating industrial work tasks have concluded that the time-weighted average work rate per day approximates 35 percent $\dot{V}O_2$ max to ensure continuous worker productivity throughout the year. Technology has made the routine production line jobs easier to do. However, emergency personnel continue to need a relatively higher grade of fitness.

Endurance exercise-trained elite athletes, marathon runners, cross-country skiers, ultra-marathoners, long-distance swimmers, and tour racing bicyclists can maintain steady-state work rates of 85 to 90 percent for a number of hours without increases in blood lactate concentrations. In ultra-marathon runners attempting to perform a 24-hour race, the %$\dot{V}O_2$ max declined from 90 to 50 percent during the last hour of the race.

Cardiovascular Drift Is a Phenomenon of Prolonged Submaximal Exercise

In all submaximal exercises requiring greater than 50 percent $\dot{V}O_2$ max work intensity that is extended beyond 30 minutes to 1 hour or more, a phenomenon of

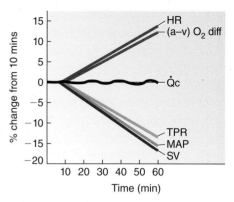

FIGURE 10.16 Cardiovascular drift. Hemodynamic changes associated with 1 hour of 65 percent maximal oxygen uptake ($\dot{V}O_2$ max) cycling exercise in a thermoneutral environment. (Adapted from Norton, K. H., K. M. Gallagher, S. A. Smith, R. G. Querry, R. M. Welch-O'Connor, and P. B. Raven. 1999. Carotid baroreflex function during prolonged exercise. *J. Appl. Physiol.* 87:339–347.)

cardiovascular drift is observed (see Figure 10.16). After the initial onset (10–20 minutes) of dynamic exercise, prolonged steady-state exercise above 50 percent $\dot{V}O_2$ max (in this case, 65 percent $\dot{V}O_2$ max; see Figure 10.16) the cardiovascular response is characterized by a progressive redistribution of the central blood volume (CBV) to the skin circulation in response to the thermoregulatory adjustments necessary to dissipate the heat buildup. The redistribution of the CBV results in a progressive decrease in the CBV, central venous pressure, and total peripheral resistance. These changes result in a reduction in stroke volume (SV) and mean arterial pressure with a concomitant increase in HR. These changes define the responses observed in *cardiovascular drift*.

Despite a number of uniquely designed investigations, the underlying mechanisms as to why blood pressure regulation appears to be compromised during prolonged exercise remain unclear, despite the maintenance of the necessary $\dot{Q}$ to maintain O_2 delivery. The progressive increase in HR is recognized as the primary marker of cardiovascular drift and was initially thought of as a compensatory response to the progressive decrease in SV, thereby maintaining the $\dot{Q}$ constant. However, in an experiment where the CBV and SV

cardiovascular drift Occurs during prolonged (>30 minutes) submaximal exercise, resulting in reduced stroke volume (SV) and mean arterial pressure with a concomitant increase in heart rate in an attempt to maintain cardiac output constant.

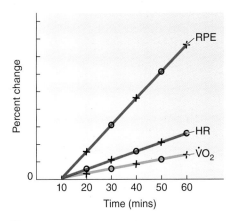

FIGURE 10.17 **Changes in psycho-physiologic variables during cardiovascular drift associated with 1 hour of 65 percent maximal oxygen uptake ($\dot{V}O_2$ max) upright cycling exercise without (X) and with (O) central blood volume (CBV) and stroke volume (SV) maintained with infusions of low-molecular-weight dextran.** (Adapted from Norton, K. H., K. M. Gallagher, S. A. Smith, R. G. Querry, R. M. Welch-O'Connor, and P. B. Raven. 1999. Carotid baroreflex function during prolonged exercise. *J. Appl. Physiol.* 87:339–347.)

were maintained constant during the prolonged exercise, the progressive increase in HR was the same as when the CBV and SV were allowed to drift downward (see Figure 10.17).

This finding suggests that as the skeletal muscle fatigues and recruitment of more muscle fibers is necessary to maintain the steady state of exercise, the increase in HR is a reflection of the progressive increase in central command that is required to increase the number of muscle fibers used (see Chapter 7 for more information on central command).

Postexercise Hypotension Is a Phenomenon of Prolonged Submaximal Exercise

A number of human and animal experiments have demonstrated that by 10 minutes after a prolonged (>30-minute) bout of submaximal exercise of greater than 50 percent $\dot{V}O_2$ max, blood pressure regulation is altered such that a **postexercise hypotension** is observed and is present for approximately 2 hours in healthy individuals and more than 12 hours in patients with hypertension. The hypotensive response of the healthy individual is a decrease in mean arterial pressure ranging from 5 to 10 mm Hg below resting baseline measures obtained before exercise (see Figure 10.18). The postexercise hypotension observed in patients with hypertension can be as large as −20 mm Hg.

Immediately after the exercise, there exists an inhibition of sympathetic activity, probably because central command is reduced during cool-down recovery or reset back to resting activity with complete cessation of exercise. Hence, the **baroreflexes** are inhibiting sympathetic outflow to peripheral vessels, allowing vasodilation returning the blood pressure back to resting pressures from the higher pressures allowed during the exercise (see Figure 10.19).

In addition, the alpha-adrenergic receptors on the vessels that are innervated by the neural sympathetic activity appear to be down-regulated (not as responsive)

postexercise hypotension A decrease in mean arterial pressure ranging from 5 to 10 mm Hg below resting baseline measures obtained before exercise in healthy individuals and up to −20 mm Hg in hypertensive patients.

arterial baroreflexes Negative feedback neural control circuits that have sensors located in the aortic arch and the carotid sinus that monitor arterial pressure and relay afferent information regarding changes in arterial pressure to the cardiovascular center in the central nervous system.

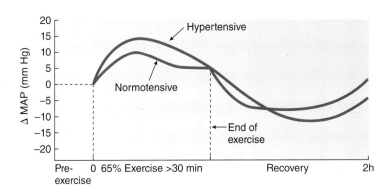

FIGURE 10.18 **Changes in mean arterial pressure (MAP) of healthy normotensive and hypertensive subjects during recovery from more than 30 minutes of 65 percent maximal oxygen uptake ($\dot{V}O_2$ max) cycling exercise.** (© Cengage Learning 2013)

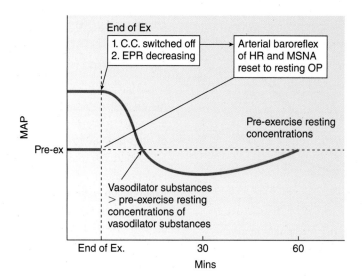

FIGURE 10.19 Schematic time course of arterial baroreflex control of sympathetic activity and exercise-related increases in vasodilator substances during recovery from exercise. (Adapted from Halliwill, J. R. 2001. Mechanisms and clinical implications of post-exercise hypotension. *Exerc. Sports Sci. Rev.* 29(2):65–70.)

and may be related to circulating vasodilator substances released into the vascular bed in response to the exercise (see Figure 10.20), such as residual nitric oxide, epinephrine (a beta-2 receptor agonist), endothelial-derived relaxing factor, histamine, and potassium ATP-sensitive channel activators.

Skeletal Muscle Resistance Vessel

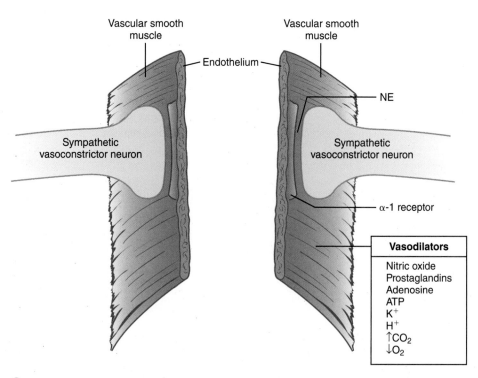

FIGURE 10.20 Schematic representation of a skeletal muscle resistance vessel and its neural and local control of the vascular smooth muscle during recovery. (Adapted from Halliwill, J. R. 2001. Mechanisms and clinical implications of post-exercise hypotension. *Exerc. Sports Sci. Rev.* 29(2):65–70.)

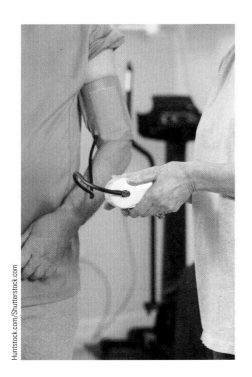

Huntstock.com/Shutterstock.com

Submaximal Exercise Tests Used for Fitness Assessments Were Based on Monitoring Heart Rate

Earlier you learned that the relationship between $\dot{Q}$ and $\dot{V}O_2$ was invariant and linear from rest to $\dot{V}O_2$ max. This relationship is expressed in the following equation:

$$\dot{Q} \text{ (L/min)} = 5.5 \, \dot{V}O_2 \text{ (L/min)} + 5.0 \text{ L/min}$$

Furthermore, in Chapter 7, you learned that $\dot{Q}$ is a product of HR and SV, and in Chapter 8, you discovered that endurance exercise training increased an individual's SV at any given workload up to maximum $\dot{Q}$ and HR. Because these relationships are consistent across a wide spectrum of fitness, a fact that was recognized very early in the development of exercise testing to determine fitness, a number of submaximal exercise tests relating HR to a given workload or $\dot{V}O_2$ were developed. The first tests developed were the "step tests." The most famous and well established of these types of tests is the Harvard step test.

Harvard Step Test

The **Harvard step test** was developed by the Harvard Fatigue Laboratory to assist army recruiters in identifying the fitness of the recruits at the recruiting stations before World War II. Subsequently, the Harvard step test was used to select men for their ability to perform hard work, evaluate the progress of endurance exercise training programs and diets, and to evaluate the fitness of schoolchildren. In this test, the individual is required to step on and off a 20-inch-high step 30 times per minute until exhaustion is reached or until 5 minutes has elapsed. Immediately after the exercise is stopped, the subject sits on the step and the recovery HR is palpated at the wrist for 30 seconds between the recovery time of 30 to 60, 90 to 120, and 150 to 180 seconds. Each of the 30-second HRs is summed together and the composite score is compared against a normative database that assigns the subjects into poor, low-average, high-average, good, and excellent fitness categories.

HOTLINK *Search the commercial site Topend Sports (http://www.topendsports.com) to learn more about administrating the Harvard step test.*

Master's Step Test

A less strenuous clinical modification of the Harvard step test known as the **Master's step test** was developed by cardiologist A. M. Master. This test could be performed in a physician's office while the patient was connected to an electrocardiogram. This test was used primarily for the evaluation of cardiac function and coronary insufficiency.

Other Aerobic Fitness Tests

Most of these progressive workload step tests have been replaced with the motor-driven treadmill or the bicycle ergometer, which can be programmed to increase the stress on the individual as per a specific stress testing protocol interfaced with a 12-lead electrocardiogram monitoring system and sometimes with imaging technology.

The step test type mass screening protocols may have disappeared, but the necessity to have a fitness evaluation test for mass screening has led to the development of timed run for distance (1 and

Master's step test A clinical version of the Harvard step test—see Rosenfeld, I. The Master Two-Step Test, 1959. *Canadian Medical Association Journal*, March 15; 80(6):480–481 for more.

Harvard step test A simple cardiorespiratory fitness test developed by the Harvard Fatigue Laboratory prior to World War II.

TABLE 10.6 Other Commonly Administered Aerobic Fitness Tests and Evaluations

YMCA cycle ergometer test
Nonexercise physical activity rating (PAR) test (University of Houston)
Distance run tests (12 minutes, 1.5 miles, 1 mile)
1-mile walking test
American College of Sports Medicine (ACSM) energy expenditure equations

© Cengage Learning 2013

1/2 mile) or distance run for time (12-minute run/walk) field tests. Table 10.6 contains several more options for aerobic fitness testing. The procedures for administering the aerobic fitness tests and the performance standards for each test listed in Table 10.6 can be found by accessing the websites listed in the Exercise Physiology Web Links or reviewing the Selected References at the end of this chapter.

Two examples of aerobic fitness tests include the 1-mile walk test and the 1.5-mile run. The 1-mile walk test is a good test for individuals who cannot run but can walk at a brisk pace. The 1.5-mile run was designed to be a maximal exertion test, and if clients cannot run the entire distance, their estimated values for $\dot{V}O_2$ max will be

much less accurate. The procedures required for using the 1.0-mile walk or the 1.5-mile run tests are provided in Figures 10.21 and 10.22.

The cardiorespiratory categories for $\dot{V}O_2$ max are listed in Table 10.7.

(What factors could influence the results of a client's performance on field tests such as the 1.5-mile run test?)

The Åstrand–Rhyming Test and the Åstrand–Åstrand Nomogram

Perhaps the most well-accepted and researched submaximal exercise test is the Åstrand–Rhyming cycle ergometer test used with the P. O. Åstrand and I. Åstrand (Rhyming) nomogram.

The **nomogram** was developed from a large number of submaximal step tests, cycle ergometer, and maximal cycle ergometer tests during which HR and $\dot{V}O_2$ were measured by electrocardiogram and the Douglas bag method, respectively. A quick method of determining an individual's predicted $\dot{V}O_2$ max using the submaximal cycle ergometer test is to select an initial work rate that is relatively low and is

1. Select the testing site. Use a 440-yard track (4 laps to a mile) or a premeasured 1.0-mile course.
2. Determine your body weight in pounds prior to the test.
3. Have a stopwatch available to determine total walking time and exercise heart rate.
4. Walk the 1.0-mile course at a brisk pace (the exercise heart rate at the end of the test should be above 120 beats per minute).
5. At the end of the 1.0-mile walk, check your walking time and immediately count your pulse for 10 seconds. Multiply the 10-second pulse count by 6 to obtain the exercise heart rate in beats per minute.
6. Convert the walking time from minutes and seconds to minute units. Because each minute has 60 seconds, divide the seconds by 60 to obtain the fraction of a minute. For instance, a walking time of 12 minutes and 15 seconds would equal 12 + (15 ÷ 60), or 12.25 minutes.
7. To obtain the estimated maximal oxygen uptake ($\dot{V}O_{2\,max}$) in mL/kg/min, plug your values in the following equation:
$\dot{V}O_{2\,max} = 88.768 - (0.0957 \times W) + (8.892 \times G) - (1.4537 \times T) - (0.1194 \times HR)$

Where:

W = Weight in pounds
G = Gender (use 0 for women and 1 for men)
T = Total time for the one-mile walk in minutes (see item 6)
HR = Exercise heart rate in beats per minute at the end of the 1.0-mile walk

Example: A 19-year-old female who weighs 140 pounds completed the 1.0-mile walk in 14 minutes 39 seconds with an exercise heart rate of 148 beats per minute. Her estimated $\dot{V}O_{2\,max}$ would be:

W = 140 lbs
G = 0 (female gender = 0)
T = 14:39 = 14 + (39 ÷ 60) = 14.65 min
HR = 148 bpm
$\dot{V}O_{2\,max} = 88.768 - (0.0957 \times 140) + (8.892 \times 0) - (1.4537 \times 14.65) - (0.1194 \times 148)$
$\dot{V}O_{2\,max} = 36.4$ mL/kg/min

FIGURE 10.21 Procedure for the 1.0-mile walk test. (From Hoeger, W. W. K., and S. A. Hoeger. 2010. Figure 6.2 in *Lifetime physical fitness & wellness*, 11th ed. Belmont, CA: Brooks/Cole-Cengage Learning.) Source byline: Dolgener et al. 1994. "Validation of the Rockport fitness walking test in college males and females," *Research Quarterly for Exercise and Sport* 65: 152–158.

Time	$\dot{V}O_{2\,max}$ (mL/kg/min)	Time	$\dot{V}O_{2\,max}$ (mL/kg/min)	Time	$\dot{V}O_{2\,max}$ (mL/kg/min)
6:10	80.0	10:30	48.6	14:50	34.0
6:20	79.0	10:40	48.0	15:00	33.6
6:30	77.9	10:50	47.4	15:10	33.1
6:40	76.7	11:00	46.6	15:20	32.7
6:50	75.5	11:10	45.8	15:30	32.2
7:00	74.0	11:20	45.1	15:40	31.8
7:10	72.6	11:30	44.4	15:50	31.4
7:20	71.3	11:40	43.7	16:00	30.9
7:30	69.9	11:50	43.2	16:10	30.5
7:40	68.3	12:00	42.3	16:20	30.2
7:50	66.8	12:10	41.7	16:30	29.8
8:00	65.2	12:20	41.0	16:40	29.5
8:10	63.9	12:30	40.4	16:50	29.1
8:20	62.5	12:40	39.8	17:00	28.9
8:30	61.2	12:50	39.2	17:10	28.5
8:40	60.2	13:00	38.6	17:20	28.3
8:50	59.1	13:10	38.1	17:30	28.0
9:00	58.1	13:20	37.8	17:40	27.7
9:10	56.9	13:30	37.2	17:50	27.4
9:20	55.9	13:40	36.8	18:00	27.1
9:30	54.7	13:50	36.3	18:10	26.8
9:40	53.5	14:00	35.9	18:20	26.6
9:50	52.3	14:10	35.5	18:30	26.3
10:00	51.1	14:20	35.1	18:40	26.0
10:10	50.4	14:30	34.7	18:50	25.7
10:20	49.5	14:40	34.3	19:00	25.4

1. Make sure you qualify for this test. This test is contraindicated for unconditioned beginners, individuals with symptoms of heart disease, and those with known heart disease or risk factors.
2. Select the testing site. Find a school track (each lap is one-fourth of a mile) or a premeasured 1.5-mile course.
3. Have a stopwatch available to determine your time.
4. Conduct a few warm-up exercises prior to the test. Do some stretching exercises, some walking, and slow jogging.
5. Initiate the test and try to cover the distance in the fastest time possible (walking or jogging). Time yourself during the run to see how fast you have covered the distance. If any unusual symptoms arise during the test, do not continue. Stop immediately and retake the test after another 6 weeks of aerobic training.
6. At the end of the test, cool down by walking or jogging slowly for another 3 to 5 minutes. Do not sit or lie down after the test.
7. According to your performance time, look up your estimated maximal oxygen uptake ($\dot{V}O_{2\,max}$) in Table 6.2.

Example: A 20-year-old male runs the 1.5-mile course in 10 minutes and 20 seconds. Table 6.2 shows a $\dot{V}O_{2\,max}$ of 49.5 mL/kg/min for a time of 10:20. According to Table 6.8 (page 187), this $\dot{V}O_{2\,max}$ would place him in the "good" cardiorespiratory fitness category.

● FIGURE 10.22 Procedure and estimated maximal oxygen uptake ($\dot{V}O_2$ max) for the 1.5-mile run test. (From Hoeger, W. W. K., and S. A. Hoeger. 2010. Figure 6.1 in *Lifetime physical fitness & wellness*, 11th ed. Belmont. CA: Brooks/Cole-Cengage Learning.) Source: Adapted from K.H. Cooper. 1978. "A means of assessing maximal oxygen uptake" *JAMA* 203: 201–204; M. L. Pollock. J. H. Wilmore, and S. M. Fox III. 1978. *Health and fitness through physical activity*. New York: John Wiley & Sons; and Wilmore, J. H. and D. L. Costill. 1988. *Training for sport and activity*. Dubuque, IA: Wm. C. Brown Publishers.

● TABLE 10.7 Cardiorespiratory Fitness Categories according to Maximal Oxygen Uptake

Sex	Age	Fitness Category (based on $\dot{V}O_2$ mm in mL/kg/min)				
		Poor	Fair	Average	Good	Excellent
Men	<29	<24.9	25–33.9	34–43.9	44–52.9	>53
	30–39	<22.9	23–33.9	31–41.9	42–49.9	>50
	40–49	<19.9	20–28.9	27–38.9	39–44.9	>45
	50–59	<17.9	18–24.9	26–37.9	38–42.9	>43
	60–69	<15.9	16–22.9	23–35.9	36–40.9	>41
	≥70	≤12.9	13–20.9	21–32.9	33–37.9	≥38
Women	<29	<23.9	24–30.9	31–38.9	39–48.9	>49
	30–39	<19.9	20–27.9	28–36.9	37–44.9	>45
	40–49	<16.9	17–24.9	25–34.9	35–41.9	>42
	50–59	<14.9	15–21.9	22–33.9	34–39.9	>40
	60–69	<12.9	13–20.9	21–32.9	33–36.9	>37
	≥70	≤11.9	12–19.9	20–30.9	31–34.9	≥35

From Hoeger, W. W. K., and S. A. Hoeger. 2010. Table 6.8 in *Lifetime physical fitness & wellness*, 11th ed. Belmont, CA: Brooks/Cole-Cengage Learning.

TABLE 10.8 Nomogram for Estimating Maximal Oxygen Uptake ($\dot{V}O_2$ max) Estimates in L/min for the Åstrand–Rhyming Test

Heart Rate	Men Workload 300	600	900	1200	1500	Women Workload 300	450	600	750	900
120	2.2	3.4	4.8			2.6	3.4	4.1	4.8	
121	2.2	3.4	4.7			2.5	3.3	4.0	4.8	
122	2.2	3.4	4.6			2.5	3.2	3.9	4.7	
123	2.1	3.4	4.6			2.4	3.1	3.9	4.6	
124	2.1	3.3	4.5	6.0		2.4	3.1	3.8	4.5	
125	2.0	3.4	4.4	5.9		2.3	3.0	3.7	4.4	
126	2.0	3.4	4.4	5.8		2.3	3.0	3.6	4.3	
127	2.0	3.1	4.3	5.7		2.2	2.9	3.5	4.2	
128	2.0	3.1	4.2	5.6		2.2	2.8	3.5	4.2	4.8
129	1.9	3.0	4.2	5.6		2.2	2.8	3.4	4.1	4.8
130	1.9	3.0	4.1	5.5		2.1	2.7	3.4	4.0	4.7
131	1.9	2.9	4.0	5.4		2.1	2.7	3.4	4.0	4.6
132	1.8	2.9	4.0	5.3		2.0	2.7	3.3	3.9	4.5
133	1.8	2.8	3.9	5.3		2.0	2.6	3.2	3.8	4.4
134	1.8	2.8	3.9	5.2		2.0	2.6	3.2	3.8	4.4
135	1.7	2.8	3.8	5.1		2.0	2.6	3.1	3.7	4.3
136	1.7	2.7	3.8	5.0		1.9	2.5	3.1	3.6	4.2
137	1.7	2.7	3.7	5.0		1.9	2.5	3.0	3.6	4.2
138	1.6	2.7	3.7	4.9		1.8	2.4	3.0	3.5	4.1
139	1.6	2.6	3.6	4.8		1.8	2.4	2.9	3.5	4.0
140	1.6	2.6	3.6	4.8	6.0	1.8	2.4	2.8	3.4	4.0
141		2.6	3.5	4.7	5.9	1.8	2.3	2.8	3.4	3.9
142		2.5	3.5	4.6	5.8	1.7	2.3	2.8	3.3	3.9
143		2.5	3.4	4.6	5.7	1.7	2.2	2.7	3.3	3.8
144		2.5	3.4	4.5	5.7	1.7	2.2	2.7	3.2	3.8
145		2.4	3.4	4.5	5.6	1.6	2.2	2.7	3.2	3.7
146		2.4	3.3	4.4	5.6	1.6	2.2	2.6	3.2	3.7
147		2.4	3.3	4.4	5.5	1.6	2.1	2.6	3.1	3.6
148		2.4	3.2	4.3	5.4	1.6	2.1	2.6	3.1	3.6
149		2.3	3.2	4.3	5.4		2.1	2.6	3.0	3.5
150		2.3	3.2	4.2	5.3		2.0	2.5	3.0	3.5
151		2.3	3.1	4.2	5.2		2.0	2.5	3.0	3.4
152		2.3	3.1	4.1	5.2		2.0	2.5	2.9	3.4
153		2.2	3.0	4.1	5.1		2.0	2.4	2.9	3.3
154		2.2	3.0	4.0	5.1		2.0	2.4	2.8	3.3
155		2.2	3.0	4.0	5.0		1.9	2.4	2.8	3.2
156		2.2	2.9	4.0	5.0		1.9	2.3	2.8	3.2
157		2.1	2.9	3.9	4.9		1.9	2.3	2.7	3.2
158		2.1	2.9	3.9	4.9		1.8	2.3	2.7	3.1
159		2.1	2.8	3.8	4.8		1.8	2.2	2.7	3.1
160		2.1	2.8	3.8	4.8		1.8	2.2	2.6	3.0
161		2.0	2.8	3.7	4.7		1.8	2.2	2.6	3.0
162		2.0	2.8	3.7	4.6		1.8	2.2	2.6	3.0
163		2.0	2.8	3.7	4.6		1.7	2.2	2.6	2.9
164		2.0	2.7	3.6	4.5		1.7	2.1	2.5	2.9
165		2.0	2.7	3.6	4.5		1.7	2.1	2.5	2.9
166		1.9	2.7	3.6	4.5		1.7	2.1	2.5	2.8
167		1.9	2.6	3.5	4.4		1.6	2.1	2.4	2.8
168		1.9	2.6	3.5	4.4		1.6	2.0	2.4	2.8
169		1.9	2.6	3.5	4.3		1.6	2.0	2.4	2.8
170		1.8	2.6	3.4	4.3		1.6	2.0	2.4	2.7

From Hoeger, W. W. K., and S. A. Hoeger. 2010. Table 6.5 in *Lifetime physical fitness & wellness,* 11th ed. Belmont, CA: Brooks/Cole-Cengage Learning. And adapted from Åstrand, I. 1960. *Acta Physiologica Scandinavica* 49 (Suppl.169):45–60.

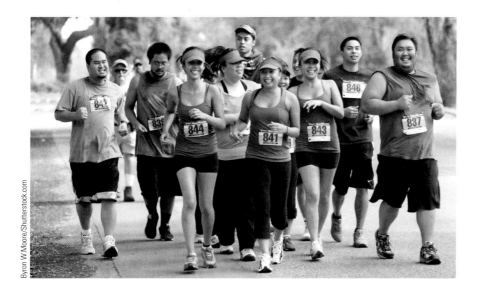

Byron W. Moore/Shutterstock.com

gradually increased until steady-state HRs achieve approximate values of 140 beats/min. The RPE of this work should be approximately 14. By extrapolating a line between the work rate and the steady-state HR on the Åstrand–Åstrand nomogram the individual's $\dot{V}O_2$ max can be predicted. Note that the nomogram has been developed for both men and women using either a cycle ergometer or a stepping bench. However, over time, the extrapolation procedure to obtain the $\dot{V}O_2$ max value has been simplified to provide the numerical data in Table 10.8. Further work on the submaximal cycle ergometer test prediction of $\dot{V}O_2$ max enabled the development of an age correction factor for ages 14 to 65 years (see Table 10.9).

TABLE 10.9 Age-Based Correction Factors for Maximal Oxygen Uptake ($\dot{V}O_2$ max)

Age	Correction Factor	Age	Correction Factor	Age	Correction Factor
14	1.11	32	.909	50	.750
15	1.10	33	.896	51	.742
16	1.09	34	.883	52	.734
17	1.08	35	.870	53	.726
18	1.07	36	.862	54	.718
19	1.06	37	.854	55	.710
20	1.05	38	.846	56	.704
21	1.04	39	.838	57	.698
22	1.03	40	.830	58	.692
23	1.02	41	.820	59	.686
24	1.01	42	.810	60	.680
25	1.00	43	.800	61	.674
26	.987	44	.790	62	.668
27	.974	45	.780	63	.662
28	.961	46	.774	64	.656
29	.948	47	.768	65	.650
30	.935	48	.762		
31	.922	49	.756		

From Hoeger, W. W. K., and S. A. Hoeger. 2010. Table 6.6 in *Lifetime physical fitness & wellness*, 11th ed. Belmont, CA: Brooks/Cole-Cengage Learning. And adapted from Åstrand, I. 1960. *Acta Physiologica Scandinavica* 49 (Suppl. 169):45–60.

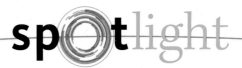

An Expert on Exercise Laboratory Measurements: Per Olof Åstrand, M.D., Ph.D.

Per Olof (P.O.) Åstrand, M.D., Ph.D., was born in 1922 and became one of the most famous Swedish and world-renowned exercise physiologists; he excelled in exercise testing, measurement, and work performance. He graduated from the College of Physical Education, Stockholm, in 1946, and completed his medical training and doctoral work at the Karolinska Institute-Medical School, Stockholm, in 1952. Åstrand taught in the Department of Physiology at the College of Physical Education from 1947 to 1977, and became department head and a professor at the Karolinska Institute from 1977 to 1987. Currently, he is retired.

Åstrand was mentored by Erik-Hohwü Christensen, who influenced him to study physical work capacity and the various measurement techniques required to understand the physiologic responses to exercise. Åstrand's dissertation involved the study of the working capacity of healthy male and female individuals ages 4 to 33. He and his wife (Irma Rhyming) published numerous studies together in the 1950s and developed the famous Åstrand–Åstrand (née Rhyming)

submaximal cycle test to estimate oxygen uptake that is still used worldwide. Dr. Åstrand's research interests included work physiology and the oxygen-transporting system in humans, limiting factors like aging that influence maximal oxygen uptake, environmental factors and exercise, physical performance in relation to sex and age, health and fitness, preventive medicine, and rehabilitation.

Åstrand is the lead author of one of the classic modern textbooks, *Textbook of Work Physiology: Physiological Bases of Exercise*, first published in 1970. He worked with many world-class exercise physiologists, such as Drs. Bengt Saltin and Björn Ekblom, who are considered among the best ever in their research areas (focused on heart and skeletal muscle physiology), and they, too, have influenced exercise physiologists internationally. Åstrand holds numerous honorary degrees, received the 1973 American College of Sports Medicine Honor Award, and has contributed to more than 200 publications.

in*Practice*

Examples of Measurement of Common Cardiorespiratory Responses to Exercise

The following subsections provide some practical examples of how physiologic measures and exercise are related to your area of interest (review the future career table from Chapter 1).

Health/Fitness: It is important for health/fitness professionals not only to understand how to effectively measure aerobic and anaerobic performance characteristics, but also how to interpret them and to develop appropriate training programs to help clients achieve their individual goals. For example, if a client's goal is to complete their first 10-kilometer (10K) run in 60 minutes, you would most likely need to measure or estimate the client's baseline $\dot{V}O_2$ max or endurance capacity to develop an appropriate plan for

success. To run a 10K in 60 minutes, your client will need to run each mile just below 10 min/mile and maintain an estimated energy expenditure (or O_2 consumption) of approximately 33 ml · kg^{-1} · min^{-1} (based on running prediction equations). As you have learned, a trained runner can usually work at least at 85 to 95 percent of their $\dot{V}O_2$ max for a 10K race; thus, your client would need to have or increase her $\dot{V}O_2$ max to a level approximately 39 ml · kg^{-1} · min^{-1} to have a realistic chance at meeting her goal.

Medicine: Graded exercise testing (GXT) has been a widely accepted effective clinical tool for the diagnostic screening for coronary heart disease since the early 1960s. Typically, a client can undergo GXT on a treadmill, cycle, or rowing ergometer, whereas the exercise physiologist and physician (as required by pretest health screening; see Chapter 2 for more information) can select a specific protocol based on the client's needs (that is, more gradually changing protocol for elderly subjects). In diagnostic testing, the exercise physiologist would usually measure the following variables during the test: heart rate, blood pressure, rating of perceived exertion, the electrocardiogram (ECG), exertional symptoms, and reason for stopping. An exercise physiologist can interpret the GXT measurements (with physician input, as needed) to determine the client's exercise risk stratification, and a follow-up plan can be developed.

Athletic Performance: Coaches should always use aerobic and anaerobic measurements to help their athletes achieve their goals and determine successful training progress. Unless you are a very lucky coach who recruits lots of highly talented athletes, you will need to help develop talent in your athletes over time, which requires regular performance evaluations. For example, football coaches should test their athletes before the beginning of the season to determine their ability to perform. What tests would you use to assess football players at the beginning of the season? Remember, several factors would need to be considered such as the experience level of the players (for example, middle school, high school), how much time you have, and testing equipment available. Common tests that are often used for football include a combination of tests (combine) that can

be modified for experience level, such as the 40-yard dash, vertical jump, standing long jump, agility test, and relative strength test (how many repetitions a given weight can be lifted). The results of combine tests can be used to help coaches access the readiness and physical abilities of their athletes and help them do individual goal setting to help improve performance over time. It is important to understand that testing should always be conducted but is fairly meaningless unless the tests are explained to the athlete in a timely and understandable manner.

Rehabilitation: One of the main daily job duties for physical therapists and athletic trainers is the measurement of their client's physical abilities. For example, a physical therapist who is working with clients who are beginning their rehabilitation from anterior cruciate ligament surgery would need to conduct a preliminary assessment of knee range of motion for both the injured and the healthy knee. Therapists should also standardize their testing so that as their clients' rehabilitation progresses, they can be evaluated with the same standardized protocol to ensure that improvements are due to actual improvements and not measurement errors. Once therapists interpret the results of their range-of-motion evaluations, they should provide clients with feedback about their clinical status and progress. This information then can be used by the therapist and client to set goals for rehabilitation before the next scheduled range-of-motion assessment.

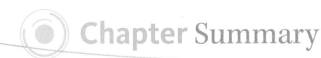

Chapter Summary

- A variety of physiologic factors (variables) can influence exercise abilities along a physical performance continuum. It is important for you to understand these factors to help your clients achieve long-term functional health and their potential for peak performance, if so desired.

- Exercise physiology–related tests generally fall into the categories of laboratory tests (very controlled, usually focused on one client at a time, and performances are commonly directly measured) and field tests (conducted in more practical settings where multiple clients can often be tested at one time and performances are often estimated form indirect physiologic measures).

- Effective anaerobic and aerobic assessments require valid, reliable, and objective measurements.

- Anaerobic performance depends heavily on an individual's ability to recruit, rate code, and synchronize a large num-

ber of fast-twitch fibers rapidly. Limiting factors associated with anaerobic performance include the individual's genetic predisposition to the amount of fast-twitch fibers they posses in a given muscle group.

- A number of practical and physiologic considerations are involved in determining an individual's $\dot{V}O_2$ max using the general principle of progressively increasing workloads and measuring the increase in oxygen uptake ($\dot{V}O_2$) until a plateau of $\dot{V}O_2$ is achieved.

- Practical considerations for $\dot{V}O_2$ testing include duration of the test protocol, type of exercise, performance testing, and the age activity level and health status of the client being tested.

- Ratings of perceived exertion (RPE) are valuable measures related to central command and the cardiovascular and respiratory systems.

- Oxygen deficit is the difference between the $\dot{V}O_2$ in the initial minutes of the exercise and the $\dot{V}O_2$ required to perform the exercise. Excess postexercise oxygen consumption (EPOC) refers to the body's gradual recovery from exercise.
- Cardiovascular drift refers to reduction to stroke volume and mean arterial pressure, with concomitant increase with heart rate during prolonged periods of exercise. After prolonged bouts of submaximal exercise, clients may often experience postexercise hypotension.
- A variety of submaximal exercise tests can used to estimate $\dot{V}O_2$ max and fitness including the Harvard step test, the Master's step test, and the Åstrand–Rhyming cycle test.

Exercise Physiology Reality

CENGAGE brain.com   To reinforce the exercise physiology concepts presented in above, complete the laboratory exercises for Chapter 10. To access labs and other course materials for this text, please visit www.cengagebrain.com. See the preface on page xiii for details. Once you complete the exercises, have your instructor evaluate your work. Remember to use your lab experience to help guide you toward future success in exercise physiology.

Exercise Physiology Web Links

Access the following websites for further study of topics covered in this chapter:

- Find updates and quick links to sites related to the measurement of common anaerobic abilities and cardiorespiratory responses related to exercise at our website. To access the course materials and companion resources for this text, please visit www.cengagebrain.com. See the preface on page xiii for details.
- Search for information about exercise testing at the American College of Sports Medicine (ACSM) website: http://www.acsm.org.

- Search for more information about exercise testing at the National Strength and Conditioning Association (NSCA) website: http://www.nsca-lift.org.
- See the following website for procedures for exercise physiology laboratory measures: http://ston.jsc.nasa .gov/collections/TRS/_techrep/TM-1998-104826.pdf.
- Search for more information about anaerobic exercise tests at the following commercial websites: http://www .exrx.net, http://www.brianmac.co.uk, or http://www.topendsports.com.
- Search YouTube© for video clips that depict poor and better examples of exercise testing.

Study Questions

Review the Warm-Up Pre-Test questions you were asked to answer before reading Chapter 10. Test yourself once more to determine what you know now that you have completed the chapter.

The questions that follow will help you review this chapter. You will find the answers in the discussions on the pages provided.

1. List and describe two commonly used tests of anaerobic power and anaerobic capacity conducted by exercise physiologists. *pp. 338, 340*

2. What is the difference between a laboratory test and a field test? *p. 336*

3. What are three practical considerations related to anaerobic exercise testing of clients? *pp. 346–347*

4. Is the plateau of oxygen uptake a reality? *p. 344*

5. Explain oxygen deficit. *pp. 351–352*

6. Describe the process of postexercise oxygen consumption. *pp. 352–353*

7. Define cardiovascular drift and explain how it occurs. *p. 354*

8. Describe the Harvard step test and how it works. *p. 357*

9. Describe the Åstrand–Rhyming cycle ergometer test. *pp. 358–361*

10. List and describe three other commonly administered aerobic fitness tests. *p. 358*

 # Selected References

American College of Sports Medicine (ACSM). 2010. *ACSM's guidelines for exercise testing and prescription,* 8th ed. Philadelphia: Lippincott Williams & Wilkins.

Åstrand, P-O., and K. Rodaahl. 1986. *Textbook of work physiology: Physiological basis of exercise,* 3rd ed. New York: McGraw-Hill.

Bar-Or, O. 1987. The Wingate anaerobic test: An update on methodology, reliability, and validity. *Sports Med.* 4:381–394.

Baumgartner, T. A., A. S. Jackson, M. T. Mahar, and D. A. Rowe. 2006. *Measurement and evaluation in physical education and exercise science,* 8th ed. Boston: WCB/McGraw-Hill.

Halliwill, J. R. 2001. Mechanisms and clinical implications of post-exercise hypotension. *Exerc. Sports Sci. Rev.* 29(2):65–70.

Hawkins, M. N., P. B. Raven, P. G. Snell, J. Stray-Gundersen, and B. D. Levine. 2007. Maximal oxygen uptake as a parametric measure of cardiorespiratory capacity. *Med. Sci. Sports Exerc.* 39(1):103–107.

Maud, P., and C. Foster, editors. 2006. *Physiological assessment of human fitness,* 2nd ed. Champaign, IL: Human Kinetics.

McDougall, J. D., H. A. Wenger, and H. J. Green. 1991. *Physiological testing of the high performance athlete,* 2nd ed. Champaign, IL: Human Kinetics.

Mitchell, J. H., B. J. Sproule, and C. B. Chapman. 1957. The physiological meaning of the maximal oxygen intake test. *J. Clin. Invest.* 37:538–547.

Taylor, H. L., E. Buskirk, and A. Henschel. 1955. Maximal oxygen intake as an objective measure of cardio-respiratory fitness. *J. Appl. Physiol.* 8:73–80.

Wasserman, K., J. E. Hansen, D. Y. Sue, and B. J. Whipp. 1987. *Principles of exercise testing and interpretation.* Philadelphia: Lea & Febiger.

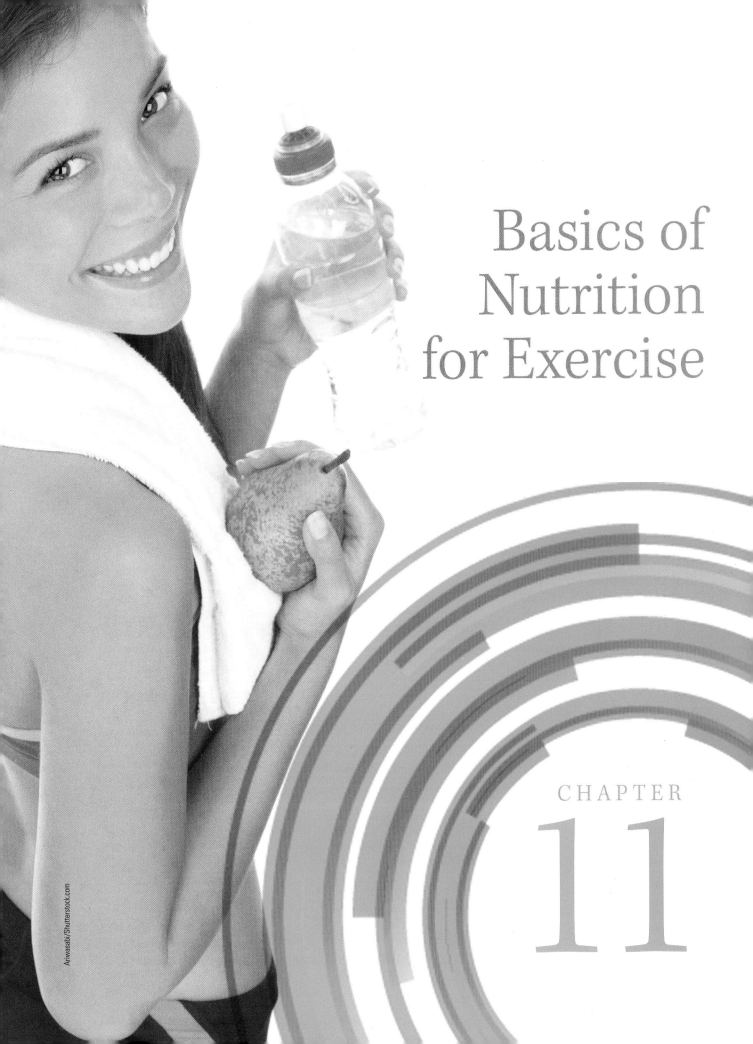

Basics of Nutrition for Exercise

CHAPTER

11

Ariwasabi/Shutterstock.com

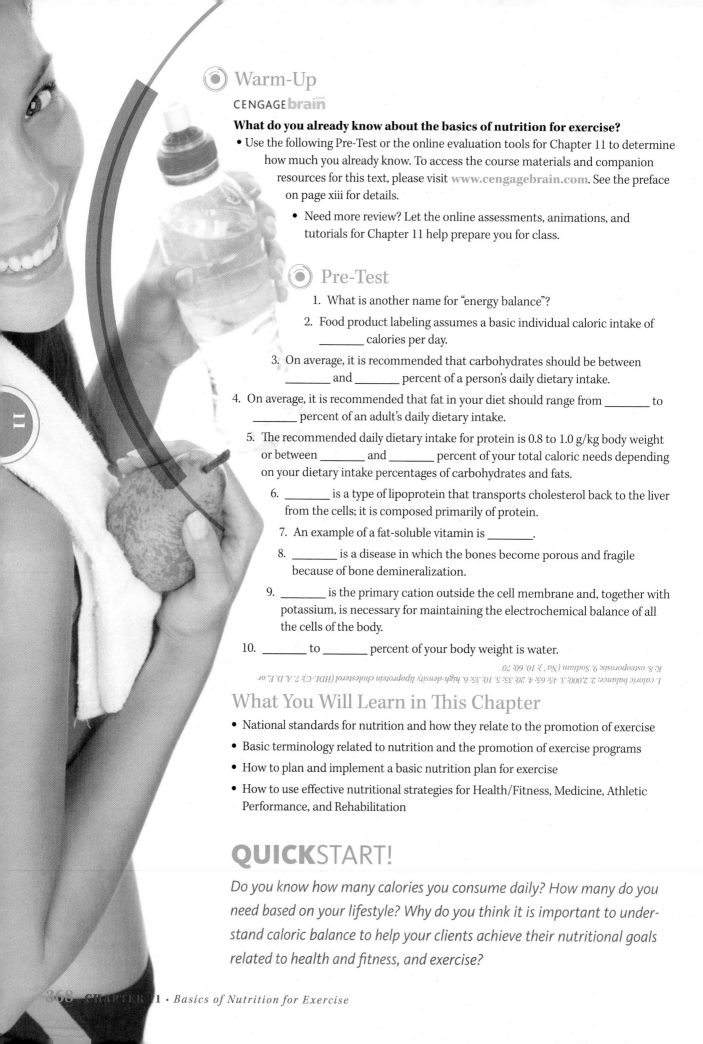

◉ Warm-Up

What do you already know about the basics of nutrition for exercise?

• Use the following Pre-Test or the online evaluation tools for Chapter 11 to determine how much you already know. To access the course materials and companion resources for this text, please visit **www.cengagebrain.com**. See the preface on page xiii for details.

• Need more review? Let the online assessments, animations, and tutorials for Chapter 11 help prepare you for class.

◉ Pre-Test

1. What is another name for "energy balance"?

2. Food product labeling assumes a basic individual caloric intake of _____ calories per day.

3. On average, it is recommended that carbohydrates should be between _____ and _____ percent of a person's daily dietary intake.

4. On average, it is recommended that fat in your diet should range from _____ to _____ percent of an adult's daily dietary intake.

5. The recommended daily dietary intake for protein is 0.8 to 1.0 g/kg body weight or between _____ and _____ percent of your total caloric needs depending on your dietary intake percentages of carbohydrates and fats.

6. _____ is a type of lipoprotein that transports cholesterol back to the liver from the cells; it is composed primarily of protein.

7. An example of a fat-soluble vitamin is _____.

8. _____ is a disease in which the bones become porous and fragile because of bone demineralization.

9. _____ is the primary cation outside the cell membrane and, together with potassium, is necessary for maintaining the electrochemical balance of all the cells of the body.

10. _____ to _____ percent of your body weight is water.

1. caloric balance; 2. 2,000; 3. 45: 65; 4. 20: 35; 5. 10: 35; 6. high-density lipoprotein cholesterol (HDL-C); 7. A, D, E, or K; 8. osteoporosis; 9. Sodium (Na⁺); 10. 60: 70

What You Will Learn in This Chapter

• National standards for nutrition and how they relate to the promotion of exercise

• Basic terminology related to nutrition and the promotion of exercise programs

• How to plan and implement a basic nutrition plan for exercise

• How to use effective nutritional strategies for Health/Fitness, Medicine, Athletic Performance, and Rehabilitation

QUICKSTART!

Do you know how many calories you consume daily? How many do you need based on your lifestyle? Why do you think it is important to understand caloric balance to help your clients achieve their nutritional goals related to health and fitness, and exercise?

Introduction to the Basics of Nutrition for Exercise

Chapters 4, 5, 6, 6A, and 6B explained energy metabolism and how fuels are utilized during participation in exercise. In this chapter, you will learn about the basics of nutrition and how you can apply the concepts to optimize the exercise goals of your clients. **Nutrition** is the science of foods and the nutrients and other substances they contain. In addition, the study of nutrition involves understanding the actions within the body that enable us to make use of our food. These actions include ingestion, digestion, absorption, transport, metabolism, and exertion.

The foundation for the study of the science of nutrition is based on your ability to understand principles from biology, biochemistry, and chemistry. Until recently, nutritional information related to exercise was largely based on anecdotal or testimonial information. Because of the complex nature of the field of nutrition, the undertaking of nutritional study interventions designed to impact our eatinxg and exercise behaviors can be challenging because many variables can influence the results. Controlling extraneous variables that affect nutrition interventions is often difficult or impossible to do, and contributes to nutritional fallacies, misconceptions, and misinterpretations by the public and even healthcare professionals. Therefore, it is important for you to apply the concepts of scientific inquiry as they relate to nutrition and exercise, to acquire accurate information that you can share with your clients (see Chapter 1).

The future nutrition recommendations you provide clients should be based on the results from large-scale studies with treatment and control groups that include placebos and double-blind studies. In double-blind studies, both the investigator and the subjects are unaware of what is being tested. All such studies should be peer-reviewed and replicated. As an exercise science professional, you should understand that even a mastery of your exercise physiology course does not necessarily make you an expert (or professionally certified) in the field of nutrition. You should not claim to be a nutritionist just because you have done well in a few courses related to nutrition. However, the basic nutrition knowledge you acquire from this chapter will provide you with the foundational knowledge required to interact with nutritional experts. Nutritional experts—individuals such as registered dietitians who undergo standardized training via the American Dietetic Association—can help you counsel clients in the areas of Health/Fitness, Medicine, Athletic Performance, and Rehabilitation.

In this chapter you will learn about the nutritional concepts required for a basic understanding of the following:

1. **The U.S. Dietary Guidelines**
2. **Energy (caloric) balance**
3. **Nutrient (carbohydrates, fats, proteins) balance**
4. **Vitamin balance**
5. **Mineral balance**
6. **Fluid balance**

Remember, diet can affect all of the following:

- Strength
- Speed
- Stamina
- Mental concentration
- Mood
- Recovery

HOTLINK *Access the following websites to review or update your fundamental understanding of nutrition for exercise:* **http://healthypeople2020.gov**, **http://www.choosemyplate.gov**, *and* **http://www.nutrition.gov**.

(What are three specific key recommendations from the 2010 Dietary Guidelines for Americans?)

nutrition The science of foods and the nutrients and other substances they contain. In addition, the study of nutrition involves understanding the actions within the body that enable us to make use of our food.

U.S. Dietary Guidelines The *Dietary Guidelines for Americans, 2010* provides evidence-based nutrition information and advice for people age 2 and older. They serve as the basis for federal food and nutrition education programs.

energy (caloric) balance The balance of caloric intake (kcals) and caloric expenditure (kcals) associated with the maintenance of homeostasis and a healthy body weight.

nutrient (carbohydrates, fats, proteins) balance Consuming the appropriate amounts of carbohydrates, fats, and proteins to maintain energy balance based on the U.S. Dietary Guidelines.

vitamin balance Consuming the appropriate amounts of vitamins to maintain energy balance based on the U.S. Dietary Guidelines.

mineral balance Consuming the appropriate amounts of minerals to maintain energy balance based on the U.S. Dietary Guidelines.

fluid balance Consuming the appropriate amounts and types of fluids to maintain normal hydration and homeostasis.

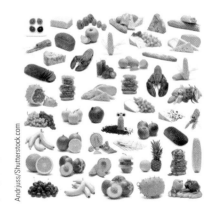

Andrjuss/Shutterstock.com

Energy (Caloric) Balance for Exercise

energy balance equation The relationship between energy intake and energy expenditure.

You learned in Chapter 1 about the importance of energy expenditure and the number of kilocalories (kcals) that one expends (energy expenditure; Figure 11.1).

The basic **energy balance (or caloric balance) equation** is based on the first law of thermodynamics: Energy is neither created nor destroyed. The relationships shown in Figure 11.1 appear to be quite simple to incorporate in our daily living. For example, if you want to lose weight, you need to take in fewer calories, expend more, or do both. However, it is obvious from the increase in the incidence of obesity in our children and adults that simple things are difficult to accomplish.

A bomb calorimeter can be used to estimate the potential energy of foods (see Figure 11.2). Direct calorimetry is a technique that measures heat released from the body and is similar to the process of the bomb calorimeter, but the chemical bonds

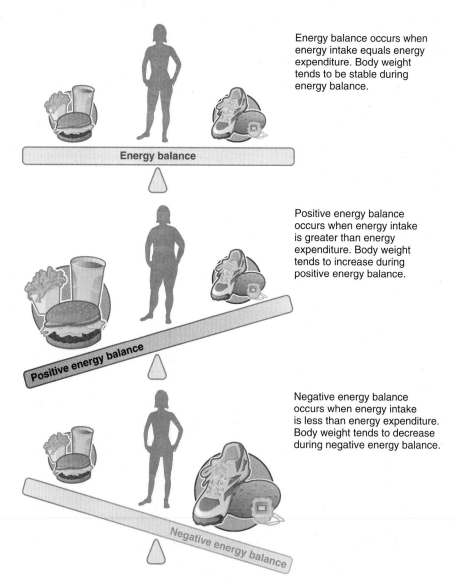

Energy balance occurs when energy intake equals energy expenditure. Body weight tends to be stable during energy balance.

Energy balance

Positive energy balance occurs when energy intake is greater than energy expenditure. Body weight tends to increase during positive energy balance.

Positive energy balance

Negative energy balance occurs when energy intake is less than energy expenditure. Body weight tends to decrease during negative energy balance.

Negative energy balance

● **FIGURE 11.1 Energy (caloric) balance equation.** (From McGuire, M., and K. A. Beerman. 2009. Figure 8.1 in *Nutritional sciences*, 2nd ed. Belmont, CA: Brooks/Cole-Cengage Learning.)

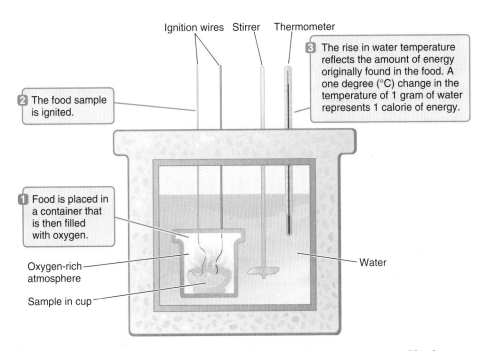

Ignition wires Stirrer Thermometer

2 The food sample is ignited.

3 The rise in water temperature reflects the amount of energy originally found in the food. A one degree (°C) change in the temperature of 1 gram of water represents 1 calorie of energy.

1 Food is placed in a container that is then filled with oxygen.

Oxygen-rich atmosphere

Sample in cup

Water

FIGURE 11.2 Bomb calorimetry used to determine the energy content of food. (From McGuire, M., and K. A. Beerman. 2009. Figure 1.3 in *Nutritional sciences*, 2nd ed. Belmont, CA: Brooks/Cole-Cengage Learning.)

of foods consumed yield energy and produce heat, which can be measured as kilocalories. Indirect calorimetry (Figure 11.3) is a technique that measures the amount of oxygen consumed. Both direct and indirect calorimetry can be used to estimate **thermogenesis**, which is the amount of heat generated by the body.

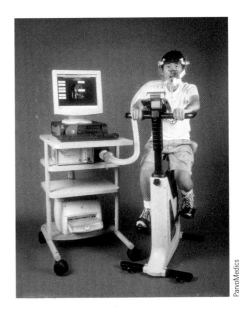

ParvoMedics

FIGURE 11.3 An open circuit metabolic measurement system (indirect calorimetry). (From Dunford, M., and J. A. Doyle. 2007. Figure 2.15 in *Nutrition for sport and exercise*. Belmont, CA: Wadsworth.)

HOTLINK *See Chapter 13 for more information about caloric intake and caloric expenditure for effective weight management.*

Unfortunately, the energy balance equation becomes more complex when you consider all the physiologic factors that can influence both energy intake and energy expenditure. To achieve energy balance, the body responds to a mixture of signals with regard to energy intake and energy expenditure. For energy intake, these include, but are not limited to, the following:

1. The five senses
2. **Satiation**: feeling of satisfaction and fullness that occurs during a meal and halts eating
3. **Satiety**: feeling of satisfaction that occurs after a meal and inhibits eating until the next meal
4. Hunger signals: the control center or hypothalamus integrates energy intake, expenditure, and storage based on the absence or presence of nutrients in the small intestines
5. Hormones and changes in substrates: influence hunger such as increased **ghrelin** and **neuropeptide Y** (hormones that stimulate appetite) concentrations and reduced **leptin**

thermogenesis The amount of heat generated by the body; used as an index of how much energy the body is expending.

satiation The feeling of satisfaction and fullness that occurs during a meal and halts eating.

satiety The feeling of satisfaction that occurs after a meal and inhibits eating until the next meal.

ghrelin A protein by the stomach cells that enhances appetite and decreases energy expenditure.

neuropeptide Y A chemical produced in the brain that stimulates appetite, diminishes energy expenditure, and increases fat storage.

leptin A protein produced by fat cells that decreases appetite and increases energy expenditure.

(hormone that suppresses appetite) and blood glucose concentrations

6. Cognitive influences: the gastric (stomach) stretch receptors and hormones like **cholecystokinin**, insulin, and leptin signal satiety and inhibit further food intake

7. Environmental influences: other factors such as portion size (normal versus "supersized"), ethnic and cultural standards, as well as socioeconomic status (financial ability, as well as having access to purchase a variety of foods) also have powerful effects on client's energy intake

Figure 11.4 shows the relative contribution of the components of **total energy expenditure (TEE)** spent in a day for an average sedentary 25-year-old adult.

Basal metabolism accounts for 60 to 75 percent of the total energy expenditure, whereas the thermic effect of the

⊚ **FIGURE 11.4 Components of total energy expenditure (TEE) for a sedentary individual.** (From Dunford, M., and J. A. Doyle. 2007. Figure 2.21 in *Nutrition for sport and exercise*. Belmont, CA: Wadsworth.)

process of digestion is about 10 percent. The amount of time spent in voluntary exercise represents the greatest variability depending on the individual activity patterns. The influence of adaptive thermogenesis or metabolic efficiency is real, but it is difficult to measure and can account for interindividual differences in energy expenditure.

Basal metabolic rate (BMR) is a measure of baseline metabolism conducted under standardized conditions (for example, quiet room; lying still; following 5-hour fast; the avoidance of caffeine, nicotine, and alcohol for 4 hours; and abstaining from exercise for at least 2 hours). Basal metabolism accounts for about two thirds of your body's energy expenditure each day and supports resting metabolic activities. **Resting metabolic rate (RMR)** is slightly higher than the BMR because it is usually measured or estimated while sitting at rest. Table 11.1 summarizes factors that influence the BMR.

The BMR is highest in clients who are growing (children and pregnant women) and those who have high amounts of lean body mass. Clients who have altered normal health status (such as fever, high stress, and hyperthyroidism) also have high BMRs, whereas individuals who have lost lean body mass or who are fasting or malnourished have lower BMRs. Before the development of blood tests, measuring BMR was the only method used to diagnose impaired metabolism. Notably, even if an individual is obese, the actual process of dieting and exercising as part of a weight-loss program causes the BMR to decrease.

(What is a possible genetic factor that may explain the difficulty that comes with controlling weight?)

Physical activity and exercise are the most variable and most changeable components of energy expenditure. As you have learned, you expend approximately 1 kcal/min of

Factor	Effect on BMR
Age	After physical maturity, BMR decreases with age.
Sex	Males have higher BMR than do females of equal size and weight.
Growth	BMR is higher during periods of growth.
Body weight	BMR increases with increased body weight.
Body shape	Tall, thin people have higher BMRs than do short, stocky people of equal weight.
Body composition	Because muscle requires more energy to maintain than does adipose tissue, people with lean tissue have higher BMRs than do people of equal weight with more adipose tissue.
Body temperature	Increased body temperature causes a transient increase in BMR.
Stress	Stress increases BMR.
Thyroid function	Elevated levels of thyroid hormones increase BMR, whereas low levels decrease BMR.
Energy restriction	Loss of body tissue associated with fasting and starvation decreases BMR.
Pregnancy	BMR increases during pregnancy.
Lactation	Milk synthesis increases BMR.

BMR, basal metabolic rate.
Source: McGuire, M., and K. A. Beerman. 2009. Table 8.3 in *Nutritional sciences*, 2nd ed. Belmont, CA: Brooks/Cole-Cengage Learning.

energy when sitting at rest, whereas various levels of exercise require 3 to 20⁺ kcal/min. Figure 11.5 shows the total energy expenditure for three different levels of exercise. Remember that the FITT (frequency, intensity, time, and type) of exercise influences energy expenditure, whereas the longer, more frequent, and more intense the activity, the more kilocalories will be expended.

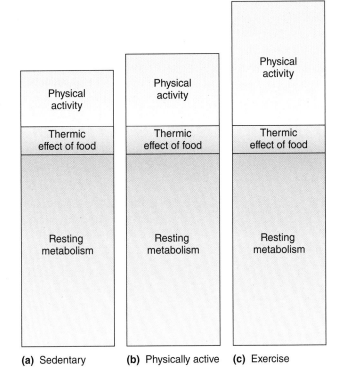

● **F I G U R E 11.5** **Total energy expenditure for three different levels of exercise.** (From Dunford, M., and J. A. Doyle. 2007. Figure 2.25 in *Nutrition for sport and exercise*. Belmont, CA: Wadsworth.)

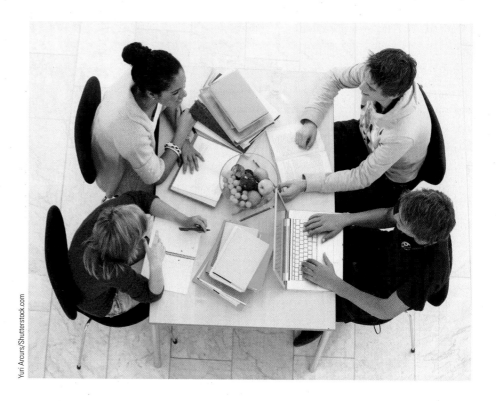

Yuri Arcurs/Shutterstock.com

HOTLINK *See the "Measurement of Moderate Physical Activity" symposium of papers in Medicine and Science in Sports and Exercise 32 (Suppl. 9), September 2000, for more information about physical activity/exercise and energy expenditure.*

thermic effect of food An estimate of the energy required to process food.

adaptive thermogenesis Adjustments to thermogenesis due to factors like environmental stress (hot or cold), injury, or changes in hormone regulation.

metabolic efficiency Primarily refers to the ability of the body to use fat and carbohydrates as fuel for energy expenditure.

The process of consuming food stimulates the RMR because of digestion and absorption. The acceleration of the RMR requires energy and produces heat; this is called the **thermic effect of food**. The thermic effect of food represents about 10 percent of energy intake and is influenced by factors such as meal size and frequency. The thermic effect of food may be accelerated if you consume several smaller meals per day versus one or two larger meals per day of equal total kilocalories, which means that skipping meals may not be an effective strategy for weight loss.

The additional energy spent when a client is adapting to change (such as beginning an exercise program, extreme cold, mental stress, trauma) or when the client expends energy more or less efficiently than others is termed **adaptive thermogenesis**, or **metabolic efficiency**. This component is variable and specific to each client, and is difficult to measure or estimate without highly controlled laboratory procedures.

Figure 11.6, as compared with Figure 11.1, shows a more realistic and complex example of the energy balance equation based on what you have learned. Based on the complexity of maintaining caloric intake and caloric expenditure, it is no wonder that healthy weight control can become a lifelong challenge for many adults (see Chapter 13 for more information).

Why does eating food affect an individual's BMR?

Energy storage

| Energy intake | Energy expenditure |

Influencing factors

Cognitive
Sensory
Food quality
Hunger signals
Satiety signals
Environment

Timing
Metabolic efficiency
Hormonal responses
Fatigue/recovery factors
Built environment

FIGURE 11.6 The simple energy (caloric) balance equation and various influencing factors. (© Cengage Learning 2013)

Estimating Energy Requirements

How many kilocalories does a competitor need to consume in a 4- to 6-hour leg of the Tour de France to maintain energy balance? You might be surprised, but it has been estimated as high as 9,000 kcal/day. It is no wonder that in extreme conditions (high heat and humidity) cyclists can "hit the wall" or "bonk" if they become dehydrated or cannot maintain their energy needs. How much energy can a trained cyclist store? Most can store approximately 2,000 kilocalories as glycogen, or stored carbohydrate (which is expended at approximately 1,000+ kcal/hour during a Tour de France stage) in the liver and muscle. This stored glycogen can become easily depleted if cyclists do not constantly replace their carbohydrate needs during the race stage.

To maintain the increased energy requirements of your clients as they start or maintain their exercise programs, you will need to ensure that they are getting the appropriate amount of total kilocalories per day, as well as the appropriate portion of nutrients as a percentage of their daily intake. Clients who do not meet their energy requirements (for example, 60 grams carbohydrate per hour depending on body weight) can become glycogen depleted and can develop the symptoms of overtraining.

Table 11.2 provides some examples of the total caloric intake needs of different individuals participating in various levels of exercise. The estimates for daily caloric intake in Table 11.2 are only estimates, but they provide specific examples of how the daily caloric needs of your clients can vary dramatically based on the intensity and duration of an exercise program. By understanding energy balance, you can help your clients understand their energy needs and how they can balance those needs.

TABLE 11.2 Total Energy Requirements of Individuals at Varying Amounts of Exercise

Individual	Total Daily Calories for Energy Balance
25-year-old healthy sedentary man	~2,400 kcal
25-year-old healthy sedentary woman	~2,000 kcal
25-year-old healthy active man	~3,000 kcal
25-year-old healthy active woman	~2,400 kcal
25-year-old male professional boxer	~5,000 kcal
25-year-old female collegiate dancer	~3,000 kcal
25-year-old female elite marathoner	~3,500 kcal
25-year-old male elite marathoner	~5,000 kcal
25-year-old male Tour de France cyclist	~9,000 kcal

Estimates from http://www.choosemyplate.gov. "Measurement of Moderate Physical Activity." 2000. *Medicine and Science in Sports and Exercise*, 32(9), S439–S516.

Nutrient Balance

Nutrient balance involves ensuring that your clients try to consume the appropriate amounts (as a percentage of total caloric intake or in grams) of carbohydrates, fats, and proteins. Nutrition experts have produced standards that define the amounts of energy, nutrients, vitamins, minerals, and fluids that help promote functional health. The recommendations are called the **dietary reference intakes (DRIs)** and are designed for healthy people.

The DRIs include the **recommended daily allowances (RDA)**. The RDA is the average daily amount of a nutrient for dietary intake by an individual. The RDA is set within a range of appropriate and reasonable

dietary reference intake (DRI) A set of nutrient intake values for healthy people in the United States and Canada.

recommended daily allowances (RDA) A goal for dietary intake of various nutrients based on the U.S. Dietary Guidelines.

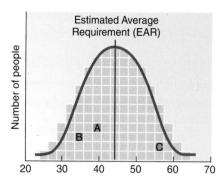

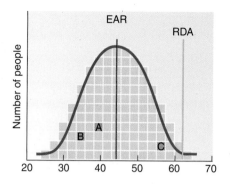

The Estimated Average Requirement (EAR) for a nutrient is the amount that covers half of the population (shown here by the red line).

The Recommended Dietary Allowance (RDA) for a nutrient (shown here in green) is set well above the EAR, covering about 98% of the population.

FIGURE 11.7 **Comparison of recommended intakes of nutrients and energy.** (From Whitney, E. N., and S. R. Rolfes. 2010. Figure 1.5 in *Understanding nutrition*, 12 ed. Belmont, CA: Wadsworth.)

adequate intake The average daily amount of a nutrient that is thought to be adequate to maintain a healthy criterion level if the RDA is not known.

complex carbohydrate Consist of large molecules composed of chains of monosaccharides called *polysaccharides* (these include glycogen, starches, and fibers). Examples of complex carbohydrates include vegetables, breads, cereals, pasta, rice, and beans.

intakes between toxicity and deficiency. Sometimes the DRI committee sets an **adequate intake** instead of an RDA because there may not be enough scientific evidence for a specific nutrient to determine an RDA. Figure 11.7 presents examples of the comparison of recommended intakes of nutrients and energy.

Oftentimes when individuals (for example, athletes) engage in exercise, they think that they need to consume far more than the RDA levels for various nutrients because they are expending more energy than sedentary individuals. In reality, if your clients develop and use a dietary plan based on the principles of the Center for Nutrition Policy and Promotion, an organization of the U.S. Department of Agriculture (http://www.choosemyplate.gov), all they need to do is consume more calories to meet their nutrition needs even if they are very active.

Little scientific evidence has been reported to support that dietary supplements (powders, shakes, vitamins, and so on) improve performance in athletes or others engaged in high intensities and long durations of their exercise.

Carbohydrates

Carbohydrates are sugars, starches, and fibers found in food. **Simple carbohydrates** include the monosaccharides (that is,

simple sugars such as glucose, fructose, and galactose) and disaccharides (such as maltose, sucrose, and lactose). Examples of simple carbohydrates include fruits, candy, cookies, and sodas. In contrast, the **complex carbohydrates** consist of large molecules composed of chains of monosaccharides called *polysaccharides* (these include glycogen, starches, and fibers). Examples of complex carbohydrates include vegetables, breads, cereals, pasta, rice, and beans. You have already studied the metabolism of carbohydrates in Chapters 4 and 5. Also, review Figure 2.2 for the various contributions of energy sources to muscle activity during different levels of intensity and recovery from exercise.

As discussed earlier, carbohydrates provide the primary fuel for your body to form glucose and store glycogen. Carbohydrates are important for proper nutrition for the following reasons:

Prime energy source: On average, it is recommended that carbohydrates should be between 45 and 65 percent of a person's daily dietary intake. As mentioned previously, you can store approximately 2,000 kilocalories glucose and glycogen, which makes carbohydrate a prime energy source because it provides fuel to your anaerobic and aerobic energy pathways. The actual percentage may vary

simple carbohydrate Include the monosaccharides (that is, simple sugars such as glucose, fructose, and galactose) and disaccharides (such as maltose, sucrose, and lactose).

depending on the FITT and amount of exercise a client does. For example, an endurance athlete (who expends approximately 3,000–5,000 kcal/day at high intensities) will need higher percentages of carbohydrate (60–65 percent) as compared with an individual who may be trying to add mass by participating solely in resistance training (45–50 percent). The ability to replenish glycogen is also important for the restoration process. Often coaches and other exercise professionals forget that clients who participate in anaerobic activities also have to worry about depleting their glycogen stores. Usually they are aware that this is a constant problem for endurance athletes, but research also shows that participating for 1 hour in activities that have a majority of anaerobic exercise can significantly lower (not necessarily deplete) glycogen stores.

Drive metabolism: Consuming adequate amounts of carbohydrate spares the breakdown of protein for energy and is the only fuel that can be used to generate ATP both from anaerobic and aerobic metabolism (see Figure 11.8). Although protein can be converted metabolically to produce glucose, if needed, it can be used by the body for tissue building and maintenance. In athletes who train in excess of their energy intake or under starvation conditions, as well as in anorexics who also practice bulimia, the breakdown of protein results in a negative nitrogen balance resulting in a loss of muscle and bone mass. In the athlete, this will result in stress fractures in the bones

that receive the greatest wear and tear. Furthermore, if too little carbohydrate is available to drive metabolism, fat is not metabolized effectively and produces fat fragments that form ketone bodies, which accumulate in the blood causing **ketosis** (an acid–base imbalance). This is a common comorbid metabolic condition of individuals with type 1 diabetes. Consuming too much carbohydrate in terms of total required daily calories can result in the conversion of carbohydrates to fat, which is stored in the adipose tissue of the body. Clearly, this is one of the primary factors in the increase in our population's obesity, especially in our children.

Maintain homeostasis: All the cells in your body depend on glucose (carbohydrate) as a fuel, and the brain and central nervous system depend almost exclusively on glucose for energy (see Chapters 4 and 5). More recently, another source of carbohydrate for the brain is lactate, especially in high rates of energy usage such as the endurance events of rowing, swimming, running, and bicycling. A new avenue of research identifies that endurance performances can be limited by the brain becoming fatigued (known as *central fatigue*) because of a lack of carbohydrate being available. If the blood glucose concentrations decline to less than normal concentrations, you will feel dizzy and weak and you may faint (syncope). If glucose concentrations

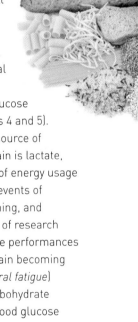

ketosis High concentration of ketone bodies associated with incomplete fat metabolism that can lower pH and produce acid–base imbalances.

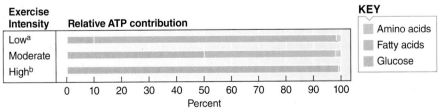

Exercise Intensity	Relative ATP contribution

KEY
- Amino acids
- Fatty acids
- Glucose

Low[a]
Moderate
High[b]

0 10 20 30 40 50 60 70 80 90 100
Percent

[a]Aerobic pathways predominate
[b]Anaerobic pathways predominate

FIGURE 11.8 Relative contributions of energy sources to varying intensities of exercise. (From McGuire, M., and K. A. Beerman. 2006. Figure 5 in *Nutritional sciences.* Belmont. CA: Brooks/Cole-Cengage Learning.)

glycemic index A way of classifying
foods according to their potential to
increase blood glucose (generally the
lower the index, the better the glucose
control).

increase above normal, it can cause
you to feel fatigued. Figure 11.9 shows
how blood glucose homeostasis is
primarily maintained by the hormones
insulin and glucagon. When blood
glucose regulation fails (too high or too
low), two conditions can result:
diabetes or hypoglycemia. Eating
balanced meals at regular intervals
throughout the day helps your body
maintain glucose homeostasis. A diet
rich in complex carbohydrates,
including fibers, and small amounts of
fat helps slow digestion and the
absorption of carbohydrates so that
glucose enters the blood more

gradually. This can help prevent
self-induced hypoglycemia. Paying
attention to the **glycemic index** of the
types of foods you consume can also be
helpful in preventing surges in blood
glucose absorption. The glycemic index
is a way of classifying foods according
to their potential to increase blood
glucose (generally the lower the index,
the better the glucose control). Figure
11.10 illustrates the ranking of selected
foods by their glycemic index.

HOTLINK *Review Chapters 6A and 6B for
detailed discussions on maintaining metabolic
homeostasis.*

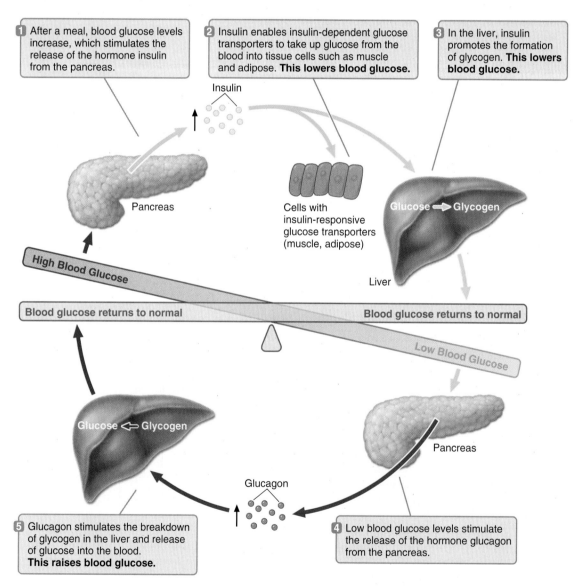

FIGURE 11.9 Hormonal regulation of glucose. (From McGuire, M., and K. A. Beerman. 2009. Figure
4.18 in *Nutritional sciences*, 2nd ed. Belmont, CA: Brooks/Cole-Cengage Learning.)

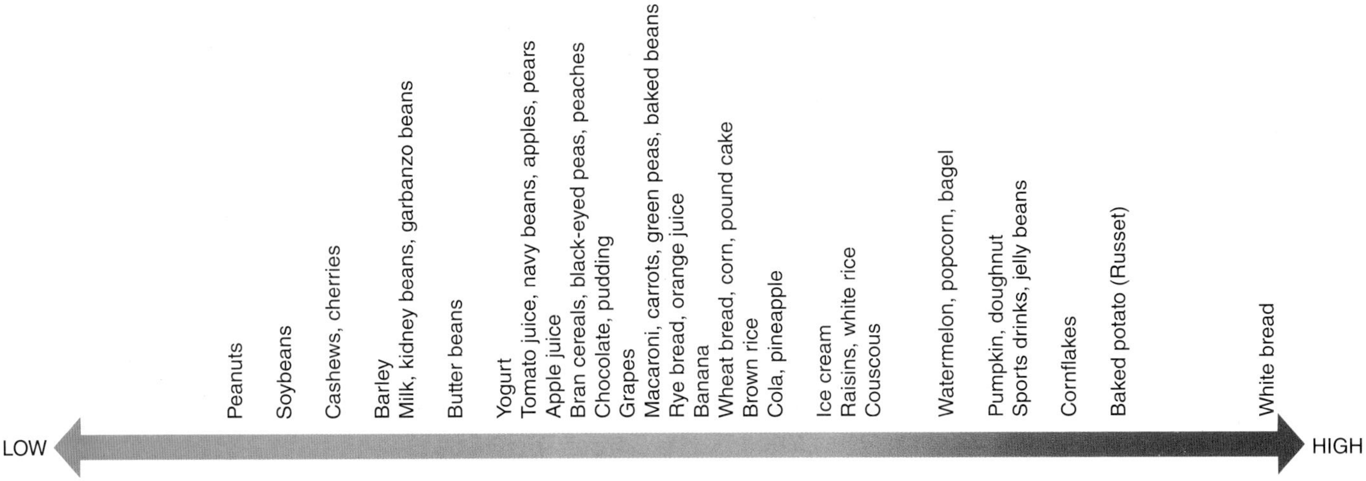

LOW ← → **HIGH**

Glycemic index of selected foods (from low to high): Peanuts; Soybeans; Cashews, cherries; Barley; Milk, kidney beans, garbanzo beans; Butter beans; Yogurt; Tomato juice, navy beans, apples, pears; Apple juice; Bran cereals, black-eyed peas, peaches; Chocolate, pudding; Grapes; Macaroni, carrots, green peas, baked beans; Rye bread, orange juice; Banana; Wheat bread, corn, pound cake; Brown rice; Cola, pineapple; Ice cream; Raisins, white rice; Couscous; Watermelon, popcorn, bagel; Pumpkin, doughnut; Sports drinks, jelly beans; Cornflakes; Baked potato (Russet); White bread.

FIGURE 11.10 Glycemic index of selected foods. (From Whitney. E. N., and S. R. Rolfes. 2010. Figure 4.13 in *Understanding nutrition*, 12 ed. Belmont, CA: Wadsworth.)

Other General Recommendations for Carbohydrate Intake

It is best to consume more complex carbohydrates than simple ones because they are absorbed more slowly by your body and contain more vitamins. The following list contains foods high in carbohydrates from a variety of sources:

Grains	Fruits	Vegetables	Milk Sources
Bagels	Apples	Carrots	Yogurt
Bread	Bananas	Corn	Milk (2 percent or less)
Cereals	Fruit juices	Green beans	Cheese
Pasta noodles	Oranges	Potatoes	Pudding
Popcorn	Pears	Broccoli	

Dietary fiber (like grains, stems, roots, nuts, seeds, and fruit coverings) is found in complex carbohydrates and is important and healthy for you to consume for good digestive health. The current recommended dietary intake is 14 g/1,000 kcal, and like all nutrition recommendations, the concept of "more is better" may only be good up to a point because excessive fiber intake can cause gastrointestinal distress and limit absorption of nutrients. However, diets rich in dietary fiber have been shown to have a number of beneficial health effects, as highlighted in the *2010 Dietary Guidelines for Americans*. In summary, adequate fiber intake can:

- Foster weight management
- Decrease blood cholesterol
- Help prevent colon cancer
- Help prevent and control diabetes
- Help prevent and alleviate hemorrhoids
- Help prevent appendicitis and diverticulosis

Finally, diets that are high in the consumption of added sugars can promote dental caries and can make it more difficult for your clients to consume enough nutrients daily without gaining weight.

Fats

Fats or lipids are triglycerides (fats and oils), phospholipids, and sterols found in food and in the body. **Triglycerides** are the chief form of fat in the diet and the major storage form of fat in the body. Triglycerides are stored in adipose tissue, liver, and skeletal muscle. They are composed of a molecule of glycerol with three fatty acids attached, which may contain a mixture of more than one type of fatty acid. Depending

triglyceride Lipid-containing glycerol bonded to three fatty acids; the chief form of fat in the diet and the major storage form of fat in the body.

saturated fat A fat that contains no double bonds between carbons.

monounsaturated fat A fat containing only one double bond between carbons. Olive oil is an example.

polyunsaturated fat A fatty acid with two or more double bonds between carbons.

omega-3 fat A polyunsaturated fatty aid in which the first double bond is three carbons away from the methyl (CH₃) end of carbon chain.

omega-6 fat A polyunsaturated fatty aid in which the first double bond is six carbons away from the methyl (CH₃) end of carbon chain.

trans fat Fatty acids with hydrogens on opposite sides of the double bonds.

phospholipid A fat that is similar to a triglyceride but contains phosphate.

sterol A fat whose core structure contains four rings.

lecithin A phospholipid important for cell membrane function.

on the number of double bonds between carbon atoms, fatty acids may be:

Saturated fat (no double bonds)

Monounsaturated fat (one double bond)

Polyunsaturated fat (more than one double bond, depending on the location of the double bonds): Polyunsaturated fats may be:

   Omega-3 fats (first double bond 3 carbons away from methyl end)

   Omega-6 fats (first double bond 6 carbons away from methyl end)

Trans fat: a monounsaturated fat that is formed by hydrogenation or the adding of hydrogen atoms to solidify or harden soft fats or oils.

Figure 11.11 compares these dietary fats.

Phospholipids and **sterols** make up only 5 percent of the lipids in the diet. **Lecithin** is the best known phospholipid, and like other phospholipids, it is important for cell membrane structure. Sterols have a multiple-ring structure that differs from

the structure of other lipids. Cholesterol is the most commonly known sterol, but others include the bile acids, testosterone, cortisol, and vitamin D. Only foods derived from animal sources and high in saturated fat contain cholesterol (like meats, eggs, fish, poultry, and dairy products). Cholesterol is produced metabolically in the body, as well as ingested in the diet. The importance of blood cholesterol concentrations and the association with the development of atherosclerosis is discussed later in this section.

Fat metabolism was discussed in Chapters 4 and 5. As you may remember, fats are an important fuel for your body because they yield 9 kcal/g. Fats are important for proper nutrition for the following reasons:

Energy source: On average, it is recommended that fat in your diet should range from 20 to 35 percent of an adult's daily dietary intake. This percentage varies slightly for teenagers and young adults (see *the 2010 Dietary*

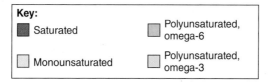

Animal fats and the tropical oils of coconut and palm are mostly **saturated** fatty acids.

| Coconut oil |
| Butter |
| Beef tallow |
| Palm oil |
| Lard |

Some vegetable oils, such as olive and canola, are rich in **monounsaturated** fatty acids.

| Olive oil |
| Canola oil |
| Peanut oil |
| Safflower oil |

Many vegetable oils are rich in **polyunsaturated** fatty acids.

| Flaxseed oil |
| Walnut oil |
| Sunflower oil |
| Corn oil |
| Soybean oil |
| Cottonseed oil |

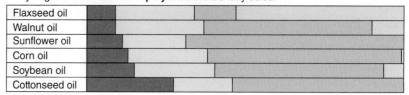

FIGURE 11.11 Comparison of dietary fats. (From Whitney, E. N., and S. R. Rolfes. 2010. Figure 5.6 in *Understanding nutrition,* 12 ed. Belmont, CA: Wadsworth.)

Guidelines for Americans for specifics). The actual percentage may vary depending on the FITT and amount of exercise a client performs, as well as the client's goals, such as a desire to reduce risk for a second heart attack or to generally improve health. For example, individuals who have had a previous heart attack should do all they can to reduce their saturated fat intake, and may even be encouraged by their physician to limit their fat intake to 10 to 15 percent of their daily caloric intake, as recommended in the popular Pritikin diet plan. Clients who are just trying to improve their general health and who are at low risk for chronic disease would be best advised to aim for a 20 to 35 percent goal for the daily intake of fat.

Often athletes or those interested in high levels of performance (where the performance is very dependent on weight carried because excess fat would limit performance in dance, gymnastics, or running) will try to limit their daily fat intake to 20 percent or less to minimize their body weight (body fat). Although this might appear to be an effective strategy, it may actually reduce the client's testosterone levels, which are dependent on daily fat intake. Athletes, or those interested in high-performance exercise, would be best advised to consume at least 25 percent of their daily caloric needs in the form of fat.

Unlike carbohydrate, you can store approximately 100,000 kilocalories fat as triglycerides in adipose tissue depending on your body size and the percentage of body fat that you have (normally about 15 percent for 21-year-old men and about 25 percent for 21-year-old women). A pound of body fat provides 3,500 kilocalories energy. Therefore, theoretically, if you burn 100 kcal/mile run (average), you would have to run 35 miles to burn a pound of fat, which illustrates that trying to lose weight just by increasing energy expenditure may not be effective for most individuals. If you diet by starving yourself, the stored body fat becomes the main source of energy. In addition, unless there is a source of carbohydrate metabolism, the overutilization of fat as fuel causes ketosis. The presence of high concentrations of ketoacids in the blood can be injurious to brain function because the brain's main source of energy is carbohydrate. This can be a problem to a tightly regulated type 1 diabetic.

Insulator/Protection: Subcutaneous fat helps insulate the body against extreme cold temperatures and provides protection to your vital organs. When body fat exceeds average values (about 15 percent for 21-year-old men and about 25 percent for 21-year-old women), it inhibits heat release and presents several physical challenges such as reduced range of motion, decreased speed, as well as health problems such as hypertension, sleep apnea, increased risk for type 2 diabetes, and heart disease. For example, investigators wanting to develop an animal model of type 2 diabetes, or non–insulin-dependent diabetes, for the study of exercise responses use a super-high-fat diet. Within 1 to 2 weeks, the muscle uptake of glucose in response to insulin released from the pancreas becomes impaired. Over the next few weeks, more and more insulin is released to enable the muscle to take up glucose from the blood. Soon the production of insulin from the Islet cells is fatigued (reduced) and exhausted, which leads to type 2 diabetes. In this way, investigators have produced fat rats, rabbits, dogs, and pigs for the study of type 2 diabetes. In contrast, increased subcutaneous fat can help long-distance swimmers maintain their core temperature in cold water, which can actually improve performance.

Recently, the topic of overweight adolescent U.S. football players has been highlighted by the national media because many athletes are trying to increase their mass significantly (≥300 pounds), perhaps in response to the increased size of many professional football players (numerous linemen now weigh more than 400 pounds). The rationale is linked to the concept that the more mass one has, the stronger one is and the additional mass will improve performance and enhance the chances of receiving a collegiate scholarship. Realistically, however, only about 1 percent of all high-school football players receive collegiate scholarships, which means that many athletic adolescents are becoming overweight and obese prematurely, and are at risk for type 2 diabetes. As you have learned, carrying too much body fat (obesity) is a current worldwide health challenge for exercise science professionals.

(Explain the explosive population growth of people with type 2 diabetes.)

Vitamin carrier and satiety factor: Dietary fat is important for the absorption of fat-soluble vitamins (A, D, E, and K) and helping us feel satisfied or full after eating. If clients limit their dietary fat intake to less than the recommended levels (20–35 percent), they may increase their risk for vitamin deficiency and affect their feelings of satiety.

Other General Recommendations for Fat Intake

Dietary therapy and recommendations for increased physical activity or exercise have been used as effective strategies to positively influence plasma lipids and lipoproteins since the early 1960s. As early as 1961, an ad hoc committee of the American Heart Association released an updated report about the possible relation of dietary fat to heart attacks and stroke that provided the following recommendations:

- Overweight persons should decrease their caloric intake and attempt to achieve a desirable body weight.
- The composition of the diet should be altered by reducing intakes of total fats, saturated fats, and cholesterol, and by increasing intakes of polyunsaturated fats.
- Weight reduction should be facilitated by regular moderate exercise.
- Men at increased risk for coronary heart disease should pay particular attention to dietary alteration.
- For those at high risk, dietary changes should be carried out with medical supervision.

With the increased public awareness of the importance of controlling lipids and lipoproteins, manufacturers have eagerly made nutritional and exercise claims about how their products help reduce or control cholesterol concentrations in the blood. These claims are often reported in various media formats, and may or may not be accurate in regard to cholesterol regulation. Many of your future clients will be concerned about their blood cholesterol, as well as the amount of body fat they are carrying. The following section highlights general information about how compliance with recommended dietary and exercise guidelines can positively influence the functional health of your clients.

HOTLINK *See Chapter 13 for more information on the link between dietary guidelines, exercise, and weight control.*

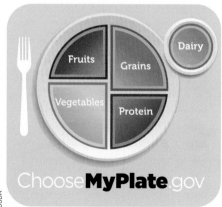

The manipulation of lipids and lipoproteins has become the major established treatment for atherosclerosis since the 1990s. For example, many of your clients will be taking prescribed cholesterol-lowering medications (like statins), which can influence how you will manage their exercise programs. Yet, numerous unresolved issues remain about how changes in the diet and/or exercise patterns can favorably alter lipid and lipoprotein values.

The major plasma lipids, including cholesterol and triglycerides, are transported in the form of lipoprotein complexes. The plasma lipoproteins transport both endogenously synthesized products and exogenously ingested dietary lipids. The **plasma lipoproteins** are clusters of lipids associated with proteins that serve as transport vehicles for lipids in the lymph and blood. They can be classified into the following classes by their gravitational density, size, and composition. These classifications are shown in Figure 11.12:

Chylomicrons: transport lipids from the intestinal cells to the rest of the body

Very-low-density lipoprotein cholesterol (VLDL-C): made primarily by liver cells to transport lipids to various tissues in the body and are composed primarily of triglycerides

Low-density lipoprotein cholesterol (LDL-C): type of lipoprotein that is derived from VLDLs as VLDL

plasma lipoprotein Clusters of lipids associated with proteins that serve as transport vehicles for lipids in the lymph and blood.

chylomicron Type of lipoprotein that transfers lipids from the intestinal cells to the rest of the body.

very-low-density lipoprotein cholesterol (VLDL-C) Type of lipoprotein made primarily by liver cells to transport lipids to various tissues in the body; composed primarily of triglycerides.

low-density lipoprotein cholesterol (LDL-C) Type of lipoprotein that is derived from VLDLs as VLDL triglycerides are removed and broken down; composed primarily of cholesterol.

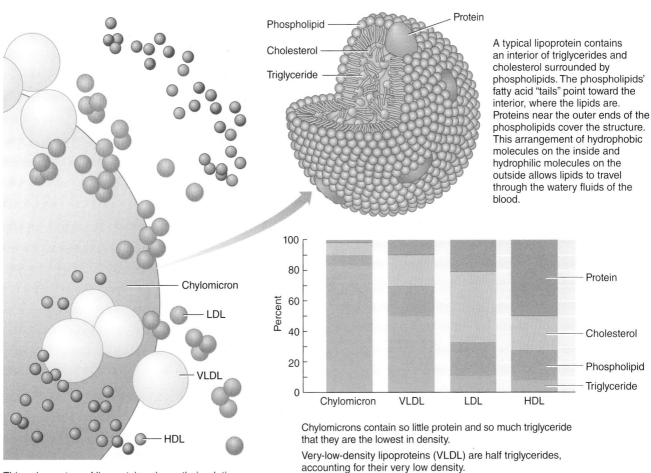

A typical lipoprotein contains an interior of triglycerides and cholesterol surrounded by phospholipids. The phospholipids' fatty acid "tails" point toward the interior, where the lipids are. Proteins near the outer ends of the phospholipids cover the structure. This arrangement of hydrophobic molecules on the inside and hydrophilic molecules on the outside allows lipids to travel through the watery fluids of the blood.

This solar system of lipoproteins shows their relative sizes. Notice how large the fat-filled chylomicron is compared with the others and how the others get progressively smaller as their proportion of fat declines and protein increases.

Chylomicrons contain so little protein and so much triglyceride that they are the lowest in density.

Very-low-density lipoproteins (VLDL) are half triglycerides, accounting for their very low density.

Low-density lipoproteins (LDL) are half cholesterol, accounting for their implication in heart disease.

High-density lipoproteins (HDL) are half protein, accounting for their high density.

FIGURE 11.12 Sizes and comparisons of lipoproteins. (From Whitney. E. N., and S. R. Rolfes. 2010. Figure 5.18 in *Understanding nutrition,* 12 ed. Belmont, CA: Wadsworth.)

triglycerides are removed and broken
down; composed primarily of cholesterol

**High-density lipoprotein cholesterol
(HDL-C)**: type of lipoprotein that
transports cholesterol back to the liver
from the cells; composed primarily of
protein

Four major enzymes that significantly influence lipid metabolism are:

Lipoprotein lipase: a lipolytic enzyme
that controls triglyceride hydrolysis and
is the rate-limiting step in the uptake of
lipoprotein, triglyceride, and free fatty
acids into adipose tissue and muscle

Hepatic lipase: interacts with lipoproteins in the liver and may play a role in
the reconversion of HDL-C

Cholesterol ester transfer protein: has
been linked to HDL particles and is one
of several transfer proteins that
mediates the transfer of esterified
cholesterol from HDL-C to VLDL and is
involved in the formation of a subfraction of HDL-C

Lecithin cholesterol acetyltransferase:
catalyzes esterified cholesterol while
binding to HDL

Apolipoproteins are also important to the
understanding of plasma lipid and lipoprotein metabolism. The apolipoproteins
regulate biochemical reactions by stabilizing lipoprotein particles, providing recognition sites for cell membranes and by acting
as cofactors for enzymes. The apolipoproteins determine the structure and regulatory functions of lipoproteins. Most apolipoproteins are synthesized by the liver or
intestines.

The LDL-C supplies cholesterol to extrahepatic cells where it is used for cell
membrane and steroid hormone synthesis.
Some of the LDL-C is degraded by scaven-
ger cells, which help control high plasma
concentrations. The liver removes the remaining circulating LDL-C. Thus, the LDL-
C concentration depends on the balance
between the liver's production of VLDL-C,
the partitioning of VLDL-C between hepatic
removal and conversion to LDL-C, as well
as the activity of LDL-C receptors.

It is thought that HDL-C serves as the
cholesterol acceptor in reverse transport
and excretion of cholesterol from the tissues. Direct production of HDL-C occurs in
both the liver and the intestine. The HDL-C
binds unesterified cholesterol and delivers
cholesterol esters to the liver and VLDL-
C. Some of the cholesterol is delivered to
the liver by HDL-C and is excreted into the
gallbladder as bile. HDL-C can be subdivided into numerous subfractions.

Low concentrations of HDL-C (<35 mg/
dl) are as predictive for coronary heart
disease as high blood pressure, cigarette
smoking, or diabetes. The major causes of
reduced HDL-C include cigarette smoking,
obesity, lack of exercise, androgenic and
related steroids (that is, anabolic steroids),
beta-adrenergic blocking agents, hypertriglyceridemia, and genetic factors.

A variety of genetic disorders in lipoprotein metabolism have been identified.
These include abnormal functions with all
the apolipoproteins and enzymes, as well
as certain cell surface receptors that bind
apolipoproteins. Most of these disorders
are fairly rare, but they are of clinical significance because they can produce severe
hyperlipidemia and predispose individuals
to premature coronary heart disease.

The aging process itself decreases the
activity of LDL-C receptors and causes
the Total cholesterol and LDL-C plasma
levels to increase. The mechanism for the
increases in LDL-C as we get older is currently unknown, but it may be because of
cellular aging or a decrease in the body's
overall metabolic rate.

Lipid/lipoprotein metabolism is regulated by a variety of physiologic variables
that can affect the synthesis and catabolism of the various particles. These variables include aging, genetics, hormones,
diet composition, calorie intake, alcohol
consumption, cigarette smoking, medication, body composition, and exercise.

Diet modification and regular exercise
are typically recommended by physicians
as important steps for adults to reduce
triglycerides and LDL-C initially, or as an
adjunct to lipid-lowering medications.
The rationale for this advice is based on

epidemiologic evidence, which indicates that there is a direct correlation between total cholesterol values and coronary heart disease. When total cholesterol level exceeds 240 mg/dl, an individual has approximately a twofold increase in coronary heart disease risk.

Reducing the LDL-C level in men can reduce coronary heart disease incidence and actually has been found to slow or produce a regression in coronary atherosclerosis. Women are also at high coronary heart disease risk when LDL-C concentrations are increased, but before menopause their LDL-C values are lower than those found for men. After menopause, their risk for coronary heart disease increases because of the loss of their estrogen-stimulated LDL receptor activity.

An 8 to 9 percent reduction in total cholesterol is required to significantly reduce the incidence of coronary heart disease mortality. If cholesterol level is decreased by 10 to 15 percent with diet, exercise, and medications, coronary heart disease risk can be reduced by 20 to 30 percent. Men and women who have total cholesterol level greater than 240 mg/dl and who engage in regular exercise have significantly reduced mortality for coronary heart disease than those who are less fit.

Dietary modification and regular exercise (which can raise HDL-C) provide the foundation for initial and long-term interventions for hyperlipidemia, because they can have significant positive affects on lipid and lipoprotein metabolism, and positively influence the metabolic syndrome. For most Americans, diet modification and regular exercise can help reduce cholesterol, and thus coronary heart disease risk, even when they are used as adjunct therapy to medication. Diet modification and exercise are also more economical than medication therapy and may help reduce the dosage of medication required for effectiveness.

(How does participating in a regular exercise program help control abnormal lipid levels?)

Protein

Proteins are compounds composed of carbon, hydrogen, oxygen, and nitrogen atoms arranged into amino acids linked in a chain. Some amino acids also contain sulfur atoms. Amino acids are the building blocks for proteins that provide vital structural and working substances in all cells, not just muscle cells. Protein is an important nutrient, but only one of those needed to maintain good health.

Nonessential amino acids (about 11) are those that the body can synthesize itself from foods consumed or from metabolic action. **Essential amino acids** (9) are those that the body cannot synthesize in sufficient quantity to meet its needs. Protein is the primary fuel for your body to grow, repair, or replace tissue. Proteins are versatile and sometimes are used by our body to facilitate or regulate, and other times are used to provide structure. The primary functions of proteins in the body are summarized in Table 11.3.

General Recommendations

The recommended daily dietary intake for protein is 0.8 g/kg body weight or between 10 and 35 percent of your total caloric needs depending on your dietary intake percentages of carbohydrates and fats. High-quality proteins provide all the essential amino acids needed to support your body's needs, whereas low-quality proteins do not. Protein quality is influenced by the protein's digestibility and its amino acid composition. Table 11.4 contains the recommended protein intake for active individuals such as athletes.

Generally, foods derived from animals (meat, fish, poultry, cheese, eggs, yogurt, and milk) provide high-quality proteins, whereas proteins from plant sources (vegetables, nuts, seeds, grains, and legumes) are more diverse in quality and usually lack one or more essential amino acids. Vegetarians can receive all the amino acids they need over the course of a day if they eat a variety of grains, legumes, seed, nuts, and vegetables. However, they can develop protein deficiency if they rely too much on

nonessential amino acid Amino acids that the body can synthesize itself from foods consumed or from metabolic action.

essential amino acid Amino acid that the body cannot synthesize in sufficient quantity to meet its needs.

TABLE 11.3 Functions of Proteins

Growth and maintenance	Proteins form integral parts of most body structures such as skin, tendons, membranes, muscles, organs, and bones. As such, they support the growth and repair of body tissues.
Enzymes	Proteins facilitate chemical reactions.
Hormones	Proteins regulate body processes. (Some, but not all, hormones are proteins.)
Fluid balance	Proteins help to maintain the volume and composition of body fluids.
Acid–base balance	Proteins help to maintain the acid–base balance of body fluids by acting as buffers.
Transportation	Proteins transport substances, such as lipids, vitamins, minerals, and oxygen, around the body.
Antibodies	Proteins inactivate foreign invaders, thus protecting the body against diseases.
Energy and glucose	Proteins provide some fuel, and glucose if needed, for the body's energy needs.

Source: Whitney, E. N., and S. R. Rolfes. 2010. *Understanding nutrition*, 12 ed. Belmont, CA: Wadsworth.

fruits and vegetables and do not diversify their protein intake.

A key point concerning the recommended daily dietary intake of protein is to encourage athletes and nonathletes alike to consume the appropriate amount of high-quality proteins without having to rely on supplemental sources or megadoses to enhance muscle development (see Chapter 12 for more information on ergogenic aids).

Vitamin Balance

Vitamins are essential nutrients required in small amounts to perform specific functions that promote growth, reproduction, or the maintenance of health and life. Vitamins do not contain calories and, therefore, do not provide your body with energy. However, they are also important in disease prevention based on their bioavailability or

rate at which they can be absorbed and used. Vitamin deficiencies can occur over time but are rare in the industrialized nations, and typically are seen only in starvation or disease states. However, in nations that have poor availability of dietary proteins from animal meat and fish, vitamin deficiency diseases remain prevalent.

HOTLINK *See Chapter 12 for more information on vitamin supplementation.*

Vitamins are classified as fat-soluble or water-soluble. **Fat-soluble vitamins** are carried by fat in your food and can be stored in large quantities. The fat-soluble vitamins are A, D, E, and K. **Water-soluble vitamins** include the B complex vitamins and vitamin C. They need to be replaced regularly by consuming nutritious foods.

Table 11.5 summarizes the major functions of vitamins in the body. Notice that

fat-soluble vitamin Vitamins carried by fat in your food and can be stored in large quantities. The fat-soluble vitamins are A, D, E, and K.

water-soluble vitamin Those that include the B complex vitamins and vitamin C. They need to be replaced regularly by consuming nutritious foods.

TABLE 11.4 Recommended Daily Intake of Protein

	Recommendations (g/kg/day)	Protein Intakes (g/day)	
		Males	Females
RDA for adults	0.8	5.6	44
Recommended intake for power (strength or speed) athletes	1.2–1.7	84–119	66–94
Recommended intake for endurance athletes	1.2–1.4	84–98	66–77
U.S. average intake		102	70

Daily protein intakes are based on a 70-kilogram (154-pound) man and 55-kilogram (121-pound) woman.
Source: Whitney, E. N., and S. R. Rolfes. 2010. Table 14.5 in *Understanding nutrition*, 12 ed. Belmont, CA: Wadsworth.

TABLE 11.5 Major Functions of Vitamins

Nutrient	Good Sources	Major Functions	Deficiency Symptoms
Vitamin A	Milk, cheese, eggs, liver, yellow and dark green fruits and vegetables	Required for healthy bones, teeth, skin, gums, and hair; maintenance of inner mucous membranes, thereby increasing resistance to infection; adequate vision in dim light.	Night blindness; decreased growth; decreased resistance to infection; rough, dry skin
Vitamin D	Fortified milk, cod liver oil, salmon, tuna, egg yolk	Necessary for bones and teeth; needed for calcium and phosphorus absorption.	Rickets (bone softening), fractures, muscle spasms
Vitamin E	Vegetable oils, yellow and green leafy vegetables, margarine, wheat germ, whole-grain breads and cereals	Related to oxidation and normal muscle and red blood cell chemistry.	Leg cramps, red blood cell breakdown
Vitamin K	Green leafy vegetables, cauliflower, cabbage, eggs, peas, potatoes	Essential for normal blood clotting.	Hemorrhaging
Vitamin B_1 (Thiamin)	Whole-grain or enriched bread, lean meats and poultry, fish, liver, pork, poultry, organ meats, legumes, nuts, dried yeast	Assists in proper use of carbohydrates, normal functioning of nervous system, maintaining good appetite.	Loss of appetite, nausea, confusion, cardiac abnormalities, muscle spasms
Vitamin B_2 (Riboflavin)	Eggs, milk, leafy green vegetables, whole grains, lean meats, dried beans and peas	Contributes to energy release from carbohydrates, fats, and proteins; needed for normal growth and development, good vision, and healthy skin.	Cracking of the corners of the mouth, inflammation of the skin, impaired vision
Vitamin B_6 (Pyridoxine)	Vegetables, meats, whole grain cereals, soybeans, peanuts, potatoes	Necessary for protein and fatty acids metabolism and for normal red blood cell formation.	Depression, irritability, muscle spasms, nausea
Vitamin B_{12}	Meat, poultry, fish, liver, organ meats, eggs, shellfish, milk, cheese	Required for normal growth, red blood cell formation, nervous system and digestive tract functioning.	Impaired balance, weakness, drop in red blood cell count
Niacin	Liver and organ meats, meat, fish, poultry, whole grains, enriched breads, nuts, green leafy vegetables, dried beans and peas	Contributes to energy release from carbohydrates, fats, and proteins; normal growth and development; and formation of hormones and nerve-regulating substances.	Confusion, depression, weakness, weight loss
Biotin	Liver, kidney, eggs, yeast, legumes, milk, nuts, dark green vegetables	Essential for carbohydrate metabolism and fatty acid synthesis.	Inflamed skin, muscle pain, depression, weight loss
Folic acid	Leafy green vegetables, organ meats, whole grains and cereals, dried beans	Needed for cell growth and reproduction and for red blood cell formation.	Decreased resistance to infection
Pantothenic acid	All natural foods, especially liver, kidney, eggs, nuts, yeast, milk, dried peas and beans, green leafy vegetables	Related to carbohydrate and fat metabolism.	Depression, low blood sugar, leg cramps, nausea, headaches
Vitamin C (Ascorbic acid)	Fruits, vegetables	Helps protect against infection; required for formation of collagenous tissue, normal blood vessels, teeth, and bones.	Slow-healing wounds, loose teeth, hemorrhaging, rough scaly skin, irritability

Source: Hoeger, W. W. K., and S. A. Hoeger. 2010. Table 3.4 in *Lifetime physical fitness & wellness*, 11th ed. Belmont, CA: Brooks/Cole-Cengage Learning.

the fat-soluble vitamins can be toxic to the body if high dosages are absorbed, which reinforces the biological principle mentioned previously that "more is not always better" when it comes to nutrition and optimizing exercise performance. The toxicity of the water-soluble vitamins is much less because they cannot be stored and need to be replenished more often, because the excess quantities are excreted from your body.

Antioxidant vitamins are another class of vitamins that helps scavenge the free radicals from many metabolic and inflammatory reactions. A free radical is a molecule

antioxidant vitamin Another class of vitamins that helps scavenge the free radicals from many metabolic and inflammatory reactions.

with one or more unpaired electrons; it is highly unstable and reactive. Many exercise science professionals believe that the production of free radicals in the body may increase the risk for chronic diseases such as cancer, atherosclerosis, and premature aging. Vitamins C, E, and beta-carotene are examples of antioxidant vitamins and are discussed further in Chapter 12.

Mineral Balance

Minerals are chemical elements that are important for the body's structure, function, and regulation of metabolism. Major minerals are found in larger quantities in the body, whereas trace minerals are found in smaller amounts. Minerals bind with other substances or interact with other minerals. When bound with other substances or minerals, their absorption is limited. Deficiencies in mineral absorption are most often associated with electrolyte imbalances (for example, sodium, potassium, magnesium). Deficiencies are easily avoided with proper hydration and dietary practices. Table 11.6 summarizes the major functions of minerals.

(Do your clients need vitamin and mineral supplementation? Why or why not?)

Four minerals that are particularly important to appropriate nutrition and optimizing exercise are calcium, iron, potassium, and sodium. A diet rich in these and other minerals can help your clients avoid electrolyte imbalances and health challenges associated with low mineral intake or absorption.

TABLE 11.6 **Major Functions of Minerals**

Nutrient	Good Sources	Major Functions	Deficiency Symptoms
Calcium	Milk, yogurt, cheese, green leafy vegetables, dried beans, sardines, salmon	Required for strong teeth and bone formation; maintenance of good muscle tone, heartbeat, and nerve function.	Bone pain and fractures, periodontal disease, muscle cramps
Copper	Seafood, meats, beans, nuts, whole grains	Helps with iron absorption and hemoglobin formation; required to synthesize the enzyme cytochrome oxidase.	Anemia (although deficiency is rare in humans)
Iron	Organ meats, lean meats, seafoods, eggs, dried peas and beans, nuts, whole and enriched grains, green leafy vegetables	Major component of hemoglobin; aids in energy utilization.	Nutritional anemia, overall weakness
Phosphorus	Meats, fish, milk, eggs, dried beans and peas, whole grains, processed foods	Required for bone and teeth formation and for energy release regulation.	Bone pain and fracture, weight loss, weakness
Zinc	Milk, meat, seafood, whole grains, nuts, eggs, dried beans	Essential component of hormones, insulin, and enzymes; used in normal growth and development.	Loss of appetite, slow-healing wounds, skin problems
Magnesium	Green leafy vegetables, whole grains, nuts, soybeans, seafood, legumes	Needed for bone growth and maintenance, carbohydrate and protein utilization, nerve function, temperature regulation.	Irregular heartbeat, weakness, muscle spasms, sleeplessness
Sodium	Table salt, processed foods, meat	Needed for body fluid regulation, transmission of nerve impulses, heart action.	Rarely seen
Potassium	Legumes, whole grains, bananas, orange juice, dried fruits, potatoes	Required for heart action, bone formation and maintenance, regulation of energy release, acid–base regulation.	Irregular heartbeat, nausea, weakness
Selenium	Seafood, meat, whole grains	Component of enzymes; functions in close association with vitamin E.	Muscle pain, possible deterioration of heart muscle, possible hair loss and nail loss

Source: Hoeger, W. W. K., and S. A. Hoeger. 2010. Table 3.5 in *Lifetime physical fitness & wellness*, 11th ed. Belmont, CA: Brooks/Cole-Cengage Learning.

Calcium

If calcium (Ca^{++}) together with phosphorus (P) is poorly absorbed from your diet, you may be at greater risk for osteoporosis. Osteoporosis is a disease in which the bones become porous and fragile because of bone demineralization. Calcium balance in the body is a complex phenomenon and is influenced by many more factors than just calcium intake. Participation in regular exercise and the proper balance of steroid hormones, such as estrogen and testosterone, are also important in maintaining calcium balance. One of the biggest challenges for long-term spaceflight, such as a trip to Mars (approximately 3 years), is the fact that the microgravity (Zero G) or weightlessness leads to calcium reabsorption from bone and results in the astronauts being at risk for kidney stone formation and osteoporosis.

Another example of an activity-related calcium imbalance is prevalent in female athletes: together with their high-intensity and duration training, they reduce their body fat by dietary restriction. The loss of body fat reduces the body's estrogen storage capacity and results in loss of calcium from the bones. This osteoporotic condition manifests itself as stress fractures and is often seen in female athletes suffering from the condition identified as the "female athlete's triad."

HOTLINK *See Chapter 12 for more information on preventing osteoporosis and the female athlete's triad.*

Figure 11.13 shows how calcium balance is regulated, in part, by vitamin D and the two hormones calcitonin and parathyroid. A low calcium intake and low amounts of participation in exercise are associated with the development of lower bone mass and density in adolescence and early adulthood.

All adults lose bone mass as they grow older, beginning between the ages of 30 and 40. If you can encourage your younger clients to consume appropriate amounts of daily calcium and engage in regular exercise, they will increase their bone mass significantly and reduce their risk for osteoporosis. The risk for osteoporosis typically increases for women at menopausal age (about 45–55 years) and men at the age of climacteric (about 65–70 years). Figure 11.14 shows the phases of bone development and loss in an average person.

Perhaps one of the least studied questions of the utmost importance to achieving lifelong bone health is whether weight training before and during pubescence provides a stronger stimulus for increases in bone mass. It is well known that the age-related loss in bone mass is relatively constant; if your bones have greater mass at the start of the age-related bone loss, it will take longer for the bone to exhibit osteoporosis.

Iron

Iron is important for the formation of hemoglobin in the red blood cells and myoglobin in the muscle cells. Iron is part of the porphyrin ring embedded in the hemoglobin molecule, and accepts the oxygen and carries it from the lung, then releases the oxygen from the porphyrin ring to the tissues. In the tissues, it is the myoglobin molecule, which also contains iron, that enables the transfer of oxygen from the surface of the muscle fibers into the mitochondria where the metabolic processes are performed. This transfer of oxygen from the lung via the blood to the tissues via its combination with hemoglobin requires a high-to-low gradient of partial pressures of oxygen. This was explained in greater detail in Chapter 9.

Iron balance poses a health challenge to many people because they do not eat enough food rich in iron (red meats and green leafy vegetables), whereas others absorb too much, which can cause toxicity. Recently, athletes using high-altitude living and low-altitude endurance exercise (Hi-Lo) training to improve endurance performances were able to improve their performances only if they had normal values of iron in their blood. Those athletes who had low iron values, primarily female athletes, were unable to gain the benefits of the Hi-Lo training. To some, this type of training is thought of as a natural way of blood doping (see Chapter 14 for more).

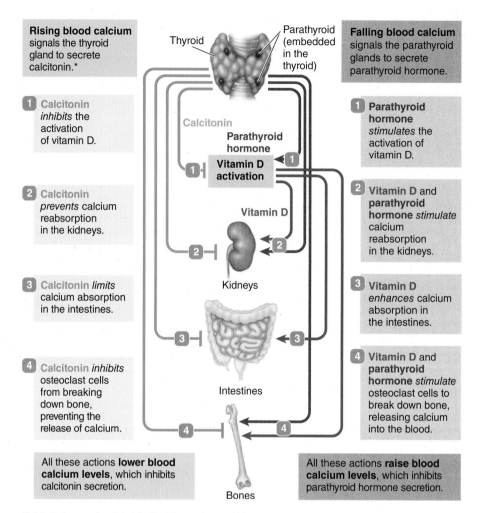

Rising blood calcium signals the thyroid gland to secrete calcitonin.*

1 Calcitonin *inhibits* the activation of vitamin D.

2 Calcitonin *prevents* calcium reabsorption in the kidneys.

3 Calcitonin *limits* calcium absorption in the intestines.

4 Calcitonin *inhibits* osteoclast cells from breaking down bone, preventing the release of calcium.

All these actions **lower blood calcium levels**, which inhibits calcitonin secretion.

Thyroid

Parathyroid (embedded in the thyroid)

Calcitonin

Parathyroid hormone

Vitamin D activation

Vitamin D

Kidneys

Intestines

Bones

Falling blood calcium signals the parathyroid glands to secrete parathyroid hormone.

1 Parathyroid hormone *stimulates* the activation of vitamin D.

2 Vitamin D and parathyroid hormone *stimulate* calcium reabsorption in the kidneys.

3 Vitamin D *enhances* calcium absorption in the intestines.

4 Vitamin D and parathyroid hormone *stimulate* osteoclast cells to break down bone, releasing calcium into the blood.

All these actions **raise blood calcium levels**, which inhibits parathyroid hormone secretion.

*Calcitonin plays a major role in defending infants and young children against the dangers of rising blood calcium that can occur when regular feedings of milk deliver large quantities of calcium to a small body. In contrast, calcitonin plays a relatively minor role in adults because their absorption of calcium is less efficient and their bodies are larger, making elevated blood calcium unlikely.

FIGURE 11.13 Calcium balance. (From Whitney, E. N., and S. R. Rolfes. 2010. Figure 12.12 in *Understanding nutrition*, 12 ed. Belmont, CA: Wadsworth.)

ferritin A protein that helps receive iron from food and helps in its storage.

transferrin Important protein for iron transport in the body.

Ferritin is a protein that helps receive iron from food and helps in its storage. **Transferrin** is another important protein for iron transport in the body. Both blood ferritin and transferrin concentrations, together with blood hemoglobin concentrations, are used as measures to help identify clients who may suffer from iron deficiency anemia. Iron deficiency anemia is a condition in which severe depletion of the iron stores reduces hemoglobin concentrations. Depending on the severity of the anemia, an individual's ability to perform optimal activity in a program of exercise is impaired in direct relation to the degree of anemia.

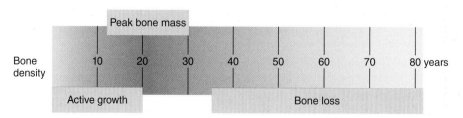

FIGURE 11.14 Phases of bone development throughout life. (From Whitney, E. N., and S. R. Rolfes. 2010. Figure 12.16 in *Understanding nutrition*. 12 ed. Belmont, CA: Wadsworth.)

(How can you help prevent iron deficiency anemia in your clients?)

HOTLINK *See Chapter 13 on weight control to learn more about iron deficiency anemia.*

Potassium

Potassium (K^+), like sodium and chloride, is an electrolyte that is important for maintaining fluid balance and is extremely important in maintaining the electrochemical balance of the body's cells. This electrochemical balance between potassium and sodium is an integral part of neural and muscular action potentials, the body's way of signaling information from the brain to the muscles.

Hypokalemia (low potassium) and hyperkalemia (high potassium) can be life-threatening. Potassium deficiency is common and can occur because of diabetic acidosis, dehydration, or prolonged vomiting or diarrhea; it is associated with the early symptom of muscle weakness. The Dietary Approaches to Stop Hypertension (DASH, search at http://www.nutrition.gov for more about DASH) eating plan recommends foods rich in potassium, such as fresh fruits and vegetables, especially bananas and tomatoes, to help reduce and control blood pressure. It is unwise to advise your clients to take potassium pills because high concentrations of potassium will interfere with a cell's electrochemical balance and, in the case of the heart, cause arrhythmias that can be fatal. Potassium is the lethal ingredient contained in the drug cocktail used in carrying out the death penalty.

Sodium

Sodium (Na^+) is the primary cation outside the cell membrane, and together with potassium, it is necessary for maintaining the electrochemical balance of all the cells of the body. In addition, it is a primary electrolyte influencing fluid balance. Sodium deficiencies are rare, but the typical daily dietary intake of sodium in the United States is high. The high sodium intake in many individuals may create sodium sensitivity that can increase blood pressure because of fluid retention. As sodium is absorbed, water is retained by the kidneys and the body to balance this effect. It appears that those with a genetic predisposition (salt-sensitive gene) for hypertension, those with type 2 diabetes, and those who are overweight are at greater risk for development of sodium sensitivity. It is recommended that salt restriction diets be encouraged for those at greater risk for hypertension or for those who have hypertension. The DASH eating plan provides key recommendations and practical examples for those clients who may fall into this category. For those clients with hypertension, endurance exercise training has been found to reduce hypertension; however, it does not appear to decrease the blood pressure of those with normal pressures.

Fluid Balance

Human fluid balance obviously involves daily water intake and excretion, as well as the maintenance of electrolyte balance. Some 60 to 70 percent of your body weight is water. The more lean, or muscle, mass you have, the more water you will contain. Water makes up three fourths of the weight of lean tissue (like muscle) and one fourth the weight of fat. Females, obese individuals, and the elderly have smaller amounts of water in their bodies because of lower amounts of lean tissue. Water is an essential nutrient for life. Without water, death occurs within 6 to 7 days. Water in the body fluids is the primary influence on fluid balance for the following reasons:

- Water carries nutrients and waste products throughout the body.
- It maintains the structure of large molecules such as proteins and glycogen.
- It participates in metabolic reactions.
- It serves as the solvent for minerals, vitamins, amino acids, glucose, and many small molecules so that they can participate in metabolic activities.

● **TABLE 11.7 Water Balance**

Water Sources	Amount (mL)	Water Sources	Amount (mL)
Liquids	550–1,500	Kidneys (urine)	500–1,400
Foods	700–1,000	Skin (sweat)	450–900
Metabolic water	200–300	Lungs (breath)	350
		GI tract (feces)	150
Total	1,450–2,800	Total	1,450–2,800

For perspective, 100 milliliters is a little less than ½ cup and 1,000 milliliters is a little more than 1 quart (1 ml = 0.33 ounces).
Source: Whitney, E. N., and S. R. Rolfes. 2010. Table 12.3 in *Understanding nutrition,* 12 ed. Belmont, CA: Wadsworth.

- It acts as a lubricant and cushion around joints and inside the eyes, the spinal cord, and in pregnancy, the amniotic sac surrounding the fetus in the womb.

- It aids in regulation of normal temperature (see Chapter 14 for more information about temperature regulation during exercise).

- It maintains blood volume.

Table 11.7 contains the daily major sources for water intake, as well as the sources for losses for water balance.

It is important to encourage your clients to maintain water and fluid balance by eating healthy and consuming 2 to 3 liters water per day (based on a person who expends 2,000 kcal/day). People who expend more energy daily (especially in hot/humid conditions) need to consume much more water and fluids to maintain their body's hydration status. Table 11.8 summarizes the common signs of dehydration and the percentage of body weight (via sweating) represented by fluid loss.

An important consideration for you and your clients to understand is that average adult sweat rates are between 1 and 1.5 L/hour. Highly conditioned endurance athletes may sweat 3 to 4 L/hour, which represents a 6- to 8-pound weight loss. In contrast, a person may reabsorb only about 3/4 of a liter of fluid immediately after exercise. This fact means they are going to have to consume fluids for several hours after completing exercise to regain fluid balance (see fluid intake recommendations later in this section). It is easy to see that if a client becomes even slightly dehydrated daily, over the course of a few days while engaging in exercise, they can increase their risk for suffering a heat injury. One practical way to observe this is for an athletic trainer, coach, teacher, personal trainer, or the client themselves to record their body weight each morning before exercise or eating. Dramatic reductions in weight can be a sign of dehydration.

HOTLINK *See Chapter 14 for a more detailed discussion of heat stress.*

Hydration Concerns

Thirst and satiety influence water intake in response to sensors in the mouth and regulation by the hypothalamus and nerves.

● **TABLE 11.8 Common Signs of Dehydration**

Body Weight Lost (%)	Symptoms
1–2	Thirst, fatigue, weakness, vague discomfort, loss of appetite
3–4	Impaired physical performance, dry mouth, reduction in urine, flushed skin, impatience, apathy
5–6	Difficulty concentrating, headache, irritability, sleepiness, impaired temperature regulation, increased respiratory rate
7–10	Dizziness, spastic muscles, loss of balance, delirium, exhaustion, collapse

The onset and severity of symptoms at various percentages of body weight lost depend on the activity, fitness level, degree of acclimation, temperature, and humidity. If not corrected, dehydration can lead to death.
Source: Whitney, E. N., and S. R. Rolfes. 2010. Table 12.1 in *Understanding nutrition,* 12 ed. Belmont, CA: Wadsworth.

TABLE 11.9 **Percentage of Water in Selected Foods**

100%	Water
90–99%	Fat-free milk, strawberries, watermelon, lettuce, cabbage, celery, spinach, broccoli
80–89%	Fruit juice, yogurt, apples, grapes, oranges, carrots
70–79%	Shrimp, bananas, corn, potatoes, avocados, cottage cheese, ricotta cheese
60–69%	Pasta, legumes, salmon, ice cream, chicken breast
50–59%	Ground beef, hot dogs, feta cheese
40–49%	Pizza
30–39%	Cheddar cheese, bagels, bread
20–29%	Pepperoni sausage, cake, biscuits
10–19%	Butter, margarine, raisins
1–9%	Crackers, cereals, pretzels, taco shells, peanut butter, nuts
0%	Oils, sugars

Source: Whitney, E. N., and S. R. Rolfes. 2010. Table 12.2 in *Understanding nutrition*, 12 ed. Belmont, CA: Wadsworth.

Thirst drives a person to drink, but it lags behind the body's need for fluid. Table 11.9 lists the percentage of water in selected foods, which can be helpful when making fluid balance recommendations to your clients.

Some general recommendations that you should consider for fluid balance are as follows:

• Drink plenty of fluids before, during, and after exercise.

  • *Before exercise:* Consume between 1 1/2 and 2 1/2 cups of cold water 10 to 20 minutes before participating in exercise. Encourage your clients to *drink before they become thirsty* or they will most likely already be dehydrated (and thus at risk for heat injury).

  • *During exercise:* During physical activity in the heat, have your clients attempt to match fluid loss with fluid intake. An example would be to consume approximately 1 cup of water every 10 to 15 minutes.

  • *After exercise:* Have your clients continue drinking water afterward even if they do not feel thirsty. It may take up to 12 hours to achieve complete fluid replacement after strenuous exercise in the heat.

For most situations, water works as well as any beverage in preventing dehydration

(loss of fluids) for activities lasting about 30 minutes. For exercise periods lasting longer than 30 to 60 minutes, you can also choose one of the many sports drinks on the market. It is best to choose one with a label indicating that it has 5 to 8 percent carbohydrate sugar in it. Avoid beverages that are carbonated or contain caffeine, or both. Such beverages are absorbed at a much slower rate than plain water and can cause you to become dehydrated. Other excellent sources that provide recommendations regarding fluid balance can be found via the National Athletic Trainer's Association and the Gatorade Sports Science Institute.

How can you help prevent dehydration in your clients?

HOTLINK *See the National Athletic Trainer's Association at http://www.nata.org for more about roper fluide hydration in athletes.*

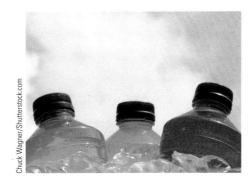

Chuck Wagner/Shutterstock.com

in*Practice*

Examples of Nutrition Tips for Optimizing Exercise

This section provides some practical examples of how providing accurate nutritional advice can optimize exercise related to your area of interest (review the future career table from Chapter 1).

Health/Fitness: Based on what you have learned thus far, what nutrition strategies would you apply if you were the personal trainer for a 40-year-old male sedentary client who was instructed by his physician to start an exercise program to lose weight and to reduce his risks for metabolic syndrome? There are many possible strategies you might consider, but you should initially review your client's health history and medical assessments and recommendations conducted by his physician. You then should inquire about the types of medications he is currently taking and how they may affect your client's exercise physiologic responses. Once you have these baseline data, you and a dietitian could interact with your client to determine how he can meet his new nutritional needs, based on the increased amount of activity in your plan for exercise. Remember, this process requires gathering and analyzing nutritional data from your client about his specific dietary guideline needs, energy balance, nutrient balance, vitamin balance, mineral balance, and fluid balance.

Medicine: If you had a client who has been diagnosed with hypercholesterolemia, specifically high low-density lipoprotein cholesterol (LDL-C) and low high-density lipoprotein cholesterol (HDL-C), how much could your client expect to change her lipid levels by diet and exercise interventions alone? Obviously, the answer to this question is highly variable based on how compliant your client can be and how fast she expects to see changes. As you will learn in Chapter 13, decreasing LDL-C and increasing HDL-C effectively over 12 weeks requires clients to reduce their saturated fat intake, an increase in exercise (equivalent to jogging about 5 miles/hour for 12 miles/week), and significant weight loss ($\geq$10 percent).

Athletic Performance: What nutritional and exercise advice would you give to an inquiring parent whose 15-year-old son, who is 5 feet 4 inches tall (parents are both 5 foot 5 inches tall), wants to take supplemental protein (powders, shakes, etc.) to get bigger? As you will learn in Chapter 12, protein supplementation is effective in some cases but may not be needed (beyond following the dietary guidelines and based on individual energy balance) if a sensible nutritional plan based on the nutritional concepts you learned is followed. However, specific exercise training programs that emphasize regular resistance training and strategies to increase weight gain (1/2 lb/week on average) have been recommended by exercise professionals as effective strategies to improve performance.

Rehabilitation: How could you use the Center for Nutrition Policy and Promotion materials found at http://www.choosemyplate.gov and your exercise knowledge to help optimize the rehabilitation of a sedentary 50-year-old woman with carpal tunnel syndrome who also suffers from osteoporosis? After you have received written directions from her physician as to what type and intensity of exercise has been prescribed, one example might include the following strategies:

Have your client go online (or teach her how to, if necessary) to the http://www.choosemyplate.gov website. Then have her evaluate whether she is meeting her basic nutritional needs according to her specific dietary guideline needs, energy balance, nutrient balance, vitamin balance, mineral balance, and fluid balance. You should also evaluate her current intensity of exercise and make specific recommendations based on what you learned in Chapters 1 and 2. Work with your client to develop and individualize a program that can help her maintain her bone mass and optimize her daily calcium intake needs.

inRETROSPECT

Healthy People 2020 Nutrition and Weight Status Objectives

Healthy People 2020 builds on the past national recommendations that were reported in the 1979 Surgeon General's Report, *Healthy People, Healthy People 2000,* and *Healthy People 2010:* National Health Promotion and Disease Prevention Objectives.

Table 11.10 lists the *Healthy People 2020* Nutrition and Overweight Objectives, which have been revised based on the national 1979 and 2000 goals and outcomes.

● **TABLE 11.10** *Healthy People 2020* **Nutrition and Weight Status**

Number	Objective Short Title
Healthier Food Access	
NWS-1	State nutrition standards for child care
NWS-2	Nutritious foods and beverages offered outside of school meals
NWS-3	State-level incentive policies for food retail
NWS-4	Retail access to foods recommended by Dietary Guidelines for Americans
Health Care and Worksite Settings	
NWS-5	Primary care physicians who measure patients' body mass index (BMI)
NWS-6	Physician office visits with nutrition or weight counseling or education
NWS-7	Worksite nutrition and weight management classes and counseling
Weight Status	
NWS-8	Healthy weight in adults
NWS-9	Obesity in adults
NWS-10	Obesity in children and adolescents
NWS-11	Inappropriate weight gain
Food Insecurity	
NWS-12	Food insecurity among children
NWS-13	Food insecurity among households
Food and Nutrient Consumption	
NWS-14	Fruit intake
NWS-15	Vegetable intake
NWS-16	Whole grain intake
NWS-17	Solid fat and added sugar intake
NWS-18	Saturated fat intake
NWS-19	Sodium intake
NWS-20	Calcium intake
Iron Deficiency	
NWS-21	Iron deficiency in young children and in females of childbearing age
NWS-22	Iron deficiency in pregnant females

Healthy People 2020: *Improving the Health of Americans.* http://www.healthypeople.gov/2020/topicsobjectives2020/objectiveslist.aspx?topicId=29(7/11/11).

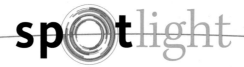

An Expert on Biochemistry, Nutrition, and Exercise: John Ivy, Ph.D.

Dr. John Ivy is an exercise physiologist who has combined the areas of biochemistry, nutrition, and exercise into his distinguished teaching and research career, which led to his recognition in 2005 by the American College of Sports Medicine as a Citation Award Winner. He is currently the Margie Gurley Seay Centennial Professor and Chair of the Kinesiology and Health Education Department in the College of Education, and the College of Pharmacy, Division of Pharmacology, at the University of Texas at Austin.

Ivy earned his B.S. degree in physical education in 1970 from Old Dominion University. He then attended the University of Maryland, where he earned his M.A. (1974) and Ph.D. in exercise physiology (1976). He served as a Postdoctoral Fellow in Physiology with Dr. John Holloszy at the Washington University School of Medicine from 1978 to 1980.

Ivy has conducted research with both animal and human models. His research focuses on the acute and chronic effects of exercise on muscle metabolism, with special emphasis on carbohydrate regulation and type 2 diabetes.

He was the first to demonstrate that exercise training could attenuate the muscle insulin resistance state and determined the mechanism by which it occurs. His research involved the regulation and expression of the glucose transporter GLUT4. Ivy has also investigated the effects of ergogenic aids on physical performance and recovery, and he was one of the first to use the term lactate threshold.

In addition, Ivy has established strategies for the rapid recovery of muscle glycogen (stored glucose) immediately after exercise and has demonstrated the beneficial effects of rapidly resynthesizing the muscle glycogen stores on subsequent exercise performance. Ivy and his colleagues have authored more than 100 peer-reviewed research articles and numerous book chapters and review articles; he also has made abstract/free communication contributions at exercise science and sports medicine professional conferences.

CONCEPTS, challenges, & controversies

Vitamin Supplementation

Do you or your friends consume a daily vitamin supplement? If you do, you certainly are not alone, at least not in the United States. It is estimated that about one third of all adults in the United States take vitamin or mineral supplements, or both, daily. How effective are vitamin or mineral supplements?

It depends on who you ask. A wealth of testimonial evidence supports vitamin and mineral supplementation with common claims that it helps prevent blood clots (thromboses), boosts the immune system, and gives individuals more energy. However, if one reviews the currently available scientific literature, such as that found at www.mypyramid.gov and www.nutrition.gov, there is little support for the benefits of supplementation in the absence of following a healthy eating plan as detailed in the *2010 Dietary Guidelines for Americans* and in the Center for Nutrition Policy and Promotion materials found at http://nutrition.gov and http://www.choosemyplate.gov.

Chapter Summary

- Nutrition is the science of foods and the nutrients and other substances they contain and of their actions within the body, including ingestion, digestion, absorption, transport, metabolism, and exertion.

- The following topics provide the basics of nutrition with regard to exercise: dietary guidelines, energy (caloric) balance, nutrient (carbohydrates, fats, proteins) balance, vitamin balance, mineral balance, and fluid balance.

- Websites such as the Center for Nutrition Policy and Promotion at http://nutrition.gov and http://www.choose myplate.gov provide excellent links to the *2010 Dietary Guidelines for Americans.*

- The basic energy balance equation is based on the first law of thermodynamics: Energy is neither created nor destroyed. The basic energy balance equation appears to be quite simple; however, it can become quite complicated.

- To maintain the increased energy requirements of your clients as they start or maintain their exercise programs, you will need to ensure that they are getting the appropriate amount of total kilocalories per day, as well as the appropriate portion of nutrients as a percentage of their daily intake.

- Nutrient balance involves ensuring that your clients try to consume the appropriate amounts (as a percentage of total caloric intake or in grams) of carbohydrates, fats, and proteins.

- Vitamins are essential nutrients required in small amounts to perform specific functions that promote growth, reproduction, or the maintenance of health and life.

- Four minerals that are particularly important to appropriate nutrition and optimizing exercise are calcium, iron, potassium, and sodium. A diet rich in these and other minerals can help your clients avoid electrolyte imbalances and health challenges associated with low mineral intake or absorption.

- Human fluid balance involves daily water intake and excretion, as well as the maintenance of electrolyte balance.

- The linkages between biochemistry, nutrition, and exercise are important for future exercise physiologists to consider as we all try to serve the needs of our clients.

Exercise Physiology Reality

CENGAGE brain To reinforce the exercise physiology concepts presented in above, complete the laboratory exercises labeled for Chapter 11. To access labs and other course materials for this text, please visit www.cengagebrain.com. See the preface on page xiii for details. Once you complete the exercises, have your instructor evaluate your prescriptions. Remember to use your lab experience to help guide you toward future success in exercise physiology.

Exercise Physiology Web Links

Access the following websites for further study of topics covered in this chapter:

- Find updates and quick links to sites related to the basics of nutrition for exercise and exercise physiology at our website. To access the course materials and companion resources for this text, please visit www.cengagebrain .com. See the preface on page xiii for details.

- Search for further information about nutrition and exercise at the Centers for Disease Control and Prevention (CDC) website: http://www.cdc.gov.

- Search for information about nutrition and exercise and the American College of Sports Medicine website: http://www.acsm.org.

- Search for more information about nutrition and exercise at: http://www.choosemyplate.gov and http://www.nutrition.gov.

- Search for more information about nutrition and exercise at the U.S. government health information website: http://www.healthierUS.gov.

- Search for more information about nutrition and exercise at the American Society for Nutrition website: http://www.nutrition.org.

- Search for information about exercise and fluid balance at the National Athletic Trainer's Association website: http://www.nata.org.

- Search for information about exercise and fluid balance at the Gatorade Sports Science Institute website: http://www.gssiweb.com.

 Study Questions

Review the Warm-Up Pre-Test questions you were asked to answer before reading Chapter 11. Test yourself once more to determine what you know now that you have completed the chapter.

The questions that follow will help you review this chapter. You will find the answers in the discussions on the pages provided.

1. Define the term *nutrition* and how the discipline relates to the field of exercise physiology. *p. 369*

2. List three specific key recommendations from the *2010 Dietary Guidelines for Americans*? *p. 369*

3. How do hormones influence your hunger signals? *pp. 370–371*

4. Describe the meaning of the "thermic effect of food." *p. 371*

5. How can you estimate the daily caloric needs of your clients with regard to their participation in exercise? *pp. 372–375*

6. What is the difference between simple and complex carbohydrates? *pp. 376–379*

7. How does an inadequate daily intake of carbohydrate influence your body's homeostasis? *pp. 377–378*

8. What are the major plasma lipoproteins and their functions? *pp. 383–384*

9. How does sodium intake influence clients with hypertension? How can they modify their diets? *p. 391*

10. List four general recommendations for helping your clients maintain fluid daily balance while engaging in regular exercise. *pp. 391–393*

 Selected References

American Heart Association Nutrition Committee, Lichtenstein, A. H., L. J. Apple, M. Brands, M. Carnethon, S. Daniels, H. A. Franch, B. Franklin, P. Kris-Etherton, W. S. Harris, B. Howard, N. Karanja, M. Lefevre, L. Rudel, F. Sacks, L. Van Horn, M. Winston, and J. Wylie-Rosett. 2006. Diet and lifestyle recommendations revision 2006: A scientific statement from the American Heart Association Nutrition Committee. *Circulation* 114:82–96.

Appel L. J., T. J. Moore, E. Obarzanek, W. M. Vollmer, L. P. Svetkey, F. M. Sacks, G. A. Bray, T. M. Vogt, J. A. Cutler, M. M. Windhauser, P. H. Lin, and N. Karanja. 1997. A clinical trial of the effects of dietary patterns on blood pressure. DASH Collaborative Research Group. *N. Engl. J. Med.* 336:1117–1124.

Appel, L. J., P. M. Sacks, V. J. Carey, E. Obarzanek, J. F. Swain, E. R. Miller 3rd, P. R. Conlin, T. P. Erlinger, B. A. Rosner, N. M. Laranjo, J. Charleston, P., L. M. Bishop, and Collaborative Research Group. 2005. The effects of protein, monosaturated fat, and carbohydrate intake on blood pressure and serum lipids: Results of the OmniHeart randomized trial. *JAMA* 294:2455–2464.

Centers for Disease Control and Prevention. National Center for Health Statistics. FastStats A to Z. Available at: http://cdc.gov/nchs/fastfacts/Default.htm. Accessed January 2007.

Expert Panel on Detection, Evaluation, and Treatment of High Blood Cholesterol in Adults. 2001. Executive summary of the third report of the National Cholesterol

Education Program (NCEP) Expert Panel on Detection, Evaluation, and Treatment of High Blood Cholesterol in Adults (Adult Treatment Panel III). *JAMA* 285:2486–2497.

Gidding, S. S., B. A. Dennison, L. L. Birch, S. R. Daniels, M. W. Gillman, A. H. Lichtenstein, K. T. Rattay, J. Steinberger, N. Stettler, L. Van Horn; American Heart Association; American Academy of Pediatrics. 2005. Dietary recommendations for children and adolescents: A guide for practitioners: Consensus statement from the American Heart Association. *Circulation* 112:2061–2075.

U.S. Department of Health and Human Services. 1988. *Nutrition and health: A report of the surgeon general* (DHHS publication no. 88-50210). Rockville, MD: U.S. Department of Health and Human Services, Public Health Service.

U.S. Department of Health and Human Services. 1996. *Physical activity and health: A report of the surgeon general.* Atlanta, GA: U.S. Department of Health and Human Services, Centers for Disease Control and Prevention, National Center for Chronic Disease Prevention and Health Promotion.

U.S. Department of Health and Human Services and U.S. Department of Agriculture. 2005. *Dietary guidelines for Americans, 2005,* 6th ed. Washington, D.C.: U.S. Government Printing Office.

Whitney, E., and S. R. Rolfes. 2007. *Understanding nutrition,* 11th ed. Belmont, CA: Thomson/Wadsworth Publishing.

Nutritional Strategies and Ergogenic Aids to Enhance Exercise

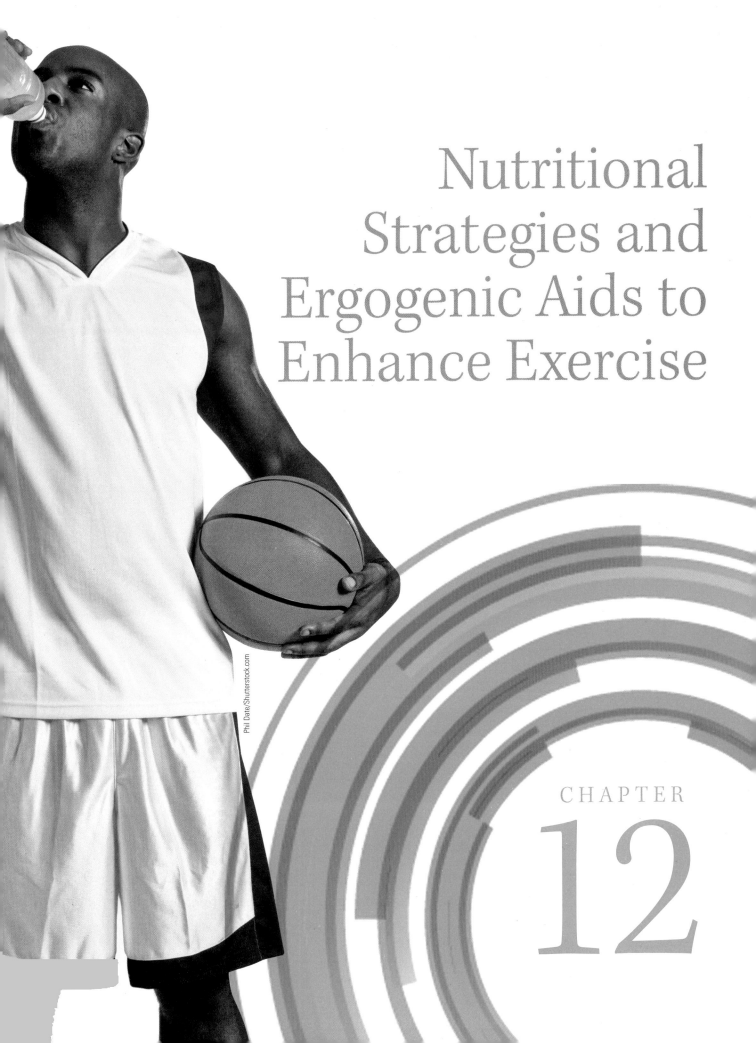

CHAPTER

12

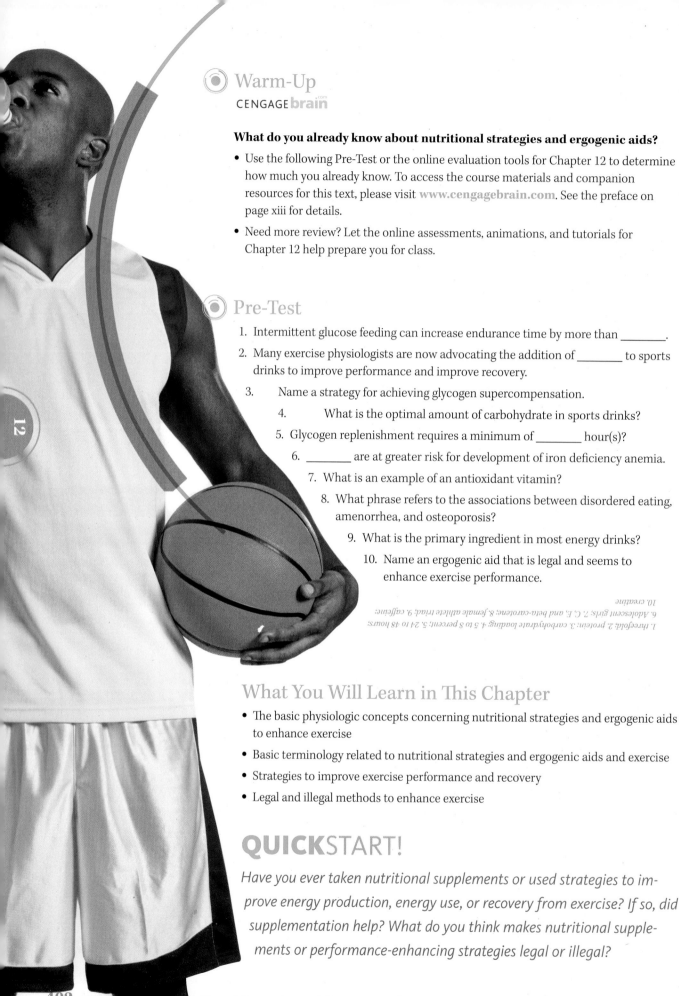

Warm-Up

CENGAGE **brain**

What do you already know about nutritional strategies and ergogenic aids?

- Use the following Pre-Test or the online evaluation tools for Chapter 12 to determine how much you already know. To access the course materials and companion resources for this text, please visit www.cengagebrain.com. See the preface on page xiii for details.

- Need more review? Let the online assessments, animations, and tutorials for Chapter 12 help prepare you for class.

Pre-Test

1. Intermittent glucose feeding can increase endurance time by more than _____.
2. Many exercise physiologists are now advocating the addition of _____ to sports drinks to improve performance and improve recovery.
3. Name a strategy for achieving glycogen supercompensation.
4. What is the optimal amount of carbohydrate in sports drinks?
5. Glycogen replenishment requires a minimum of _____ hour(s)?
6. _____ are at greater risk for development of iron deficiency anemia.
7. What is an example of an antioxidant vitamin?
8. What phrase refers to the associations between disordered eating, amenorrhea, and osteoporosis?
9. What is the primary ingredient in most energy drinks?
10. Name an ergogenic aid that is legal and seems to enhance exercise performance.

1. threefold; 2. protein; 3. carbohydrate loading; 4. 5 to 8 percent; 5. 24 to 48 hours; 6. Adolescent girls; 7. C, E, and beta-carotene; 8. female athlete triad; 9. caffeine; 10. creatine.

What You Will Learn in This Chapter

- The basic physiologic concepts concerning nutritional strategies and ergogenic aids to enhance exercise
- Basic terminology related to nutritional strategies and ergogenic aids and exercise
- Strategies to improve exercise performance and recovery
- Legal and illegal methods to enhance exercise

QUICKSTART!

Have you ever taken nutritional supplements or used strategies to improve energy production, energy use, or recovery from exercise? If so, did supplementation help? What do you think makes nutritional supplements or performance-enhancing strategies legal or illegal?

Introduction to Nutritional Strategies and Ergogenic Aids

According to the U.S. Food and Drug Administration, at least 50 percent of the U.S. general population has reported using dietary supplements. **Dietary supplements** are defined by the U.S. Dietary Supplement Health and Education Act as something added to the diet, mainly vitamins, minerals, amino acids, herbs or botanicals, metabolites/constituents/extracts, or a combination of any of these ingredients. **Ergogenic aids**, in contrast, can be defined as substances, devices, or strategies to improve an individual's energy use, production, or recovery. Examples of ergogenic aids that have been reported in the scientific literature to enhance exercise performance, at least in part, include stretching, weight training, visualization, anabolic steroid use, nutritional and vitamin supplementation, and blood doping.

It has been reported that 76 to 100 percent of athletes in many sports use dietary supplements and/or ergogenic aids to enhance their exercise performances. New products appear on the market virtually every week that claim to enhance exercise performance, control body weight, improve appearance, increase energy, and so on. Because the selling and distribution of many dietary supplements is fairly unrestricted, it can be difficult for experts in nutrition and exercise physiology to familiarize themselves with all the new products available. As an exercise leader, you will need to be concerned with how these products affect exercise performance, negatively or positively, what negative side effects they may cause, and whether the supplement is considered legal or illegal to use in regulated sport competitions.

In Chapter 11, you learned the basic relationships between nutrition and exercise. In this chapter, you will learn specific nutritional strategies to enhance exercise performance, as well as information about legal and illegal ergogenic aids that are commonly used by consumers with mixed results to enhance exercise performance. For additional information on dietary supplements and ergogenic aids, consult the Selected References at the end of this chapter, namely, Ahrendt (2001), Williams (2004), and Yesalis (2000).

HOTLINK *For more information about dietary supplements and ergogenic aids, access the following U.S. federal guide offering access to all government websites with reliable and accurate information on nutrition and dietary guidance:* **http://www.nutrition.gov**.

dietary supplements Defined by the U.S. Dietary Supplement Health and Education Act as something added to the diet, mainly vitamins, minerals, amino acids, herbs or botanicals, metabolites/constituents/extracts, or a combination of any of these ingredients.

ergogenic aids Substances, devices, or strategies to improve an individual's energy use, production, or recovery.

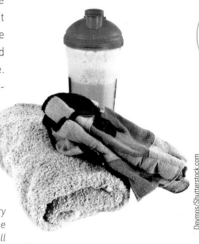

● **Numerous dietary supplements and ergogenic aids are available to consumers, but most are not regulated by the U.S. Food and Drug Administration (FDA).**

Specific Nutritional Strategies to Enhance Exercise Performance

Some examples of nutritional strategies that might be used to enhance exercise performance include:

1. Ingestion of carbohydrates for homeostasis during the performance of a prolonged steady-state exercise

2. Carbohydrate loading or glycogen loading before starting the prolonged exercise

3. Recovery from prolonged exercise and glycogen uptake/replenishment/ storage; tissue repair and mainte-

nance of immune function after prolonged exercise

4. Prevention of iron deficiency exercise training for prolonged performance

5. Protein (amino acid) supplementation and/or vitamin supplementation

6. Understanding and combating the medical consequences of the female athletic triad

7. Energy drinks for combating fatigue or to increase performance

8. Rehydration drinks for the prevention of heat cramps, heat stress, heat stroke, and death

You will learn how to develop nutritional strategies to meet the physiologic challenges listed above. However, you will need to continue expanding your knowledge of exercise physiology to prepare yourself and your clients for other nutritional and exercise performance challenges that both of you may encounter.

(Define the terms *dietary supplements* and *ergogenic aids,* and explain how they may influence exercise.)

Carbohydrates Can Be Ingested to Improve Exercise Performance

The carbohydrate stores of the body are finite, and in the fasted state, their depletion represents one limiting factor for prolonged exercise. This limitation can be circumvented to some extent by carbohydrate ingestion. In 1932, Bruce Dill and his colleagues, working in the Harvard Fatigue Laboratory, demonstrated the important role carbohydrate ingestion can play in exercise tolerance by showing that intermittent glucose feeding (20 g/hour) in the exercising dog increases endurance time by more than threefold. Since then, numerous experiments have also demonstrated the potential importance of glucose ingestion

in exercising humans. The mechanism by which carbohydrate ingestion delays fatigue is related to an increased availability of glucose to the working muscle and prevention of the effects of a decline in blood glucose.

In the early 1970s, Jere Mitchell, M.D., organized a closed-door symposium at the University of Texas (UT) Southwestern Medical Center in Dallas on carbohydrate metabolism during exercise (see Selected References at end of this chapter). At this symposium, Professors Bergstrom and Sjostrand presented a study that helped establish a fundamental tenet of exercise physiology. They used multiple serial muscle biopsy sampling of the quadriceps during exhaustive cycling exercise to determine the cause of muscular fatigue. It took both the heroic efforts of the volunteer subjects and the insight of the investigators to find that muscular fatigue is linked to the amount of glycogen (carbohydrate) stored in the muscle: When carbohydrate stores are exhausted, physical activity of the muscle cannot continue.

Subsequently, it has been found that the development of even moderate hypoglycemia may contribute to glycogen depletion by accentuating the exercise-induced increases in the release of glucagon and catecholamines. These hormonal changes, in turn, accelerate glycogen breakdown. What, in effect, may occur is a self-propagating cycle that is triggered during prolonged exercise by diminished glycogen stores that results in a reduction of blood glucose. This reduction then elicits a neuroendocrine response that further accelerates glycogen depletion.

This self-propagating cycle can be broken by supplementation with ingested glucose. The effectiveness with which carbohydrate feeding maintains glucose availability to the working muscle depends on the amount and form of the ingested glucose. Moreover, the timing of glucose ingestion with respect to exercise is a key factor. Although conflicting evidence remains, Dr. John Ivy (see Spotlight feature in Chapter 11) and his colleagues have

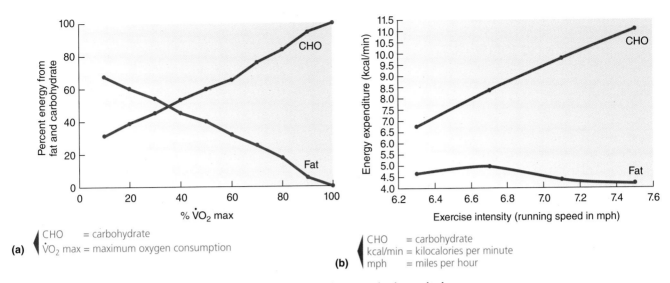

(a)

CHO = carbohydrate
$\dot{V}O_2$ max = maximum oxygen consumption

(b)

CHO = carbohydrate
kcal/min = kilocalories per minute
mph = miles per hour

● **FIGURE 12.1** **(a) Percentage of fat and carbohydrate used as exercise intensity increases. (b) Absolute fat and carbohydrate oxidation.** (From Dunford, M., and J. A. Doyle. 2007. Figures 6.10 and 6.11 in *Nutrition for sport and exercise.* Belmont, CA: Wadsworth.)

reported that the metabolic window (or timing for replenishing valuable nutrients depleted or lowered with high-intensity exercise) begins to close within 45 minutes after exercise. They have also reported that a delay in nutrient supplementation of up to 3 hours can dramatically decrease important anabolic activities, including glycogen storage and protein balance (see Figures 12.4 through 12.6 for more information on the timing of fluids, glucose, and protein ingestion).

In addition, the duration and intensity of exercise will, to a large extent, determine the contribution of ingested glucose to exercise metabolism. Figures 12.1 and 12.2 illustrate the contributions of carbohydrates and fats as fuels for the performance of exercise (see Chapters 4 and 5). Figures 12.1 and 12.2 also identify the effects of glycogen depletion that occurs with increased exercise intensity over time and the dependence on fat as a primary fuel at prolonged, lower intensity exercise.

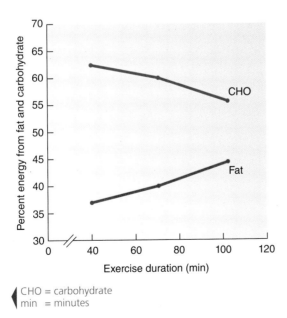

CHO = carbohydrate
min = minutes

● **FIGURE 12.2** **Percentage of fat and carbohydrate used as exercise duration increases.**
(From Dunford, M., and J. A. Doyle. 2007. Figure 6.12 in *Nutrition for sport and exercise.* Belmont, CA: Wadsworth.)

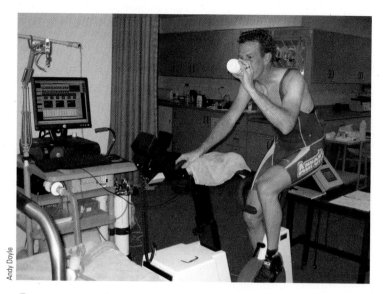
An experimental study of carbohydrate consumption and endurance cycling performance.

Why are carbohydrate stores important for prolonged participation in exercise?

Factors That Determine Gastrointestinal Absorption of Ingested Carbohydrate

Because exercise causes a reduction in gut blood flow, it was thought that ingested glucose might not be absorbed effectively. It appears, however, that ingested glucose is readily available during submaximal exercise. The effectiveness with which ingested glucose enters the blood is determined, in part, by the time ingested glucose spends in the gastrointestinal tract, or its "transit time." The longer the transit time, the greater is the time available for gastrointestinal absorption. The rate of gastric emptying into the small intestine is a key factor in determining transit time. Exercise causes an increase in intestinal transit time, which may effectively counterbalance the reduction in blood flow to the gut, allowing efficient nutrient absorption.

The precise metabolic availability of ingested carbohydrate depends on many factors related to the composition and quantity of carbohydrate. In addition, exercise parameters (that is, work rate, duration, modality) are also important determinants of how readily ingested glucose will be made available. During very light rates of exercise, there is probably little difficulty in delivering adequate amounts of ingested glucose to the working muscle. As exercise intensity and glucose oxidation by the working muscle increase, it may no longer be possible to absorb adequate amounts of ingested glucose from the gastrointestinal tract. The chief limitation for the oxidation of ingested glucose during light work rates is the low muscle metabolic rate requirement to perform the activity, which is more efficiently met by fat metabolism (see Chapters 4 and 5).

At higher work rates, absorption from the gastrointestinal tract is apt to be limiting. As exercise intensity increases to about 50 percent of the maximum oxygen uptake, the oxidation of ingested glucose increases proportionally. Total carbohydrate oxidation continues to increase with further increases in exercise intensity; however, oxidation of ingested glucose increases no further. This suggests that, at this point, the rate that glucose is made available from the gastrointestinal tract has become limiting.

One approach for increasing the amount of carbohydrate that enters the blood from the gut is simply to increase the mass of ingested glucose. Although this is an effective approach in increasing the absolute amount of glucose that is metabolically available, the fraction of the ingested glucose that is made available for metabolism is actually decreased. The reason for the decreased percentage of metabolized glucose with larger amounts of ingested glucose is that more glucose remains in the gastrointestinal tract. The decreased percentage of ingested glucose that is oxidized when larger quantities of glucose are consumed orally suggests that one or more steps involved in the intestinal absorption of glucose have become saturated. This saturation can be circumvented and more carbohydrates can be metabolically available by using different sugar types.

A greater percentage of ingested sugar is oxidized during exercise if it is given as a combination of glucose and fructose rather than in one form or the other. It is important to recognize that carbohydrate ingestion may result, in some instances, in a paradoxical decrease in plasma glucose, which is counterproductive for work performance. This typically will occur if glucose ingestion precedes exercise by an interval (about 45 minutes) that causes the onset of exercise to coincide with peak postprandial insulin concentrations.

Ingestion of glucose polymers (such as commercial sports drinks) has been frequently used during exercise. The basis for consuming this form of sugar is that the osmolarity of the ingested solution will be reduced, thereby decreasing the movement of water and electrolytes into the gastrointestinal tract.

Once in the small intestine, the glucose polymers are rapidly hydrolyzed to free glucose and absorbed in this form. Therefore, on absorption from the gastrointestinal tract, they are metabolized with the same efficiency as that of ingested glucose. Sucrose ingestion has been used as a source of substrate during exercise with similar effectiveness to ingested glucose. This is not surprising because, again, the hydrolysis of this sugar leads to the entry of glucose into the circulation.

In the 1990s, the consensus among most exercise physiologists was that water was the best fluid to recommend for consumption before participating in exercise, to consume during exercise, and to encourage for continued consumption after exercise and leading up to the next bout of exercise. Since 2000, it has become accepted practice for exercise physiologists to recommend the consumption of sports drinks with 5 to 8 percent solution of glucose and isotonic (consistent with normal bodily fluids) concentrations of electrolytes (for example, sodium, potassium). In 2004, some exercise scientists began recommending the addition of protein (approximately 2–3 percent solution), vitamins, and minerals to the traditional sports drink recipe to enhance glycogen replenishment, initiate tissue repair, and maintain the body's immune function. Although this last recommendation

continues to cause controversy in the current exercise literature, it appears that the high levels of interest in determining the precise prescription for legal manipulation involving this nutritional strategy will keep it at the forefront of further investigation. Table 12.1 contains some of the common commercially available sports drinks, soft drinks, fruit juices, and energy drinks, as well as their contents.

> In 1995, what do you think was considered the best fluid to consume during or after exercise? How has the recommendation changed?

Effect of Carbohydrate Ingestion on Body Fuel Stores

Carbohydrate ingestion is accompanied by hormonal and metabolic changes that impact the fuel supply to the working muscle. Carbohydrate ingestion usually slows the rate of decline of circulating glucose that generally occurs with prolonged exercise or leads to an overt increase in circulating glucose. At least two important endocrine changes accompany the increase in glucose availability.

The exercise-induced decline in insulin and increase in glucagon are attenuated or eliminated altogether. The higher insulin level will suppress both the mobilization of nonesterified fatty acids (NEFA) from adipose tissue and glucose from the liver, whereas a reduction in glucagon will reduce the latter. Insulin will, of course, stimulate glucose transport at the working muscle, a process that may also be increased by a reduction in NEFA concentrations. Insulin suppresses muscle glycogen breakdown. However, multiple signals act on the working muscle (for example, epinephrine or calcium), and the antiglycogenolytic effects of insulin are counterbalanced by the release of these other substances (see Chapter 6).

TABLE 12.1 Composition of Selected Beverages

Beverage	Serving Size (oz)	Energy (kcal)	CHO (g)	CHO (source)	CHO (%)	Cations (mg)	Caffeine (mg)	Other
Carbohydrate-electrolyte beverages (4–7% carbohydrate)								
Hydrade	8	55	10	HFCS	4	Na$^+$: 91 K$^+$: 77	0	5.1% glycerol; some vitamin C
Gatorade Original Thirst Quencher	8	50	14	Sucrose syrup; glucose–fructose syrup	6	Na$^+$: 110 K$^+$: 30	0	
Gatorade Endurance Formula	8	50	14	Sucrose syrup; glucose–fructose syrup	6	Na$^+$: 200 K$^+$: 90	0	Some calcium and magnesium
Accelerade	8	80	14	Sucrose, maltodextrin, fructose	6	Na$^+$: 133 K$^+$: 43		Some magnesium, vitamin C, E; 5 g protein
All Sport Body Quencher	8	60	16	HFCS	7	Na$^+$: 55 K$^+$: 50	0	Vitamin C; some B vitamins
POWERade	8	64	17	HFCS, glucose polymers	7	Na$^+$: 53 K$^+$: 32	0	Some B vitamins
Lightly sweetened waters with vitamins added								
Propel Fitness Water	8	10	3	Sucrose syrup	1	Na$^+$: 35 K$^+$: 0	0	Some B vitamins; may have added calcium; contains sucralose*
Vitamin water	8	50	13	Fructose	5.5	Na$^+$: 0 K$^+$: 0	0	Vitamins A, C, and some B vitamins; lutein
Soft drinks								
Coca Cola	8	97	27	HFCS	11	Na$^+$: 33 K$^+$: 0	23	
Pepsi	8	100	27	HFCS and/or sugar	11	Na$^+$: 25 K$^+$: 10	25	
Mountain Dew	8	110	31	HFCS, orange juice concentrate	13	Na$^+$: 50 K$^+$: 0	37	
Fruit juices								
Orange juice	8	110	27	Sucrose, fructose, glucose	11	Na$^+$: 15 K$^+$: 450	0	Naturally occurring vitamins and minerals
Unsweetened apple juice	8	116	28	Primarily fructose, some glucose and sucrose	11.5	Na$^+$: 8 K$^+$: 296		Naturally occurring vitamins and minerals
Energy drinks								
AMP Energy Drink	8	110	29	HFCS and/or sugar	12.5	Na$^+$: 65 K$^+$: 7	71 (guarana)	Some B vitamins, taurine, ginseng
Red Bull	8.3	110	28	Sucrose, glucose, glucuronolactone	11	Na$^+$: 200	80	Some B vitamins
Rock Star Energy	8	140	31	Surcose, glucose	13	Na$^+$: 40	80 (25 mg guarana)	Some B vitamins, taurine, herbs (for example, milk thistle, ginseng, ginkgo)
SoBe Adrenaline Rush	8.3	140	37	HFCS	15	Na$^+$: 115 K$^+$: 20	86 (50 mg guarana)	Vitamin C; 50 mg ginseng
Venom Energy Drink	8.3	130	29	HFCS	11.5	Na$^+$: 10 K$^+$: 28	~ 100 (250 mg mate 50 mg guarana)	Vitamin C, some B vitamins, taurine, bee pollen, ginseng
Other								
Extran	6.75	320	80	Glucose syrup	42	Na$^+$: 20 K$^+$: 50		Concentrated CHO source for ultradistance events

Nutrient information obtained from company websites and product labels.

CHO, carbohydrate; HFCS, high-fructose corn syrup; Na$^+$, sodium; K$^+$, potassium.

*Sucralose (Splenda) is an artificial sweetener.

From Dunford, M., and J. A. Doyle. 2007. Table 7.2 in *Nutrition for sport and exercise.* Belmont, CA: Wadsworth.

The effects of carbohydrate ingestion on muscle glycogen breakdown during exercise have yielded conflicting results. Glucose ingestion has been shown both to attenuate glycogen breakdown during exercise and to have no effect. These conflicting results may be caused by differences in exercise intensity and duration or by other differences because of research methodology. The decreased availability of circulating NEFA with glucose ingestion may require continued utilization of muscle glycogen that, in some cases, may offset the effects of insulin and glucose on muscle glycogen breakdown.

Glucose ingestion reduces liver glycogen breakdown during exercise. Furthermore, it inhibits gluconeogenesis during prolonged exercise. The potent effect of carbohydrate ingestion at the liver is probably mediated, in large part, by highly sensitive glucagon responses. Liver and muscle glucose uptake after ingestion of carbohydrate are both increased after exercise. The improved ability of the liver and muscle to extract glucose from the blood is due, in part, to an increase in insulin sensitivity after exercise. The glucose taken up by the liver, like the glucose taken up by muscle, is largely used to replenish tissue glycogen stores. Glycogen replenishment, which requires 24 to 48 hours, is facilitated after exercise by an increased capacity for intestinal glucose absorption of ingested glucose.

(What is the difference between the classical and modified methods of carbohydrate loading?)

inRETROSPECT

Classical Exercise Physiology History

Carbohydrate loading (defined in Chapter 5) or **glycogen loading** is a training and dietary technique developed by Bergstrom and Hultman in the 1960s to achieve precompetition muscle glycogen supercompensation. Glycogen supercompensation has been shown to increase exercise time to exhaustion and has commonly been used since the 1980s by distance runners, cyclists, triathletes, and other endurance performers to enhance their exercise performance.

Two methods of carbohydrate loading have been described in the literature: the classical method and the modified method. Figure 12.3 illustrates the classical and modified method of how glycogen compensation can be achieved; they produce similar results.

The **classical method** requires clients to prepare for 7 days before a competition by depleting their glycogen stores on day 1 by engaging in 90 minutes or more of endurance exercise followed by 3 days of a low-carbohydrate (<15–25 percent) and high-protein/high-fat diet, while continuing to train as tolerated because of decreased glycogen stores. On days 4 to 7, clients begin consuming a diet of 90 percent carbohydrate while participating in minimal exercise. Although the classical method of glycogen loading is effective at increasing endurance time, it is not easy for clients to comply with because of the psychological stress and the low energy capacity associated with days 1 to 3.

The **modified method** is an effective alternative to the classical method and has been advocated since the early 1980s. In the modified method, clients engage in an exercise taper, where they engage in more than 40 to 90 minutes of endurance exercise on day 1 while consuming a mixed diet of 50 percent carbohydrates for 4 days. Clients then reduce their exercise gradually on days 2 to 4 to about 20 minutes, and on days 5 to 7 increase their dietary carbohydrate intake to 75 percent with a day of rest before competition.

glycogen loading Another term for carbohydrate loading.

classical method Method of carbohydrate loading that requires a glycogen depletion bout of exercise on day 1 followed by a low carbohydrate diet for 3 days, and then a diet rich in carbohydrates for next 4 days.

modified method Effective alternative to classic method that requires an exercise taper followed by mixed diet of carbohydrates (50%) for 3 days, and then a diet rich in carbohydrates for next 4 days.

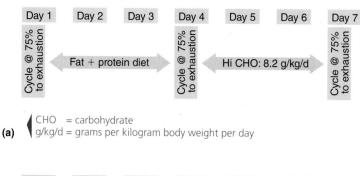

(a)

CHO = carbohydrate
g/kg/d = grams per kilogram body weight per day

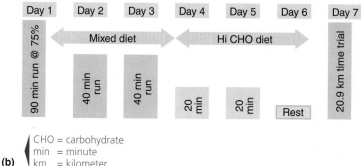

(b)

CHO = carbohydrate
min = minute
km = kilometer

FIGURE 12.3 (a) "Classical" carbohydrate-loading protocol. (b) "Modified" carbohydrate-loading protocol. (From Dunford, M., and J. A. Doyle. 2007. Figures 4.13 and 4.14 in *Nutrition for sport and exercise*. Belmont, CA: Wadsworth.)

The carbohydrate loading nutritional strategies are probably most effective for use with recreational athletes or clients who are average competitors (maximal oxygen uptake [$\dot{V}O_2$ max] ≤ 55 ml/kg · min^{-1}, >3 hours for the marathon distance). The more elite endurance performers are usually in a constant state (daily) of carbohydrate depletion and loading because of high training loads. Elite performers should be consuming ≥ 60 to 75 percent carbohydrates in their daily diet to maintain glycogen stores. Therefore, they can achieve glycogen supercompensation by tapering training intensities for 2 to 3 days before a competition and by consuming their usual high-carbohydrate diet (≥ 70 percent).

One of the main complications with the classical method of carbohydrate loading strategies is that for every mole of glycogen stored, there are 5 moles of water stored with it. This usually results in competitors feeling bloated and uncomfortable at the beginning of the race. If the competitors can get through the first part of the race by ignoring the bloated feeling as the glycogen stores are diminished, the stored water is released and may help in maintaining hydration. However, in many cases, competitors may need to take an unwanted stop to empty their bladders. This complication has probably had much to do with the development of the modified method of carbohydrate loading.

Optimizing Recovery Strategies from Exercise Has Become Increasingly Important

Since the 1980s, many exercise scientists have studied legal means and strategies to enhance recovery from exercise to provide alternatives for optimizing performance without consuming illegal ergogenic aids. Dr. John Ivy at the University of Texas and his colleagues have suggested that the following challenges must be achieved to optimize recovery from exhaustive exercise

so that one can engage in high-intensity regular, daily, vigorous activities:

- Replace fluid/electrolyte
- Stimulate insulin release within 20 to 45 minutes after exercise
- Increase and maintain muscle blood flow in recovery
- Replenish glycogen stores
- Initiate tissue repair and stimulate protein synthesis
- Minimize muscle damage while stimulating the immune system

To optimize recovery from high-intensity exercise within 24 to 48 hours, Dr. Ivy and his colleagues have recommended strategies as illustrated in Figures 12.4 through 12.6. Nutritional timing and dosage is important to the recovery process.

Fluid/electrolyte replacement

- Water by itself is not good enough!
- Consume .3 to .5 grams of sodium chloride per liter of water
- This maintains drive to drink
- Reduces urine loss and promotes rapid fluid replacement
- Need to replace 125 to 150% of water lost to fully rehydrate

FIGURE 12.4 Fluid/electrolyte replacement. (From Ivy, J., and R. Portman. 2004. *Nutrient timing*. North Bergen, NY: Basic Health Publications.)

Glycogen replenishment

- Considerations—significantly decreased after 1 and 1/2 hours of high intensity exercise, requires 24 hours to replenish
- Consume 1.2 to 1.5 grams of CHO per Kg body weight (154 lbs = 70 kg = 84 to 105 grams) and .3 to .5 grams of protein per Kg body weight (154 lbs = 70 kg = 21 to 35 grams)
- Consume carbos/protein (meal or fluids) immediately post (within 30 minutes) and every 2 hours afterwards

FIGURE 12.5 Glycogen replenishment. (From Ivy, J., and R. Portman. 2004. *Nutrient timing*. North Bergen, NY: Basic Health Publications.)

Initiation of tissue repair

- Considerations—prevent protein degradation
- Increased protein synthesis
- Insulin and amino acids can work together to increase protein synthesis and stimulate tissue repair
- Insulin can also slow protein degradation
- Consuming a CHO/PRO (2.5 to 1 ratio) supplement immediately post-exercise will reduce protein breakdown, increase protein synthesis, and produce a net positive protein balance. This will result in a faster training adaptation

FIGURE 12.6 Initiation of tissue repair. (From Ivy, J., and R. Portman. 2004. *Nutrient timing*. North Bergen, NY: Basic Health Publications.)

By optimizing recovery from exercise, you can help your high-performing clients effectively achieve their goals while minimizing the effects of overtraining and risks for injury. This type of recovery strategy has become important for the track and field athletes who compete in major events, such as the Olympics and world championships, where many repetitive performances are required in a short period. In addition, professional team sports players, such as basketball and ice hockey players who are asked to compete on back-to-back nights or with only one day in between competition, benefit from these nutritional (ergogenic) recovery strategies. Although specific recovery strategies are just beginning to be developed and published for various modes of exercise (for example, anaerobic versus aerobic activities), many recommendations are controversial and will require further inquiry to determine their true effectiveness.

What specific strategies can you provide to your clients to optimize their recovery from high-intensity exercise?

HOTLINK *See Chapter 11 for more information on fluid balance.*

Monitoring Diet Can Help Prevent Iron Deficiency Anemia

Iron deficiency anemia refers to the severe depletion of iron stores that reduces hemoglobin concentration. Iron deficiency (with or without anemia) affects more women than men because of women's habitually low intakes of iron-rich foods and their high iron losses through menstruation. However, men can also become iron deficient, especially if they are vegetarian and do not address their dietary iron needs. In addition, the constant pounding on hard pavement endured by distance runners, both men and women, has been shown

iron deficiency anemia Refers to the severe depletion of iron stores that reduces hemoglobin concentration.

to mechanically disrupt and break the red blood cells (RBCs) in the small blood vessels of the foot, resulting in iron loss.

Adolescent girls are particularly vulnerable to iron deficiency anemia if they are vegetarians and do not select good dietary sources of iron (for example, fortified cereals, legumes, nuts, and seeds). If you have clients who have recently shown signs of iron deficiency anemia (for example, lethargy, decreased aerobic performances because of decreased hemoglobin), you should encourage them to follow up with their personal physician who can test their blood hemoglobin and ferritin levels for further diagnosis.

As long as athletes on a vegetarian diet consume enough calories that are nutrient dense, they can perform as well as all other athletes. However, if you have a client with iron deficiency anemia, identification of the problem early by a healthcare professional will minimize the time lost for treatment that might be used to develop and sustain regular exercise.

HOTLINK *See Chapter 11 for more information about iron.*

Vitamin Supplementation May or May Not Improve Performance

In general, active individuals who eat well-balanced meals need no vitamin supplementation. However, some individuals who do not have a well-balanced eating plan can balance their nutrient intake by consuming an inexpensive daily vitamin supplement that does not negatively affect exercise performance. Vitamin supplementation can provide some dietary reassurance for your clients who do not regularly eat fresh fruits and vegetables, but you should remember to encourage your clients to adopt recommendations from the 2010 Dietary Guidelines for Americans.

Antioxidant vitamin supplementation (vitamin C, vitamin E, and beta-carotene) has been advocated by some sports nutritionists for those who engage in exercise in extreme environmental conditions

(heat, cold, altitude). Experimental scientific evidence suggests that antioxidant supplementation may protect against exercise-induced stress that can cause cell membrane damage because of the release of free radicals. However, little evidence has been reported that antioxidants can improve performance, although more studies are needed to clarify the issue. The idea of antioxidant supplementation as a nutritional strategy during recovery as a means of reducing exercise-induced inflammation, that is, muscle soreness, is an active area of investigation.

(*Should you recommend vitamin supplementation to your clients? Defend your answer.*)

HOTLINK *See Chapter 14 for more details about environmental challenges and exercise.*

The Female Athlete Triad Must Be Recognized and Treated Properly

Disordered eating, amenorrhea, and osteoporosis resulting in multiple stress fractures typify the **female athlete triad**. This syndrome affects those women (and some men) in physical activities and sports such as dance, gymnastics, wrestling, figure skating, endurance running, and cheerleading (flyers). To be successful, these physical activities and sports often require participants to train excessively hard and to maintain extremely low body fat percentages and high ratios of strength to lean body mass. Figure 12.7 illustrates the female athlete triad and contributing factors such as restrictive dieting, high intensities of exercise, weight loss, and lack of body fat.

Amenorrhea (absence or cessation of menstruation) is common among premenopausal women and **secondary amenorrhea** (the absence of three to six consecutive menstrual cycles in previously menstruating women) can be associated with excessive training, depleted body fat,

female athlete triad A combination of interrelated conditions like disordered eating, amenorrhea, and increased risk of osteoporosis.

amenorrhea Absence or cessation of menstruation.

secondary amenorrhea The absence of three to six consecutive menstrual cycles in previously menstruating women.

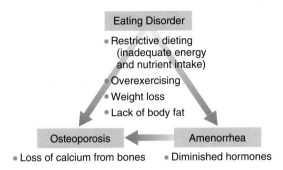

Eating Disorder
- Restrictive dieting (inadequate energy and nutrient intake)
- Overexercising
- Weight loss
- Lack of body fat

Osteoporosis
- Loss of calcium from bones

Amenorrhea
- Diminished hormones

FIGURE 12.7 The female athlete triad. (From Whitney E. N., and S. R. Rolfes. 2010. Figure H8.1 in *Understanding nutrition*, 12th ed. Belmont, CA: Wadsworth.)

low body weight, and inadequate nutrition. The loss of body fat has been linked to a reduced storage of the estrogen precursors, which results in the amenorrhea and subsequent bone demineralization.

The female athlete triad involves the combination of physiologic and psychological stressors that can increase the risks for osteoporosis, stress fractures, and eating disorders. These eating disorders can begin with bulimia 2 to 3 days before competition, thereby maintaining lean body mass while rapidly losing water weight to increase strength-to-weight ratios. This practice enables gymnasts and cheerleaders to perform strength-related activities, wrestlers to change weight wrestling categories, and jockeys to carry a lighter weight. Unfortunately, the practice of bulimia can, and often does, result in anorexia nervosa, which sometimes results in severe dehydration, cardiac myopathy, and death.

It is important to understand the components of the female athlete triad so you can help your clients who might be at risk seek appropriate follow up from their personal healthcare professionals. Many underweight young (and at-risk) athletes have bones that are low in mineral content, similar to postmenopausal women, and may never recover from their bone loss without proper diagnosis and treatment.

How can you help identify someone who might be at risk for the female athlete triad?

HOTLINK *See the American College of Sports Medicine website (http://www.acsm.org) for more information on the female athlete triad.*

Energy Drinks Have Adverse Effects That Can Hinder Performance

Energy drinks have become popular throughout the world and have been in North America since the 1980s when Jolt Cola was first introduced. Energy drinks are typically loaded with corn syrup, amino acids, and caffeine (see Table 12.1 for examples). Numerous brands of energy drinks are available for consumers, but all contain caffeine as their most active ingredient. Although some experimental research supports the concept that caffeine can enhance endurance by stimulating the use of fatty acids and sparing glycogen utilization, too much caffeine ingestion has numerous adverse effects. It can also be illegal in regulated national and international competitions.

Overconsumption of caffeine can cause nausea, diarrhea, indigestion, irregular heart rhythms, irregular respiration, lightheadedness, jitteriness, and frequent urination. Energy drinks often exceed the current recommendations of the U.S. Food and Drug Administration (FDA) of no more than 5 g caffeine per 12 ounces of fluid. In fact, many energy drinks contain as much as four times the recommended caffeine dosage and vary greatly in other ingredients from brand to brand. The overconsumption of energy drinks (and caffeine) can inhibit exercise by causing dehydration, cramping, fatigue, sleeplessness, and nervousness.

> What advice do you have for an athlete who is consuming six energy drinks per day?

Heat Cramping Can Be Prevented

Muscle cramping is a result of muscle fatigue, salt loss, sodium/potassium imbalance, and dehydration. Active clients who sweat heavily and cake their workout clothes with salt may be at greater risk for muscle cramping. Clients who cramp often lose excessive amounts of sodium while working out and may avoid dietary salt for health reasons (to maintain or lower their blood pressure), or they do not realize they need more in their diets. You can help prevent cramping in your higher risk athletic clients by encouraging them to follow the National Athletic Trainers' Association (NATA) recommendations referred to in Chapter 11. More information on the prevention of dehydration caused by exercise in the heat is presented in Chapter 14.

Common Ergogenic Aids and Exercise

High levels of socioeconomic success in our modern society are often associated with individuals who are highly motivated, who work hard, who have the ability to change and adapt to new paradigms, and who are willing to assume some risk. This description may also be applicable when we describe individuals who use common legal and illegal ergogenic aids. Although athletes receive a lot of media attention when they are suspected of using or are found to have used illegal ergogenic aids (for example, baseball players or track and field champions), recreational users of ergogenic aids also generate millions of dollars annually for advertisers and manufacturers.

Because employers want some assurance that employees are alert and safe on the job, random drug testing has become a regular part of many workplaces. In recent years, random drug testing in schools for illegal drugs and ergogenic aids (such as steroids) has also become more prevalent. In conjunction with educational interventions, random drug testing has become a popular model for drug use prevention. As an exercise science professional, you may become the "local expert" in your workplace regarding ergogenic aids, drugs, and drug testing just because you have, or are expected to have, some knowledge of exercise and supplement use. To feel more comfortable with this potential professional challenge, you may want to become more familiar with the resources listed at the end of the chapter regarding the topics of ergogenic aids, drugs, and drug testing.

The following section provides an overview of commonly used ergogenic aids that are promoted regularly by various media sources. The development of new ergogenic aids and the claims about their effectiveness at enhancing exercise grows daily. It is difficult even for experts in the exercise science field to keep up with the list of new products. It is also difficult to determine which exercise-enhancing claims by advertisers of ergogenic aids actually have merit.

A final consideration regarding supplement use to enhance exercise is the lack of regulation of quality control by the FDA for advertisers or manufacturers of various products. Research has shown that the actual ingredients described on the labels of exercise-enhancing supplements often are different in quantity and quality when the product is chemically analyzed. In many cases, the chemical analyses of supplemental products indicates that the ingredients are contaminated with substances not listed and/or that are unsafe and illegal.

As an exercise science professional, you should rely on scientific inquiry to help guide you in making decisions about whether to advise clients to acquire and consume supplements. You should also remember that it is unethical to recommend items like ergogenic aids to clients if those aids are not safe or if they are illegal for possession or use, or both.

The dietary strategies and ergogenic aids that have been found to be most effective via scientific inquiry are usually evaluated by researchers using controlled double-blind crossover experimental design studies (where the researcher and subjects do not know which group is receiving the treatment at any given time, while all groups receive the treatment during the course of the study). Although this research design is an accepted rigorous model by exercise scientists, many advertisers and manufacturers of exercise-enhancing supplements rely more on individual testimonials, rather than independent research findings, to promote their products.

HOTLINK *See the Office of National Drug Control Policy website (*http://www.whitehouse-drugpolicy.gov*) for more information on U.S. drug policies.*

Anabolic Steroids Increase Strength and Endurance but Have Serious Adverse Effects

Anabolic steroids are derived from the hormone testosterone, and their ingestion in combination with exercise promotes male characteristics, increases muscle mass, and decreases recovery time from vigorous exercise. Anabolic steroids are illegal and are designed for medical use only. In the United States, state and federal laws prohibit possession, dispensing, delivering, or administering anabolic steroids. Table 12.2 contains a list of commonly used anabolic steroids or agents and common sources. Anabolic steroids are usually taken orally or by intramuscular injection as listed in Table 12.3. More recently, anabolic creams have been developed and used by individuals in their efforts to avoid detection of drug use.

Although anabolic steroids have been condemned by many professional organizations, such as the American College of Sports Medicine, and outlawed by the International Olympic Committee and all national governing bodies of a multitude of sports and athletic activities, synthetic derivatives have been used and abused for decades by those (athletes and nonathletes

anabolic steroids Drugs derived from the hormone testosterone; their ingestion in combination with exercise promotes male characteristics, increases muscle mass, and decreases recovery time from vigorous exercise.

TABLE 12.2 Examples and Sources of Anabolic Steroids

Examples*		
Testosterone	Methandienone	Tetrahydrogestrinone (THG)
Oxandrolone	Fluoxymesterone	Dehydroepiandrosterone (DHEA)
Oxymesterone	Nandrolone	Mesterolone
Methyltestosterone	Androstenedione (Andro)	Danazol
Norethandrolone	Trenbolone	Stanozolol
Boldenone	Methenolone	Clostebol
Oxymetholone	Drostanolone	
Sources†		
Physicians	Pharmacists	Veterinarians
Dentists	Athletic trainers	Physical therapists
Sport coaches	Conditioning coaches	Nutrition consultants

*Source: World Anti-Doping Agency. 2003. WADA Statistics. Available at: http://www.wada-ama.org/en/tl.asp. Available online at http://www.wada-ama.org/en/Anti-Doping-Community/Anti-Doping-Laboratories/Laboratory-Statistics/Archived-Laboratory-Statistics/.
†Source: Adapted from Bahrke, M. S., and C. E. Yesalis. 2002. *Performance-enhancing substances in sport and exercise.* Champaign, IL: Human Kinetics.
Yesalis *Research Digest* article (www.fitness.gov), March 2005. Available online at President's Council on Physical Fitness and Sports: www.fitness.gov.

TABLE 12.3 Examples of Oral and Injectable Anabolic Steroids

Steroid	Oral*	Injectable†
Testosterone cypionate		X
Nandrolone decanoate		X
Stanozolol	X	X
Methandienone	X	
Mesterolone	X	
Boldenone undecylenate		X
Tetrahydrogestrinone (THG) (may also be a gel or injectable)	X	X
Methyltestosterone	X	
Methenolone acetate	X	
Methenolone enanthate		X
Oxandrolone	X	
Androstenedione (Andro)	X	
Clostebol acetate	X	X
Fluoxymesterone	X	
Danazol	X	
Oxymetholone	X	
Dehydroepiandrosterone (DHEA)	X	
Norethandrolone	X	
Drostanolone propionate	X	X
Oxymesterone	X	
Trenbolone acetate	X	X

*Adverse effects of oral steroids: liver disease, decreased high-density lipoprotein, increased low-density lipoprotein.

†Adverse effects of injecting anabolic steroids (that is, "needle sharing"): infections, AIDS, hepatitis.

Sources: Adapted from Llewellyn, W. 2000. *Anabolics.* Aurora, CO: Anabolics.com, Inc., 2000; Grunding, P., and M. Bachmann. 1995. *World anabolic review, 1996.* Houston, TX: MB Muscle Books; and Phillips, W. N. 1991. *Anabolic reference guide,* sixth issue. Golden, CO: Mile High Publishing.

Yesalis *Research Digest* article (www.fitness.gov), March 2005.

Source: Adapted from Bahrke, M. S., and C. E. Yesalis. 2002. *Performance-enhancing substances in sport and exercise.* Champaign, IL: Human Kinetics. Available online at President's Council on Physical Fitness and Sports: www.fitness.gov.

The urge for quick gains in strength and power by using anabolic steroids is tempting for many.

alike) who want to enhance exercise success, their physical physique, or both. Indeed, the ancient Olympic Games were discontinued because of professionalism and drug use problems. In the Soviet Union (and particularly the Eastern bloc countries, like East Germany) during the 1950s and into the 1970s, anabolic steroids (as well as creatine supplementation and blood doping techniques; see later in this chapter) were administered (often involuntarily) to athletes (especially strength and power event participants) who often won international success at the time. The Soviet research on these ethically questionable practices of enhancing athletic performance remained relatively secret until 2002.

From 2005 to 2007, many states, including Texas, passed laws to test athletes in public high schools as a deterrent to steroid use. Table 12.4 lists the documented side acute or reversible effects and adverse or irreversible long-term reactions that consuming or injecting steroids may cause.

The research surveys that have been used to study the prevalence of steroid use are limited. Little is known about the actual frequency of use and abuse of steroids. Because there are individual variations on how testosterone affects a person, the signs or side effects exhibited by steroid users vary greatly. Table 12.5 provides some signs that can help you recognize that someone is abusing steroids.

TABLE 12.4 Anabolic Steroids: Side Effects and Adverse Reactions

Mind

- Extreme aggression with hostility ("steroid rage"); mood swings; anxiety; dizziness; drowsiness; unpredictability; insomnia; psychotic depression; personality changes, suicidal thoughts

Face and Hair

- Swollen appearance; greasy skin; severe, scarring acne; mouth and tongue soreness; yellowing of whites of eyes (jaundice)
- In females, male-pattern hair loss and increased growth of face and body hair

Voice

- In females, irreversible deepening of voice

Chest

- In males, breathing difficulty, breast development
- In females, breast atrophy

Heart

- Heart disease; elevated or reduced heart rate; heart attack; stroke; hypertension; increased low-density lipoprotein; reduced high-density lipoprotein

Abdominal Organs

- Nausea; vomiting; bloody diarrhea; pain; edema; liver tumors (possibly cancerous); liver damage, disease, or rupture leading to fatal liver failure; kidney stones and damage; gallstones; frequent urination; possible rupture of aneurysm or hemorrhage

Blood

- Blood clots; high risk for blood poisoning; those who share needles risk contracting HIV (the AIDS virus) or other disease-causing organisms; septic shock (from injections)

Reproductive System

- In males, permanent shrinkage of testes; prostate enlargement with increased risk for cancer; sexual dysfunction; loss of fertility; excessive and painful erections
- In females, loss of menstruation and fertility; permanent enlargement of external genitalia; fetal damage, if pregnant

Muscles, Bones, and Connective Tissues

- Increased susceptibility to injury with delayed recovery times; cramps; tremors; seizurelike movements; injury at injection site
- In adolescents, failure to grow to normal height

Other

- Fatigue; increased risk for cancer

Source: Whitney E. N., and S. R. Rolfes. 2010. Table 14. in *Understanding nutrition*, 12th ed. Belmont, CA: Wadsworth.

Strong scientific evidence has been reported that anabolic steroids increase body weight and also increase muscular strength and endurance. However, the long-term use of these agents, although poorly documented in large, controlled studies, has been associated with increased chronic health risks, such as heart disease, liver disease, elevated lipids, increased blood pressure, a multitude of cancers, and mental problems.

In recent years, researchers have reported an increase in steroid use and abuse in adolescents, women, and recreational athletes. A strong body of older research literature is available that documents the benefits and adverse effects of anabolic steroid use, whereas more recent research studies in the United States have focused on the various dose–response effects used over time, such as the effects of stacking and cycling.

HOTLINK *For more information on the effects of steroid abuse see the article "A Guide for Understanding Steroids and Related Substances" posted on the Drug Enforcement Administration website (*http://www.deadiversion.usdoj.gov/pubs/brochures/steroids/professionals/index.html*).*

Future exercise professionals will need to understand and optimize effective drug testing models for steroids while also using effective educational programs to prevent use and abuse.

● **TABLE 12.5** **Common Signs Associated with Steroid Abuse**

Men	Women	Both Men and Women
Baldness	Growth of facial hair	Jaundice (yellowing of skin)
Development of breasts	Deepened voice	Swelling of feet and ankles
Impotence	Breast reduction	Rapid lean muscle weight gain (25–40 pounds)
		Bad breath
		Mood swings
		Nervousness
		Trembling
		Acne (back of arms)

© Cengage Learning 2013

(How would you identify someone who might be using anabolic steroids?)

HOTLINK *Search the Internet to find more information about the research-based educational steroid use prevention programs entitled ATLAS and ATHENA. See* **http://www.ohsu.edu/ xd/education/schools/school-of-medicine/ departments/clinical-departments/medicine/ divisions/hpsm/research/atlas-and-athena -program.cfm** *for more.*

Human Growth Hormone Increases Muscle Mass but Is Also Linked to Many Serious Health Problems

Human growth hormone (HGH) is produced by the pituitary gland and has been used since the 1950s to help children with growth problems. Biosynthetic HGH has been developed and can be injected to stimulate growth. Researchers report in the exercise science literature that athletes in power sports such as weight lifting and bodybuilding have used HGH, just as they have used anabolic steroids, to increase muscle mass but without the dangerous adverse effects.

A dose of HGH is expensive, and regular ingestion has been associated with cancer development in mice. Taken in large quantities, HGH can cause acromegaly (abnormal growth of body parts like the hands

and feet). In addition, excessive HGH intake has been linked to diabetes, thyroid disorders, heart disease, menstrual irregularities, diminished sex drive, and shortened life span. The use of HGH is considered illegal unless prescribed by a physician for hormonal deficiencies.

Protein and Amino Acid Supplementation

Exercise scientists have estimated that protein contributes between 2 and 3 percent to a maximum of 10 percent of the energy needs of exercising subjects in endurance activities or high-intensity/high-volume resistance training sessions. The maximum daily protein requirement for athletes in training is between 1.2 and 1.7 g/kg body weight (0.55–0.77 g/lb) according to the American Dietetic Association, Dietitians of Canada, and the American College of Sports Medicine (2000).

Aspiring teens or athletes, or both, often engage in protein supplementation to increase muscle growth by purchasing and consuming essential amino acids because they assume that because amino acids are the building blocks of proteins, they will be absorbed and metabolized more effectively than protein found in foods. This has not been supported by research studies, and it has been reported that excessive amino acid supplementation may cause dehydration and reduce normal carbohydrate intake, which could challenge the maintenance of normal energy balance.

human growth hormone (HGH) Hormone produced by the pituitary gland and initially used in the 1950s to help children with growth problems. HGH has been synthetically produced and used/abused by those interested in enhancing speed, strength, and power performances.

Most well-controlled studies show that, by increasing dietary intake of protein (via food intake versus supplements) to meet the caloric demands of daily exercise, even the most active athletes can optimize their protein intake without supplementation. An exception to this statement is covered in optimizing recovery strategies detailed earlier in this chapter, whereas protein supplementation helps glycogen replenishment and promotes tissue growth. There is also emerging evidence that some protein supplementation, discussed in the next section of the chapter, can benefit exercise performances.

Branched-Chain Amino Acids, beta-Hydroxy-beta-methylbutyrate, Whey Protein, beta-Alanine, and Other Protein Supplements

Leucine, isoleucine, and valine are three amino acids known as the branched-chain amino acids (BCAAs); they serve as precursors for the amino acids glutamine and alanine. Isoleucine and valine are used as direct energy sources during intense exercise, and some studies suggest that they may help prevent fatigue, whereas leucine has been reported to help activate protein resynthesis related to muscle growth. The positive effects of BCAA supplementation are debatable, as many well-controlled studies have shown no effect on performance.

Beta-Hydroxy-beta-methylbutyrate (HMB) is a metabolite of leucine and has been reported to increase muscle size and strength. Some research has also shown that HMB reduces muscle breakdown after exercise without side effects. The effect of HMB supplementation also remains debatable.

Whey protein is a popular protein supplement because it is processed from milk, absorbed quickly, easily digestible, and high in BCAAs. Whey protein is popular with athletes because it is inexpensive and is used in current strategies (commercially available products) to increase protein synthesis after exercise. Casein protein is another amino acid processed from milk, but it is slower acting (absorbed slower) than whey protein; both are often combined in protein supplement products to take advantage of both their fast and slower absorption rates.

Beta-Alanine is the rate-limiting precursor of carnosine, which is found in fast-twitch muscle and accounts for about 10 percent of a muscle's ability to buffer H^+ ions (help maintain blood pH) during high-intensity exercise. beta-Alanine supplementation has been shown in recent studies to increase muscle carnosine content significantly, which may offer athletes an alternative to an older, little used bicarbonate/citrate loading procedure to increase buffers for high-intensity exercise, such as running the 800-meter dash.

HOTLINK *Use your favorite Internet search engine to find out more about the bicarbonate/citrate loading procedure described in the older ergogenic aid literature (specifically the benefits and limitations of the procedure). See the following link as one example:* http://www.ncbi.nlm.nih.gov/pub med/19255457.

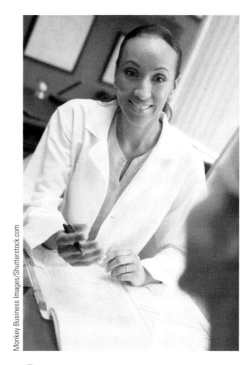

Monkey Business Images/Shutterstock.com

● **A board-certified specialist in sport dietetics can help those seeking high levels of performance develop a diet plan to match their training needs.**

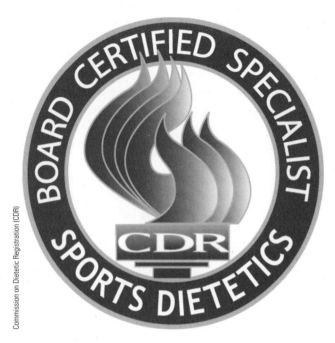

Commission on Dietetic Registration (CDR)

● **This logo indicates an individual is a registered dietitian who is board certified in sports medicine.** (From Dunfold, M., and J. A. Doyle. 2007. *Nutrition for sport and exercise.* Belmont, CA: Wadsworth.)

Many other popular protein supplements currently are commercially available and marketed to enhance exercise performance. However, most products have limited or no published scientific evidence to support the manufacturer claims. When considering or recommending protein supplementation (as well as other ergogenic aid strategies), you should look for a body of scientific evidence that supports the effectiveness of a product or technique, before exposing yourself or your clients to it.

Creatine Supplementation Is Common, Legal, and May Improve Performance

Creatine is primarily associated with the skeletal muscle and the high-energy compound phosphocreatine, which can help enhance the synthesis of ATP. Oral creatine supplementation has become a common practice for strength and power athletes, and it has been anecdotally reported that athletes as young as 9 and 10 years are using creatine regularly.

Theoretically, creatine supplementation improves the recovery time from high-intensity bouts of exercise. Scientific evidence supports the fact that creatine supplementation increases creatine stores by as much as 20 percent. In many individuals, creatine supplementation in combination with resistance training has been associated with gains in strength. Creatine supplementation also causes weight gain, which may be good or bad depending on the sport, but most of the weight gain has been attributed to water retention in the muscles.

Creatine supplementation may help vegetarians increase their resting muscle creatine stores the most because the consumption of red meat in the diet is a prime source of creatine. Many routines have been reported about how to optimize creatine supplementation, including loading doses, maintenance doses, and cycling on and off usage. However, it appears that quality creatine can be purchased inexpensively at large supercenter outlets and that a standard dosage of 2 g/day is enough to maximize the effects of creatine in most individuals. The potential benefits of creatine supplementation are significant and may help provide those interested in high levels of strength and power development with a legal and apparently safe way to improve performance. Creatine is legal for use in regulated sports.

creatine A nitrogen-containing compound that combines with phosphate to form the high-energy compound creatine phosphate.

> What advice can you provide a client who is thinking about starting creatine supplementation?

Ephedrine Has Been Used as an Ergogenic Aid but May Also Be Harmful

Ephedrine, pseudoephedrine, phenylpropanolamine, and herbal ephedrine (ma huang) are sympathomimetics. These substances simulate the sympathetic nervous system's physiologic effects, such as increased heart rate, blood pressure, and so on. They have reportedly been used as dietary supplements and ergogenic aids to increase energy, decrease appetite, and increase metabolism without exercise.

The use of ephedrine (and ephedrine-related products) is banned in regulated sports and has been associated with restlessness, nervousness, tachycardia, arrhythmias, hypertension, and even death. Because it is one of the fundamental chemicals in the distilling of methamphetamine (speed), the FDA has required all medicines (decongestants) that contain ephedrine, pseudoephedrine, or phenylpropanolamine to be removed from the over-the-counter shelves of drugstores and pharmacies.

Hi-Lo Altitude Training: Is It Blood Doping?

Perhaps one of the most recently accepted, yet controversial, training practices for endurance athletes is the idea of high-altitude living; that is, living at 7,000 feet or more while training at low altitude (≤4,000 feet). This practice was devised based on one idea that worked and another that did not. Both ideas are based on the concept of increasing erythropoietin (EPO) concentrations in the blood by ascending to altitude (adaptation to altitude increases RBC mass) and stimulating RBC production, that is, natural **blood doping** (often defined as transfusion, storage, and reinfusion of RBCs or the supplemental use of the hormone EPO to increase RBCs).

In the 1960s and 1970s, the work of Dr. Jack Daniels, a U.S. Olympic silver medalist in the pentathlon, identified that when athletes trained at high altitude, they were unable to perform the training intensities necessary to increase their sea-level performances, even though residing at altitude increased their RBC mass.

In 1972, Dr. Bjorn Ekblom, a Swedish investigator at the Karolinska Institute in Stockholm, Sweden, increased RBC mass by transfusing the subjects own blood after storage, and demonstrated that the increased RBC mass increased the oxygen-carrying capacity of the blood; that is, it increased $\dot{V}O_2$ max (see Chapter 7). After this work was published, a number of reports began to surface that Olympic performances and tour cycling performances were being assisted by the practice of blood doping (blood transfusions). Unfortunately, at that time, there was no criterion to test whether blood doping had occurred.

In the 1980s and 1990s, Drs. Ben Levine and Jim Stray-Gundersen at the Institute of Exercise and Environmental Stress at UT Southwestern Medical Center/Presbyterian Hospital in Dallas convincingly demonstrated that, by living at high altitudes (7,000 feet) and training at low altitudes (4,000 feet), the RBC mass, $\dot{V}O_2$ max, and 10,000-meter performance times can be improved. These findings have resulted in the development of portable nitrogen tents, which can be used at sea level to dial in an altitude for the athletes to live and sleep in while training at sea level. Indeed, many of the Scandinavian countries have built nitrogen houses for their endurance ski teams to use year round.

See Chapter 14 for more about acclimatization to altitude with exercise training. This concept has been challenged by the World Anti-Doping Authority on the basis that it provides the economically advantaged countries an unfair advantage.

blood doping Often defined as transfusion, storage, and reinfusion of RBCs or the supplemental use of the hormone EPO to increase RBCs.

ephedrine Substance that simulates the sympathetic nervous system to cause physiologic effects like increased heart rate and blood pressure.

12

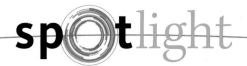

spotlight

An Expert on Nutritional Strategies and Ergogenic Aids Related to Exercise: Kristine Clark, Ph.D.

Dr. Kristine Clark earned her undergraduate degree in Nutrition and Diabetes from the Viterbo College in LaCrosse, Wisconsin. She earned her M.S. in Health Education at the University of Wisconsin, and her Ph.D. in Nutrition Science from Penn State University. Dr. Clark is also a registered dietitian. She is currently the Director of Sport Nutrition for Penn State University's Athletic Department, where she counsels more than 800 varsity athletes from 29 teams and advises head coaches, team physicians, athletic trainers, strength and conditioning coaches, and athletic administrators about eating disorders, weight management, and supplement use among athletes.

Clark is a past president of the American Dietetic Association's practice group of Sports Medicine and is a regular lecturer at national health, fitness, and nutrition conferences across the United States. She also holds a faculty position as an assistant professor in the Department of Nutrition at Penn State University, where she teaches a course entitled "Nutrition for Exercise and Sport."

Clark is a Fellow of the American College of Sports Medicine and has served as a Board Trustee. Her research interests include food choices, timing of eating, athletic performance, and weight management. In addition, Dr. Clark serves as a spokesperson for the International Food Information Council and provides advice about nutrition, exercise, and fitness to the media on a daily basis.

erythropoietin (EPO) Hormone that stimulates the formation of red blood cells (RBCs).

CONCEPTS, challenges, & controversies

EPO and Blood Doping in Cyclists

The synthetic hormone **erythropoietin (EPO)** was developed separately as a medical treatment to increase the RBC mass in patients with anemia and in patients with renal dialysis and cancer who sometimes have anemia. This development led to the illegal use of EPO as another method of increasing an athlete's RBC mass. However, in some cases, the increase in RBC mass was excessive, and in exhaustive endurance and heat stress conditions, the blood of the athletes became so thick that circulation through the heart and brain was impaired, causing death. Whether EPO injections remain in use is not known, but any sudden increase in an athlete's RBC mass to more than 17 g/dl is grounds for suspension. Numerous cyclists since 2000 who have competed in the Tour de France have been accused of and/or caught (via random drug testing) using EPO to improve performance. The use of EPO by cyclists is considered illegal and has resulted in lifetime bans from competition for some athletes.

Many Other Ergogenic Aids Are Also Used

Table 12.6 lists other selected ergogenic aids that have been reported, at least anecdotally, to improve exercise when used. Table 12.6 includes the name of the ergogenic aid, a brief description, the basic claims for improving exercise, the available scientific evidence to support the claims (if any), any side effects, and the legality of use.

HOTLINK *See the U.S. Olympic Committee website (http://www.usoc.org; search under "U.S. Anti-Doping Agency") for more information about legal and illegal nutritional supplements and ergogenic aids.*

TABLE 12.6 Other Selected Ergogenic Aids

Name	Description	Claims Related to Exercise	Evidence	Side Effects	Legality
Alcohol	Ethanol beverage	Decreases anxiety, relaxes	No benefits	Yes, serious	Banned for some sports*
Amphetamines	Pep pills; central nervous system (CNS) stimulant	Increases arousal and decreases fatigue	Mixed, with some positive	Yes, serious	Illegal
Aspirin	Pain reliever	Decreases pain and muscle fatigue	Limited positive benefit	Yes, mild	Legal
Beta-blockers	Reduces heart rate and blood pressure	Decreases anxiety	Positive on motor function, but reduced aerobic function	Yes, serious	Banned by some sports bodies*
Beta-2 agonists	Relaxes bronchiolar smooth muscle	Increases lean muscle mass	Mixed with no effects from inhalers	Yes, mild	Banned unless prescribed
Branched-chain amino acids	Precursors for the amino acids	Decreases mental fatigue	Mixed to negative	Yes, mild	Legal
Caffeine	CNS stimulant	Increases muscle contractility, aerobic endurance, and increased fat metabolism	Lower versus higher amounts produce best benefits	Yes, serious	Banned by some sports bodies*
Carnitine	Derived amino acid involved in energy production	Increases fat metabolism, spares glycogen	No benefits	None	Legal
Chromium	Trace mineral	Increases lean muscle mass	No benefits unless deficient	None	Legal
Diuretics	Increase fluid excretion	Decreases body mass	Limited benefit (dehydration)	Yes, serious	Banned by some sports bodies*
Ephedrine	CNS stimulant	Increases energy level and delays fatigue	No benefit or limited	Yes, serious	Banned by many sports bodies*
Erythropoietin	Red blood cell stimulant	Increases aerobic capacity	Positive benefit	Yes, serious	Illegal
Magnesium	Major mineral (electrolyte)	Enhances muscle growth	No benefits unless deficient	Yes, mild	Legal
Sodium bicarbonate	Baking soda	Buffer of lactic acid that delays fatigue	Positive benefit in events <3 minutes in duration	Yes, mild to serious	Legal
Vitamin B_{12} (cyanocobalamin)	Coenzyme involved in metabolism	Increases energy production	Mixed to negative	None	Legal

*See specific sport governing body information for more on banned substances.
© Cengage Learning 2013

in*Practice*

Examples of Nutritional Strategies and Ergogenic Aids to Enhance Exercise

The following examples are related to the use of nutritional strategies and ergogenic aids to enhance exercise performance. The considerations for each specific recommendation are based on the most current understanding of the link between the topics of nutrition and exercise physiology, which is continuing to evolve.

Health/Fitness: David is a 25-year-old college student who is a recreational power lifter who religiously works out three to five times a week in the weight room for 11 months of the year. He has recently started taking creatine so he can get bigger and increase his muscular strength. What advice can you give David to optimize his creatine supplementation experience if he asks for your expertise?

First, let him know that he can purchase creatine inexpensively at a large supercenter outlet and should be able to get a quality product if he reads the labeling. If he takes 2 g/day (and not more), he may see some additional muscle mass gain in addition to what is normal with lifting and growth and development at his age. Although David may see some increase in muscular strength, remember that the main advantage of taking creatine is that it helps to improve muscular endurance; most of the increases in muscle size are from fluid retention by the muscle.

He should maintain normal hydration while taking creatine and may want to cycle on and off the product as part of normal periodization. He does not need to do the loading dose or strategies that suggest higher amounts (which can cause headache, diarrhea, and other adverse affects); 2 g/day is safe and effective. Lastly, it is important to remember that it would be unethical to encourage (or give formal professional advice) to individuals younger than 18, yet you will undoubtedly be asked such questions by youths or their parents about creatine because of its popularity.

Medicine: Karen is a 26-year-old woman who runs on the collegiate cross-country team, and she has recently reported feeling tired all the time. Her running performance has dropped off considerably even though she has continued to train hard. She has recently adopted a vegetarian diet so she can remain lean. If Karen's coach asked you as an exercise professional for advice about her problem, what information could you provide?

You would probably guess that Karen might be suffering from iron deficiency anemia based on her complaints. To rule out iron deficiency anemia, Karen should be encouraged to visit her personal physician and initially have her blood hemoglobin evaluated. If it is below normal limits (12–15 mg/dl) or at the lower limits of normal ($\leq$11 mg/dl), she may need to follow up with a sports hematologist for serum ferritin testing and further evaluation.

If Karen were found to have iron deficiency anemia, she would most likely be prescribed iron supplements. Prevention and early diagnosis of iron deficiency are important because effective treatment can last 2 to 3 months, which means an athlete is out for all or most of a competitive season.

Athletic Performance: Renee is a 22-year-old woman who is majoring in dance at her university and dances 1 to 2 hours daily. Renee has a history of stress fractures in both her lower legs since she was in high school and participated on the school and club drill teams. Renee only eats one meal a day but snacks regularly on candy to keep her energy up. She also has secondary amenorrhea and has not had a menstrual cycle for 5 months.

After the first 3 weeks of the fall semester, she has noticed that her right front lower leg is aching consistently, and her therapy of applying ice and taking anti-inflammatory drugs is not helping to relieve the pain. What advice might you provide Renee if she asked for your help?

Do you think Renee might have the symptoms of a stress fracture? You may even think she is at risk for the female athlete triad based on her profile. Individuals who are at risk for the female athlete triad are often restrictive eaters, have low bone mineral content, and have diminished hormone levels, all of which increase their risk for stress fractures. It would be in Renee's best interest to visit with a sports medicine physician who has experience with diagnosing and treating the female athlete triad.

Rehabilitation: Matt is a 25-year-old male collegiate volleyball player who is recovering from a grade 2 ankle sprain that he suffered 3 weeks ago. His initial rehabilitation went well, and now he has been instructed by the athletic trainer to ride a stationary cycle daily for 30 minutes as part of his recovery routine. Unfortunately, Matt has been struggling to do even 5 to 10 minutes of cycling without getting extreme muscle cramping in his left calf. The athletic trainer has had Matt cycling outside by the sand volleyball court where the daily temperature and humidity have been high. The trainer has also noticed that Matt sweats heavily, and his shirt is caked with salt after just a few minutes of exercise. Matt

does not have close access to fluids by the volleyball court. What might be contributing to Matt's cramping problem?

Matt probably is not consuming enough fluids, sodium, or both, which contributes to cramping. To help Matt prevent the cramping that is interfering with his rehabilitation, his trainer should make sure he has easy access to fluids and make sure he is getting enough sodium in his diet, as per the National Athletic Trainers' Association.

 # **Chapter** Summary

- Ergogenic aids are defined as substances, devices, or strategies to improve an individual's energy use, production, or recovery. It has been reported in the exercise sports science literature that from 76 to 100 percent of athletes in some sports use dietary supplements or ergogenic aids, or both, to enhance their exercise performances.

- The carbohydrate stores of the body are finite, and in the fasted state, their depletion represents one limiting factor for prolonged exercise. The limitations posed by the exhaustible carbohydrate stores of the body can be circumvented to some extent by carbohydrate ingestion.

- Since 2004, some exercise scientists began recommending the addition of protein (approximately 2–3 percent solution), vitamins, and minerals to the traditional sports drink recipe to enhance glycogen replenishment, initiate tissue repair, and maintain the body's immune function.

- Carbohydrate loading or glycogen loading is a training and dietary technique that Bergstrom and Hultman developed in the 1960s to achieve precompetition muscle glycogen supercompensation.

- Adolescent girls are particularly vulnerable to iron deficiency anemia if they are vegetarians and do not select good dietary sources of iron (fortified cereals, legumes, nuts, and seeds). If you have clients who have recently shown signs of iron deficiency anemia (for example, lethargy, decreased aerobic performances caused by reduced hemoglobin level), you should encourage them to follow

up with their personal physicians who can test their blood hemoglobin and ferritin levels for further diagnosis.

- Since the 1980s, the incidence of disordered eating and those with distorted body image perceptions has increased as more people have become preoccupied with food, dieting, exercise, weight loss, and weight gain.

- Amenorrhea (absence or cessation of menstruation) is common among premenopausal women, and secondary amenorrhea (the absence of three to six consecutive menstrual cycles) can be associated with excessive training, depleted body fat, low body weight, and inadequate nutrition.

- Overconsumption of caffeine can cause one to experience nausea, diarrhea, indigestion, irregular heart rhythms, irregular respiration, light-headedness, jitteriness, and frequent urination.

- Anabolic steroids are derived from the hormone testosterone, and their ingestion in combination with vigorous exercise promotes male characteristics, increases muscle mass, and decreases recovery time from vigorous exercise.

- The potential benefits of creatine supplementation are significant and may help provide those interested in high levels of strength and power development with a legal and apparently safe way to improve performance. Creatine is legal for use in regulated sports.

 # **Exercise Physiology** Reality

CENGAGE brain To reinforce the exercise physiology concepts presented above, complete the laboratory exercises for Chapter 12. To access labs and other course materials for this text, please visit www.cengagebrain.com. See the preface on page xiii for details. Once you complete the exercises, have your instructor evaluate your prescriptions. Remember to use your lab experience to help guide you toward future success in exercise physiology.

Exercise Physiology Web Links

Access the following websites for further study of topics covered in this chapter:

- Find updates and quick links to nutritional strategies, ergogenic aids, and exercise physiology–related sites at our website. To access the course materials and companion resources for this text, please visit www.cengagebrain.com. See the preface on page xiii for details.

- Search for further information about nutritional strategies and ergogenic aids to enhance exercise at the U.S. Olympic Committee Anti-Doping Agency website: http://www.usoc.org.

- Search for information about nutritional strategies and ergogenic aids to enhance exercise at the American College of Sports Medicine website: http://www.acsm.org.

- Search for more information about nutritional strategies and ergogenic aids to enhance exercise at the following U.S. federal guide website: http://www.nutrition.gov.

- Search for more information about nutritional strategies and ergogenic aids to enhance exercise at the U.S. Government Office of National Drug Control Policy website: www.whitehousedrugpolicy.gov.

Study Questions

Review the Warm-Up Pre-Test questions you were asked to answer before reading Chapter 12. Test yourself once more to determine what you know now that you have completed the chapter.

The questions that follow will help you review this chapter. You will find the answers in the discussions on the pages provided.

1. Define the terms *dietary supplements* and *ergogenic aids,* and how they may influence exercise. *p. 405*

2. Why are carbohydrate stores important for prolonged participation in exercise? *pp. 406–411*

3. In the 1990s, what was considered the best fluid to consume during or after exercise? How has the recommendation changed? *pp. 409–413*

4. What is the difference between the classical and modified methods of carbohydrate loading? *pp. 411–412*

5. What specific strategies can you provide to your clients to optimize their recovery from high-intensity exercise? *pp. 412–413*

6. Should you recommend vitamin supplementation to your clients? Defend your answer. *p. 414*

7. How can you help identify someone who might be at risk for the female athlete triad? *pp. 414–415*

8. What advice do you have for an athlete who is consuming six energy drinks per day? *pp. 415–416*

9. How would you identify someone who might be using anabolic steroids? *pp. 417–420*

10. What advice can you provide to a client who is thinking about starting creatine supplementation? *p. 422*

Selected References

Ahrendt, D. M. 2001. Ergogenic aids: Counseling the athlete. *Am. Fam. Physician* 63:913–922.

Dunford, M., and J. A. Doyle. 2008. *Nutrition for sport and exercise.* Belmont, CA: Thomson/Wadsworth Publishing.

Hobart, J. A., and D. R. Smucker. 2000. The female athlete triad. *Am. Fam. Physician* 61:3357–3364.

Ivy, J., and R. Portman. 2004. *Nutrient timing.* North Bergen, NY: Basic Health Publications.

Reents, S. 2000. *Sport and exercise pharmacology.* Champaign, IL: Human Kinetics.

Whitney, E., and S. Rady Rolfes. 2007. *Understanding nutrition,* 11th ed. Belmont, CA: Thomson/Wadsworth Publishing.

Williams, M. H. 2004. *Nutrition for health, fitness, and sports.* Boston: McGraw-Hill.

Williams, M. H. 1998. *The ergogenics edge: Pushing the limits of sports performance.* Champaign, IL: Human Kinetics.

Yesalis, C. E. 2000. *Anabolic steroids in sport and exercise,* 2nd ed. Champaign, IL: Human Kinetics, 2000.

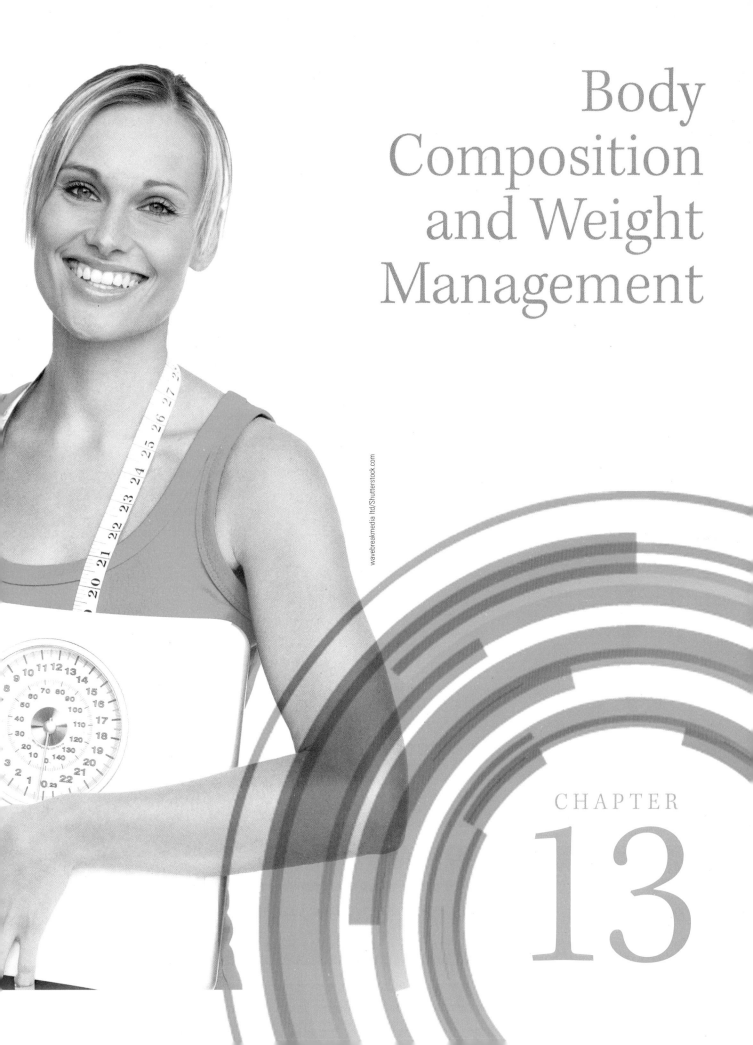

Body Composition and Weight Management

CHAPTER

13

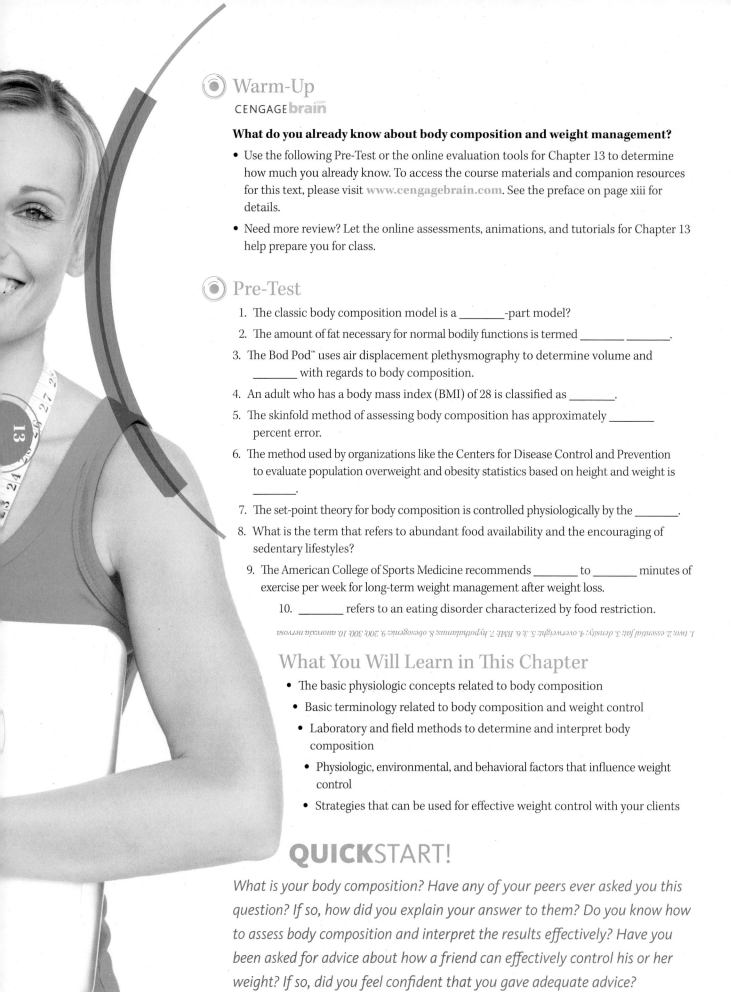

Warm-Up

CENGAGE**brain**.com

What do you already know about body composition and weight management?

- Use the following Pre-Test or the online evaluation tools for Chapter 13 to determine how much you already know. To access the course materials and companion resources for this text, please visit www.cengagebrain.com. See the preface on page xiii for details.

- Need more review? Let the online assessments, animations, and tutorials for Chapter 13 help prepare you for class.

Pre-Test

1. The classic body composition model is a _____-part model?
2. The amount of fat necessary for normal bodily functions is termed _____ _____.
3. The Bod Pod™ uses air displacement plethysmography to determine volume and _____ with regards to body composition.
4. An adult who has a body mass index (BMI) of 28 is classified as _____.
5. The skinfold method of assessing body composition has approximately _____ percent error.
6. The method used by organizations like the Centers for Disease Control and Prevention to evaluate population overweight and obesity statistics based on height and weight is _____.
7. The set-point theory for body composition is controlled physiologically by the _____.
8. What is the term that refers to abundant food availability and the encouraging of sedentary lifestyles?
9. The American College of Sports Medicine recommends _____ to _____ minutes of exercise per week for long-term weight management after weight loss.
10. _____ refers to an eating disorder characterized by food restriction.

1. two; 2. essential fat; 3. density; 4. overweight; 5. 3; 6. BMI; 7. hypothalamus; 8. obesogenic; 9. 200; 300; 10. anorexia nervosa

What You Will Learn in This Chapter

- The basic physiologic concepts related to body composition
- Basic terminology related to body composition and weight control
- Laboratory and field methods to determine and interpret body composition
- Physiologic, environmental, and behavioral factors that influence weight control
- Strategies that can be used for effective weight control with your clients

QUICKSTART!

What is your body composition? Have any of your peers ever asked you this question? If so, how did you explain your answer to them? Do you know how to assess body composition and interpret the results effectively? Have you been asked for advice about how a friend can effectively control his or her weight? If so, did you feel confident that you gave adequate advice?

Introduction to Body Composition and Weight Management

The health benefits for adults of participating in regular exercise and eating healthy are well documented, and these behaviors can help reduce the risks associated with becoming overweight or obese and decrease the risks for incurring many chronic diseases associated with aging, such as cardiovascular disease, colon cancer, hypertension, non–insulin-dependent diabetes mellitus, and osteoporosis (for more information, see the *2008 Physical Activity Guidelines for Americans* available online at: http://www.health.gov/paguidelines). Although overweight- and obesity-related problems are reported mostly in adults, important health problems also occur in children and adolescents who are overweight. Overweight children and adolescents are more likely than normal weight children and adolescents to become overweight or obese adults. Overweight children and adolescents are developing the adult health problems associated with obesity. These problems include type 2 diabetes, high blood lipids, hypertension, early maturation in females, orthopedic problems, and a multitude of cancers and psychosocial problems, such as depression and social discrimination.

Although it is difficult to determine an optimal weight or body composition that is consistent with optimizing exercise, substantial scientific evidence is available for you to use and learn more about body composition and weight control.

In Chapters 6, 6A, 6B, and 11, you have learned about the current significant societal challenges of overweight, obesity, metabolic syndrome (increased girth, elevated blood pressure, abnormal lipids, and abnormal blood glucose and insulin concentrations), and non–insulin-dependent diabetes mellitus (adult-onset diabetes) that we all face. In this chapter, you will learn about the physiologic concepts that influence body composition and how to effectively measure it.

Body composition is defined as the distribution of fat, lean mass (muscle and bone), and minerals in the body. **Weight management** refers to understanding the physiologic influences, environmental challenges, and behavioral strategies that all impact the ability to maintain a healthy weight for functional health and wellness. It is important for you to learn about a variety of strategies to help your clients achieve effective weight control for Health/Fitness, Medicine, Athletic Performance, and Rehabilitation.

HOTLINK *For more information about national weight management goals, see the* Healthy People 2020 *Objectives for overweight and obesity at:* http://www.healthypeople.gov.

> What do the terms *body composition* and *weight management* refer to and how do you think they influence exercise prescription for your clients?

Body Composition Models

Various direct measuring models have been proposed for determining body composition based on the chemical analyses of human body organs and whole cadavers. Theoretical and scientific indirect models derived from anthropometric data and reference bodies of population examples, such as infants, adolescents, and adults, have been developed to analyze body composition. Anthropometric measures (for example, weight-to-height ratios, limb and torso circumferences, and skinfold thickness) are

body composition The distribution of fat, lean mass (muscle and bone), and minerals in the body.

weight management Understanding the physiologic influences, environmental challenges, and behavioral strategies that all impact the ability to maintain a healthy weight for functional health and wellness.

13

field measures that are typically validated against indirect laboratory methods to predict body composition. Although field measures of body composition are less complex than laboratory measures, and are commonly used in clinical settings and epidemiologic surveys, they produce greater errors of estimate than laboratory methods. For a more thorough review of body composition determination, see the references at the end of the chapter for Baumgartner and colleagues (2007), Ellis (2000), and Going (2006).

Compartment models have been developed to evaluate body composition in laboratory settings that range from the basic and classic two-compartment (2-C) model to the complex multicompartment model with five or more compartments ranging from elements, molecular, cellular, functional, and whole-body compartments, as shown in the example in Figure 13.1.

The 2-C model includes: (a) the body fat compartment, and (b) all other body tissues labeled as fat-free mass (FFM). Once FFM is known, percentage body fat can be calculated by subtracting FFM from total body weight. For example, if a 200-pound individual has 20 percent body fat, they would have an FFM of 200 − (0.2 × 200 pounds), or 160 pounds.

The 2-C model is most frequently based on the measurement of total body density, which is the proportion of body weight that is FFM (the higher the FFM, the higher the body density). Conversion factors for total body water (TBW) are then used from reference subjects to determine body composition.

Primary Considerations before Accessing Body Composition

You should consider two primary questions before measuring a client's body composition. The first question is, "Why are you measuring the body composition of your client?" Is it to improve his health, control disease, rehabilitation, or to improve athletic performance? How will you interpret the results and provide your client with clear messages about how to maintain or change her body composition? The second question is, "Which method should you use?" The method will be based on the cost of the procedure, the procedure's ease of use, the accuracy of the procedure, and whether the procedure measures fat distribution.

Although body composition analysis can become quite complex, you can get a rough

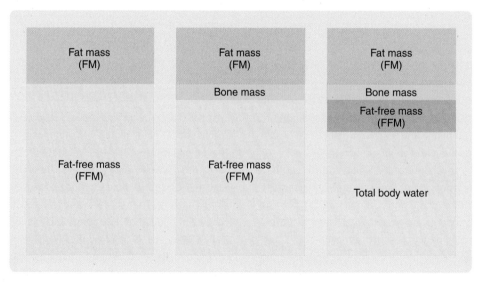

● FIGURE 13.1 Two-, three-, and four-compartment models of body composition. (From Dunford, M., and J. A. Doyle. 2007. Figure 11.2 in *Nutrition for sport and exercise*. Belmont, CA: Wadsworth.)

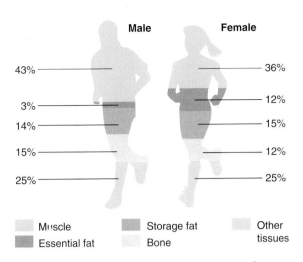

	Male		Female
43%			36%
3%			12%
14%			15%
15%			12%
25%			25%

Muscle   Storage fat   Other tissues

Essential fat   Bone

FIGURE 13.2 Typical body composition of an adult man and woman. (From Hoeger, W. W. K., and S. A. Hoeger. 2010. Figure 4.1 in *Lifetime physical fitness & wellness*, 11th ed. Belmont, CA: Brooks/Cole-Cengage Learning.)

estimate of your client's body composition by performing visual inspection and generally determining your client's body type classification. By performing visual inspection, you can often readily determine whether people are very lean, are in a normal range for their weight, or whether they need to lose weight. Further analyses using various body composition techniques can provide you with more precise information for developing strategies for determining a healthy or more optimal body weight for your clients.

Essential fat is the amount of fat necessary for normal bodily functions. Essential fat includes fat in and around the nervous system, heart, lungs, kidneys, spleen, intestines, and muscles. The lower limit of essential fat for men has been estimated to be approximately 3 percent of body weight and approximately 12 percent of body weight for women (see Figure 13.2). When an individual's essential body fat is too low, her health risks for chronic disease and adverse immune reactions increases.

Ideal body fat and **ideal body weight** are terms often used to describe the hypothetical optimal percentage of body fat or body weight that a person should have. The values for ideal body fat and ideal body weight are highly arbitrary, as you will learn later in this chapter with regard to factors such as age, sex, individual goals, behaviors, and required educational message.

Figure 13.3 illustrates various silhouettes of various body types, or somatotypes, with body mass index (BMI) labels (see Body Mass Index section later in this chapter for an explanation of BMI). The female and male silhouettes on the far left are representative of the ectomorph body type.

The **ectomorph** body type is associated with low body fat, small bone mass, and a small amount of muscle mass and size. The **mesomorph** body type (see center female and male silhouettes of Figure 13.3) is characterized by a low-to-medium body fat and medium-to-large bone size, and is muscular and well proportioned. The **endomorph** body type (see female and male in the far right silhouettes of Figure 13.3) is characterized by large quantities of body fat and large bone size, and is muscular but not as well proportioned as the mesomorphs.

(What is essential fat and why is it important?)

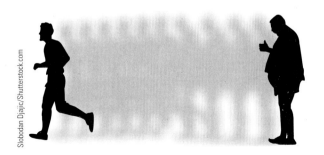

ectomorph Body type associated with low body fat, small bone mass, and a small amount of muscle mass and size.

mesomorph Body type characterized by a low-to-medium body fat and medium-to-large bone size, and is muscular and well proportioned.

essential fat The amount of fat necessary for normal bodily functions. Essential fat includes fat in and around the nervous system, heart, lungs, kidneys, spleen, intestines, and muscles.

endomorph Body type characterized by large quantities of body fat and large bone size, and is muscular but not as well proportioned as the mesomorphs.

ideal body fat Term often used to describe the hypothetical optimal percentage of body fat a person should have.

ideal body weight Term often used to describe the hypothetical optimal body weight a person should have.

Women

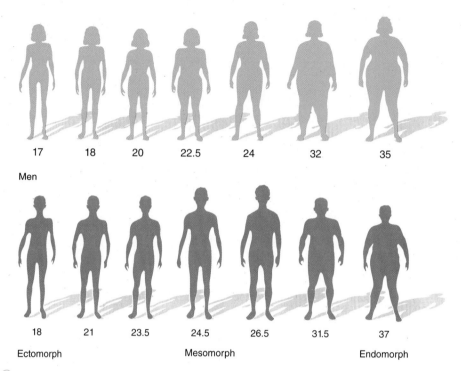

17   18   20   22.5   24   32   35

Men

18   21   23.5   24.5   26.5   31.5   37

Ectomorph   Mesomorph   Endomorph

FIGURE 13.3 Silhouettes of various body types and BMIs (From Whitney, E. N., and S. R. Rolfes. 2010. Back Inside Cover in *Understanding nutrition*, 12 ed. Belmont, CA: Wadsworth.)

Body Composition and Client Health

Body weight, and thus body composition, can be influenced by a variety of factors that affect energy intake and energy expenditure. Strong epidemiologic research exists that indicates strong relationships between body weight and body composition levels and health risks. For example, all-cause mortality (or overall health risk) is highly related to measures of body composition that are weight related. Figure 13.4 shows the relationship between all-cause mortality and BMI.

Underweight individuals (less than approximately 3 percent of body weight for men and less than approximately 12 percent of body weight for women) are at high risk for immune system deficiencies that can increase their mortality risk because of development of chronic disease processes such as diabetes, certain cancers, and eating disorders. Overweight individuals (greater than approximately 28 percent of body weight for men and greater than

approximately 32 percent of body weight for women) are at increased mortality risk from diabetes, hypertension, cardiovascular disease, sleep apnea, osteoarthritis, some cancers, gallbladder disorders, and respiratory problems.

Most likely, you will spend a lot of your professional work time counseling clients about how best to manage their body weight and body composition to achieve or maintain their desired health status (that is, athlete, middle-aged adult, post–heart attack patient). For additional information on factors that influence body composition, see the weight management section later in this chapter.

HOTLINK *See Figure 11.4 (Components of Total Energy Expenditure (TEE)) for a sedentary individual and Figure 11.5 (Total Energy Expenditure) for three different levels of exercise. Also see Chapter 11 to review the variety of factors that can affect weight gain, weight loss, and weight maintenance.*

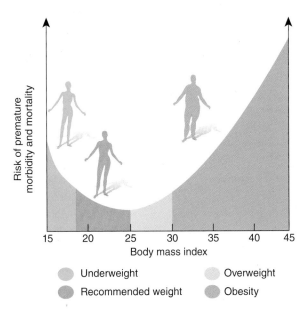

Underweight   Overweight

Recommended weight   Obesity

FIGURE 13.4 Mortality risk versus body mass index. (From Hoeger. W. W. K., and S. A. Hoeger. 2010. Figure 4.4 in *Lifetime physical fitness & wellness*, 11th ed. Belmont, CA: Brooks/Cole-Cengage Learning.)

Laboratory and Field Models to Evaluate Body Composition

Laboratory and field methods have been developed by exercise physiologists and other exercise scientists for more than 50 years to determine the body composition of individuals based on assumed chemical relationships among various body components. Laboratory methods involve attempts by the physiologists to control as many conditions in the laboratory setting as possible, such as temperature, the participant's activities, and the protocol used for measurement. The accuracy of laboratory assessments of body composition varies with the underlying assumptions from which the various methods have been developed. For example, traditional 2-C models developed by Siri (1956) and Brozek and colleagues (1963), as per references at the end of this chapter, were developed on adults and assume that there is little change in chemical body composition after early childhood. If the models of Siri and Brozek and colleagues are applied to other populations, such as adolescents, additional error is introduced that can make the new, alternative techniques less accurate.

Field methods for measuring body composition measurement are less controlled than laboratory tests and are simpler to use for measuring large numbers of clients quickly. Field methods are usually validated against laboratory methods and are easier to perform than laboratory procedures, but they yield a minimum of 3 to 4 percent measurement error.

HOTLINK *See* http://ston.jsc.nasa.gov/collections/TRS/_techrep/TM-1998-104826.pdf *for access to a laboratory book, "Procedures for Exercise Physiology Laboratories—NASA," for more about how to perform body composition measures.*

Laboratory Models to Evaluate Body Composition

The most common laboratory methods for measuring body composition are **densitometry**, **hydrometry**, and **dual-energy X-ray absorptiometry (DEXA)**. Densitometry is the estimation of body composition from body density, which is determined from body mass and volume. Hydrometry is the measurement of TBW, which can be determined from stable isotope dilution techniques. (Stable isotopes are a stable form of an element that contains additional neutrons.) DEXA uses two low doses of X-rays that differentiate between total body bone mineral, lean soft tissue, and fat in a 3-C model.

densitometry The estimation of body composition from body density, which is determined from body mass and volume.

hydrometry The measurement of TBW, which can be determined from stable isotope dilution techniques.

dual-energy X-ray absorptiometry (DEXA) Uses two low doses of X-rays that differentiate between total body bone mineral, lean soft tissue, and fat in a 3-C model.

Densitometry

Underwater weighing or hydrostatic weighing, until recently, has been the most common laboratory method and the accepted gold standard for determining body composition by exercise physiologists. Figure 13.5a illustrates the technique of hydrostatic weighing, which is based on Archimedes' principle, that is, "a body immersed in a fluid is buoyed up by a force equal to the weight of the displaced fluid."

By measuring a person's weight both in and out of water, a person with more fat (lower density) will be buoyed up more than a leaner person (higher density) and will weigh less underwater. Hydrostatic weighing requires that subjects blow out as much air as possible from their lungs before submerging and remaining motionless for several seconds. Therefore, hydrostatic weighing can be difficult for some subjects to perform. The residual lung volume of an individual can cause large errors in measurement if it is not measured. Residual volume can be measured, but it requires additional laboratory equipment and time, and many exercise physiologists instead now use age, height, and weight normative estimations of residual volume. If residual volume is measured during hydrostatic weighing, the method has a 1 to 3 percent measurement error when

compared with the measures of body composition with the newer technologies, such as whole body DEXA. If the residual volume is not measured in conjunction with hydrostatic weighing, the errors of the method are higher, ranging from 3 to 6 percent. An effective operational hydrostatic tank system costs about $10,000 to $15,000 and requires regular hygiene maintenance.

Recently, air displacement plethysmography (measurement of change in volume) has become a commonly used laboratory method (via the Bod Pod™) to determine volume and density. Figure 13.5b shows the air displacement technique. This technique is easy to administer, but it is expensive (about $30,000 to $40,000) and has an approximate measurement error of 3 percent when compared with the DEXA technique.

Hydrometry

The measurement of TBW using stable isotopes is a laboratory method usually used to determine body composition in the more rigorous exercise science research studies. A common TBW technique is the doubly labeled water method, which requires a subject to drink two forms of water that have been labeled with stable isotopes. This technique has become the standard for estimating total energy expenditure by measuring the elimination of oxygen and

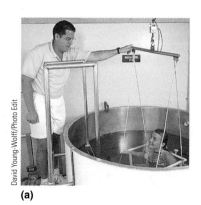
(a)

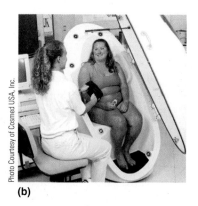
(b)

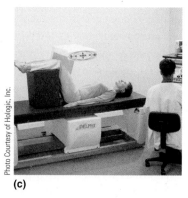
(c)

● **FIGURE 13.5** (a) Hydrodensitometry measures body density by weighing the person first on land and then again while submerged in water. The difference between the person's actual weight and underwater weight provides a measure of the body's volume. A mathematical equation using the two measurements (volume and actual weight) determines body density, from which the percentage of body fat can be estimated. (b) Air displacement plethysmography estimates body composition by having a person sit inside a chamber while computerized sensors determine the amount of air displaced by the person's body. (c) Dual-energy X-ray absorptiometry (DEXA) uses two low-dose X-rays that differentiate among fat-free soft tissue (lean body mass), fat tissues, and bone tissue, providing a precise measurement of total fat and its distribution in all but extremely obese subjects. (Adapted from Whitney, E. N., and S. R. Rolfes. 2010. Figure 8.10 in *Understanding nutrition*, 12 ed. Belmont, CA: Wadsworth.

hydrogen isotopes from the body as water and carbon dioxide.

Once the TBW is known, body density estimates using the underwater weighing or air volume displacement methods can be added to provide a 3-C or 4-C model. The combination of these measurement methods provides a more precise measurement of body composition than the 2-C methods. However, because of the increased cost of measurement and time required of the subjects and technicians, this combination of techniques is used only when the increased precision provides a more definitive answer to a very important (usually clinical) question.

Dual-Energy X-ray Absorptiometry

The DEXA whole body technique has become the current gold standard for exercise physiologists in the laboratory measurement of body composition. Figure 13.5c shows the DEXA body composition technique.

DEXA scanning is done while a person is lying supine on a table without movement while X-ray beams are emitted and data can be differentiated into fat mass, FFM, and skeletal (bone) mass in a two-dimensional display.

The DEXA technique not only provides precise information about a person's percentage of body fat, but also provides bone mineral density data. DEXA technology is expensive (about $100,000 for a full-body scan device), yet has minimal error (about 1 percent) when compared with other, even more precise assessment methods, like computed tomography (CT) and magnetic resonance imaging (MRI). Because of the additional expense of the CT and MRI techniques (about $1,000/scan or about $1,000,000 for purchase of the scanning device), their use is currently limited to research and medical diagnostic tools.

Because the DEXA can provide bone density and body composition measures, many weight management clinics use DEXA in their clinical and research assessments.

Field Models to Evaluate Body Composition

The most common field methods for measuring body composition include:

1. Weight-to-height ratios
2. Circumferences or girths
3. Skinfold measurements

Field measures of body composition are the most commonly used methods that the Centers for Disease Control and Prevention (CDC) recommends for population

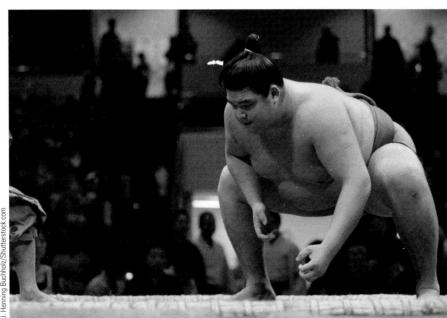

J. Henning Buchholz/Shutterstock.com

studies to determine whether adults, children, and adolescents are underweight, overweight, or obese.

- **Underweight** refers to low weight for a given height.
- **Overweight** refers to excess weight for a given height.
- **Obesity** refers to the excessive accumulation of body fat.

Body Mass Index

The most commonly used measurement in a physician's office is the weight-to-height ratio measurement, and it is used to calculate a BMI. The BMI measurement is used in public health settings as a large population assessment tool and is used by life insurance companies to assess risk for morbidity and mortality.

BMI is equal to one's weight in kilograms divided by one's height in meters squared:

$$\text{BMI} = \text{weight (kg)} \div \text{height (m}^2)$$

Table 13.1 contains the BMI calculations and classifications of underweight, healthy weight, overweight, and obese for adults.

The CDC and other U.S. national organizations classify adults with BMIs between 18.5 and 24.9 as normal weight, whereas those with BMIs less than 18.5 are classified as underweight. Adults with BMIs between 25 and 29.9 are classified as overweight, and those with BMIs greater than 30 are classified as obese. Currently, adults with a BMI greater than 40 are considered at high health risk and are generally referred (if financially feasible) for surgical treatments for obesity.

underweight Low weight for a given height.

overweight Excess weight for a given height.

obesity Excessive accumulation of body fat.

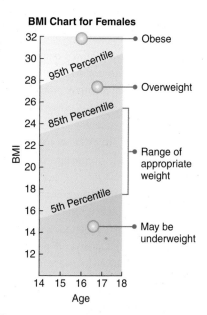

BMI Chart for Females

● **FIGURE 13.6 Body mass index chart for 14- to 18-year-old girls.** (Based on Centers for Disease Control values at: http://apps.nccd.cdc.gov/dnpabmi/.)

Figure 13.6 contains an example of the BMI calculations and classifications for underweight, healthy weight, overweight, and obese 14- to 18-year-old girls.

When classifying children and adolescents based on BMI, the CDC (and others) recommends that BMI calculators (see later Hotlink) be used that integrate the factors of age and sex into consideration relative to growth and developmental factors. The CDC classifies children and youths (ages 2 to 19) for BMI generally as follows:

- Underweight: BMI <5th percentile for age and sex
- Normal weight: BMI between >5th and <85th percentile for age and sex
- Overweight: BMI >85th and <95th percentile for age and sex
- Obese: BMI >95th percentile for age and sex

BMI is a better indicator of obesity than weight alone, requires minimal cost, and can be used to predict percentage of body fat, but it has a larger measurement error (approximately 6 percent). However, BMI does not consider a person's body type

● **TABLE 13.1 Weight Classifications Using Body Mass Index (BMI)**

Body Mass Index (kg/m²)	Classification
<18.5	Underweight
18.5–24.9	Healthy weight
25.0–29.9	Overweight
30	Obese

Source: McGuire, M., and K. A. Beerman. 2009. Back Inside Cover in *Nutritional sciences*, 2nd ed. Belmont, CA: Brooks/Cole-Cengage Learning.

(ectomorph, mesomorph, or endomorph) or the amount of lean tissue a person has. Therefore, athletes or your more muscular clients can easily be misclassified as being overweight or obese. You should consider using additional body composition methods that partition lean body mass versus fat weight to effectively evaluate your adult athlete or your more muscular clients. Partly because of growth and development factors for athletic children and adults, no currently published body composition criterion evaluation methods or nationally recognized guidelines effectively evaluate athletes or your more muscular youth clients.

HOTLINK *Access the Centers for Disease Control and Prevention website (http://www.cdc.gov) and search under BMI calculators for more information.*

Body Circumferences or Girths
Clinically, the most common current methods of evaluating body circumferences are the measurements of waist circumference in adults and youths, and the measurement of the waist-to-hip ratio in adults. Waist circumference provides the most practical measure of abdominal fat for adults and youth. Carrying more upper body fat is associated with having an "apple shape" versus the "pear shape" associated with carrying more fat on the lower body (see Figure 13.7).

Excessive upper body fat, like abdominal fat, is associated with an increased risk for the development of the chronic disease processes such as heart disease, stroke, diabetes, the metabolic syndrome, and some types of cancer. You should measure an adult client's waist circumference using a cloth measuring tape, if possible (low-cost device), as shown in Figure 13.8, and record the girth in centimeters (or inches).

After recording the client's waist circumference, you can use the evaluation guidelines in Table 13.2 to determine the client's clinical health risk. Recently, waist circumference reference data for children and adolescents (ages 2–18) have been

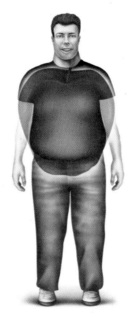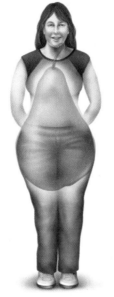

Upper-body fat is more common in men than in women and is closely associated with heart disease, stroke, diabetes, hypertension, and some types of cancer.

Lower-body fat is more common in women than in men and is not usually associated with chronic diseases.

FIGURE 13.7 Comparison of "apple" and "pear" body shapes. (Adapted from Whitney, E. N., and S. R. Rolfes. 2010. Figure 8.9 in *Understanding nutrition,* 12 ed. Belmont, CA: Wadsworth.)

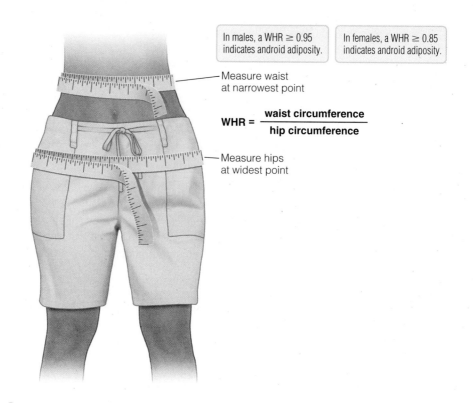

In males, a WHR ≥ 0.95 indicates android adiposity.

In females, a WHR ≥ 0.85 indicates android adiposity.

Measure waist at narrowest point

$$WHR = \frac{waist\ circumference}{hip\ circumference}$$

Measure hips at widest point

FIGURE 13.8 Waist-to-hip ratio: an indication of body fat distribution. (From McGuire, M., and K. A. Beerman. 2006. Figure 9.9 in *Nutritional sciences.* Belmont, CA: Brooks/Cole-Cengage Learning.)

published for African American, European American, and Mexican American youths (Fernandez et al., 2004). Once you have measured a younger client's waist circumference, you can use the appropriate ethnic/race data from Table 13.3 to evaluate the waist circumference and health risk.

Youths are classified by waist girth in Tables 13.3a–c as being in the 10th percentile through the 90th percentile. Although there is not a current national consensus for health considerations (reducing the risks for chronic disease processes as an adult), a general recommendation that you might use with your younger clients is to encourage them (and their parents)

to maintain their girth as close to the 50th percentile as they can. If a youngster has a high BMI (>85th percentile for age and sex) and a waist girth in the 90th percentile or greater, they probably should not try to gain more weight. And if a youngster has a low BMI (<5th percentile for age and sex) and a waist girth in the 10th percentile or less, they probably should not try to lose any more weight.

The waist-to-hip ratio (see Figure 13.8) can also be used to simply evaluate the distribution of body fat in adults. Health risk increases as waist-to-hip ratio increases and standards vary by age and sex. Young adult men and women should have ratios lower than 0.95 and 0.86, respectively, to be categorized as low health risk. Older adult men and women (ages 60–69) should have ratios of lower than 1.03 and 0.90, respectively, to be classified as having a low health risk.

Skinfolds

The measurement of skinfold thickness is a popular method of determining body composition, and it has been used by exercise

TABLE 13.2 Disease Risk according to Waist Circumference in Inches

Men	Women	Disease Risk
<35.5	<32.5	Low
35.5–40.0	32.5–35.0	Moderate
>40.0	>35.0	High

Source: Hoeger, W. W. K., and S. A. Hoeger. 2010. Table 4.8 in *Lifetime physical fitness & wellness,* 11th ed. Belmont, CA: Brooks/Cole-Cengage Learning.

Age (y)	Percentile for Boys					Percentile for Girls				
	10th	25th	50th	75th	90th	10th	25th	50th	75th	90th
2	17.00	17.55	18.26	19.09	19.68	16.92	17.55	18.11	18.77	19.72
3	17.63	18.22	19.01	19.96	20.94	17.55	18.22	18.93	19.92	21.18
4	18.22	18.89	19.72	20.82	22.20	18.14	18.89	19.76	21.02	22.63
5	18.85	19.56	20.47	21.69	23.46	18.77	19.56	20.59	22.12	24.05
6	19.44	20.23	21.22	22.55	24.72	19.37	20.23	21.45	23.22	25.51
7	20.07	20.90	21.92	23.42	26.02	19.99	20.94	22.28	24.33	26.96
8	20.66	21.57	22.67	24.29	27.28	20.62	21.61	23.11	25.47	28.42
9	21.29	22.20	23.38	25.15	28.54	21.22	22.28	23.97	26.57	29.84
10	21.88	22.87	24.13	26.02	29.80	21.85	22.95	24.80	27.67	31.29
11	22.51	23.54	24.88	26.88	31.06	22.44	23.62	25.62	28.77	32.75
12	23.11	24.21	25.59	27.75	32.32	23.07	24.29	26.49	29.88	34.21
13	23.74	24.88	26.33	28.62	33.58	23.70	24.96	27.32	31.02	35.62
14	24.33	25.55	27.04	29.48	34.84	24.29	25.62	28.14	32.12	37.08
15	24.96	26.22	27.79	30.35	36.10	24.92	26.29	28.97	33.22	38.54
16	25.55	26.88	28.54	31.22	37.36	25.51	26.96	29.84	34.33	39.99
17	26.18	27.55	29.25	32.08	38.66	26.14	27.67	30.66	35.43	41.41
18	26.77	28.22	29.99	32.95	39.92	26.77	28.34	31.49	36.57	42.87

Source: Fernández, J. R., D. T. Redden, A. Pietrobelli, and D. B. Allison. 2004. Waist circumference percentiles in nationally representative samples of African-American, European-American, and Mexican-American children and adolescents. *J. Pediatr.* 145:439–444.

● TABLE 13.3B Estimated Values for Waist Circumference (in inches) by
Percentile for European American Children and Adolescents, according to Sex

Age (y)	Percentile for Boys					Percentile for Girls				
	10th	25th	50th	75th	90th	10th	25th	50th	75th	90th
2	16.88	18.46	18.54	19.13	19.92	16.96	17.75	18.66	19.52	20.66
3	17.59	19.21	19.37	20.15	21.25	17.59	18.42	19.40	20.43	21.81
4	18.30	19.92	20.19	21.18	22.59	18.22	19.09	20.15	21.33	22.91
5	19.01	20.66	20.98	22.24	23.93	18.85	19.76	29.90	22.24	24.05
6	19.72	21.27	21.81	23.26	25.27	19.48	20.39	21.65	23.14	25.19
7	20.43	22.12	22.63	24.29	26.61	20.11	21.06	22.40	24.05	27.08
8	21.14	22.87	23.46	25.31	27.95	20.74	21.73	23.14	24.96	27.44
9	21.85	23.58	24.29	26.37	29.25	21.37	22.40	23.89	25.86	28.58
10	22.55	24.33	25.07	27.40	30.59	22.00	23.07	24.60	26.77	29.72
11	23.26	25.03	25.90	28.42	31.92	22.63	23.70	25.35	27.67	30.82
12	23.97	25.78	26.73	29.48	33.62	23.26	24.37	26.10	28.58	31.96
13	24.68	26.53	27.55	30.51	34.60	23.89	25.03	26.85	29.48	33.11
14	25.39	27.24	28.38	31.77	35.94	24.52	25.70	27.59	30.39	34.21
15	26.10	27.99	29.17	32.59	37.28	25.15	26.37	28.24	31.29	35.35
16	26.81	28.70	29.99	33.62	38.62	25.78	27.00	29.09	32.20	36.49
17	27.51	29.44	30.82	34.64	39.96	26.41	27.67	29.84	33.11	37.59
18	28.22	30.19	31.65	35.66	41.29	27.04	28.34	30.59	34.01	38.74

Source: Fernández, J. R., D. T. Redden, A. Pietrobelli, and D. B. Allison. 2004. Waist circumference percentiles in nationally representative samples of African-American, European-American, and Mexican-American children and adolescents. *J. Pediatr.* 145:439–444.

TABLE 13.3C Estimated Values for Waist Circumference by Percentile for Mexican American Children and Adolescents, according to Sex

	Percentile for Boys					Percentile for Girls				
Age (y)	10th	25th	50th	75th	90th	10th	25th	50th	75th	90th
2	17.48	17.92	18.74	19.60	20.95	17.51	17.99	18.89	19.68	21.06
3	18.14	18.70	19.60	20.66	22.32	18.11	18.66	19.72	20.70	22.32
4	18.81	19.44	20.47	21.77	23.70	18.70	19.37	20.55	21.73	23.58
5	19.48	20.19	21.51	22.83	25.03	19.29	20.07	21.33	22.75	24.80
6	20.15	20.94	22.16	23.89	26.41	19.88	20.74	22.16	23.77	26.04
7	20.82	21.69	23.03	24.96	27.79	20.47	21.45	22.99	24.80	27.32
8	21.49	22.44	23.89	26.06	29.17	21.06	22.16	23.77	25.82	28.58
9	22.16	23.18	24.76	27.12	30.55	21.65	22.83	24.60	26.85	29.84
10	22.83	23.93	25.62	28.18	31.88	22.24	23.54	25.43	27.87	31.06
11	23.50	24.68	26.45	29.29	33.26	22.87	24.25	26.22	28.89	32.32
12	24.17	25.43	27.32	30.35	34.64	23.46	24.96	27.04	29.92	33.58
13	24.84	26.18	27.79	31.41	36.02	24.05	25.62	27.87	30.94	34.84
14	25.51	26.92	29.05	32.51	37.40	24.64	26.33	28.70	31.96	36.10
15	26.18	27.67	29.92	33.58	38.74	25.23	27.04	29.48	32.99	37.32
16	26.85	28.42	30.74	34.64	40.11	25.82	27.71	30.31	34.01	38.58
17	27.51	29.17	31.61	35.70	41.49	26.41	28.42	31.14	35.03	39.84
18	28.18	29.92	32.48	36.81	42.87	27.00	29.13	31.92	36.06	41.10

Source: Fernández, J. R., D. T. Redden, A. Pietrobelli, and D. B. Allison. 2004. Waist circumference percentiles in nationally representative samples of African-American, European-American, and Mexican-American children and adolescents. *J. Pediatr.* 145:439–444.

scientists for many years to estimate body composition based on population-specific and generalized equations. Skinfold measurements are based on the concept that approximately 50 percent of body fat is subcutaneous tissue, and that by measuring numerous body sites, body composition can be calculated from a number formulae that require an estimate of the sum of skinfold thickness, age, and sex.

Many of the skinfold equations include three or more sites. The equations that use the three skinfold sites have been determined to be more generalizable to specific populations than those that require only one or two site measures.

Skinfold measurements are highly correlated with hydrostatically determined body density, as well as other more currently precise methods, such as DEXA. The accuracy of skinfold measurements are approximately ±3.5 percent, and errors can be minimized by using quality commercially available calipers (like Lange, Harpenden, and Lafayette; cost of device

is about $250–$400) and by training evaluators in proper site selection and proper measurement techniques. Figure 13.9 shows a typical skinfold measurement of the suprailium. The Exercise Physiology Reality feature at the end of this chapter provides the specific instructions and illustrations for performing multisite skinfold measurements for adults and youth.

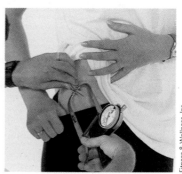

FIGURE 13.9 Skinfold pressures estimate body fat by using a caliper to gauge the thickness of a fold of skin on the back of the arm (over the triceps), below the shoulder blade (subscapular), and in other places (including lower body sites), and then comparing these measurements with standards.

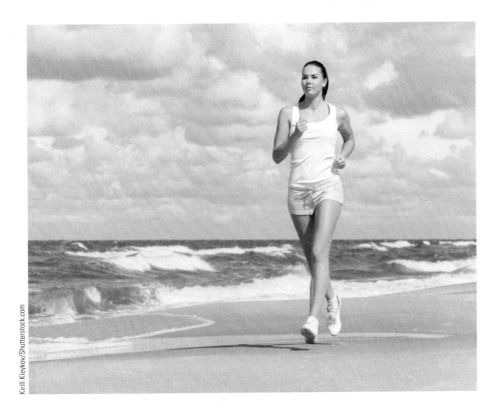

Kirill Kleykov/Shutterstock.com

More than 100 skinfold prediction equations for determining body composition have been published; thus, it is often difficult to determine which one to use with your clients. It is important to consider the following items when deciding which skinfold equation to use:

- What type of client is being measured? (Athlete or nonathlete? Adult or child?)

- Is the equation based on a large representative study sample?

- How has the equation been validated?

- Has the equation been cross-validated across laboratories and investigators?

- How accurate is the equation compared with other methods?

Generalized skinfold equations for adults like those developed by A. S. Jackson and Mike Pollock (1978) and Jackson et al. (1980) have become commonly used by exercise science professionals because they were developed on heterogeneous samples that vary considerably by age and body fatness. Initially, Jackson and Pollock developed skinfold predictions based on measuring the sum of seven skinfolds (chest,

axilla, triceps, abdomen, subscapular, suprailium, and thigh) and age. Because of the potential embarrassment associated with measuring certain sites, the sum of three sites and age are now more commonly recommended for use based on sex. The sum of three sites for men, are chest, abdomen, and thigh, whereas those for women are triceps, suprailium, and thigh. Once the sum of three skinfold sites is measured and the age of your client has been determined, you can use Tables 13.4a–c to obtain the estimated percentage of body fat.

If you are ever required to measure skinfolds in specialized populations, like athletes, it may be easier to initially measure and record the sum of the skinfolds gathered, then just compare the sum over time instead of trying to select a specific prediction equation. The sum of skinfolds measured over time can be used to determine changes in fitness or the maintenance of body composition that are consistent with good health.

HOTLINK *See the Exercise Physiology Reality feature at the end of this chapter for more on acquiring the sum of three skinfolds.*

TABLE 13.4A Skinfold Thickness Technique: Percent Fat Estimates for Women Calculated from Triceps, Suprailium, and Thigh

Sum of 3 Skinfolds	Age at Last Birthday								
	22 or Under	23 to 27	28 to 32	33 to 37	38 to 42	43 to 47	48 to 52	53 to 57	58 and Over
23–25	9.7	9.9	10.2	10.4	10.7	10.9	11.2	11.4	11.7
26–28	11.0	11.2	11.5	11.7	12.0	12.3	12.5	12.7	13.0
29–31	12.3	12.5	12.8	13.0	13.3	13.5	13.8	14.0	14.3
32–34	13.6	13.8	14.0	14.3	14.5	14.8	15.0	15.3	15.5
35–37	14.8	15.0	15.3	15.5	15.8	16.0	16.3	16.5	16.8
38–40	16.0	16.3	16.5	16.7	17.0	17.2	17.5	17.7	18.0
41–43	17.2	17.4	17.7	17.9	18.2	18.4	18.7	18.9	19.2
44–46	18.3	18.6	18.8	19.1	19.3	19.6	19.8	20.1	20.3
47–49	19.5	19.7	20.0	20.2	20.5	20.7	21.0	21.2	21.5
50–52	20.6	20.8	21.1	21.3	21.6	21.8	22.1	22.3	22.6
53–55	21.7	21.9	22.1	22.4	22.6	22.9	23.1	23.4	23.6
56–58	22.7	23.0	23.2	23.4	23.7	23.9	24.2	24.4	24.7
59–61	23.7	24.0	24.2	24.5	24.7	25.0	25.2	25.5	25.7
62–64	24.7	25.0	25.2	25.5	25.7	26.0	26.2	26.4	26.7
65–67	25.7	25.9	26.2	26.4	26.7	26.9	27.2	27.4	27.7
68–70	26.6	26.9	27.1	27.4	27.6	27.9	28.1	28.4	28.6
71–73	27.5	27.8	28.0	28.3	28.5	28.8	29.0	29.3	29.5
74–76	28.4	28.7	28.9	29.2	29.4	29.7	29.9	30.2	30.4
77–79	29.3	29.5	29.8	30.0	30.3	30.5	30.8	31.0	31.3
80–82	30.1	30.4	30.6	30.9	31.1	31.4	31.6	31.9	32.1
83–85	30.9	31.2	31.4	31.7	31.9	32.2	32.4	32.7	32.9
86–88	31.7	32.0	32.2	32.5	32.7	32.9	33.2	33.4	33.7
89–91	32.5	32.7	33.0	33.2	33.5	33.7	33.9	34.2	34.4
92–94	33.2	33.4	33.7	33.9	34.2	34.4	34.7	34.9	35.2
95–97	33.9	34.1	34.4	34.6	34.9	35.1	35.4	35.6	35.9
98–100	34.6	34.8	35.1	35.3	35.5	35.8	36.0	36.3	36.5
101–103	35.2	35.4	35.7	35.9	36.2	36.4	36.7	36.9	37.2
104–106	35.8	36.1	36.3	36.6	36.8	37.1	37.3	37.5	37.8
107–109	36.4	36.7	36.9	37.1	37.4	37.6	37.9	38.1	38.4
110–112	37.0	37.2	37.5	37.7	38.0	38.2	38.5	38.7	38.9
113–115	37.5	37.8	38.0	38.2	38.5	38.7	39.0	39.2	39.5
116–118	38.0	38.3	38.5	38.8	39.0	39.3	39.5	39.7	40.0
119–121	38.5	38.7	39.0	39.2	39.5	39.7	40.0	40.2	40.5
122–124	39.0	39.2	39.4	39.7	39.9	40.2	40.4	40.7	40.9
125–127	39.4	39.6	39.9	40.1	40.4	40.6	40.9	41.1	41.4
128–130	39.8	40.0	40.3	40.5	40.8	41.0	41.3	41.5	41.8

Body density is calculated based on the generalized equation for predicting body density of women developed by A. S. Jackson, M. L. Pollock, and A. Ward and published in *Medicine and Science in Sports and Exercise* 12 (1980): 175–182. Percent body fat is determined from the calculated body density using the Siri formula.
Source: Hoeger, W. W. K., and S. A. Hoeger. 2010. Table 4.1 in *Lifetime physical fitness & wellness*, 11th ed. Belmont, CA: Brooks/Cole-Cengage Learning.

13

TABLE 13.4B Skinfold Thickness Technique: Percentage Fat Estimates for Men Younger Than 40 Calculated from Chest, Abdomen, and Thigh

Sum of 3 Skinfolds	Age at Last Birthday							
	19 or Under	20 to 22	23 to 25	26 to 28	29 to 31	32 to 34	35 to 37	38 to 40
8–10	.9	1.3	1.6	2.0	2.3	2.7	3.0	3.3
11–13	1.9	2.3	2.6	3.0	3.3	3.7	4.0	4.3
14–16	2.9	3.3	3.6	3.9	4.3	4.6	5.0	5.3
17–19	3.9	4.2	4.6	4.9	5.3	5.6	6.0	6.3
20–22	4.8	5.2	5.5	5.9	6.2	6.6	6.9	7.3
23–25	5.8	6.2	6.5	6.8	7.2	7.5	7.9	8.2
26–28	6.8	7.1	7.5	7.8	8.1	8.5	8.8	9.2
29–31	7.7	8.0	8.4	8.7	9.1	9.4	9.8	10.1
32–34	8.6	9.0	9.3	9.7	10.0	10.4	10.7	11.1
35–37	9.5	9.9	10.2	10.6	10.9	11.3	11.6	12.0
38–40	10.5	10.8	11.2	11.5	11.8	12.2	12.5	12.9
41–43	11.4	11.7	12.1	12.4	12.7	13.1	13.4	13.8
44–46	12.2	12.6	12.9	13.3	13.6	14.0	14.3	14.7
47–49	13.1	13.5	13.8	14.2	14.5	14.9	15.2	15.5
50–52	14.0	14.3	14.7	15.0	15.4	15.7	16.1	16.4
53–55	14.8	15.2	15.5	15.9	16.2	16.6	16.9	17.3
56–58	15.7	16.0	16.4	16.7	17.1	17.4	17.8	18.1
59–61	16.5	16.9	17.2	17.6	17.9	18.3	18.6	19.0
62–64	17.4	17.7	18.1	18.4	18.8	19.1	19.4	19.8
65–67	18.2	18.5	18.9	19.2	19.6	19.9	20.3	20.6
68–70	19.0	19.3	19.7	20.0	20.4	20.7	21.1	21.4
71–73	19.8	20.1	20.5	20.8	21.2	21.5	21.9	22.2
74–76	20.6	20.9	21.3	21.6	22.0	22.2	22.7	23.0
77–79	21.4	21.7	22.1	22.4	22.8	23.1	23.4	23.8
80–82	22.1	22.5	22.8	23.2	23.5	23.9	24.2	24.6
83–85	22.9	23.2	23.6	23.9	24.3	24.6	25.0	25.3
86–88	23.6	24.0	24.3	24.7	25.0	25.4	25.7	26.1
89–91	24.4	24.7	25.1	25.4	25.8	26.1	26.5	26.8
92–94	25.1	25.5	25.8	26.2	26.5	26.9	27.2	27.5
95–97	25.8	26.2	26.5	26.9	27.2	27.6	27.9	28.3
98–100	26.6	26.9	27.3	27.6	27.9	28.3	28.6	29.0
101–103	27.3	27.6	28.0	28.3	28.6	29.0	29.3	29.7
104–106	27.9	28.3	28.6	29.0	29.3	29.7	30.0	30.4
107–109	28.6	29.0	29.3	29.7	30.0	30.4	30.7	31.1
110–112	29.3	29.6	30.0	30.3	30.7	31.0	31.4	31.7
113–115	30.0	30.3	30.7	31.0	31.3	31.7	32.0	32.4
116–118	30.6	31.0	31.3	31.6	32.0	32.3	32.7	33.0
119–121	31.3	31.6	32.0	32.3	32.6	33.0	33.3	33.7
122–124	31.9	32.2	32.6	32.9	33.3	33.6	34.0	34.3
125–127	32.5	32.9	33.2	33.5	33.9	34.2	34.6	34.9
128–130	33.1	33.5	33.8	34.2	34.5	34.9	35.2	35.5

Body density is calculated based on the generalized equation for predicting body density of men developed by A. S. Jackson and M. L. Pollock and published in the *British Journal of Nutrition* 40 (1978): 497–504. Percent body fat is determined from the calculated body density using the Siri formula.
Source: Hoeger, W. W. K., and S. A. Hoeger. 2010. Table 4.2 in *Lifetime physical fitness & wellness*, 11th ed. Belmont, CA: Brooks/Cole-Cengage Learning.

13

TABLE 13.4C Skinfold Thickness Technique: Percentage Fat Estimates for Men Older Than 40 Calculated from Chest, Abdomen, and Thigh

Sum of 3 Skinfolds	Age at Last Birthday							
	41 to 43	44 to 46	47 to 49	50 to 52	53 to 55	56 to 58	59 to 61	62 and Over
8–10	3.7	4.0	4.4	4.7	5.1	5.4	5.8	6.1
11–13	4.7	5.0	5.4	5.7	6.1	6.4	6.8	7.1
14–16	5.7	6.0	6.4	6.7	7.1	7.4	7.8	8.1
17–19	6.7	7.0	7.4	7.7	8.1	8.4	8.7	9.1
20–22	7.6	8.0	8.3	8.7	9.0	9.4	9.7	10.1
23–25	8.6	8.9	9.3	9.6	10.0	10.3	10.7	11.0
26–28	9.5	9.9	10.2	10.6	10.9	11.3	11.6	12.0
29–31	10.5	10.8	11.2	11.5	11.9	12.2	12.6	12.9
32–34	11.4	11.8	12.1	12.4	12.8	13.1	13.5	13.8
35–37	12.3	12.7	13.0	13.4	13.7	14.1	14.4	14.8
38–40	13.2	13.6	13.9	14.3	14.6	15.0	15.3	15.7
41–43	14.1	14.5	14.8	15.2	15.5	15.9	16.2	16.6
44–46	15.0	15.4	15.7	16.1	16.4	16.8	17.1	17.5
47–49	15.9	16.2	16.6	16.9	17.3	17.6	18.0	18.3
50–52	16.8	17.1	17.5	17.8	18.2	18.5	18.8	19.2
53–55	17.6	18.0	18.3	18.7	19.0	19.4	19.7	20.1
56–58	18.5	18.8	19.2	19.5	19.9	20.2	20.6	20.9
59–61	19.3	19.7	20.0	20.4	20.7	21.0	21.4	21.7
62–64	20.1	20.5	20.8	21.2	21.5	21.9	22.2	22.6
65–67	21.0	21.3	21.7	22.0	22.4	22.7	23.0	23.4
68–70	21.8	22.1	22.5	22.8	23.2	23.5	23.9	24.2
71–73	22.6	22.9	23.3	23.6	24.0	24.3	24.7	25.0
74–76	23.4	23.7	24.1	24.4	24.8	25.1	25.4	25.8
77–79	24.1	24.5	24.8	25.2	25.5	25.9	26.2	26.6
80–82	24.9	25.3	25.6	26.0	26.3	26.6	27.0	27.3
83–85	25.7	26.0	26.4	26.7	27.1	27.4	27.8	28.1
86–88	26.4	26.8	27.1	27.5	27.8	28.2	28.5	28.9
89–91	27.2	27.5	27.9	28.2	28.6	28.9	29.2	29.6
92–94	27.9	28.2	28.6	28.9	29.3	29.6	30.0	30.3
95–97	28.6	29.0	29.3	29.7	30.0	30.4	30.7	31.1
98–100	29.3	29.7	30.0	30.4	30.7	31.1	31.4	31.8
101–103	30.0	30.4	30.7	31.1	31.4	31.8	32.1	32.5
104–106	30.7	31.1	31.4	31.8	32.1	32.5	32.8	33.2
107–109	31.4	31.8	32.1	32.4	32.8	33.1	33.5	33.8
110–112	32.1	32.4	32.8	33.1	33.5	33.8	34.2	34.5
113–115	32.7	33.1	33.4	33.8	34.1	34.5	34.8	35.2
116–118	33.4	33.7	34.1	34.4	34.8	35.1	35.5	35.8
119–121	34.0	34.4	34.7	35.1	35.4	35.8	36.1	36.5
122–124	34.7	35.0	35.4	35.7	36.1	36.4	36.7	37.1
125–127	35.3	35.6	36.0	36.3	36.7	37.0	37.4	37.7
128–130	35.9	36.2	36.6	36.9	37.3	37.6	38.0	38.5

Body density is calculated based on the generalized equation for predicting body density of men developed by A. S. Jackson and M. L. Pollock and published in the *British Journal of Nutrition* 40 (1978): 497–504. Percent body fat is determined from the calculated body density using the Siri formula.

Source: Hoeger, W. W. K., and S. A. Hoeger. 2010. Table 4.3 in *Lifetime physical fitness & wellness*, 11th ed. Belmont, CA: Brooks/Cole-Cengage Learning.

Although skinfold equations have been developed to predict the body composition for children and youths, the error of such measurements for youths is higher (≥3 percent) compared with adults because of growth and development variability. The percentage of body fat for youths based on sex from the sum of a calf (or subscapular) and triceps skinfold measure can be estimated. (For more details on predicting the body composition of youths, see Lohman [1986].)

Bioelectrical Impedance

The ability of bodily tissues to conduct an electric current has been recognized by scientists for more than 100 years. A technique called **total body electrical conductivity (TOBEC)** allows body composition to be determined based on the concept that water and lean body tissue (like muscle) conducts electricity better than fat tissue. In the TOBEC method, a subject is placed in a cylindrical coil as an electric current is passed through the coil, which changes the electromagnetic field based on the person's body composition. The TOBEC technique has been shown to be reliable but is costly (several thousand dollars) and is used mainly in clinical or medical centers.

Bioelectrical impedance (BIA) is based on the concepts of TOBEC, but it is easy to use, popular, portable, noninvasive, and costs only a moderate amount to evaluate body composition (see Figure 13.10). Body composition can be estimated by the BIA method. A low-amperage electrical current is passed through surface electrodes attached to the body (often at the wrist and ankle) ostensibly to measure whole-body resistance and use basic assumptions about body shape. However, the accuracy of BIA is like skinfold methodology and is highly dependent on which device is used and which prediction equation is used to estimate body composition. The BIA has

been reported to be as accurate as skinfold measurements (3.5 percent error), but the reliability of the method can be low and is highly dependent on the following factors when measured:

- State of hydration
- Effects of recent eating
- Effects of recent drinking of fluids
- Effects of recent bouts of exercise
- Same instrument used for multiple measures

Newer BIA instruments and technologic advances have improved the effectiveness of the method. The cost of BIA instruments range from about $100 to several thousand dollars, with more expensive models yielding better measures when limitations are minimized. Simple BIA evaluations can be self-administered and require the subject to stand on a scale (the feet act as surface electrodes) or to hold electrode-like handles with a handheld device. Clients then enter their age, sex, height, and weight.

Many simple (inexpensive) BIA instruments have an internal microprocessor that uses the data entered by the subject to predict percentage body fat based on BMI (approximately 6 percent error). More sophisticated BIA devices have been developed that provide calculated data about fat mass, FFM, TBW, estimated muscle mass, and predicted ideal weight that can be printed as a record and shared with the client. Although the BIA method for evaluating body composition has emerged as a low-tech methodology, questions about the accuracy of various BIA devices remains problematic.

(Which field model of evaluating body composition has the least error?)

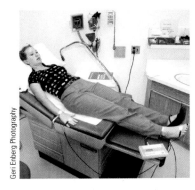

Geri Enberg Photography

FIGURE 13.10 Bioelectrical impedance measures body fat by using a low-intensity electrical current. Because electrolyte-containing fluids, which readily conduct an electrical current, are found primarily in lean body tissues, the leaner the person, the less resistance to the current. The measurement of electrical resistance is then used in a mathematical equation to estimate the percentage of body fat.

13

total body electrical conductivity (TOBEC) A method used to determine body composition based on the concept that water and lean body tissue (like muscle) conducts electricity better than fat tissue.

bioelectrical impedance (BIA) A simplified method used to evaluate body composition; based on the concepts of TOBEC.

● TABLE 13.5 Comparison of Methods Used to Estimate Body Composition

Method	Accuracy	Practicality and Portability	Ease of Use	Time	Cost	Subject Comfort and Effort	Technician Training
Underwater (hydrostatic) weighing	SEE = ±2.7%	Practical in exercise physiology laboratories or large fitness centers; not portable	Requires subject to submerge, exhale, and hold breath	~30 minutes because the procedure should be repeated 5 to 10 times	Initial purchase of equipment is expensive	Subject may be uncomfortable wearing a bathing suit, submerging in water, and exhaling air	Training is needed but is not difficult
Plethysmography	SEE = ±2.7–3.7%	Requires 8' × 8' space; can be moved with proper equipment, but takes effort	Requires subject to sit quietly	~5 minutes	Initial purchase of equipment is expensive	Subject may be uncomfortable wearing a bathing suit and cap and sitting in an enclosed space	Minimal training needed
Skinfold measurements	SEE = ±3.5%	Practical in settings that have a private area; very portable	Requires subject to be still; measurement sites must be determined and marked	<5 minutes	Initial purchase of equipment is relatively inexpensive	Subject may be uncomfortable partially disrobing; some skinfolds are difficult to grasp	Training and consistency are critical; technique improves with experience
Bioelectrical Impedance Analysis (BIA)	SEE = ±3.5%	Practical in most settings; very portable	Easy to use	<5 minutes	Initial purchase of equipment is moderately expensive	Procedure is simple but pre-measurement guidelines require substantial subject compliance	Minimal training needed
Dual-Energy X-ray Absorptiometry (DEXA)	SEE = ±1.8%; more research needed to verify SEE	Practical in imaging centers, physicians' offices, or research facilities; not portable	Easy to use	~5 to 10 minutes	Initial purchase of equipment is very expensive	Simple procedure; subject is exposed to a very small amount of radiation; use prohibited during pregnancy	Training is needed; license to operate is required
Computed Tomography Scans (CT) and Magnetic Resonance Imaging (MRI)	Not yet established	Practical in imaging centers and research facilities; not portable	Requires subject to be still throughout the entire procedure	~30 minutes	Initial purchase of equipment is very expensive	Procedure is relatively simple with some subject discomfort	Training is needed; license to operate is required

Legend: SEE = Standard Error of the Estimate
Source: Dunford, M., and J. A. Doyle. 2007. Table 11.1 in *Nutrition for sport and exercise*. Belmont, CA: Wadsworth.

13

Selecting the Appropriate Body Composition Tool and Interpretation of Body Composition

As you have learned, a variety of laboratory and field methodologies exist for you to choose from to evaluate a client's body composition. So, which is the best method to use to determine body composition for your clients? Perhaps the best answer to this question is that the best method depends on the resources you have (cost), ease of use, accuracy (amount of error of each method) required, and whether the method you choose measures fat distribution. Table 13.5 contains the advantages and disadvantages of the previously discussed laboratory and field measures of body composition. You should become familiar with all the methods discussed and be able to help your clients understand the benefits and limitations of measurements of body composition.

To interpret body composition, you will first need to understand that many ways to evaluate body composition results have been reported in the exercise science literature. Each interpretation depends on the population you are working with (for example, youth versus adults), goals of your client (health versus athleticism), and the educational messages you need to share with your client (weight loss, weight gain, weight maintenance). Table 13.6 provides

● T A B L E 13.6 Standards for Evaluating Body Composition of Adults

Body Composition Category	Age			
	<30	30–39	40–49	Over 50
Men				
High	>28%	>29%	>30%	>31%
Moderately high	22–28%	23–29%	24–30%	25–31%
Optimal range	11–21%	12–22%	13–23%	14–24%
Low	6–10%	7–11%	8–12%	9–13%
Very low	≥5%	≥6%	≥7%	≥8%
Women				
High	>32%	>33%	>34%	>36%
Moderately high	26–32%	27–33%	28–34%	29–35%
Optimal range	15–25%	16–26%	17–27%	18–28%
Low	12–14%	13–15%	14–16%	15–17%
Very low	≥11%	≥12%	≥13%	≥14%

High—Percentage fat at this level indicates the person is seriously overweight to a degree that can have adverse health consequences. The person should be encouraged to lose weight through diet and exercise. Maintaining weight at this level for a long period places the person at risk for hypertension, heart disease, and diabetes. A long-term weight-loss and exercise program should be initiated. **Moderately high**—It is likely that the person is significantly overweight, but the level could be high, in part, because of measurement inaccuracies. It would be wise to carefully monitor people in this category and encourage them not to gain additional weight. People in this category may want to have their body composition assessed by the underwater weighing method. **Optimal range**—It would be highly desirable to maintain body composition at this level. **Low**—This is an acceptable body composition level, but there is no reason to seek a lower percentage body fat level. Loss of additional body weight could have health consequences. **Very low**—Percentage fat level at this range should be reached only by high-level endurance athletes who are in training. Being this thin may carry its own additional mortality risk. Individuals, especially females, this low are at risk for having an eating disorder such as anorexia nervosa.
Source: Jackson, A. S., and R. M. Ross. 1997. Table 4.2 and Figure 4.7 in *Understanding health and fitness*, 3rd ed. Dubuque, IA: Kendall Hunt Publishing.

body composition standards for adults and the interpretation for each body composition category. You will need to search the exercise science literature for specific body composition standards and interpretations based on each of your client's needs as discussed earlier.

HOTLINK *Search the Internet for samples of reliable body composition standards and interpretations for adolescents, adult athletes, and youth athletes. For example, see the Exercise Prescription commercial website at* **http://www.exrx.net**.

What is the best way to measure body composition? Defend your answer. What factors can you use to interpret the body composition of your clients?

Weight Management

Throughout the text you have read that the prevalence of obesity and metabolic syndrome are dramatically increasing, not only in the United States, but worldwide. One of the greatest challenges you will face as a professional in the exercise science field is helping your clients control their body weight and body composition. An important weight management goal for you is to educate your clients to understand and implement behaviors that will help them control their body weight at healthy levels. The primary factors that will influence the healthy weight control for your clients will be genetic and environmental factors that affect their energy intake and energy expenditure balance. However, it is difficult to convince overweight clients to modify their exercise and eating behaviors if you yourself do not practice what you preach.

What does "practice what you preach" mean to you?

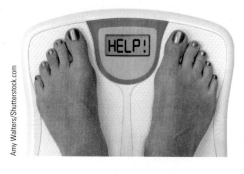

Amy Walters/Shutterstock.com

Genetic Factors

The genetics of your clients may not affect just their basal metabolic rate (BMR), the thermic effect of food intake, and their spontaneous exercise, but also their fat cell development, fat cell metabolism, and their "set point" for weight control. Genetics, as you may recall from the thrifty gene hypothesis (see Chapter 6A), suggests that people who are genetically best able to survive famine and starvation are also those most prone to gain weight when food is plentiful.

The amount of fat in an individual's body is due to both the number and size of the fat cells. The number of fat cells increases rapidly during childhood and early puberty. After growth ceases, fat cell number may continue to increase whenever energy balance is positive. Obese people have more fat cells and larger fat cells than those individuals who are at a healthy weight. When energy intake exceeds energy expenditure, fat cells accumulate triglycerides and expand in size. When fat cells enlarge, they also stimulate an increase in the number of cells again. Therefore, when individuals become obese, they may increase both the number of and size of their fat cells. When energy expenditure exceeds energy intake, fat cells decrease in size, but not number (see Figure 13.11).

Individuals with extra fat cells tend to regain lost weight more rapidly, whereas those who have a more average number of fat cells have more success at maintaining

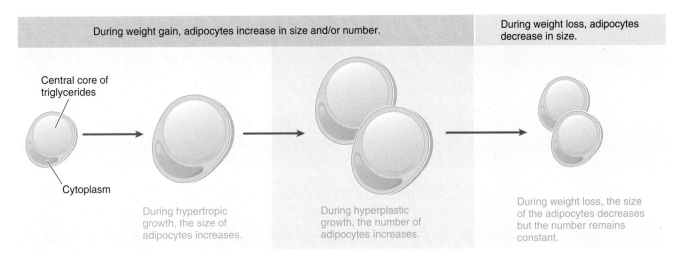

| During weight gain, adipocytes increase in size and/or number. | During weight loss, adipocytes decrease in size. |

Central core of triglycerides

Cytoplasm

During hypertropic growth, the size of adipocytes increases.

During hyperplastic growth, the number of adipocytes increases.

During weight loss, the size of the adipocytes decreases but the number remains constant.

FIGURE 13.11 Hypertrophic and hyperplastic growth of adipose tissue. The amount of adipose tissue a person has depends on the number and size of his or her adipose cells (adipocytes). (From McGuire, M., and K. A. Beerman. 2009. Figure 8.2 in *Nutritional sciences.* 2nd ed. Belmont, CA: Brooks/Cole-Cengage Learning.)

weight loss because when their cells shrink, both cell size and number become normal. The prevention of excessive weight gain between adolescence and adulthood is critical, when the fat cells are increasing in number. For grade kindergarten (K) through 12 teachers and coaches, it is of the utmost importance that the programs of exercise in the schools increase the activity of the children above moderate intensities for at least half of their physical education/sports class periods for at least 30 minutes per day. Furthermore, children at risk for being overweight in their early teens should be identified in the Pre-K years, and through parent/teacher/coach/ family physician meetings, some form of weight management plan needs to be developed. Unfortunately, recent public health surveys identify that the parents of these at-risk children are not aware of or even think that their child is overweight.

Fat cell metabolism is highly influenced by genetics based on the numerous hormone and enzymatic reactions that occur in fat oxidation. As discussed in Chapter 11, adjusting energy intake and energy expenditure factors can have positive influences on fat cell metabolism, even when controlling for genetic factors. Cellular metabolism is elevated after exercise, as measured by BMR studies. Aerobic and anaerobic (resistance training) exercise can increase fat metabolism and help maintain or increase lean body mass. However, questions remain as to how much and how long BMR is elevated after exercise.

HOTLINK *See Chapters 5, 6, 6A, and 6B for more information on fat cell metabolism.*

Set-point theory refers to the control or maintenance of a specific body weight by an individual's internal controls (primarily the hypothalamus). Although the "set point" is just a concept and perhaps not a reality, exercise scientists have confirmed that after weight gains or weight losses, the body attempts to adjust its metabolism to restore the original weight. Energy expenditure increases after weight gain and decreases after weight loss. These changes in energy expenditure are different than those expected based on body composition and may help explain why it is so difficult for an underweight person to maintain weight gain and why an overweight person fails to maintain weight loss.

It has been reported in the research literature that the "set point" for the individual's BMR can decrease after **weight cycling** (losing and then regaining the lost weight and even more) and remain low, creating a major challenge for future weight loss. Figure 13.12 shows how the devastating psychological effects of obesity and dieting perpetuate themselves.

set-point theory The control or maintenance of a specific body weight by an individual's internal controls (primarily the hypothalamus).

weight cycling Losing weight and then regaining the lost weight and even more over time.

Indeed, rapid weight cycling practiced by wrestlers, ballet dancers, gymnasts, cheerleaders, jockeys, Haute Couture models, and entertainment stars have resulted in devastating hormonal imbalances, anorexia nervosa (AN), and death. Another clinical sequela of these weight cycling paradigms is that they can lead to hypertension, which may be difficult to control with medications. Excessive weight cycling also can lead to dehydration and have negative effects on "set point" that may lead to serious health risks. Position statements from the American College of Sports Medicine and state laws have been published to limit the amount of weight wrestlers can or should lose to make weight for various weight categories during competition.

Environmental Factors

Environmental factors have become as much of an influence on weight management as the genetic factors since the 1980s. For example, the ever-changing American societal environment has become **obesogenic**; that is, it is abundant in food availability and encourages a sedentary lifestyle. Figure 13.13 demonstrates the increases in obesity prevalence in the United States since 1990.

Although public policy statements such as *Healthy People 2020* have focused on efforts to reduce overweight and obesity, the trend has been in the opposite, undesired direction. Figure 13.14 highlights several items that have been identified for modification in youth intervention studies (like HEALTHY) to control/prevent the onset of type 2 diabetes. Ongoing societal and environmental changes have created many

obesogenic An abundance in food availability and a societal environment that encourages a sedentary lifestyle.

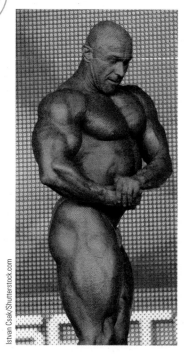

Istvan Csak/Shutterstock.com

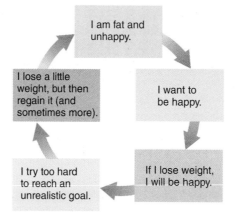

FIGURE 13.12 The psychology of weight cycling. (Adapted from Whitney, E. N., and S. R. Rolfes. 2010. Figure 9.4 in *Understanding nutrition*, 12 ed. Belmont, CA: Wadsworth.)

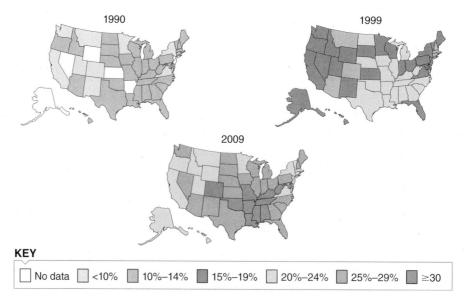

KEY

| | No data | | <10% | | 10%–14% | | 15%–19% | | 20%–24% | | 25%–29% | | ≥30 |

FIGURE 13.13 Obesity trends among U.S. adults: Behavioral Risk Factor Surveillance System 1990, 1999, and 2009. (From Centers for Disease Control and Prevention. Obesity trends among adults between 1985 and 2009. Available at: www.cdc.gov/obesity/downloads/obesity_trends_2009.pdf)

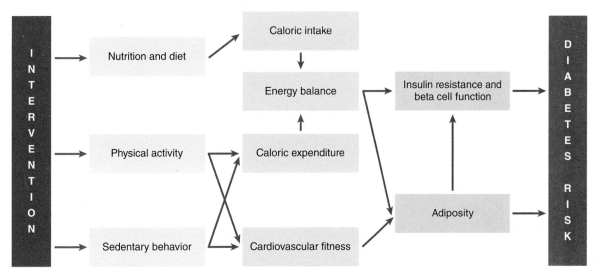

FIGURE 13.14 Relationship between intervention and diabetes risk. (From HEALTHY Coordinating Center. 2008. Prevention study group primary prevention trial: Protocol [version 1.4]. Available at: http://www .healthystudy.org/files/Additional%20Web%20Docs/HEALTHY%20public%20website%20protocol%20v1_4%20

barriers with regard to weight management (healthy eating and engaging in regular exercise).

HOTLINK *See the HEALTHY Study website (http://www.healthystudy.org) for more information about a national U.S. youth school-based intervention to prevent and control the development of type 2 diabetes.*

One of the most obvious influences on developing sound weight management programming is how people perceive their ideal weight or physique. Figure 13.15 illustrates the decline in weight for those who have won the Miss America title (an icon for beauty) for the past 80 years. Since the mid-1960s, most of the winners had

BMIs less than 18.5, which is considered underweight and unhealthy.

Research findings indicate that there is great disparity between reasonable weight loss or gain goals and "dream weight." Figure 13.16 shows the reasonable goals and expectations (ratings of dream, happy, acceptable, and disappointing weights) of a group of obese women before engaging in a weight-loss program.

Close to one year later, the group lost an average of 35 pounds, although about half of the women did not even reach their "disappointing weight." Although most of the women were not happy with a 16 percent weight loss, they reported positive

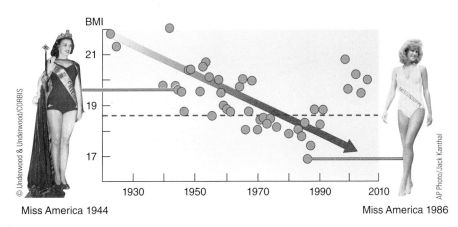

Miss America 1944

Miss America 1986

FIGURE 13.15 The declining weight of Miss America. (Adapted from Whitney, E. N., and S. R. Rolfes. 2010. Figure 8.5 in *Understanding nutrition.* 12 ed. Belmont, CA: Wadsworth.)

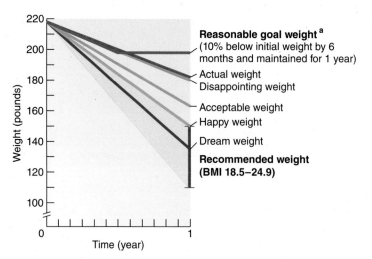

FIGURE 13.16 **Comparison of reasonable weight goals and expectations.** (Adapted from Whitney, E. N., and S. R. Rolfes. 2010. Figure 9.6 in *Understanding nutrition*, 12 ed. Belmont, CA: Wadsworth.)

physical, social, and psychological benefits of weight loss. This example reinforces the concept that you must help your clients establish realistic goals for effective weight management.

HOTLINK *See Chapter 1 for more information on setting behavioral goals.*

(What does the term *obesogenic* mean and how does it contribute to effective weight management?)

Dr. John C. Peters, who is an expert in biochemistry and nutrition and cofounder of Colorado on the Move and America on the Move (campaigns that promote choosing healthy lifestyles), has suggested that social changes are required to prevent the current obesity crisis. He has proposed several causal factors that are driving our current society to eat more and move less. Figure 13.17 highlights some of the environmental factors that Dr. Peters believes that we need to consider as professionals interested in developing effective weight management strategies. Although

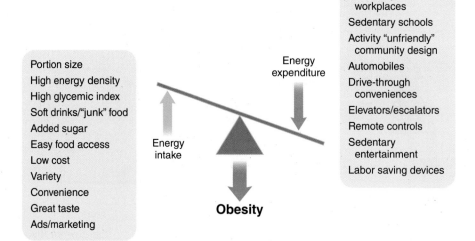

FIGURE 13.17 **Environmental factors hypothesized to promote excess energy intake and reduced energy expenditure.** (From Peters, J. C. 2006. Societal factors related to promoting obesity. *Exerc. Sport Sci. Rev.* 34:4–9.)

many of the factors shown in Figure 13.17 are consistent markers of a successful society as a whole, the "good life" produced by our societal technological advances may also carry unwanted health consequences.

(What are three environmental factors that can affect successful weight management for your clients?)

Developing an Effective Weight Management Plan

The first step in developing a weight management program for your clients is to help them generate an effective plan based on realistic goals and your professional input. An effective weight management program should consider the following client factors:

- Current body composition
- Current eating and exercise behaviors
- Environmental lifestyle
- Personal goals
- Mental stress
- Occupation
- Recreational behaviors
- BMR
- Genetics
- Self-esteem
- Body image
- Peer influences

In addition, the weight management plan for your clients should include strategies for education and behavioral adaptations for adjusting caloric intake and caloric expenditure once realistic goals have been set.

According to the *Physical Activity Guidelines Advisory Committee Report, 2008* (available at: http://www.health.gov/paguidelines), **weight loss** has been defined as at least a 5 percent loss of body weight (clinically significant). **Weight maintenance** (or weight stability) has been defined as a weight change of less than 3 percent, and **prevention of weight**

regain would be consistent with a change in weight of 3 percent to less than 5 percent. Table 13.7 provides general guidelines for weight management and specific guidelines for effective weight loss and prevention of weight regain that you should consider using to educate your clients as they develop their weight management plan.

In addition, the following list contains realistic and healthy tips to help your clients reach their goals:

- Have your clients check with their physicians or healthcare professionals to verify that their weight management goals are realistic and not unhealthy.

- Check your client's BMI, waist circumference, and percentage of body fat to help them determine a healthy goal weight.

- Use the *2010 Dietary Guidelines for Americans* for healthy eating.

- Adjust calorie intake and energy expenditure depending on your client's needs such as their BMI, waist circumference, and percentage of body fat (see Table 13.8).

- Engage in 200 to 300 minutes of exercise for long-term maintenance.

- Allow plenty of time (20–30 weeks) for long-term results and educate your clients that after achieving success, they need to be prepared for normal behavioral relapse, and yet develop strategies to return to an effective weight management plan as soon as possible.

weight loss At least a 5 percent loss of body weight (clinically significant).

weight maintenance A weight change of less than 3 percent. Also known as *weight stability*.

prevention of weight regain Consistent with a change in weight of 3 percent to less than 5 percent.

● **T A B L E 13.7 Weight Management Strategies**

In General

- Focus on healthy eating and activity habits, not on weight losses or gains.
- Adopt reasonable expectations about health and fitness goals and about how long it will take to achieve them.
- Make nutritional adequacy a high priority.
- Learn, practice, and follow a healthful eating plan for the rest of your life.
- Participate in some form of physical activity regularly.
- Adopt permanent lifestyle changes to achieve and maintain a healthy weight.

For Weight Loss

- Energy out should exceed energy in by about 500 kcalories/day. Increase your physical activity enough to spend more energy than you consume from foods.
- Emphasize foods with a low energy density and a high nutrient density.
- Eat small portions. Share a restaurant meal with a friend or take home half for lunch tomorrow.
- Eat slowly.
- Limit high-fat foods. Make legumes, whole grains, vegetables, and fruits central to your diet plan.
- Limit low-fat treats to the serving size on the label.
- Limit concentrated sweets and alcoholic beverages.
- Drink a glass of water before you begin to eat and another while you eat. Drink plenty of water throughout the day.
- Keep a record of diet and exercise habits: it reveals problem areas, the first step toward improving behaviors.
- Learn alternative ways to diet with emotions and stresses.
- Attend support groups regularly or develop supportive relationships with others.

For Weight Gain

- Energy in should exceed energy out by at least 500 kcalories/day. Increase your food intake enough to store more energy than you expend in exercise. Exercise and eat to build muscles.
- Expect weight gain to take time (1 pound per month would be reasonable).
- Emphasize energy-dense foods.
- Eat at least three meals a day.
- Eat large portions of foods and expect to feel full.
- Eat snacks between meals.
- Drink plenty of juice and milk.

Source: Whitney, E. N., and S. R. Rolfes. 2010. Table 9.6 in *Understanding nutrition*, 12 ed. Belmont, CA: Wadsworth.

- Retest BMI, waist circumference, and percentage of body fat every 3 months.

- Develop incentives for your clients to help them meet their individual needs.

Have your clients keep a log/journal to track their progress and reevaluate their plan every 3 months.

(What are five client-specific factors that can affect successful weight management?)

Dieting

Although many dietitians and other health professionals encourage their clients not to diet, but to just eat healthy according to various guides like the *2010 Dietary Guidelines for Americans*, a majority of your

clients (usually recreational or school/club athletes) will most likely be following some type of diet for weight loss or weight gain. Many weight-loss diets are indeed successful, at least initially, although dieting without regular exercise does not allow lean muscle mass to be maintained, so fat loss is also accompanied with muscle mass loss. Long-term diets usually fail because they are not sustainable for clients.

HOTLINK *See the U.S. Department of Agriculture website at* **http://www.cnpp.usda.gov/dietaryguidelines.htm** *to review the 2010 Dietary Guidelines for Americans.*

Weight-gain programs can be effective if the goal weight increase is reasonable (1/2 lb/week) and regular resistance training (two to three times per week) is included in your client's plan to maintain lean body mass. Genetic factors can significantly limit the ability of the clients to gain excessive

TABLE 13.8 Possible Caloric Intake and Caloric Strategies for Weight Management

	Underweight BMI <18.5	Normal BMI 18.5–24.9	Overweight BMI 25–29.9	Obese BMI >30
Caloric Intake	Use Dietary Guidelines for Americans 2010 Increase intake 200–500 kcal/day	Use 2010 DGA	Use 2010 DGA and reduce intake 200–300 kcal/day*	Consult physician and registered dietitian Follow 2010 DGA Reduce intake by 500 calories per day*
Caloric Expenditure	Become or remain physically active Use 2008 Physical Activity Guidelines for Americans Do not try to lose more weight!	Become or remain physically active Follow 2008 PAGA	Become or remain physically active Follow 2008 PAGA Guidelines Expend 200–300 kcal per day minimum in exercise	Become or remain physically active Follow 2008 PAGA Guidelines Go slowly and try to expend 500 kcal/day in exercise

*Never reduce dietary intake to below 2000 kcal/day unless under medical supervision.
It is best not to reduce dietary intake to below 2,000 kcal/day unless under the care of your physician.
© Cengage Learning 2013

lean muscle mass, and yet behavioral and environmental factors can help them optimize their individual potentials.

The majority of weight management challenges you will encounter in the next 5 to 10 years will involve clients trying to achieve effective weight loss. Dieting for weight loss may be an important first step for your clients who are 20 to 50 pounds overweight because they can probably expect to see significant weight loss (even without doing much exercise) in the first 4 to 8 weeks before hitting a weight-loss plateau. Although the weight-loss plateau may be a normal outcome or transition, you will need to help your clients with developing new goals and plans for future success.

So, which diet strategy is the best or most effective? The current research literature suggests that many dietary strategies (for example, Mediterranean diet, the Atkins diet, the Zone diet, South Beach diet, Weight Watchers) work at varying levels but depend on your client's ability to tolerate and adhere to the requirements of each plan. As long as the plan does not jeopardize your client's good health, it may be helpful for initial weight loss and success. However, after initial weight loss via dieting, you will probably need to educate your clients about how to adopt a physically active lifestyle (to expend additional calories and increase/maintain lean muscle mass) and to adopt eating behaviors like those in the *2010 Dietary Guidelines for Americans*.

> How effective are dieting strategies for long-term weight management? Why?

Medications and Bariatric Surgery/Banding

Because of the increasing incidence of obesity, many of your future clients may be undergoing aggressive treatments such as taking weight-loss drugs or preparing/recovering from **bariatric** surgery/banding. (Bariatric refers to the treatment of obesity or obesity-related problems.) Individuals who have BMIs greater than 35 to 40 are considered candidates for aggressive weight loss because these individuals either have metabolic syndrome or will develop it without treatment.

One method of aggressive treatment is with drugs used to produce appetite suppression (sibutramine) or to inhibit fat absorption (orlistat). Other drug therapies include the combination of appetite suppressants and metabolism-boosting agents. Although some new medications have had limited success (for example, weight loss of 10–20 pounds in obese subjects), many undesirable side effects are associated with drug use, including gas, frequent bowel movements, reduced vitamin absorption, rapid heart rate, and increased blood pressure.

bariatric Refers to the treatment of obesity or obesity-related problems.

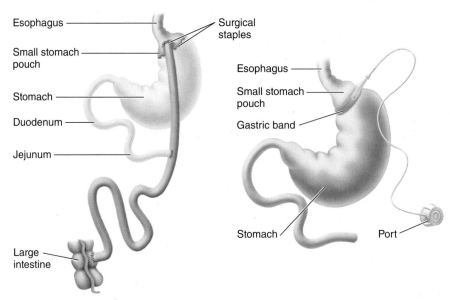

Esophagus

Surgical staples

Small stomach pouch

Stomach

Duodenum

Jejunum

Large intestine

Esophagus

Small stomach pouch

Gastric band

Stomach

Port

In gastric bypass, the surgeon constructs a small stomach pouch and creates an outlet directly to the small intestine, bypassing most of the stomach, the entire duodenum, and some of the jejunum. (Dark areas highlight the flow of food through the GI tract; pale areas indicate bypassed sections.)

In gastric banding, the surgeon uses a gastric band to reduce the opening from the esophagus to the stomach. The size of the opening can be adjusted by inflating or deflating the band by way of a port placed in the abdomen just beneath the skin.

● FIGURE 13.18 Gastric surgery used in the treatment of severe obesity. (Adapted from Whitney, E. N., and S. R. Rolfes. 2010. Figure 9.5 in *Understanding nutrition,* 12 ed. Belmont, CA: Wadsworth.)

13

CONCEPTS, challenges, controversies

Benefits of Bariatric Surgery

Long-term success data on large numbers of bariatric patients are not currently available, but many successful published clinical case studies have concluded that for many patients, their metabolic syndrome symptoms improve after treatment. Although risky, bariatric surgeries are on the rise, and for many obese individuals, this type of treatment may be their last chance to lose weight and adopt a healthy lifestyle. To maintain long-term success, bariatric surgery patients will still need to adopt a lifestyle that includes healthy eating and a regular program of exercise.

The National Institutes of Health has recommended bariatric surgery for obese people with a BMI of at least 40 and for people with a BMI of 35 and serious coexisting medical conditions such as diabetes. Bariatric surgery can be an excellent alternative for people who cannot lose significant weight through exercise and dieting, and whose general health is compromised.

Bariatric surgery has been associated with reversing type 2 diabetes, curbing sleep apnea, improving hypertension (blood pressure), reducing cholesterol levels, and reducing risk for coronary artery disease and some cancers. The long-term effects (like weight regain prevalence and economic insurance impact) remain to be determined.

Another aggressive treatment for obesity that has increased dramatically for youths and adults since 2004 is bariatric surgery and bariatric banding (also called *gastric banding*). These two procedures are shown in Figure 13.18 and are considered by many to be a last alternative for many obese individuals who cannot lose weight via normal behavioral change strategies or medication.

Bariatric bypass surgery alters the digestive tract so that only small amounts of food can be consumed or digested. Bariatric bypass reduces the stomach pouch and a connection is formed to the small intestine, bypassing some of the small intestine, thus limiting digestion and absorption. **Bariatric banding surgery**, or stapling, makes the stomach very small and increases the level of satiety for individuals, although they are consuming much less food. This type of treatment means that patients need to be careful to not overeat and to eat foods that are easy to chew completely before swallowing.

Both types of bariatric procedures have numerous specific adverse effects including nausea and diarrhea, and approximately 20 percent of people who have the procedures experience complications. In addition, bariatric surgeries carry an approximately 1 to 3 percent death rate depending on an individual's age, sex, and health status.

What is the difference between bariatric bypass surgery and banding? What type of clients do you think would typically undergo these procedures?

A Regular Program of Exercise

As you might have guessed, for effective long-term weight management success, the exercise science literature supports the need for regular amounts of exercise, even with successful dietary changes. Figure 13.19 illustrates the caloric intake and expenditures between those who are physically active and those who are sedentary. The active person has a more variable energy allowance, which allows for some leverage when one is trying to achieve weight management.

Self-reported data from studies where weight management failed indicate that the cessation of exercise by the study subjects is often to blame. Adherence to exercise should be a critical factor in any plan for successful weight management, and you will need to able to provide your clients with many options and plans for them to acquire regular exercise in their daily lives.

bariatric bypass surgery A procedure that alters the digestive tract so that only small amounts of food can be consumed or digested.

bariatric banding surgery A procedure that makes the stomach very small and increases the level of satiety for individuals, although they are consuming much less food.

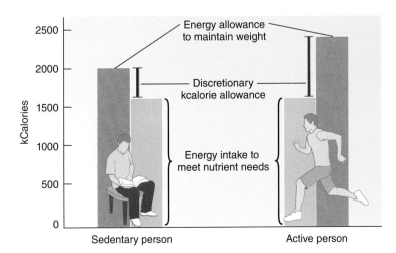

FIGURE 13.19 Influence of physical activity on discretionary kilocalorie allowance.
(Adapted from Whitney, E. N., and S. R. Rolfes. 2010. Figure 9.8 in *Understanding nutrition*, 12 ed. Belmont, CA: Wadsworth.

Eating Disorders and Body Image Disorders

You no doubt have known or currently know someone who has abnormal eating behaviors or someone who feels uncomfortable about her body image. Since the 1980s, the incidence of disordered eating and those with distorted body image perceptions has increased as more people have become preoccupied with food, dieting, exercise, weight loss, and weight gain. **Disordered eating** includes a variety of eating patterns that are irregular, or excessive, or too sparse. Although disordered eating may be normal, particularly during times of stress or illness, these patterns may turn into full-blown **eating disorders** over time that can result in serious physical and psychological consequences.

The American Psychiatric Association (APA) has classified eating disorders into the categories of **anorexia nervosa (AN)**, **bulimia nervosa (BN)**, eating disorders not otherwise specified, binge-eating disorder (BED), and restricted eating. Table 13.9 contains the criteria used by the APA to classify behaviors associated with eating disorders.

Significant behavioral overlap exists between the eating disorders; therefore, clinical diagnostic guidelines have also been developed by the APA and are listed in Table 13.10.

As an exercise science professional, you will not have the clinical skills or credentials to treat clients with eating disorders or body image problems, but you do have a duty to understand the health challenges of these problems, and you should encourage individuals with symptoms to seek professional help for treatment.

Anorexia nervosa is an eating disorder characterized by excessive fear of gaining weight or becoming obese. People with AN can have one of two types: restricting (food restriction) or **binge-eating/purging** type (food restriction as well as bingeing and/or purging). Table 13.11 lists the signs, symptoms, and health consequences associated with AN.

Bulimia nervosa is an eating disorder characterized by repeated cycles of bingeing and purging. Individuals with BN eat large quantities of food and then vomit and/or misuse laxatives, diuretics, and/or enemas. Table 13.12 lists the signs, symptoms, and health consequences associated with BN.

Individuals with eating disorders not otherwise specified, BEDs, and restricted eating do not have specific diagnostic criteria as for AN or BN, but include multiple combinations of AN and BN behaviors that are serious and can disrupt daily life.

disordered eating Includes a variety of eating patterns that are irregular, excessive, or too sparse.

eating disorder Abnormal eating behaviors that compromise a person's physical and/or psychological health.

anorexia nervosa (AN) Eating disorder where a person refuses to maintain a minimally normal body weight and has a distorted view of their body shape and weight.

bulimia nervosa (BN) Eating disorder where a person has repeated episodes of binge eating, usually followed by self-induced vomiting, misuse of laxatives or diuretics, or engaging in excessive exercise.

binge eating/purging Eating extreme amounts at one meal/self-induced vomiting.

◉ TABLE 13.9 Behaviors Associated with Different Eating Disorders

Type of Eating Disorder	Food Restriction	Purging*	Binging	Excessive Exercise
Anorexia nervosa, restricting type				
Anorexia nervosa, binge eating/ purging type				
Bulimia nervosa, purging type				
Bulimia nervosa, nonpurging type				
Binge-eating disorder				
Restrained eating				

"Blue" indicates primary behavior associated with a specific eating disorder, whereas "Yellow" indicates that behavior occurs to a lesser extent.
*Refers to self-induced vomiting and for the misuse of laxatives, diuretics, or enemas.
© Cengage Learning 2013

● TABLE 13.10 Classification and Diagnostic Criteria for Eating Disorders

Anorexia Nervosa

A. Refusal to maintain body weight at or above a minimally normal weight for age and height.

B. Intense fear of gaining weight or becoming fat, even though underweight.

C. Disturbance in body weight or shape is experienced, or denial of the seriousness of the current low body weight.

D. In postmenarchal females, the absence of at least three consecutive menstrual cycles.

Two types:

- Restricting type: The person has not regularly engaged in binge eating or purging behavior.
- Binge-eating/purging type: The person has regularly engaged in binge eating and purging behavior.

Bulimia Nervosa

A. Recurrent episodes of binge eating. An episode of binge eating is characterized by both of the following: (1) eating, in a discrete period of time, an amount of food that is definitely larger than most people would eat during a similar period of time and under similar circumstances, and (2) a sense of lack of control over eating during the episode.

B. Recurrent compensatory behavior to prevent weight gain, such as self-induced vomiting, misuse of laxatives, diuretics, enemas, or other medications; fasting or excessive exercise.

C. The binge eating and inappropriate compensatory behaviors both occur, on average, at least twice a week for three months.

D. Self-evaluation is unduly influenced by body shape and weight.

E. The disturbance does not occur exclusively during episodes of anorexia nervosa.

Two types:

- Purging type: The person has regularly engaged in self-induced vomiting or the misuse of laxatives, diuretics, or enemas.
- Nonpurging type: The person has used inappropriate compensatory behaviors, such as fasting or excessive exercise, but has not regularly engaged in self-induced vomiting or the misuse of laxatives, diuretics, or enemas.

Eating Disorders Not Otherwise Specified

Includes disorders of eating that do not meet the criteria for any specific eating disorder.

A. The criteria for anorexia nervosa are met except the individual has regular menses.

B. The criteria for anorexia nervosa are met except that, despite significant weight loss, the individual's current weight is in the normal range.

C. The criteria for bulimia nervosa are met except that the binge eating and inappropriate compensatory mechanisms occur at a frequency of less than twice a week or for a duration of less than three months.

D. The regular use of inappropriate compensatory behavior by an individual of normal body weight after eating small amounts of food.

E. Repeatedly chewing and spitting out, but not swallowing large amounts of food.

F. Binge-eating disorder: recurrent episodes of binge eating in the absence of the regular use of inappropriate compensatory behaviors characteristic of bulimia nervosa.

Diagnostic and Statistical Manual of Mental Disorders, 4th ed. (DSM-IV). Washington, DC: American Psychiatric Association Press, 2004.
Source: Reprinted with permission from *The Diagnostic and Statistical Manual of Mental Disorders,* Text Revision, Fourth edition (Copyright 2000). American Psychiatric Association.

Individuals with a BED have at least two binges per week for at least six months but do not purge. Individuals with a BED who avoid eating for periods between binges are identified as restrained eaters.

HOTLINK *To learn more about eating disorders, see the National Eating Disorders Association website* (**http://www.edap.org**).

The most common subgroups at risk for eating disorders are adolescent girls and young women. The APA has estimated that more than 8 million girls and young women in the United States battle eating disorders. Although little is known about the incidence of eating disorders in men, the APA has estimated that men account for 10

TABLE 13.11 Signs, Symptoms, and Health Consequences Associated with Anorexia Nervosa

Signs and Symptoms	Health Consequences
• Rigid dieting resulting in dramatic weight loss • At or below 15% of an ideal body weight • Diets or restricts food even though he or she is not overweight • Complains of being fat when he or she is thin • Preoccupied with food, calories, nutrition, and/or cooking • Denial of hunger • Exercises obsessively • Weighs self frequently • Complains about feeling bloated when eating • Complains of feeling cold • Irregular or cessation of menstruation • Food rituals such as excessive chewing or cutting food into small pieces • Restricts amount and types of food consumed • Maintains rigid schedule and routine • Tendency toward perfectionism	• Dry skin, dry hair, thinning hair, hair loss • Fainting, fatigue, overall weakness • Intolerance to cold • Formation of fine hair on the body (lanugo) • Significant loss of fat and lean body mass • Reproductive problems • Loss of bone mass • Electrolyte imbalance • Irregular heartbeat • Bruises • Injuries such as stress fractures • Impaired iron status • Impaired immune status • Slow heart rate and low body pressure

Source: McGuire, M., and K. A. Beerman. 2009. Table 3 in *Nutritional sciences*, 2nd ed. Belmont, CA: Brooks/Cole-Cengage Learning.

bigorexia Lay term for muscle dysmorphia.

muscle dysmorphia Body image disorder where individuals think that their muscles are too small and they workout excessively to obtain a "perfect" physique.

percent of the people with AN and 15 percent of the people with BN. The risk factors for eating disorders include sociocultural factors, family dynamics, personality traits, and biological (genetic) factors.

Although not necessarily associated with eating disorders, a variety of body image problems such as muscle dysmorphia, or **bigorexia**, have been identified in men and women. **Muscle dysmorphia** affects individuals who think that their muscles are too small and they workout excessively to obtain a "perfect" physique. People with muscle dysmorphia believe that bigger is better. Dissatisfaction with body image and body weight are often linked to other personality problems, such as low self-esteem, lack of self-confidence, obsessiveness, anxiety, depression, and feelings of hopelessness.

TABLE 13.12 Signs, Symptoms, and Health Consequences of Bulimia Nervosa

Signs and Symptoms	Health Consequences
• Responds to emotional stress by overeating • Feels guilt or shame after eating • Obsessive concerns about weight • Repeated attempts at food restriction and dieting • Frequent use of bathroom during and after meals • Feels out of control • Moodiness and depression • Fluctuations in body weight • Swollen or puffy face • Teeth may appear eroded • Odor of vomit on breath or in bathroom • Frequent purchase of laxatives • Fear of not being able to stop eating voluntarily • Disappearance of food	• Erosion of tooth enamel and tooth decay from exposure to stomach acid • Electrolyte imbalances that can lead to irregular heart function and possible sudden cardiac arrest • Inflammation of the salivary glands • Irritation and inflammation of the esophagus that could lead to hemorrhaging and bleeding during vomiting • Irregular bowel function • Dehydration

Source: McGuire, M., and K. A. Beerman. 2009. Table 4 in *Nutritional sciences*, 2nd ed. Belmont, CA: Brooks/Cole-Cengage Learning.

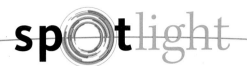

spotlight

An Expert on Body Composition Issues Related to Exercise: A. S. "Tony" Jackson, Ph.D.

A. S. "Tony" Jackson grew up in Minnesota and earned his undergraduate degree in physical education from St. Cloud State College, his master's in physical education from the University of Minnesota, and his P.E.D. in measurement and research design from Indiana University. Tony taught and served as Professor of Physical Education at the University of Houston (1977–2007) and as adjunct professor in the Department of Medicine at Baylor College of Medicine (1985–2007). He retired in 2007.

Tony played football as an undergraduate and was elected to the St. Cloud State University Athletic Hall of Fame in 1985. In his academic life, he, together with colleague Michael Pollock, became well known for their seminal work in the evaluation of body composition using skinfold measurements to predict percentage of body fat. He also has helped develop research methods and statistical models to study exercise science questions related to business and industry, epidemiology, exercise physiology, and NASA and the U.S. space program.

Jackson is a Fellow of the Research Council of the American Alliance of Health, Physical Education, the American College of Sports Medicine, and the American Academy of Physical Education. Jackson also has been recognized for his scientific measurement expertise by authoring numerous books, including *Measurement for Evaluation in Physical Education and Exercise Science*, 8th edition, and more than 200 articles in scientific journals on body composition, strength, and other exercise science issues. Jackson currently serves as professor emeritus at the University of Houston. He is founder and president of the Udde Rowing Club in Onalaska, Texas.

13

in*Practice*

Examples of Body Composition and Weight Management

The following examples are related to the measurement of body composition, advice for weight control, and exercise considerations for weight management, and are based on the most current understanding of the link between the topics of body composition and weight management, which are continuing to evolve.

Health/Fitness: Luke is a 25-year-old college student who has a BMI of 28. His percentage of body fat, as measured in his exercise physiology laboratory with three-site skinfolds, is 24 percent. How you would you interpret his body composition data based on his primary goal of maintaining good health? What body composition goals can you provide Luke to improve his future health risks?

One way to evaluate Luke's body composition measures is to recognize that both his BMI and percentage of body fat are higher than they should be for good health. If his BMI was high and his percentage of body fat lower (in the optimal range), he might be carrying more muscle mass, which is not identified with BMI measures. For good health, Luke should try to lower his BMI to the 18.5 to 25 range and reduce his percentage of body fat to a level between 11 and 21 percent.

Medicine: Harold is a 27-year-old man who has been overweight since childhood with a current BMI of 42 and a waist circumference of 44 inches. His general physician has referred him as a good candidate for gastric banding, because his most recent physical examination revealed that he has some of the symptoms of metabolic syndrome (increased girth, elevated blood pressure, abnormal lipids, and abnormal glucose/insulin levels). As part of the lead-up process, before the banding procedure, Harold is required to visit with an exercise science professional like you to discuss his current exercise levels and future exercise plan. What type of advice can you provide Harold to help him control his body composition in the future?

It certainly would be important that Harold understand that the gastric banding procedure may be his last chance for effective weight loss, which can help him prevent the development of problems associated with chronic metabolic syndrome. Although the gastric banding procedure has become popular and has helped many individuals lose their excess weight, about 20 percent of people who undergo the procedure experience complications, and many regain the lost weight if they do not change their behaviors. For Harold to achieve and maintain success with weight management, you will need to help him develop a short-term and a long-term exercise plan that can improve his quality of life.

Athletic Performance: Jeanette is a 22-year-old collegiate cross-country runner who has run 5:00 minutes for the mile and 10:05 for 2 miles. Her percentage of body fat, as measured with three-site skinfolds by her coach, is 12 percent. Many of Jeanette's friends and competitors have asked her if she is anorexic because she looks so lean. She has become concerned about all the questions she has gotten, and although she feels fine and is competing well, she wants advice from an exercise science professional about her current body composition.

One way to evaluate Jeanette's low percentage of body fat is to remind her that the best distance runners carry less weight, and yet, when individuals become too lean they can compromise their immune function and increase their health risks for upper respiratory infections and the negative effects of the female athletic triad. It would be important to explain to Jeanette the significance of maintaining energy balance, that is, to take in enough calories to offset those expended, and she should not try to lose more weight.

Rehabilitation: Kristin is a 45-year-old woman who is recovering from anterior cruciate ligament surgery to her right knee performed 10 months ago. Her current BMI is 28, and her percentage of body fat is 32 percent as measured with a dual-energy X-ray absorptiometry (DEXA) scan. Kristin does have some pain and swelling when she stands for long periods at work or if she walks for more than 10 minutes. She is frustrated because she does not feel that she has rehabbed her knee effectively, although she worked with a physical therapist for 3 months after surgery. She feels that if she could manage her weight better that she might be able to engage in more regular exercise, to improve the functional ability of her knee. What advice might you provide her to help her improve her knee rehabilitation?

Kristin needs someone to help her understand the concept of "weight cycling" (see Figure 13.12) that was discussed earlier in this chapter. She needs an effective short-term and long-term weight management plan with effective exercise strategies that will allow her to expend additional calories while eating a healthy diet that is approximately 200 to 300 calories below her normal energy intake. She may need to try cycling or water moderate-to-vigorous physical activity as alternatives to walking/standing activities and have an exercise professional help her develop range-of-motion activities in the water specifically for her knee.

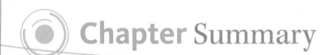

Chapter Summary

- In this chapter, you learned about the physiologic concepts that influence body composition, how to effectively measure it, and the specific strategies for weight management.

- The two-compartment (2-C) model consists of two parts. One part includes body fat; the other includes all other body tissues and is labeled fat-free mass (FFM). Once FFM is known, percentage body fat can be calculated by subtracting FFM from total body weight.

- Although body composition analysis can become quite complex, you can get a good start for body composition analyses by performing visual inspection and generally determining your client's body type classification.

- The general classifications of body types are ectomorph, mesomorph, and endomorph.

- Laboratory methods to evaluate body composition include densitometry, hydrometry, dual-energy X-ray absorptiometry (DEXA), and computed tomography (CT) and magnetic resonance imaging (MRI) scans.

- Field models to evaluate body composition include body mass index (BMI), girths, skinfolds, and bioelectrical impedance (BIA).

- Effective weight management is influenced by genetic and environmental factors.

- The development of effective weight management plans should be based on realistic goals, client behaviors, medical input as necessary, body composition evaluations, exercise prescription, and sound dietary strategies.

- Since the 1980s, the incidence of disordered eating and those with distorted body image perceptions has increased as more people have become preoccupied with food, dieting, exercise, weight loss, and weight gain.

Exercise Physiology Reality

CENGAGE brain To reinforce the exercise physiology concepts presented above, complete the laboratory exercises for Chapter 13. To access labs and other course materials for this text, please visit www.cengagebrain.com. See the pref-

ace on page xiii for details. Once you complete the exercises, have your instructor evaluate your prescriptions. Remember to use your lab experience to help guide you toward future success in exercise physiology.

Exercise Physiology Web Links

Access the following websites for further study of topics covered in this chapter:

- Find updates and quick links to sites related to the basics of nutrition for exercise and exercise physiology at our website. To access the course materials and companion resources for this text, please visit www.cengagebrain.com. See the preface on page xiii for details.

- Search for further information about body composition and weight control at the Centers for Disease Control and Prevention (CDC) website: http://www.cdc.gov.

- Search for information about body composition and weight control at the American College of Sports Medicine website: http://www.acsm.org.

- Search for more information about body composition and weight control at the National Institute of Diabetes and Digestive and Kidney Diseases website: http://www.niddk.nih.gov.

- Search for more information about energy balance and weight control in the *Physical Activity Guidelines Advisory Committee Report, 2008* at: http://www.health.gov/paguidelines.

- Search for more information about body composition and weight control at the U.S. government health information website: http://www.healthierUS.gov.

Study Questions

Review the Warm-Up Pre-Test questions you were asked to answer before reading Chapter 13. Test yourself once more to determine what you know now that you have completed the chapter.

The questions that follow will help you review this chapter. You will find the answers in the discussions on the pages provided.

1. Define the terms *body composition* and *weight management* and how they influence exercise prescription for your clients. *p. 431*

2. What is essential fat and why is it important? *p. 433*

3. What is the best way to measure body composition? Defend your answer. *pp. 448–450*

4. Which field model of evaluating body composition has the least error? *pp. 437–447*

5. What factors can you use to interpret the body composition of your clients? *pp. 449–450*

6. List and describe three genetic factors that can affect successful weight management for your clients. *pp. 450–451*

7. Define the term *obesogenic.* How does it contribute to effective weight management strategies? *p. 452*

8. List and describe five client-specific factors that can affect successful weight management. *p. 455*

9. How effective are dieting strategies for long-term weight management? Why? *pp. 456–457*

10. What is the difference between bariatric bypass surgery and banding? What type of client would typically undergo these procedures? *pp. 457–459*

Selected References

Baumgartner, T. A., A. S. Jackson, M. T. Mahar, and D. A. Rowe. 2007. *Measurement and evaluation in physical education and exercise science,* 8th ed. Boston: WCB/McGraw-Hill.

Brozek, J., F. Grande, and J. T. Anderson. 1963. Densitometric analysis of body composition: Revision of some quantitative assumptions. *Ann. N. Y. Acad. Sci.* 110:113–240.

Brozek, J., and A. Keys. 1951. The evaluation of leanness-fatness in man: Norms and intercorrelations. *Br. J. Nutr.* 5:194–206.

Ellis, K. J. 2000. Human body composition: In vivo methods. *Physiol. Rev.* 80:649–680.

Fernández, J. R., D. T. Redden, A. Pietrobelli, and D. B. Allison. 2004. Waist circumference percentiles in nationally representative samples of African-American, European-American, and Mexican-American children and adolescents. *J. Pediatr.* 145:439–444.

Going, S. 2008. Optimizing techniques for determining body composition. *Sports Sci. Exch.* #101, Gatorade Sports Science Institute. Available at http://www.gssiweb.com/. Accessed July 18, 2011.

Jackson, A. S., and M. L. Pollack. 1978. Generalized equations for predicting body density of men. *Br. J. Nutr.* 40(3):497–504.

Jackson, A. S., M. L. Pollack, and A. Ward. 1980. Generalized equations for predicting body density of women. *Med. Sci. Sports Exerc.* 12(3):175–181.

Lohman, T. G. 1986. Applicability of body composition techniques and constants for children and youths. *Exerc. Sport Sci. Rev.* 14:325–357.

Peters, J. C. 2006. Obesity prevention and social change: What will it take? *Exerc. Sport Sci. Rev.* 34(1):4–9.

Siri, W. E. 1956. The gross composition of the body. In *Advances in biological and medical physics* (pp. 239–280), edited by C. A. Tobias and J. H. Lawrence. New York: Academic Press.

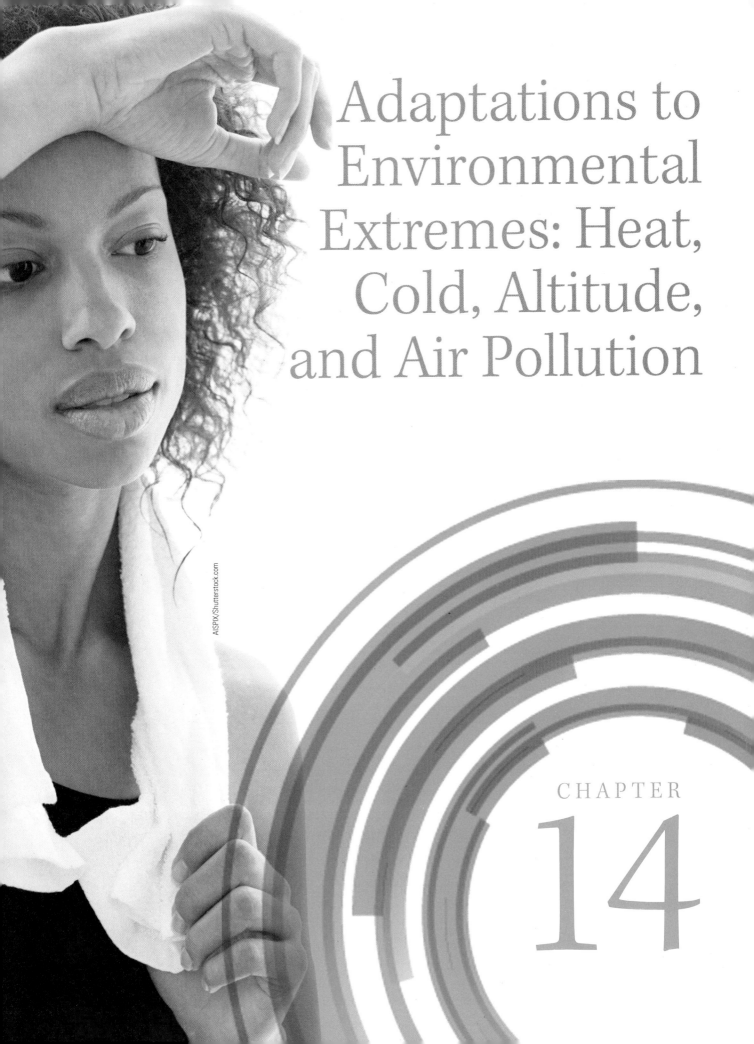

Adaptations to Environmental Extremes: Heat, Cold, Altitude, and Air Pollution

CHAPTER

14

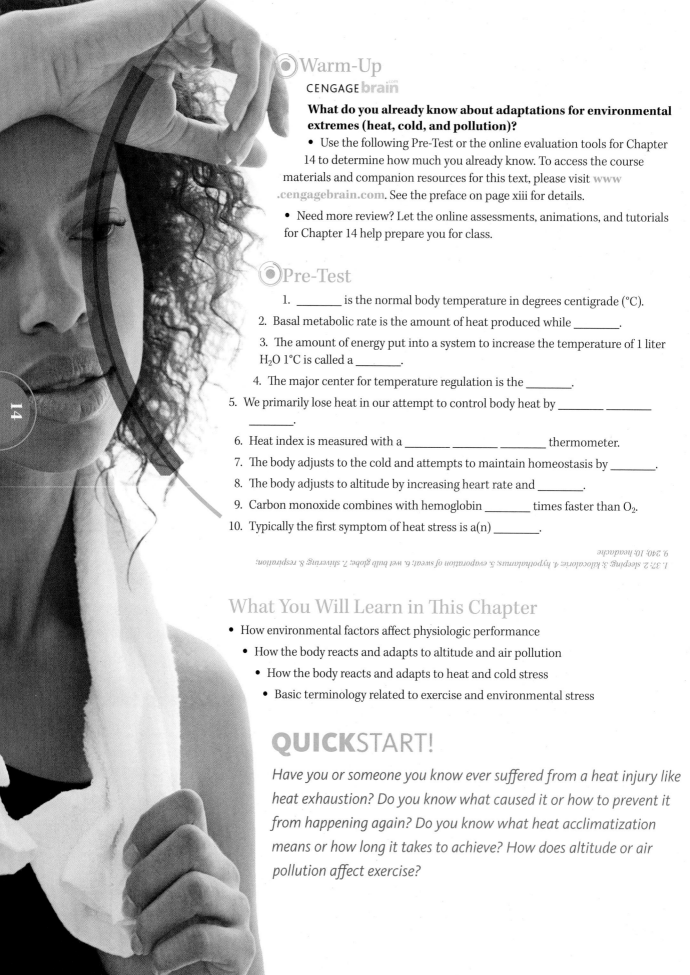

Warm-Up

CENGAGE brain.com

What do you already know about adaptations for environmental extremes (heat, cold, and pollution)?

• Use the following Pre-Test or the online evaluation tools for Chapter 14 to determine how much you already know. To access the course materials and companion resources for this text, please visit **www.cengagebrain.com**. See the preface on page xiii for details.

• Need more review? Let the online assessments, animations, and tutorials for Chapter 14 help prepare you for class.

Pre-Test

1. _____ is the normal body temperature in degrees centigrade (°C).

2. Basal metabolic rate is the amount of heat produced while _____.

3. The amount of energy put into a system to increase the temperature of 1 liter H₂O 1°C is called a _____.

4. The major center for temperature regulation is the _____.

5. We primarily lose heat in our attempt to control body heat by _____ _____ _____.

6. Heat index is measured with a _____ _____ _____ thermometer.

7. The body adjusts to the cold and attempts to maintain homeostasis by _____.

8. The body adjusts to altitude by increasing heart rate and _____.

9. Carbon monoxide combines with hemoglobin _____ times faster than O₂.

10. Typically the first symptom of heat stress is a(n) _____.

1. 37; 2. sleeping; 3. kilocalorie; 4. hypothalamus; 5. evaporation of sweat; 6. wet bulb globe; 7. shivering; 8. respiration; 9. 240; 10. headache

What You Will Learn in This Chapter

• How environmental factors affect physiologic performance

• How the body reacts and adapts to altitude and air pollution

• How the body reacts and adapts to heat and cold stress

• Basic terminology related to exercise and environmental stress

QUICKSTART!

Have you or someone you know ever suffered from a heat injury like heat exhaustion? Do you know what caused it or how to prevent it from happening again? Do you know what heat acclimatization means or how long it takes to achieve? How does altitude or air pollution affect exercise?

 CHAPTER 14 • *Adaptations to Environmental Extremes: Heat, Cold, Altitude, and Air Pollution*

Introduction to Adaptations to Environmental Extremes

Perhaps the least understood of the factors that affect physical performance are those associated with the different environments that the activity is to be performed in. Inattention to, or ignorance of, the interaction between the stress of the environment and the activity being performed, as well as the resulting challenge to the body's physiologic regulation, may result in life-threatening collapse. Teachers and coaches need to safeguard the health of their students and athletes during the course of exercise training, athletic performance, or the physical education class. For example, the idea of toughening the football athlete by refusing to allow time for rehydration during a football practice was accepted practice up to the 1970s and was the cause of many cases of debilitating heat exhaustion and sometimes death. Such catastrophes resulting from ignorance or lack of following established guidelines to protect the exerciser are inexcusable in this day and age. This chapter discusses the effects of hot and cold environments on the performance of physical activity and training, as well as the challenges created by the effects of altitude and air pollution.

Humans, like other mammals are warm-blooded, classified as homeotherms and attempt to maintain a constant body temperature over a wide range of ambient temperatures. In contrast, poikilotherms, such as lizards and snakes, are cold-blooded, and their body temperatures gain or lose heat in direct relation to the ambient temperature (see Figure 14.1).

When the ambient environment results in no physiologic adjustments to lose or gain heat, it is identified as the **thermoneutral environment**. For the naked human at rest, the thermoneutral environment ranges between 24.0°C and 26°C, or 75.2°F and 78.8°F, at a relative humidity of 50 percent and no airflow over the body (see Figure 14.2).

During exercise, the efficiency of the metabolic processes of the human to provide the energy to perform work ranges from 23 to 27 percent. Therefore, much of the energy (approximately 75 percent) generated by the metabolic processes to

thermoneutral environment The state in which the ambient environment surrounding the naked human does not activate the physiological mechanism to gain or lose body heat.

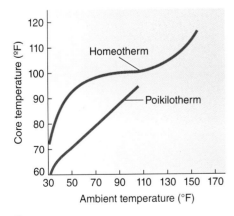

FIGURE 14.1 Changes in core temperature (°F) of homeotherms and poikilotherms in relation to a wide range of ambient temperatures (°F). (Adapted from Guyton, A. C. 1976. Figure 72-6 in *Medical physiology*. 5th ed. Philadelphia, PA: Saunders.)

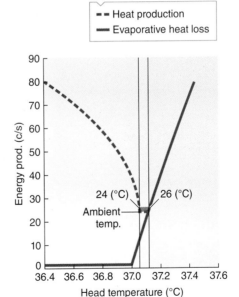

FIGURE 14.2 Relationship between energy production at rest and hypothalamic temperatures below (dashed line) and above (solid line) the set point temperature. (Modified from Guyton, A. C. 1976. Figure 72-7 in *Medical physiology*. 5th ed. Philadelphia, PA: Saunders.)

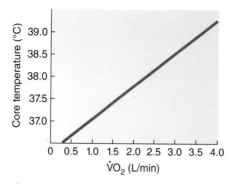

● **FIGURE 14.3** **Relationship between exercise intensity (maximal oxygen uptake [V̇O₂] in L/min) and core temperature.** (Modified from data presented in Astrand, P. O., and K. Rodahl (Eds.). 1986. Figure 5-3 in *Textbook of work physiology: Physiological bases of exercise*, 3rd ed. New York: McGraw-Hill Book Co.

perform the exercise is added to the body as a heat load. An example of this heating phenomenon is presented in Figure 14.3.

The data presented in Figure 14.3 were obtained from subjects performing 45 minutes of submaximal oxygen uptake (V̇O₂) exercise ranging from 0.75 to 3.5 liters oxygen. At 45 minutes of exercise, the core (rectal) temperature was measured and was linearly correlated to the steady-state V̇O₂.

The ambient temperature needs to be cooler than the thermoneutral environment to maintain a stable body temperature while performing heavy to maximal exercise; ambient temperature has been calculated to an optimum range from 15°C to 22°C, or 59°F to 71.6°F, depending on the clothing worn and the exercise intensity. However, regardless of the ambient temperature, it is unusual for the human to exercise without increasing the body's temperature.

We usually dress for thermal comfort, sensed primarily by the skin, at the start of the exercise; therefore, in cold ambient temperatures, we tend to overdress at the beginning of the exercise, and as the core temperature increases, we shed clothing to maintain thermal comfort. However, we have usually increased the amount of heat stored in the body, causing our core temperature to increase, and unless we reduce or stop the activity, the body's heat-loss mechanisms are not able to reduce the body's temperature.

The body redistributes its blood flow to the skin surface when the core and skin

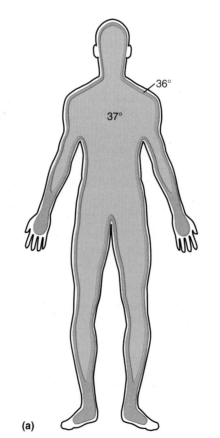

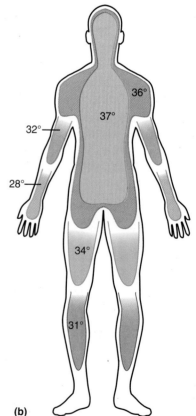

● **FIGURE 14.4** **Schematic representations of the effect of (a) increasing and (b) decreasing core and skin temperatures on blood flow distribution during rest and exercise.** (© Cengage Learning 2013)

temperatures are sensed as being hot (see Figure 14.4a). When the skin temperature senses that it is cold, it results in the body redistributing its blood flow to heart, lung, and brain circulation (see Figure 14.4b).

The maintenance of a stable **central body temperature or core temperature** at 37°C, or 98.6°F, is beneficial because it approximates the optimal temperature for enzymatic reactions involved in many of the metabolic reactions and the maintenance of cellular integrity. The normal range of body temperatures and the clinical limits of **temperature regulation** are summarized in Figure 14.5.

In general, experiments in the laboratory that involve human subjects and use heat and cold stresses to challenge the body's temperature regulation rarely allow the core temperature to exceed 39°C, or 102.2°F, or to decline to less than 35°C, or 95.5°F, respectively, especially if the measure of core temperature is changing rapidly (that is, one tenth of a °C per minute). However, it is not unusual to record temperatures of 40°C to 41°C, or 104°F to 105.8°F, for periods of 2 hours or more in competitive runners performing a marathon in warm conditions at

a pace required to complete the course in less than 3 hours.

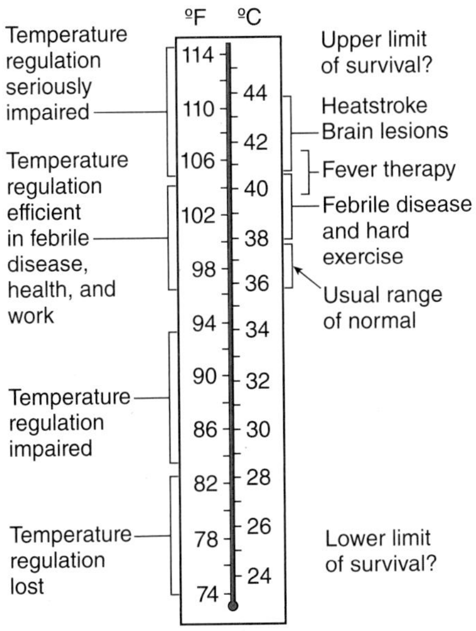

The protection offered by rehydration and heat acclimatization to these stresses is discussed later in the chapter. However, if the body's core temperature exceeds 45°C, or 113°F, it is probable that death will occur because this is the temperature at which proteins are denatured and the gastrointestinal tract begins to segment. When the temperature of the skin is increased to 45°C, or 113°F, it is felt as painful. In many countries with ambient temperatures that exceed 110°F, where outdoor activities are a part of normal daily life, individuals usually cover their skin to protect it from being burned by the sun.

If the body's core temperature is allowed to decline to less than 25°C, or 77°F, respiratory and/or circulatory failure resulting in death usually occurs. However, in some unique situations of very rapid cooling and/or incrementally slow cooling, recoveries from core temperatures of less than 20°C have been reported.

It is unusual that an individual's core temperature would reach 25°C without part of their limbs, fingers, and toes being frozen, resulting in ice crystal formation in the cells of the tissues. In Figure 14.4b, overexposures to the cold results in the body trying to preserve its heat by vasoconstriction of the peripheral blood vessels and allowing the appendages and limbs to approach the ambient temperature. The result of this physiologic response is that the body redistributes the blood to the heart, lungs, and brain, sacrificing the limbs and appendages to freezing. When ice forms in the cells, not only are there mechanical damage to the cells, but the proteins are denatured by dehydration, resulting in frostbite that rapidly results in gangrene. Once gangrene has been established, tissue salvage is difficult and usually requires cutting away the dead tissue or amputation of an appendage or limb. It is imperative when exercising in cold weather, or water, that you protect your hands and feet, limbs, and ears and nose.

In some genetically susceptible individuals, cold ambient temperatures that are not necessarily freezing may trigger an

central body or core temperature The temperature of the blood near the heart, brain, gut, or rectum.

temperature regulation The neural process by which the body senses whether it is hot or cold and reflexively activates physiologic responses to cool or heat the body, respectively.

● **FIGURE 14.5 Range of thermometer readings of core body temperatures with equivalent clinical descriptions of functional effects.** (From Guyton, A. C. 1976. Figure 72-8 in *Medical physiology.* 5th ed. Philadelphia, PA: Saunders. Adapted from Du Bois, E. F. 1948. *Fever: Regulation of body temperature.* Springfield, IL: C. C. Thomas.)

intense vasospasm in the fingers or toes, resulting in the fingers and toes feeling ice cold and losing the pink color associated with the presence of the blood circulating in the skin. This intense vasoconstriction will result in capillary congestion and fluid exudation (escaping) from the blood vessels. If untreated, the condition, known as Raynaud disease (named after the French physician who recognized it), can lead to tissue anoxia and gangrene. Raynaud disease occurs primarily in women (7 percent of women) and should not be ignored in outdoor activities in cold environments.

Even though you may be mountaineering or scuba diving in warm ambient temperatures, the higher one climbs, the colder the ambient temperature is (a loss of 2°C for each 1,000 feet climbed), and the deeper one dives, the colder the water temperature.

Physical Principles Guide the Temperature Regulatory Responses

The metabolic processes of generating energy from food and/or performing exercise causes the body to gain heat. It gains and loses heat from or to the external environment, respectively, across the skin and, in extreme conditions, the respiratory tract. When heat gain exceeds heat loss, the body temperature increases and a number of neural and hormone-mediated control mechanisms are activated to lose the excess heat. If the heat gained exceeds the ability of the body to lose heat, the extra heat is "stored" and the core temperature increases. In contrast, if the heat losses exceed the heat gained, the heat "stores" of the body decrease and the core temperature decreases. These processes are summarized in the following heat balance equation:

$$M = E \pm R \pm C \pm K \pm W \pm S \quad [14.1]$$

where M = metabolic rate; E = evaporation; R = radiation; C = convection; K = conduction; W = work; and S = storage. M (metabolism) is always a plus value (if zero or less, the individual is dead); E can

be zero, but never negative, because it is the rate of heat loss by the evaporation of sweat (1 liter = 700 kilocalories); R, C, and K can be both positive and negative, and indicate that the body can gain and lose heat by these processes. The storage term, S, is a result of whether the body is gaining or losing heat, hence it also can be positive or negative. However, storage is not an active mechanistic process in which the body gains or loses heat. Finally, the work term, W, has a positive and, in some instances, a negative (based on the concept of negative work) component. However, in general, we regard the W as always having a positive value in the heat balance equation; that is, during exercise, the mechanical energy (that is, the energy required to do the work) is being lost from the body.

At rest, the core temperature is regulated at 37°C (98.6°F) and the **mean skin temperature (or Tsk)** is regulated at 34°C (93.2°F). If, as recommended, our room temperatures in the summer are regulated at 25.6°C (78°F) and in the winter are regulated at 20.0°C (68°F), there will be a constant flux of the body's heat from the core to the skin to the room air regardless of seasons. Remember, heat flux is based on the physical principle of "heat flows from hot to cold". Figure 14.6 depicts the flow of heat within the body and out to the ambient environment at rest (Figure 14.6a) and during dynamic exercise (Figure 14.6b).

Radiation (R) occurs in the form of infrared rays (heat) and occurs by the transfer of heat from a hot surface to a cool surface without physical contact between the two surfaces. However, radiation to the skin occurs when the temperature of a heat source is hotter than the skin, for example, the radiant heat from a fire or outdoors on a cloudless day, the sun radiates its heat directly to the skin surface.

Conduction (K) is the transfer of heat from a hot surface to a colder surface while the two surfaces are in contact with each other. For example, the heat of the skin is transferred to the water of a swimming pool unless, of course, the water temperature is warmer than the Tsk of 34.0°C (that is, 93.2°F).

mean skin temperature (or Tsk) A calculated summation of different body segments (arm, legs, thorax, etc.) weighed to the ratio of the segment's surface area to the total body surface area.

radiation (R) The transfer of heat from a hot surface to a cool surface without physical contact between the two surfaces.

conduction (K) The transfer of heat from a hot surface to a colder surface while the two surfaces are in contact with each other.

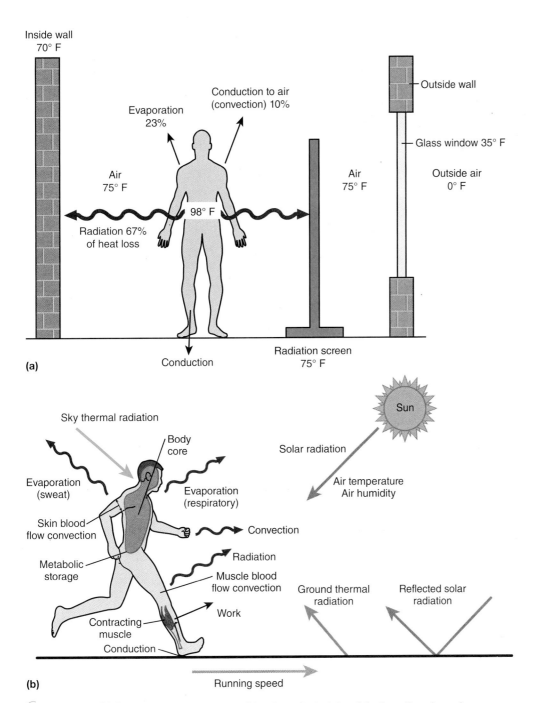

Inside wall
70° F

Evaporation
23%

Conduction to air
(convection) 10%

Air
75° F

98° F

Radiation 67%
of heat loss

Air
75° F

Outside wall

Glass window 35° F

Outside air
0° F

(a)

Conduction

Radiation screen
75° F

Sun

Sky thermal radiation

Body
core

Solar radiation

Evaporation
(sweat)

Evaporation
(respiratory)

Air temperature
Air humidity

Skin blood
flow convection

Convection

Metabolic
storage

Radiation

Muscle blood
flow convection

Ground thermal
radiation

Reflected solar
radiation

Contracting
muscle

Work

Conduction

(b)

Running speed

● F I G U R E 14.6 (a) Schematic description of the physical principles of the flow of heat from a human body to the ambient environment during rest. (Adapted from Guyton, A. C. 1976. Figure 72-3 in *Medical physiology.* 5th ed. Philadelphia, PA: Saunders.) (b) Schematic description of the physical principles of the flow of heat from a human body to the ambient environment during exercise. (From Powers, S. K., and E. T. Hauley. 2004. Figure 12-3 in *Exercise physiology: The theory and application to fitness and performance,* 5th ed. Boston, MA: McGraw-Hill Co.)

Convection (C) heat transfer requires a disturbance of a temperature gradient built up on the surface of the skin by air movement across the skin's surface. (Remember, the air nearest the skin is warmer than the next layer of air above it.) The amount of heat loss caused by convection is due to the speed of the air movement across the skin. For example, the heat loss caused by convection is greater when running at 6.0 miles/hour compared with running at 2.0 miles/hour. Because the skin can sense the difference between the chilling effect of the 6-mile/hour versus the 2-mile/hour air movement across the skin (the greater the wind speed, the greater the heat loss),

convection (C) A type of heat transfer that requires a disturbance of a temperature gradient by air or fluid flow.

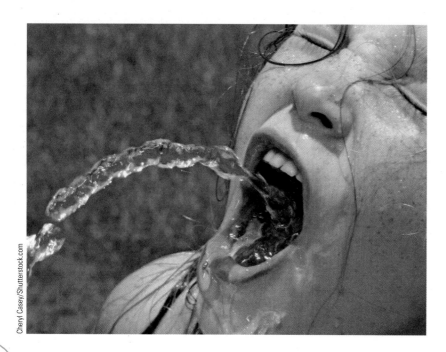
Cheryl Casey/Shutterstock.com

14

wind chill The cooling power of the environment as a function of wind velocity and ambient temperature and relates the time of cooling a given volume of water to the point of freezing.

evaporation (E) The cooling effect associated with the changing of water into vapor, or, in this case, sweat into vapor. The specific heat of sweat evaporation is a measure of the heat energy required to vaporize the sweat. About 600 calories of energy are needed for every gram of water at room temperature.

you should be able to understand the fundamental physical concept of the "**wind chill**" effect.

Evaporation (E) of sweat is the human's primary means of losing heat while exercising in the heat (1 liter sweat = 700 kilocalories). When the body temperature increases, the central nervous system signals the sweat glands to secrete sweat onto the skin surface from the pores of the skin. It is the evaporation of the sweat that provides the cooling of the skin, which, in turn, cools the hot arterial blood that has been circulated into the skin giving the skin a bright red color. The venous blood coming from the skin and returning to the central circulation is now cooler than the arterial blood and results in cooling the central circulation. This circulatory cooling process is very similar to the cooling system of a car in which the engine (the muscles) heats up the water (blood) that is pumped to the radiator (the skin) to be cooled by the air flowing across the pipes of the radiator, which is similar to the evaporation of sweat from the skin (see Figure 14.7, page 475).

When heat from the environment flows to the body (that is, adds heat) and the metabolic heat generated from exercise is being added to the body, the only avenue of heat loss is the evaporation of sweat. In very hot conditions, whole-body sweat

rates approach a maximum of 2 liters/hour, but dripping sweat is not evaporating from the body. Therefore, the cooling effect associated with the changing of water into vapor (that is, the specific heat of evaporation) is not effective. However, dripping sweat has a big effect in hastening the onset of dehydration.

Evaporation of sweat from the skin is dependent on a variety of factors:

1. The amount of the area of skin exposed to the air; the larger the surface area, the larger the amount of heat that can be lost for any given temperature gradient, and the higher the air temperature, the greater the evaporation of sweat

2. The relative humidity (water vapor pressure) of the air; the greater the relative humidity and the lower the capacity to evaporate the sweat; hence the more dripping, the less cooling

3. The rate of air flow across the body's surface; that is, convective heat loss is greater at higher wind speeds

4. The capacity of the clothes being worn to "wick" the sweat away from the skin surface to expose the sweat to the ambient conditions and allow evaporation from the surface of the clothes

Respiratory heat loss is another avenue of heat loss that is minor in hot conditions but becomes very significant during exercise in the cold and at altitude. This is because of the need for the body to warm and humidify the inspired air even though the metabolic heat production of the exercise may be increasing your core temperature and causing you to sweat. This is discussed in a later section on the effects of altitude.

In a cold environment, the body increases its metabolic heat production by shivering, and in situations where replenishment of energy by eating food is not limited, you can increase heat production using exercise. However, in survival situations and situations of limited food supply, you would be better off if you conserve your energy by not exercising.

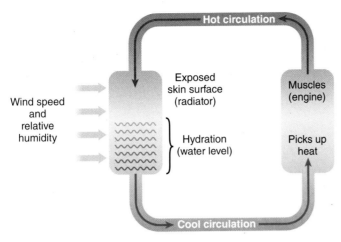

FIGURE 14.7 **Model of how the evaporation of sweat (specific heat of evaporation) from the skin surface.** The circulation is the convective means of transferring the heat produced by the exercising muscles, similar to an automobile's water cooling system convectively transferring heat from the engine to the radiator. (© Cengage Learning 2013)

> *Why would you be better off not exercising in the cold when food is not available? See the earlier heat balance equation for hints.*

HOTLINK *Visit the course materials for Chapter 14 for an animation of neural control with regard to temperature.*

Neural Control

To switch "on" and "off" the body's physiologic systems that regulate the body's temperature, we need a control system that uses negative feedback similar to the thermostat in your house (see Figure 14.8).

The human body's thermoregulatory control system generally involves the neural and endocrine systems. The neural system is the fast-response system, and the endocrine system is the slow-response system.

> *What is the physiologic meaning of the thermoneutral zone?*

In heating and cooling your room, the thermostat serves as the regulatory center and has a "**set point**," that is, the reference temperature to which all the input signals are compared. In the human body, the temperature regulatory center is located in the hypothalamus, and it attempts to maintain the body's core temperature at a set point of 37°C, or 98.6°F.

The anterior hypothalamus responds to increases in the body's heat content by turning on the heat-loss mechanisms

set point The central nervous system's temperature (similar to setting the thermostat temperature of a heating and cooling system) that is the reference temperature the core, mean body, and mean skin temperatures are compared with to activate the regulatory physiological responses if a difference between the two temperatures exists.

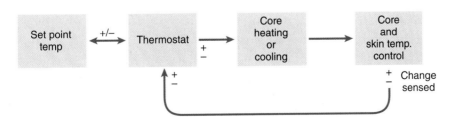

FIGURE 14.8 **Schematic example of a negative feedback system involving a thermostat that compares the core and skin temperatures with their specific set-point temperatures and controls the physiologic heating and cooling mechanisms.** (© Cengage Learning 2013)

(sweating), and the posterior hypothalamus responds to losses of body heat content by turning on the heat-generating mechanisms (shivering). **Thermal sensors or receptors**, located in the spinal cord and brain (hypothalamus) sense the core temperature. Because of the circulation of blood throughout the body, *the core temperature, Tcore,* is reflected in the blood temperature measured in the heart, brain, gut, or rectum.

The more sensitive and valid measure of core temperature is obtained from the blood within the brain and the heart. Brain blood temperature is difficult to measure in humans during exercise. In experimental situations, the temperature measured at the tympanum in the ear is the best approximation of brain blood temperature. In addition, the temperature of the blood in the heart is difficult to measure. Therefore, in the experimental situation, the **esophageal temperature (Tes)** at the level of the heart provides the best approximation of the body's blood temperature in the thorax, that is, Tcore. Both temperature measures have practical limitations and need to be made with appropriate safety precautions. A more benign technology of measuring core temperature involves the use of a radiotelemetry plastic-coated transmitter in the form of a pill that the subject swallows. After a 30-minute period in which the pill enters the small intestine, the radio signal calibrated to the temperature is acquired by a tuned recording device. Experiments can then be performed and a continuous recording of the subject's gastrointestinal temperature can be obtained safely and with minimal discomfort. The pill is discarded by flushing the feces of the subject's next bowel movement.

The temperature of the skin (both hot and cold) is sensed by thermal sensors (or receptors) within the skin. These skin sensors send neural messages to the hypothalamus and are integrated with the Tcore information and compared with the set-point temperature, and the appropriate heat-loss or heat-gain responses are initiated in an attempt to maintain the Tcore constant at the set-point temperature of 37°C. The measure of skin temperature at one particular area of the skin is fairly simple. However, because the surface area of the skin is large, a single measure of skin temperature, for example, on the forehead, would not be representative of the rest of the body's skin temperatures. A weighting factor based on the surface area represented by a single temperature measurement of the discrete area of the skin is summated for seven separate areas of the body surface and a mean Tsk is calculated (see Equation 14.2), to overcome this measurement problem.

$$Tsk = 0.07\ Tforehead + 0.36\ Tchest + \\ 0.05\ Tfinger + 0.14\ Tarm + \\ 0.05\ Ttoe + 0.13\ Tcalf + \\ 0.20\ Tthigh \qquad [14.2]$$

The set point of the Tsk is approximately 34°C, or 93.2°F. It remains a mystery as to how exactly the body senses whether it is hot or cold by comparing its sensed Tcore and/or Tsk with their set-point temperatures. However, from the representative Figure 14.4, in which the body has responded to a hot environment by whole-body vasodilatation and expansion of its shell (see Figure 14.4a) and to a cold environment (see Figure 14.4b) by vasoconstriction to maintain the core of its shell to heart, lung, and brain circulation, it is easy to imagine an engineer designing a model in which the temperature sensors in some way compare the body's average temperature (mean body temperature with the set-point temperature).

In calculating the mean body temperature, it is readily apparent that the shell of the body will have a greater weight in its calculation in a hot environment than in a cold environment (see Figure 14.4). Therefore,

Hot environment mean body
temperature = 0.35 Tsk + 0.65 Tcore
[14.3a]

Cold environment mean body
temperature = 0.20 Tsk + 0.80 Tcore
[14.3b]

inRETROSPECT

Measurement of Radiant Heat from Skin Surfaces

In a series of classical experiments by Thomas Benzinger and colleagues between the 1940s and the 1960s using a specially designed whole-body calorimeter to measure the radiant heat from the surface of humans, the integration of the Tsk and the core temperature, and their comparison with their individual set-point temperatures and the resultant physiologic responses were demonstrated.

Figure 14.9 summarizes the effect of different skin temperatures on the hypothalamic, or central, set point for sweating. The data indicate that as the skin temperature decreases, the central set point for sweating increases. In these data, the central set point was 36.7°C when the Tsk was greater than 33°C; but when the Tsk was less than 29°C, the central set point had increased to 37.4°C.

Figure 14.10 summarizes the effect of different skin temperatures on the central set point for shivering. The data indicate that as the skin temperature increases, the central set point for shivering decreases. More importantly, it demonstrates that even though our central set-point temperature may be above normal, that is, 37.2°C, a cool Tsk of 20.0°C can increase shivering markedly.

The relationship between the set-point temperatures of the skin and core, and the integration of the information whether the skin and/or core are relatively hot or cold enables the hypothalamus, analogous to a thermostat, to grade the physiologic responses accordingly (see Figures 14.8, 14.9, and 14.10).

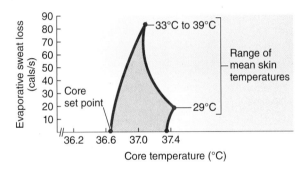

● FIGURE 14.9 Schematic summary of the effect of different skin temperatures on the hypothalamic, or central, set point for sweating. (Modified from Benzinger. T. H. 1969. Heat regulation: Homeostasis of central temperature in man. *Physiol. Rev.* 49:671–759.)

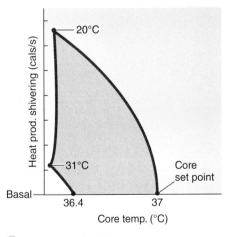

● FIGURE 14.10 Schematic summary of the effect of different skin temperatures on the hypothalamic, or central, set point for shivering. (Modified from Benzinger, T. H. 1969. Heat regulation: Homeostasis of central temperature in man. *Physiol. Rev.* 49:671–759.)

Passive Heating

When the core temperature is passively (no exercise) increased above the central set-point temperature, heat-loss mechanisms are activated via the hypothalamus for the following purposes:

1. To vasodilate the skin's circulation and maximize the skin surface area where the warm blood can be cooled directly by convective/conductive heat loss and indirectly by the evaporation of the sweat (see Figure 14.11)

2. To increase sweat released from the sweat glands

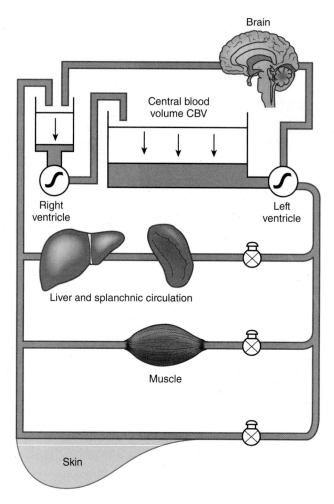

● FIGURE 14.11 Model describing the competition between the distribution of blood flow to the exercising muscles and the skin circulations, and their effect on central blood volume and the regional circulations of the splanchnic bed and the brain. (Adapted from Rowell, L. B. 1986. Figure 8-20 in *Human circulation: Regulation during physical stress.* New York: Oxford University Press.)

These responses result in a variety of cardiovascular changes, such as:

1. Increases in cardiac contractility and left ventricular systolic function, which result in maintenance of stroke volume even though ventricular filling pressures and central blood volume are reduced

2. Reductions in cerebral perfusion and orthostatic tolerance

3. Unchanged arterial baroreflex control of heart rate and muscle sympathetic nerve activity

4. Impaired arterial baroreflex control of systemic vascular resistance associated with reduced responsiveness of the cutaneous circulation

For many years, vasodilatation of the skin's blood vessels during heating was thought to occur primarily by withdrawal of the sympathetic vasoconstrictor tone; however, work over the past 20 years has demonstrated that there is an active vasodilator mechanism involving an unidentified vasodilator substance (see Figure 14.12, page 479).

Passive Cooling

When the cold receptors of the skin and hypothalamus are stimulated, either separately or together, heat gain and heat conservation mechanisms are activated. The initial responses are: (a) sympathetically mediated cutaneous vasoconstriction and piloerection of the hair covering the skin;

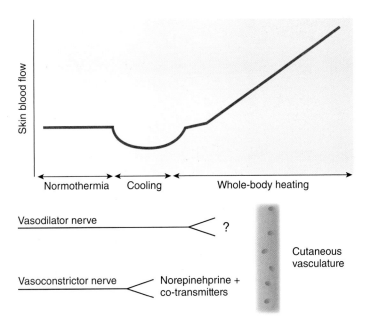

● **F I G U R E** **14.12** **Model of the skin's heating-induced vasodilator mechanism.** Previously it was thought that the skin's vasodilation in response to heating required only the withdrawal of vasoconstriction; it is now known that there exists a mechanism of active vasodilation. (© Cengage Learning 2013)

(b) followed by muscle tension, especially in the limbs; and (c) subsequently, frank shivering.

Shivering occurs when the skin is cold even if the core is warm. The piloerection observed in the human is a vestigial mechanism for increasing the outer shell of the body as a means of increasing insulation from the cold. For the human, this response is ineffective, but for an animal like the Arctic fox or the Siberian Husky, the piloerection of their fur, which traps air layers on top of each other (the warmest air being next to the skin) increases the insulation. The fluffed out fur along with their behavior of burrowing into the snow to shield the air layers from the wind enables the fox to withstand temperatures of −70°C.

HOTLINK *See the Iditarod Trail Committee website (http://www.iditarod.com) to learn more about the Iditarod Dog Sled Race.*

In humans, the muscle tension noticed before actual shivering is also thought to be a vestigial part of the nonshivering thermogenesis mechanism requiring brown fat for the production of heat via endogenous catecholamine production. This mechanism is of major importance to rodents,

marsupials, and hibernating mammals. Indeed, human infants have some vestiges of brown fat between the shoulder blades immediately after birth. This usually disappears by 4 weeks of neonatal development; however, in premature neonates, presence of brown fat may last longer than 4 weeks. At rest, the human's main heat production mechanism is via shivering thermogenesis and involves the release of thyroxine and catecholamines to increase cellular heat production (see Figure 14.13, page 480).

These responses result in a variety of cardiovascular changes related to stimulation of sympathetic and thyroid activity, such as:

1. Increased oxygen uptake
2. Increased cardiac output
3. Unchanged or decreased resting heart rate
4. Increased stroke volume
5. Increased total peripheral resistance

Shivering is the main mechanism by which the human adds heat to the body without exercising. When the cold is extreme and the consequent shivering is very hard, muscular fatigue results. Unfortunately, for the amount of energy expended, shivering has

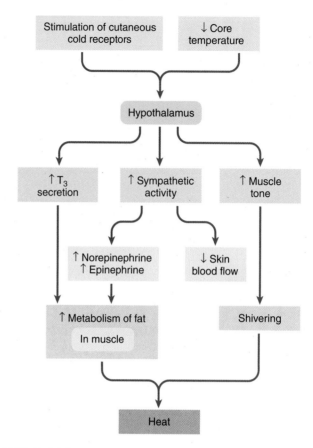

FIGURE 14.13 Model describing the role of thyroxin and catecholamines in generating heat when their release is stimulated by cold exposure. (Adapted from Sherwood, L. 2004. Figure 17-6 in *Human physiology: From cells to systems.* 5th ed. Belmont, CA: Thomson-Brooks/Cole.)

been calculated to be only 11 percent efficient in adding heat to the body. In survival situations, when food availability is limited, the human is best served by increasing insulation, reducing physical activity, and using an external heating source to maintain the body's core temperature.

HOTLINK *Access the NASA website (http:// www.NASA.gov) to find out more about the environmental challenges of spaceflight.*

Therefore, the comfortable survival of humans in extreme conditions, hot or cold, requires their engineering expertise rather than their physiologic capacities. In emergency situations when humans are exposed to extreme conditions, all available engineering aids (slight as they may be) and maximization of physiologic capacities are required for survival.

Survival from Extreme Cold

One classic example of survival in the cold was the dramatized true story of the *Apollo 13* mission to the Moon, during which an oxygen tank exploded and caused a shutdown of the main electrical power. The forced shutdown of the main power source to the *Apollo 13* "command module" left the spacecraft with the astronauts in the command module exposed to near-absolute zero (Kelvin) temperatures (−273 °Celsius)

outside the craft. To survive the subzero temperatures that existed in the spacecraft, the astronauts set up camp in the lunar module (which was designed to be used on the moon surface), dressed in their launch suits, and used the limited battery power of the lunar module to intermittently heat up the module. Unfortunately, they had to abort the moon landing; but fortunately, they returned safely for a successful landing on Earth.

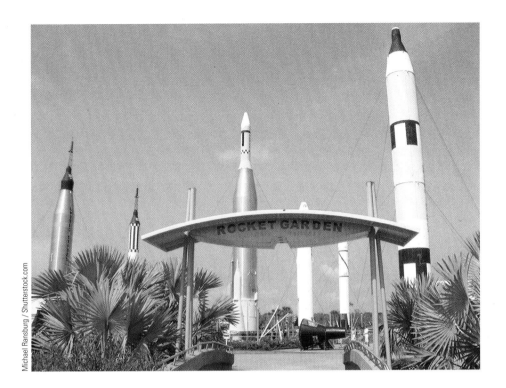

Exercise in Hot Environments

With the exception of severe hemorrhage, exercising in the heat provides the greatest challenge to the human cardiovascular system. As noted previously, muscle contraction is approximately 25 percent efficient, resulting in 75 percent of the metabolic energy used to perform exercise being added to the body as a heat load. The increased heat production resulting from muscular contraction is directly proportional to the intensity of the exercise and results in a linear increase in the active muscle's temperature and, consequently, increases in Tcore in ambient temperatures ranging from 8°C to 29°C (46.4–84.2°F; see Figure 14.3, page 470).

As you can see, these are not very hot conditions for the athlete to encounter. With increases in ambient temperatures above the higher limit of the thermoneutral environment (26°C), the challenges to the cardiovascular system are twofold:

1. It must maintain delivery of oxygen to the active muscles.

2. It must divert blood flow from the core to the skin to enable the process of evaporation of sweat to cool the blood

as it circulates through the skin (see Figure 14.14).

In Figure 14.14, the central blood volume during supine rest is maintained during the heat-induced increase in esophageal temperature even though the **forearm blood flow (FBF)** is increasing per unit increase in the Tes. However, during upright exercise in the heat, the amount of increase in FBF per degree increase in Tes is less compared with supine rest and is

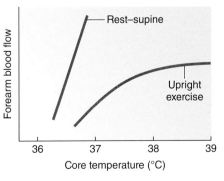

FIGURE 14.14 Redistribution of blood flow to the forearm during supine rest and upright exercise in the heat. (From Rowell, L. B. 1993. Figure 6-12 in *Human cardiovascular control.* New York: Oxford University Press.)

forearm blood flow (FBF) The blood flow measured in the forearm by invasive or non-invasive measurement techniques.

further reduced at 38°C Tes. In this experiment using leg exercise, the measurement of FBF is an index of the amount of blood being redistributed to the skin in response to the increase in core temperature. The reductions in the amount of FBF during upright exercise indicates that to maintain the blood flow to the exercising muscles (the legs), sympathetic vasoconstriction of the skin diverts the blood from the skin to the muscles. The need to provide an increase in sympathetic activity to increase vasoconstriction of the skin is thought to be a response to the decrease in central blood volume.

Because the skin's circulation is relatively slower than the muscles' circulation, the diversion of the circulation to the skin effectively reduces the filling volume of the heart. At the same time, the increases in sympathetic activity result in increases in left ventricular contractility and heart rate, which temporarily maintains, or increases, the cardiac output, exercising muscle blood flow and oxygen delivery until exhaustion. Current evidence suggests that heat stress- or dehydration-related hyperthermia increases the strain on the cardiovascular system before exhaustion. Responses identifying evidence of the cardiovascular strain during exercise in the heat related to dehydration are:

1. Reductions in cardiac output, stroke volume, and arterial pressure
2. Reductions in brain, skin, and exercising muscle blood flow

Unfortunately, the highly motivated, either by self-motivation or by external motivation (drill sergeants, coaches) can drive themselves to the point beyond the warning signs of cardiovascular strain and impending collapse, often resulting in debilitating or fatal consequences. It appears, therefore, that the voluntary, or cognitive, brain processes can override the involuntary (hypothalamic) brain processes to establish a hierarchy of physiologic responses that put the delivery of oxygen to the working muscles above the internal physiologic warning signs of impending circulatory collapse and hyperthermia (see Figure 14.15).

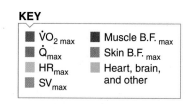

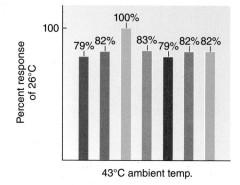

FIGURE 14.15 **Changes in maximal physiological variables during maximal effort in the heat.** Percentage decreases in maximal oxygen uptake ($\dot{V}O_2$ max), cardiac output ($\dot{Q}$max), stroke volume (SVmax), heart rate (HRmax), and muscle, skin, and brain blood flow before impending collapse associated with dehydration and exercising in 43°C heat compared with 100 percent values obtained in 26°C ambient temperature. (Adapted from Rowell, L. B. 1986. Figure 13-13 in *Human circulation: Regulation during physical stress.* New York: Oxford University Press.)

When exercising in a hot outdoor environment, the challenge is for the body's heat-loss mechanisms to equilibrate with the heat gain generated by the metabolic energy production and thereby maintain a stable core temperature (see Figure 14.16). The data presented in Figure 14.16 indicate that as the workload increases, the range of ambient temperatures at which a steady-state core temperature is maintained by physiologic temperature regulatory responses decreases.

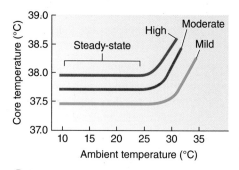

FIGURE 14.16 **Effect of ambient temperature and high, moderate, and mild exercise intensity on the human body's ability to maintain a steady-state core temperature.** (© Cengage Learning 2013)

Explain why the range
of ambient
temperatures for
maintaining the core
temperature stable
decreases with
increasing workloads.

The Need for Prevention of Heat-Related Injuries during Exercise

The primary means of preventing heat-related injuries is by understanding how the body regulates its temperature when challenged by the hot ambient environment and understanding what best practices of prevention are necessary to follow when performing exercise in hot environments.

Heat Acclimatization

More than 60 years ago, a number of investigations were performed to determine the best methods of combating the debilitating effects of hyperthermia and its resultant heat illness, heat exhaustion, heat stroke, and sometimes death. Although the concepts of preventing heat illness were established by these historic experiments, many athletes and coaches are unaware of the fact that practical information is readily available. However, the findings remain the foundation of the modern-day training programs, hydration protocols, and rehydration drinks used today.

In the early work, it was found that the ability to tolerate and perform competitive activity in the heat was improved by repeated exposures to exercising in the heat (see Figure 14.17).

Figure 14.17 summarizes the changes in Trectal (core), heart rate, and sweat loss while exercising at 50 watts for 100 minutes in a thermoneutral environment on day "0" and in a hot environment of 49°C (120°F) and 50 percent relative humidity for a subsequent 8 days. All of the soldiers completed their 100 minutes of 50-watt exercises on the first day (day 0) in the thermoneutral environment. However, during the first day of heat exposure (day 1), none of the nine soldiers was able to complete the 100 minutes of exercise because their rectal temperatures (Trectal) exceeded 39.5°C (clinical hyperthermia). By day 8 of the heat exposure (day 9), all of the soldiers were able to complete the 100-minute exercise without evidence of clinical hyperthermia.

The primary physiologic adaptations that had occurred were:

1. Increases in plasma volume
2. Increases in sweat rate
3. Decreased rise in heart rate
4. Decreased rise in Tcore

Subsequent investigations have found that with this type of **heat acclimatization** procedure, the core temperature at which the onset of sweating is observed decreases. In addition, the amount of sweat produced per degree Celsius increase of

heat acclimatization The adaptation of the physiologic responses to heat stress that occurs after repeated daily exposures to a given hot environment for a period of 8 days.

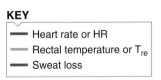

FIGURE 14.17 Physiologic changes associated with an 8-day heat acclimation protocol. (Adapted from data in Belding, H. S. 1972. Chapter 11, Biophysical principles of acclimatization to heat, in *Physiological adaptations: Desert and mountain (Environmental sciences),* edited by M. Yousef, S. M. Horvath, and R. B. Bullard. New York: Academic Press.)

Tcore is greater. It appears that the exercise stress increases the sensitivity of the sweating response of the sweat gland, whereas the heat exposure "*per se*" results in a decreased threshold of Tcore for sweating and a greater capacity of sweat production by the sweat gland.

Another important adaptation of the sweat gland resulting from the acclimatization process is that the sweat contains less sodium after acclimatization than before, thereby conserving the body's sodium stores. This increase in evaporative cooling capacity of both the skin tissue and the blood contained in the skin's circulation by the evaporation of the sweat is beneficial in a dry heat (low humidity) because it increases the core-to-skin temperature gradient, enabling a greater convective (via the circulation) and conductive (via the tissues) heat transfer from the core to the skin.

HOTLINK *See the National Athletic Trainers' Association website (http://www.nata.org) for more information on heat acclimatization.*

However, the benefits of acclimatization are not associated with a cooler skin in hot humid conditions where evaporation of sweat is minimal. The mechanism by which acclimatization to hot, humid conditions provides protection against hyperthermia remains obscure. However, partial acclimatization to hot, humid conditions can be obtained but is far less effective in combating the effects of hydration. Conditions of high humidity are more debilitating with respect to performance and dangerous with respect to health, especially for unacclimatized elderly adults. Suffice to say, acclimatization is both environment-specific and exercise workload-specific. Therefore, once you have completed an 8-day acclimatization process to a specific ambient environment and exercise workload, any increase in the exercise workload or ambient environmental conditions requires another acclimatization process. The acclimatization workloads need to progress to near maximal over an extended period to achieve maximal efforts in hot environments.

Because the acclimatization process increases the body's capacity to sweat per unit increase in Tcore, it is obvious that acclimatized individuals exercising in the heat need to begin their rehydration earlier and to take in more fluids, not less. Another important caveat for the process of acclimatization is that repeated exposures to the heat without exercise (for example, sun bathing at the side of a swimming pool or at the beach) do not provide the benefits of heat acclimatization. Furthermore, a more than 1-day layoff after the environment-specific acclimatization process has been completed results in a decrease in acclimatization.

Rehydration

Another investigation into preparing soldiers to fight in hot environments focused on the role of rehydration in the prevention of heat illness, exhaustion, and stroke. In this study, three pairs of soldiers in full battle gear were asked to walk on a treadmill at 3.5 miles/hour at a 9 percent grade in a hot (32°C, or 90°F) environment until their core temperature (Trectal) reached 39.0°C (102.2°F; see Figure 14.18).

Each soldier was weighed before beginning the walk and then again during the walk at 90, 150, 210, 270, and 320 minutes, when they were allowed to rest for 10 minutes. The first pair of soldiers performed the walk without receiving any rehydration

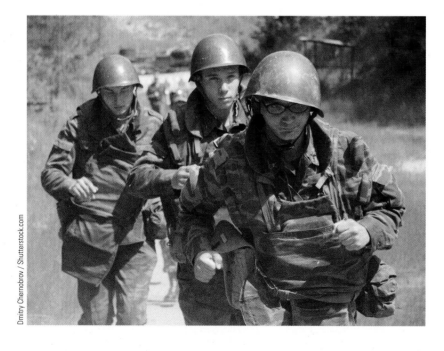

Dmitry Chernobrov / Shutterstock.com

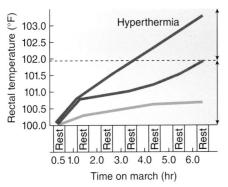
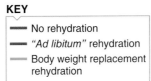

FIGURE 14.18 **Evidence of the benefits of rehydration during exercise in the heat.**

(Adapted from Johnson, R. E. 1972. Figure 1 in Chapter VII, Some nutritional and metabolic aspects of exposure to heat, in *Physiological adaptations: Desert and mountain (Environmental sciences)*, edited by M. Yousef, S. M. Horvath, and R. B. Bullard. New York: Academic Press.)

fluids and completed only approximately 3 hours of walking before their core temperatures (Trectal) exceeded 39°C.

The second pair was allowed to drink a salt solution ad libitum (as desired) during the weigh-in period and completed approximately 5 hours before their core temperature (Trectal) exceeded 39°C.

The third pair of soldiers was required to drink enough of the salt solution at each of the weigh-in periods to replace the body weight they had lost in the previous exercise period. The core temperatures (Trectal) of both these soldiers appeared to achieve a steady state after 6 hours of walking at a Trectal less than 39°C, and the experiment was concluded.

This classic experiment has formed the basis of the testing of all the **rehydration** (replenishment of fluids) drinks now on the market. Even though the formula makeup of the later drinks is more complete in providing more effective replacements of electrolytes, antioxidants, and carbohydrates, the maintenance of the body's **euhydrated** (normal-hydrated) state should remain the primary objective of all the sports drinks. From this initial experiment, the benefits of maintaining hydration in defending against hyperthermia were identified.

Another outcome of the experiments was the recognition that the psychophysical feelings of thirst can be quenched before achieving a replacement volume sufficient to maintain euhydration. The data also identified that replacing the amount of weight lost was the best means of rehydrating and protecting against hyperthermia.

Unfortunately, many of the preventative medical practices developed by this research were not transferred to the huge number of student and recreational athletes (or to their teachers and coaches) performing exercise in the heat until late in the 1970s. It was not until the advanced marketing techniques of the large sports drinks companies were used to identify the benefits that the everyday practice of rehydration during exercise was established.

Unfortunately, even today a number of preventable deaths from dehydration and deconditioning occur each year. Subsequently, it is now a recommended standard of practice for athletic trainers, coaches, and physicians to monitor their athletes' pre-practice body weights on a daily basis.

Monitoring Ambient Conditions

Regardless of whether an athlete has prepared for exercising in hot conditions by acclimatizing to the heat and understanding the practice of rehydration, the key to preventing injuries is to avoid conditions that place the individual at risk. Over the years of training recruits, the military developed a measurement of the ambient conditions known as the **wet bulb globe temperature (WBGT) index**. This index integrates the primary extrinsic risk factors of dry and wet bulb temperatures (humidity) and solar radiant energy into a practical indication of the relative risk for heat injury (see Table 14.1).

The American College of Sports Medicine Position Stand "Prevention of Thermal Injuries during Distance Running" is based on the WBGT index to provide practical guidelines for coaches, athletic trainers, athletic event directors, and physicians. A summary of the recommended

rehydration The replacement of body fluids, orally or intravenously, following heat stress dehydration, vomiting, or diarrhea.

euhydrated The normal hydrated state.

wet bulb globe temperature (WBGT) index An index that integrates the primary extrinsic risk factors of dry and wet bulb temperatures (humidity) and solar radiant energy into a practical indication of the relative risk for heat injury.

Range (°F)	Signal Flag	Activity
<64	None	Unlimited
64–76	Green	Be alert for possible increases in the wet bulb globe temperature index and for symptoms of heat stress
73–82	Yellow	Exercise activities for unacclimatized persons should be curtailed
82–85.9	Red	Exercise activities for all but well-acclimatized persons should be curtailed
≥86	Black	All exercise activities should be stopped

strategies for minimizing the risks for heat injury are:

1. Allow time for acclimatization to the heat; 10 to 14 days working out in the heat.

2. Exercise during the cooler times of the day.

3. Limit or defer to another time if the WBGT index is in the red or black zone.

4. Plan to drink fluids before, during, and after exercise in the heat. The recommended quantities of fluids are 400 to 500 milliliters before and 300 milliliters every 20 minutes during the activity.

5. Monitor training intensity to a given target heart rate because this will account for hyperthermia-induced increases in heart rate tachycardia (the use of a target heart rate to monitor the stress of the training is a quantitative way of determining the strain that is being placed on an individual's cardiovascular system). This is very important when planning a cardiac rehabilitation or weight-loss training program.

HOTLINK *See the American College of Sports Medicine (ACSM) website (http://www.acsm.org) for more details on ACSM recommendations for exercising in the heat.*

For example, in an ambient temperature of 25°C (77°F), the maximal heart rate of an individual is 180 beats/min. When the same individual exercises in any hot ambient temperature, for example, 30°C (86°F), the maximal heart rate remains at 180 beats/min; hence, any training target heart rate set at a percentage of the maximum heart rate will provide the same cardiovascular strain but will account for the difference in the heat stress between the two ambient conditions.

Temperature Regulation during Rest and Exercise in Cold Environments

The heat balance equation summarized in Equation 14.1 accounts for all the avenues of heat loss and heat gained by the body when exercising in the cold and the heat. However, in cold air, the amount of heat lost from the body is much greater in cold temperatures than is added to the body in hot temperatures.

In the cold, while at rest, unwanted heat loss is normally avoided, or reduced, by adding layers of clothing (reducing losses via radiation and convection) and keeping the skin dry. If these measures are unable to maintain the skin temperatures at or above its "set-point temperature," the skin vasoconstricts and diverts the skin blood flow inward toward the central circulation, resulting in an increase in the central blood volume and core temperature.

After a number of ground-based experiments, this normal physiologic response is consistently used by NASA during reentry and at landing of the astronauts to stave off blackout and orthostatic syncope, respectively. Just before reentry, the astronauts don an "Ice Vest," which keeps them somewhat cool during reentry and redirects the peripheral blood inward and increases the central blood volume.

As long as you provide adequate physical and mental warm-up, an individual's athletic performances are less affected by the cold. Nevertheless, cold weather can result in injury to an exercising individual, especially a cardiac-impaired individual (see later in this chapter). The effect of the cold is especially insidious during performance of exercise in cold water and at high altitudes. For the school teacher and/or coach, the underlying principles of heat loss are readily evident during swim class. For example, during a swim class, the water temperature is 80°F (26.8°C) and you notice that a young healthy lean 14-year-old girl (BMI = 15) is doing the exact same workout as a young 14-year-old boy (BMI, 25), but she is shivering very hard and is showing signs of distress. When individuals are shivering very hard during exercise in cold water, it is wise to have them exit the water and use external heating to get them warm.

What do you think is the cause of the two different responses? It has nothing to do with sex differences. Remember the principle of convective and conductive heat loss, insulation, and the concept of the Tsk "set-point" temperature (see Figure 14.10).

If cold stress is sufficiently severe, shivering will begin in an effort to add metabolic heat to the body. Exercising in the cold can be beneficial because it generates heat (remember that when a person exercises, he or she adds 75 percent of the energy used to do the exercise to the body as a heat load). However, if the replenishment energy stores are limited because the availability of food is limited, as in a survival situation, then it may be better not to exercise and instead to assume the fetal position to maximize insulation.

When exercising in cold water, the water temperature and the skin temperature are the same temperature because the specific conductivity of heat of the water is large compared with the individual's tissues, such that it is continuously fluxing heat away from the body. Survival time in cold water can be extended by not exercising and by using clothes as a flotation device and maintaining a fetal position with the nose and mouth above water.

HOTLINK *To learn more about survival in cold water, access the Canadian Red Cross website at:* http://www.redcross.ca/article.asp?id=15204&tid=024.

Acute cold exposure to temperatures as low as −20°C (−4°F) does not affect measures of maximal oxygen uptake ($\dot{V}O_2$ max) because the oxygen transport system to active muscles is not compromised. However, it has been observed that submaximal endurance performance can be reduced.

During cold exposure at rest, the increased metabolic demand for oxygen to sustain shivering is accomplished by an increase in cardiac output but at a reduced heart rate, resulting in a greater stroke volume (see Figure 14.19).

As a result of the relative bradycardia, or slower heart rate, the target heart rate for a given $\dot{V}O_2$ will be lower than predicted from the usual percentage heart rate max value. This physiologic response is important in prescribing exercise to a cardiac-compromised patient who exercises outdoors in a cold environment. However, if you adjust the target heart rate upward to account for the relative bradycardia, you will be working the heart above

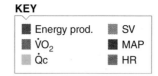

KEY

■ Energy prod.	■ SV
■ $\dot{V}O_2$	■ MAP
■ $\dot{Q}c$	■ HR

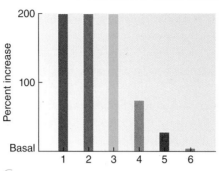

⬤ **FIGURE 14.19 Percentage change in heat production, oxygen uptake ($\dot{V}O_2$), cardiac output ($\dot{Q}c$), stroke volume (SV), and mean arterial blood pressure (MAP) after 2 hours of resting near nude in 5°C.** (Adapted from Raven, P. B., et al. 1970. Compensatory cardiovascular responses during an environmental cold stress of 5C. *J. App. Physiol.*, 29:417–421.)

that required for the training because the stroke volume has adjusted to maintain the cardiac work. It would be safer and more accurate to keep the workload of the cardiac rehabilitation patient constant to the predicted heart rate in normothermic conditions than to adjust the workload to increase the heart rate to account for cold-induced bradycardia.

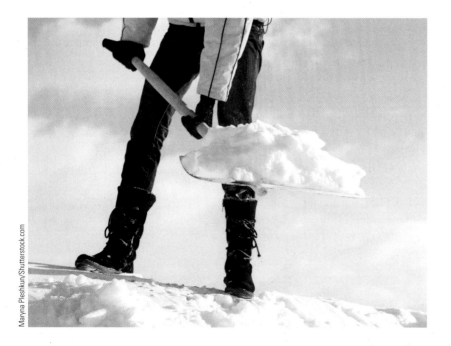

Prevention of Cold-Related Injuries during Exercise

As is evident in heat stress, the human body has the capability to acclimatize to the cold, in that it is not unusual to observe a resident of a cold geographical area withstand much colder ambient temperatures without requiring additional clothing for insulation than a resident of a warm geographical area. Consistent findings between acclimatized and unacclimatized individuals associated with changes in metabolism or cardiovascular function have been difficult to identify. However, one of the most consistent findings is the development of localized cold-induced vasodilatation of the cheeks of infants carried outdoors by the parents in a backpack and the hands of the people who fillet fish.

The effect of cold exposure on the human is one of degree and depends on air movement across the skin surface, humidity and precipitation, as well as the ambient temperature. As the temperature declines to below freezing, the humidity becomes less of a factor because the water is condensed out of the air. As the temperature decreases, the wind velocity becomes a major factor in exacerbating body heat loss because of increased convectional heat loss at the skin surface. The effect of the air-velocity factor, that is, the wind chill effect, is shown in Figure 14.20. The cold injuries to protect against during outdoor training include hypothermia and frostbite and Raynaud disease.

HOTLINK *Perform an Internet search for more information on frostbite and Raynaud disease. For example, see the National Blood and Lung Institute's Diseases and Conditions Index page for more about Raynaud disease at:* http://www.nhlbi.nih.gov/health/dci/Diseases/raynaud/ray_what.html.

Breathing cold air does not cause injury to the trachea and lung tissue because on entering the mouth, warming and humidifying begins, and by the time it reaches the bronchus, the air has been warmed and humidified. However, it may feel uncomfortable to some people. The fact that the upper respiratory tract is the avenue by which the inspired air is warmed and

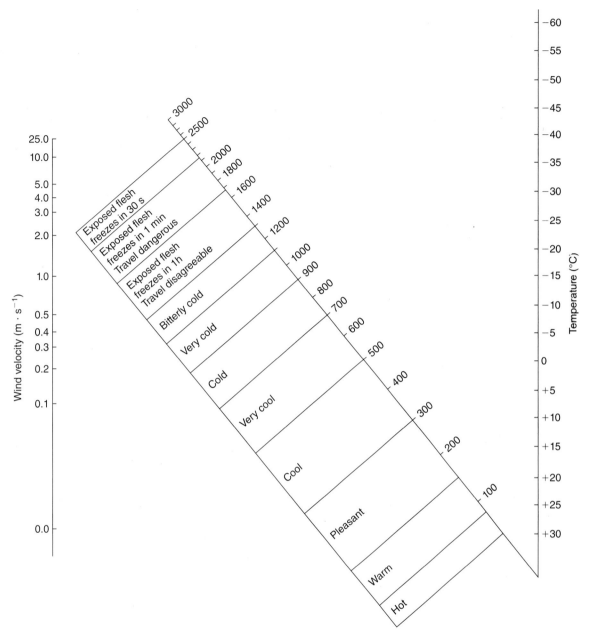

● **FIGURE 14.20 Wind chill nomogram: interrelation between ambient temperature and wind velocity, and perceptual sensations and rate of heat loss (kcal·m⁻³·h⁻³) from the skin.** Under conditions of bright sunshine, cooling is reduced by about 200 kcal·m⁻³·h⁻³. Expressions of relative comfort are based on a lightly clad, inactive individual. To convert kcal·m⁻³·h⁻³ to W·m⁻³, multiply by 1.163. (From Pandolf, K. B., M. N. Sawka, and R. R. Gonzalez, editors. 1989. Figure 9-5 in *Human performance physiology and environmental medicine at terrestrial extremes.* Dubuque, IA: Brown and Benchmark.

humidified also means that, in a cold environment, this can become a major avenue of body heat and water loss, which become substantial during exercise when the ventilation is increased. One means of reducing the discomfort and loss of heat is to breathe through a cloth bandana.

The inhalation of very cold air by cardiac patients can cause a variant of Prinzmetal's angina pectoris, that is, chest pain stemming from the heart from vasoconstriction of the coronary arteries; thus, precautions should be taken in cardiac rehabilitation programs performed outdoors.

The main risk factors for cold injury are those that affect energy metabolism or the circulation, such as fatigue, hunger, low-percent body fat (less insulation), use of tobacco and/or caffeine (vasoconstriction), and alcohol (vasodilatation). The major factor in prevention of cold injury when practicing exercise in an outdoor environment is adequate clothing. If the wind-chill temperatures are −26 to −29°C (−15 to −20°F) or lower, exposed skin such as the face, nose, ears, and hands should be adequately protected. The body should be covered with several layers of loose-fitting clothing, and layers should be removed as the body warms up to reduce the accumulation of sweat. Water conducts the cold rapidly; therefore, in wet, cold environments, an outer layer of waterproof clothing needs to be worn.

During extended periods of exercise, the intensity should be set to avoid a significant decrease toward the end of the training period to maintain the body's heat production. This phenomenon becomes a major problem in competitive running, swimming, or skiing events.

Altitude and Air Pollution

We have addressed the stress that heat and cold impose on individuals involved in exercise training programs. The following sections address the stress imposed by altitude and air pollution, and the resulting physiologic responses to exercise. Similar to stresses imposed by heat and cold, the environments of altitude and air pollution provide a major challenge to the human's regulatory control systems. For example, the effects of cold stress and wind chill, identified previously, become an additive challenge to the body's regulatory system the higher altitude one explores; that is, an individual at the peak of Mt. Everest (29,200 feet) is exposed to the winds associated with the jet stream (150 miles/hour), and for every 1,000-foot increase above sea level, the temperature decline approximates 3.5°F (2°C). In addition, severe air pollution episodes occur during temperature inversions in which a stationary mass of cold air is trapped under hot air or hot air is trapped under cold air.

Acute Exposure to Altitudes

To understand the physical challenge posed to the individual by altitude, you will need to recall from Chapter 9 the following information:

1. The ideal gas laws and their physical properties

2. The effect of changes in partial pressure of oxygen (PO_2) on the oxygen-hemoglobin saturation curve

3. The effects of hypoxia on blood gases and their effects on respiration

The fundamental property to keep in mind is that as one ascends to altitude (climbing or flying), the absolute barometric pressure becomes reduced; however, the percentage of O_2 (20.9 percent) in the air is unchanged. Therefore, by Dalton's law of partial pressures, the PO_2 of the atmosphere is less.

For example:
At sea level, where the barometric pressure is 760 mm Hg, the PO_2 is calculated as

$$760 \times 20.9/100 = 159 \text{ mm Hg}$$

At 10,000 ft (3,049 m), where the barometric pressure is 523 mm Hg, the inspired PO_2 (PiO_2) can be similarly calculated.

(Calculate the PiO_2 at 10,000 feet.)

There is a near-linear decrease in barometric pressure and its effect on PiO_2 in relation to an increase in altitude. For example, at 5,000 meters (16,400 feet), the PiO_2 is half that at sea level.

The reduction in ambient PO_2 is a hypoxic (low oxygen pressure) environment, and the resultant reduction in arterial PO_2 (that is, PaO_2, or hypoxia) is known as **hypoxic hypoxia** and distinguishes the environmentally induced hypoxia from the arterial **hypoxia** associated with chronic obstructive pulmonary disease.

hypoxic hypoxia The reduction in arterial oxygen tension (PaO_2) associated with hypoxia.

hypoxia A reduction in ambient PO_2 or a low oxygen pressure environment.

At the summit of Mt. Everest, 9,300 meters (29,200 feet), the PiO$_2$ is 30 percent of the sea level value. There is no doubt that high-altitude mountaineering and climbing require extreme physical exertion and are usually attempted by only a relatively few number of individuals; however, it is at the more moderate altitudes that everyday athletic and daily physical activity performed by the general population take place.

In Denver, at 1,600 meters (5,280 feet), the ambient PO$_2$ declines to 132 mm Hg from 159 mm Hg at sea level and is as low as 94 mm Hg at Pikes Peak, Colorado, at 4,276 meters (14,110 feet); this location annually hosts a marathon run that requires the competitors to run up and down the mountain. In Colorado alone, there are more than fifty 14,000-foot mountains, many of which have skiing resorts where the everyday skier is routinely exposed to altitudes ranging from 7,000 (2,333) to 11,000 feet (3,666 meters), and the more adventurous are sometimes exposed to altitudes of 14,000 feet (4,666 meters).

These examples of altitude exposure are described to indicate to you that altitude is not an exceptional environment, but one that is encountered daily. Indeed, the African village from which many of the elite Kenyan runners were born and raised is located at 7,000 feet (2,333 meters). The capital city of Bolivia, La Paz, is located at 13,100 feet (4,366 meters), and many silver and lead mines of the Andes are located at 17,000 feet (5,667 meters) plus. Furthermore, the usual cabin pressure for commercial airlines is 8,000 feet (2,667 meters).

Oxygen Transport in the Acute Stages of Exposure to Altitude

Because of air and car travel, the ascent to altitude locations has become a rapid process. On arrival at the moderate- to high-altitude location, acute adaptive physiologic responses occur as the body attempts to adjust to the reduced PiO$_2$.

Partial Pressure of Oxygen

Figure 14.21 describes the PO$_2$ at different distances along the oxygen transport cascade in the body from atmospheric air to its ultimate destination, the mitochondria, at sea level and at 16,500 ft (5,500 m). The

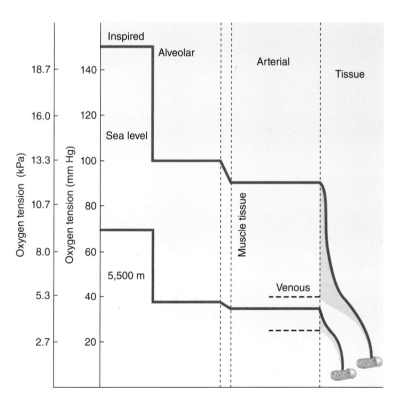

● **FIGURE 14.21** **Schematic depiction of the differences in the cascade of oxygen partial pressures from inspiration to the mitochondria at sea level and 5,500 meters (18,000 feet).** (From Astrand, P. O., and K. Rodahl. 1986. Figure 15-2 in *Textbook of work physiology: Physiological basis of exercise.* 3rd ed. New York: McGraw-Hill Book Co.)

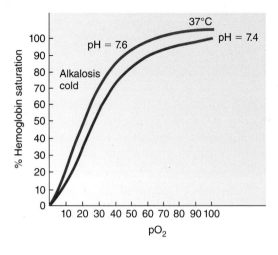

FIGURE 14.22 Representative oxyhemoglobin saturation/O$_2$ partial pressure curves at sea level and at altitude. Note the leftward shift of the oxyhemoglobin saturation/O$_2$ partial pressure curve at altitude. (Adapted from Sherwood, L. 2004. Figure 13-30 in *Human physiology: From cells to systems*, 5th ed. Belmont, CA: Thomson-Brooks/Cole.)

reduction in alveolar pressure of oxygen (P$_A$O$_2$) from 100 mm Hg at sea level to 40 mm Hg at 16,500 feet results in a reduced PaO$_2$ and oxygen delivery to the tissues.

Cardiorespiratory Responses

Immediately on arrival at 16, 500-foot altitude, the low PaO$_2$ stimulates the peripheral chemoreceptors. This stimulation of the peripheral chemoreceptors increases pulmonary ventilation, resulting in hyperventilation and respiratory alkalosis.

> Explain why hyperventilation causes alkalosis.

Hyperventilation increases the P$_A$O$_2$, but it is insufficient to reinstate a 90 to 98 percent saturation of the hemoglobin molecule. Once again, this fact reinforces the importance of the PO$_2$ and not oxyhemoglobin saturation in the regulation of ventilation.

The hyperventilation-induced alkalosis, in turn, causes a leftward shift in the oxygen-hemoglobin dissociation curve, which means that the tissue needs to be at a lower PO$_2$ to allow the oxygen to unload from the hemoglobin (see Figure 14.22).

Therefore, because of the reduced oxygen content and the tighter binding of oxygen to the hemoglobin at any given metabolic rate, the oxygen delivery to the mitochondria is reduced. Note that the major effect of the reduced barometric pressure is manifest on the PiO$_2$ and the subsequent

PaO$_2$. Therefore, at the more moderate altitudes of 3,000 to 10,000 ft, the tissue PO$_2$ is not as severely reduced. However, during 60 percent $\dot{V}O_2$max cycling exercise at a simulated altitude exposure of 3,100 m (9,400 ft), there was a 50 percent increase in ventilation ($\dot{V}e$) and a 15 percent increase in heart rate (HR). The increase in HR resulted in a 13 percent increase in the cardiac output ($\dot{Q}c$). Therefore, despite a slightly reduced stroke volume, the increase in $\dot{Q}c$ at submaximal workloads compensated for the reduced oxygen-carrying capacity of the blood. This compensatory mechanism provides sufficient oxygen delivery to support metabolism, especially at rest and during submaximal exercise (see Figure 14.23). However, at maximal exercise, the reduced

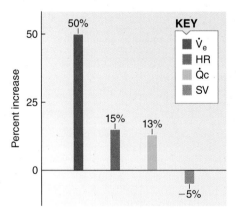

FIGURE 14.23 Summary of the cardiovascular responses during 60 percent maximal oxygen uptake ($\dot{V}O_2$ max) cycling exercise at a simulated altitude exposure of 3,100 meters (10,000 feet). (Adapted from Astrand, P. O., and K. Rodahl. 1986. Figure 15-4 in *Textbook of work physiology: Physiological basis of exercise*, 3rd ed. New York: McGraw-Hill Book Co.)

oxygen-carrying capacity reduces $\dot{V}O_2$ max despite the cardiovascular hemodynamics achieving sea level maximal values.

At altitudes as low as 3,000 feet (1,000 meters), the exercise ventilation is increased at any given workload because the reduction in PaO_2 (91 mm Hg) is sufficient to stimulate the peripheral chemoreceptors to increase ventilation despite 97 percent oxygen saturation of the hemoglobin molecules in the arterial blood (see Figure 14.24). This physiologic response emphasizes the importance of the PO_2 in the regulation of ventilation.

It is this acute hypoxic drive to hyperventilate that determines the reduction in the bicarbonate buffering capacity of the blood because of the "blow off" of CO_2 at the lungs, resulting in the leftward shift of the oxygen-hemoglobin saturation curve (see Equation 9.11). In addition, the hyperventilation results in a decrease in CO_2 and hydrogen ions in the cerebrospinal fluid (CSF) and the blood, that is, respiratory alkalosis resulting in a blood pH of 7.6. The increase in blood pH triggers the start of a process of bicarbonate excretion at the kidney to reinstate the CSF and blood pH to its normal value of 7.4. Normalization of blood pH is one measure identifying the establishment of altitude acclimatization.

Is it PaO_2 or O_2 saturation that stimulates the peripheral chemoreceptors?

Oxygen Delivery

Beginning at approximately 5,000 feet (1,525 meters) at a barometric pressure of 634 mm Hg, the $\dot{V}O_2$ max (or the circulation's maximal capacity to deliver oxygen) begins to decrease at a rate of 3 percent every 1,000 feet (300 meters) increase in altitude. As a point of reference, Denver is located at an altitude of 5,280 feet (1,600 meters) and hosts many athletic events.

At approximately 10,000 feet (3,050 meter), at a barometric pressure of 520 mm Hg, the decrease in $\dot{V}O_2$ max becomes exponentially greater, such that at the summit of Mt. Everest (29,200 feet), the $\dot{V}O_2$ max of even the most experienced mountain climbers approaches their individual resting $\dot{V}O_2$ (see Figure 14.25).

Interestingly, it was at an altitude of 10,000 feet that the air forces involved in World War II, and before cabin pressurization, identified from their research that the aircraft pilots would require supplemental oxygen to enable the pilots and crew to retain their cognitive function.

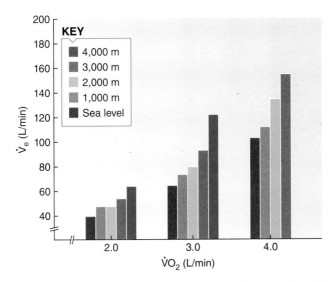

KEY
- 4,000 m
- 3,000 m
- 2,000 m
- 1,000 m
- Sea level

● **FIGURE** 14.24 **Summary of the ventilatory response to cycling exercise at 1, 2, 3, and 4 L/min oxygen uptake ($\dot{V}O_2$) at sea level and at altitudes of 1,000, 2,000, 3,000, and 4,000 meters.** Note that the 4.0 L/min $\dot{V}O_2$ workload was not completed. (Adapted from Astrand, P. O., and K. Rodahl. 1986. Figure 15-3 in *Textbook of work physiology: Physiological basis of exercise*, 3rd ed. New York: McGraw-Hill Book Co.)

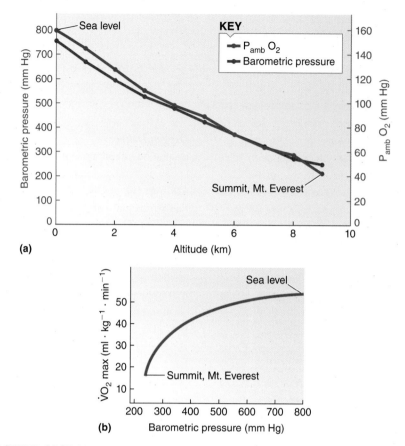

FIGURE 14.25 (a) Summary of the relationship between increasing altitude and decreasing barometric pressure and the partial pressure of O_2 in the ambient air ($P_{amb}O_2$). (b) Summary of the relationship between increasing altitude and decreasing measured maximal oxygen uptake ($\dot{V}O_2$ max). (Adapted from data in Cymerman, A., et al. 1988. Operation Everest II: Maximal oxygen uptake at extreme altitude. *J. App. Physiol.*, 64:1309–1321.)

As altitude increases, an individual's $\dot{V}O_2$ max decreases in direct proportion to the decrease in the oxygen content of the arterial blood (CaO_2). In addition, the $\dot{V}O_2$ required to perform a given amount of work (100 Watts) at altitude is the same as at sea level. Therefore, a given amount of work performed at altitude represents a greater percentage of the individual's altitude $\dot{V}O_2$ max and is reflected in a greater heart rate and cardiac output.

Even though the $\dot{V}O_2$ for a given workload is the same at altitude as it is at sea level, the individual's perception of effort to do the work is much greater. This finding has raised a complex and intriguing discussion. It is generally accepted that heart rate and $\dot{V}O_2$ are indices of changes in central command (see Chapter 7), yet at altitude, the $\dot{V}O_2$ is the same as at sea level, whereas the heart rate and perception of effort, as measured by ratings of perceived exertion, are increased. A probable

explanation is that a number of investigations have identified a close association between ventilation and perception of effort. Therefore, it is thought that it is the hypoxic drive to increase ventilation that cues the increase in an individual's rating of their perception of effort independent of changes in central command. This is important for athletes, coaches, and rehabilitation specialists because it is the individual's ventilation response to exercise that appears to be tightly coupled to the individual's perception of effort.

Metabolism

The basal metabolic rate is increased at altitude and is related to an increase in carbohydrate metabolism because of the reduced oxygen content of the blood stimulating an increase in sympathetic activity and resulting in an increased epinephrine secretion. Epinephrine stimulates glycogenolysis (breakdown of glycogen) and results in an increase in lactate production at any given $\dot{V}O_2$, or workload (see Figure 14.26). Notably, it is the increase in lactate production and not a decrease in lactate clearance mechanisms that is responsible for the increased blood lactate concentrations at any given workload at sea level.

There appears to be no independent effect of altitude on fat and protein metabolism, and it is only the increased sympathetic activity associated with altitude exposure that accelerates the glycolytic production of lactate at the submaximal workloads.

Chronic Exposure to Altitude

Chronic exposure to altitude results in a series of physiologic adaptations that become more established the longer the duration at altitude. At approximately 6,000 feet (approximately 2,000 meters; Colorado Springs, Colorado, is at an altitude of 6,035 feet), the resulting reduction in PaO_2 and oxygen content of the blood precipitates an increase in the number of red blood cells, resulting in an increase in hematocrit and total hemoglobin. This adaptation is termed **polycythemia** and is the primary adaptation of low-altitude dwellers who sojourn at altitude for long periods. Whether natives born and raised at altitude have some genetic advantages other than the

increase in the number of red blood cells has not been clearly identified. However, it does appear that the number of champion endurance performance athletes born and raised at altitude has increased as the opportunities to train and travel have increased, thereby enabling the previously geographically and economically limited athletes to attend more competitions. Prolonged exposure (months and years) maximizes the adaptations that occur; however, the sea level inhabitant's performance remains decreased at altitude even if they are well acclimatized.

Oxygen Transport after Chronic Exposure to Altitude

As noted earlier, the normalization of blood pH marks the establishment of acclimatization at a given altitude. In planning an assault on Mt. Everest, it was usual to use a 70-day trek from a low-altitude (5,000-feet) starting point to a base camp altitude of 18,000 feet to allow the climbers to acclimatize. This period of acclimatization reduced the number of climbers suffering from the many altitude illnesses, such as **acute mountain sickness (AMS)**, **high-altitude pulmonary edema (HAPE)** and **high-altitude cerebral edema (HACE)**, which sometimes can be fatal. Unfortunately, because air travel has reduced the time it takes to reach the starting altitudes of high-altitude climbing, the prevalence of altitude illnesses in mountaineers has increased.

HOTLINK *Perform an Internet search for more information on AMS, HAPE, and HACE. For example, see Pub Med website at:* http://www.ncbi.nlm.nih.gov/pubmedhealth/PMH0001190/ *for more about AMS.*

The hyperventilatory response to acute altitude exposure decreases the blood's CO_2 and results in an alkaline blood pH and excess in bicarbonate ions in the CSF and blood. The excretion of the bicarbonate at the kidney returns CSF and blood pH to normal (pH 7.4) and improves respiratory control, but reduces the buffering capacity of the blood. The normalization of the blood's pH shifts the oxyhemoglobin-saturation curve back from the left to the right.

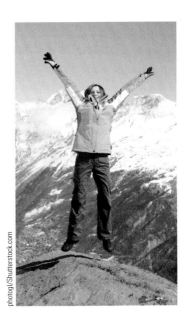

polycythemia An excess number of red blood cells above normal sea level values.

acute mountain sickness (AMS) A complex of symptoms that present acutely and include severe headache, lassitude, irritability, nausea, vomiting, anorexia, indigestion, flatus, constipation, and sleep disturbances characterized by periodic breathing.

high-altitude pulmonary edema (HAPE) A non-cardiogenic pulmonary edema that usually results 12 to 96 hours from rapid ascent to high altitude (10,000 ft). Active adults appear to be more susceptible than middle-aged and older adults. Symptoms include those of AMS, rapid and shallow breathing, rapid heart rate, and rale lung sounds.

high-altitude cerebral edema (HACE) A severe form of AMS and its symptoms with the presence of edema in the brain and is potentially fatal if left untreated.

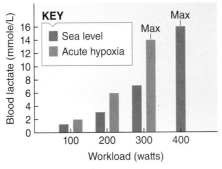

⊙ FIGURE 14.26 Increases in blood lactate concentrations during simulated acute hypoxia (4,100 meters) and sea level at any given workload. Note that submaximal blood lactate concentrations were higher in acute hypoxia but were lower at the maximal workloads achieved at sea level. (Modified from partial data presented in Wagner, P. D., and C. Lundby. 2007. The lactate paradox: Does acclimatization to high altitude affect blood lactate during exercise? *Med. Sci. Sports Exerc.* 39:749–755.)

Using the information from Chapter 9, explain how the shift in the oxyhemoglobin-saturation curve from left to right benefits the individual at altitude.

In addition, another adaptation that occurs over the first weeks at altitude is the gradual increase in the concentration of 2-3-diphosphoglycerate within the red blood cell. This molecule decreases the affinity for oxygen, causing it to unload the oxygen at higher tissue PO_2 and effectively shifting the oxyhemoglobin-saturation curve farther to the right. Above 15,000 feet (5,000 meters), this acclimatization property becomes detrimental because it impairs the hemoglobin's ability to bind with oxygen.

Oxygen Delivery

With prolonged exposure at altitude, submaximal workload heart rates return to sea level values, but because of persistent reductions in submaximal and maximal stroke volume, the submaximal and maximal cardiac output is reduced. An increase in the oxygen extraction from the blood at the tissues (calculated from the arterio-venous oxygen content difference, that is, the $(a-v)$ O_{2diff}; see Chapter 7) during submaximal workloads compensates for the reduced cardiac output ($\dot{Q}$). However, when

CONCEPTS, challenges, & controversies

The Lactate Paradox

At rest, the response of circulating lactate concentrations to altitude exposure remain unchanged over the course of acclimatization. However, the submaximal and maximal exercise blood lactate concentrations have both been reported to decrease over the period of acclimatization (see Figure 14.27, page 497).

It has generally been accepted that hypoxia stimulates cellular lactate production during exercise. Therefore, the apparent lack of an increase in anaerobic glycolysis during exercise in chronic hypoxia (altitude acclimatization) identified in Figure 14.27 has been termed the **lactate paradox**.

More recent experiments using experimental protocols to address issues of differences in the subjects' aerobic fitness and acclimatization periods have indicated that the lactate paradox was not present (see Figure 14.28, page 497).

A multitude of experiments conducted by a number of investigative groups indicate the presence of the lactate paradox. Only one set of experiments from a highly respected group of investigators indicated the absence of a lactate paradox. A collaborative compromise investigation with investigators from both points of view has been proposed but not yet enacted.

The first step in this process is to agree on the identifying questions to be asked. Perhaps underlying this first step is to realize that it may not be hypoxia per se that the lactate production identifies as being the cause, but to analyze whether the speed of glycolysis can surpass the individual's mitochondrial capacity for oxidation, especially when altitude acclimatization may decrease an individual's mitochondrial capacity and the amount of physical activity that the individual can achieve.

lactate paradox The apparent lack of an increase in anaerobic glycolysis during exercise in chronic hypoxia (altitude acclimatization).

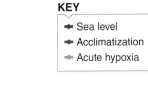

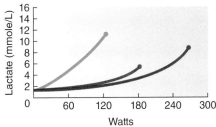

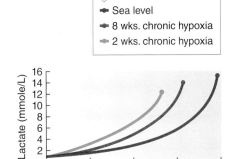

FIGURE 14.27 **The accepted view of the lactate paradox.** Many studies have found that after a period of acclimatization to altitude, the magnitude of glycolytic production of lactate for any given workload is less than observed during an acute exposure to hypoxia. In addition, the maximal lactate achieved during maximal work is reduced after acclimatization when compared with sea level and acute hypoxia. (Modified from Wagner. P. D., and C. Lundby. 2007. The lactate paradox: Does acclimatization to high altitude affect blood lactate during exercise? *Med. Sci. Sports Exerc.* 39:749–755.)

FIGURE 14.28 **A contrasting set of findings regarding the lactate paradox.** The data indicate that after 8 weeks living and training at 4,100-meter altitude, the glycolytic production of arterial blood lactate was greater than at sea level for any given submaximal workload, and at maximal workloads was not significantly less than observed at sea level. (Modified from partial data presented in Wagner. P. D., and C. Lundby. 2007. The lactate paradox: Does acclimatization to high altitude affect blood lactate during exercise. *Med. Sci. Sports Exerc.* 39:749–755.)

the extraction of O_2 is maximized resulting in approximately 3 volumes percent in the pulmonary artery, the individual's $\dot{V}O_2$ max will be less than the sea level value because of the reduced $\dot{Q}$max even though they are acclimatized to the altitude.

The reduction in stroke volume during submaximal exercise with acute and chronic exposure to altitude and the persistent reduction in submaximal and maximal stroke volume after altitude acclimatization remains a puzzle, especially because there is no evidence of a reduction in myocardial contractility. The most plausible explanation lies with the increased sympathoexcitation resulting from hypoxic stimulation of the chemoreceptors causing an increase in peripheral vasoconstriction, thereby increasing mean arterial pressure and cardiac afterload.

Another factor in the reduced stroke volume effect of altitude is that the plasma volume is reduced. This is due to a whole-body dehydration resulting from the respiratory system's need to humidify the inspired air. The higher the altitude, the colder the air, and as per the process of air conditioning, the water in the inspired air is squeezed out; therefore, during inspiration, the nasal and

pharyngeal passages have to rehumidify the air before it reaches the lung tissues. At altitude, individuals are generally unable to adjust their fluid intake to completely offset the water loss. The subsequent dehydration, together with the acclimatization-induced increase in red blood cells *(polycythemia)*, increases the blood's viscosity, that is, the blood becomes thick and sticky. This increase in blood viscosity adds to the increase in cardiac afterload, which, in turn, resists the amount of blood ejected from the heart during each beat.

Exercise Performance at Altitude

Two types of athletic events are performed at altitude: power events and endurance events. The power events primarily use anaerobic energy sources and include running; swimming and bicycling that last for less than 2 minutes; field events, such as discus, shot put, javelin, and hammer throw; all the jumping events; and gymnastics. Many winter events last less than 2 minutes and therefore can be classified as power events. The 2-minute period is based on the maximum time that the body

erythropoietin (EPO) An endogenous hormone produced by the kidney in response to low PaO$_2$ and stimulates the production of red blood cells in the bone marrow.

can operate using mechanisms for generating energy anaerobically. The major benefit afforded by altitude to the power event competitors is the reduction in the density of the ambient air.

(*Why is the density of the air less at altitude than at sea level?*)

The endurance events primarily use aerobic energy sources and include the following: track and field, swimming, bicycling, rowing, canoeing, and winter events that last longer than 2 minutes. The reduction in the cardiopulmonary system's ability to deliver oxygen to working tissues because of the reduced ambient PO$_2$ is the primary reason for the reduction in $\dot{V}O_2$ max and prolongation of performance time (see Figure 14.29).

Remember, if the event requires an animal to be the athletic competitor, for example, horse show jumping and the 3-day endurance event for horses, the same advantages and disadvantages of competing at altitude exist for the animal.

Training at Altitude for Competition

Earlier, the clinical scientists had identified hypoxia as being the stimulus for increasing red blood cell number and hemoglobin content via the upregulation of the production of **erythropoietin (EPO)** in the kidney, an endogenous hormone that stimulates the production of red blood cells in the bone marrow. When the Olympic Games were scheduled in 1960 to take place in Mexico City in 1968, at an altitude of 7,340 feet or 2,446 meters, many of the endurance athletes and their coaches set up training camps at altitude and some used altitude chambers. Others who were born and raised at altitude, such as some of the African athletes, were seen to have an advantage. However, the major practical finding that came from most of the studies of residents living below 1,000 meters (3,000 feet) who moved and trained at altitude was that the endurance athlete was unable to perform the total amount of training necessary to improve his sea level performance, even though his training and acclimatization to altitude had improved his $\dot{V}O_2$ max at that altitude by increasing the blood's oxygen-carrying capacity.

(*What do you conclude from the fact that the $\dot{V}O_2$ max was improved but the performance had decreased?*)

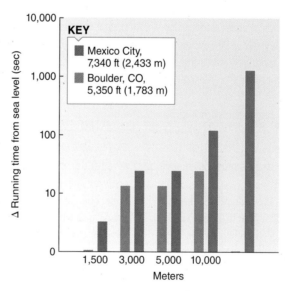

● **FIGURE 14.29 Comparison of the effect of altitude on competitive running performance times at sea level, Boulder, Colorado (5,350 meters), and Mexico City Olympics (7,340 meters).** Note the exponential "Y"-axis of time in seconds. (Modified from Reeves, J. T., P. Jokl, and J. E. Cohn. 1965. Performance of Olympic runners at altitude of 7,350 and 5,350 feet. *Am. Rev. Respir. Dis.* 92(5):813–816.)

An illustration of the lack of the beneficial effects of altitude training was evident at the Mexico City Olympic Games when the Japanese women's swimming team failed to medal, even though the team had world record holders and had trained at altitude for more than a year.

Blood Doping

The clinical treatment for patients with severe anemia or blood loss during surgery was to transfuse them with one or more units of matched blood. It did not take long after the 1968 Olympic Games for exercise scientists to determine that they could acutely boost a healthy subject's $\dot{V}O_2$ max and endurance performance by withdrawing 1.0 liter of an individual's own blood, waiting for the physiologic processes to restore the blood volume back to its original volume, and then acutely infuse their 1.0 liter stored blood just before competition (**blood doping**). These experiments were performed ethically and were conducted with the knowledge of the appropriate oversight committees. However, since the publication of the findings in the scientific literature in the early 1970s, the unethical use of blood doping before endurance competitions, especially with the increase of professionalism and the attitude of "win at all cost regardless of whether I risk my life," has increased exponentially. In addition, the development of synthetically produced EPO for the clinical use and benefit of anemic patients resulting from dialysis and other conditions has resulted in its illegal and unethical use in boosting the athlete's red cell volume. Unfortunately, in some cases, EPO use has been linked to the death of some athletes, especially during exhaustive exercise and thermal dehydration. However, the beneficial effect of using synthetic EPO to boost red blood cell volume has formed the basis of the Hi-Lo altitude training programs and the use of nitrogen tents to naturally produce increases in the synthesis of endogenous EPO (see Chapter 9) and Hi-Lo training. However, whether the "Hi-Lo altitude" training programs help to overcome the reduction in performance times at the moderate altitudes of a Denver or a Mexico City has not been delineated.

HOTLINK *Perform an Internet search for more information on blood doping tests and illegal performances in sport activities such as the Tour de France. For example, for more about blood doping associated with the Tour de France, see the ESPN Cycling and BMX website at:* http://sports.espn.go.com/espn/wire?section=cycling&id=2882358.

Air Pollution

As the population of cities increase, the number of cars and industries using fossil fuels and exhausting air pollutants and particulates into the air also increases. The concentration of the pollutants and particulates in the air are measured in parts per million (ppm). Many cities grow and develop in locations that geographically result in air stagnation and temperature inversions. For example, Los Angeles grew and developed in a location known to the Native Americans as "the valley of the smoke," because on a day in which the winds were not blowing, the smoke from the wood-burning fires hung over the valley formed by the surrounding hills and mountains. As new economies based on industrialization and transportation via the automobile emerged, the increase in numbers of industrial plants and automobile traffic worldwide produced an exponential increase in the amount of pollutants and particulates in the air. Indeed, cities of India, China, Russia, Eastern Europe, Malaysia, Japan, South America, and Australia have joined the North American and older European cities as major polluters of the atmosphere. In these cities and their surrounding suburban areas, many pollutants reach concentrations that produce significant increases in morbidity and excess deaths, reductions in functional performance, and increases in subjective feelings of malaise.

The most common air pollutants found to be harmful to an individual's cardiopulmonary system and to be performance limiting are:

1. **Oxidants** (90 percent ozone)
2. **Sulfur oxides**
3. **Particulates**
4. **Carbon monoxide (CO)**

blood doping The acute infusion of 1.0 blood just before competition.

oxidants A substance that oxidizes another substance. In air pollution, a mixture of oxidative substances and usually consists of ozone and nitrogen oxides.

sulfur oxides Result from fossil fuel combustion and include sulfur dioxide (SO_2), sulfuric acid, and sulfate. SO_2 is a soluble gas that irritates the upper respiratory tract and causes reflex bronchoconstriction.

particulates Can be a mixture of one or more pieces of soot, sand, smoke, etc., that is in the air we breathe. During inspiration, settles on lung tissue depending on the size of the particles.

carbon monoxide (CO) An odorless and colorless gas produced from combustion of fossil fuels (gasoline, oils, and coals). It has the ability to combine with the hemoglobin (Hb) in our blood 240 times stronger than oxygen.

Most of the catastrophic air pollution episodes that have occurred worldwide usually involve a combination of a high concentration of particulates and either sulfur oxides or oxidants and CO. These high concentrations usually occur during a temperature inversion (hot air trapped under cold air or cold air trapped under hot air) with no air movement. The presence of particulate matter appears to enable greater penetration of the air pollutant gases into the lung and produce severe lung tissue irritation.

Oxidant and Sulfur Oxides

The important point for teachers, coaches, parents, and athletes to remember is that all airborne pollutants exhibit a dose–response relationship summarized in the following relationship:

$$\text{Air pollutant concentration} \times \\ \text{ventilation volume (L/min)} \times \\ \text{time of exposure}$$

During an oxidant (ozone) exposure, this relationship results in a quantifiable physiologic effect on lung function (see Figure 14.30).

This fundamental relationship exists for both oxidant pollutants and sulfur dioxide (SO_2). In nonasthmatic healthy individuals, ozone is the pollutant most likely to significantly affect the individual's ventilation during exercise. For example, many trained bicyclists were unable to complete 1 hour of cycling requiring 90 to 120 L/min of ventilation in ozone concentrations of 0.12 ppm. The end point of the individual cyclist's performance was usually respiratory discomfort with substernal pain and was associated with a 16 to 30 percent increase in performance time and was associated with a 6 to 16 percent reduction in $\dot{V}O_2$ max.

In the Western industrialized nations, the air pollution controls have reduced the ambient SO_2 and acid aerosol concentrations to less than the concentrations that would affect the exercise performance or lung function of healthy individuals. This is not the case on the Asian continent. In contrast, SO_2 and acid aerosol concentrations initiate and exacerbate the bronchoconstriction of the asthmatic patient and the exercise-induced asthmatic. The prevalence of asthma in the United States is approximately 5 percent and continues to increase. In the United States, it has been found to have the greatest prevalence in Puerto Rican Hispanic and African American male children; in Australia, it approaches 10 percent in the general population.

Individuals with asthma have a greater prevalence to exercise-induced broncho-

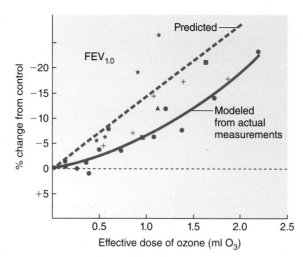

● **FIGURE 14.30** Comparison between the predicted decrease in a forced expiratory volume in 1 second (FEV 1.0) lung function measurement and the modeled response from actual measurements related to the amount of actual ozone delivered. (ozone delivered = time of exposure × concentration of O_3 in parts per million × ventilation volume)(Modified from Folinsbee, L. J., and P. B. Raven. 2001. Air pollution: Acute and chronic effects. Figure 1 in *Marathon medicine* [pp. 235–245], edited by D. Tunstall Pedoe. London: Royal Society of Medicine Press.)

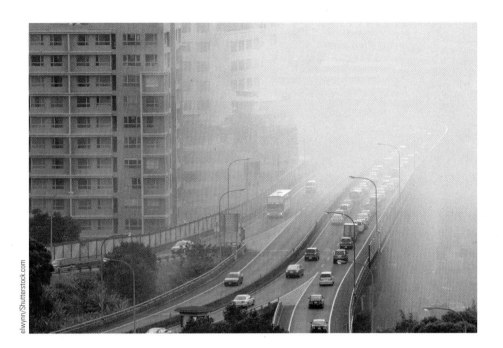

spasm; the prevalence of exercise-induced asthma among U.S. athletes approximates 10 to 20 percent, and in Australian athletes approximates 20 to 30 percent.

HOTLINK *Perform an Internet search for more information on asthma and exercise. For example, for more about exercise-induced asthma, see the Mayo Clinic website at:* http://www.mayo clinic.com/health/exercise-induced-asthma/ DS01040.

Based on relatively few experiments identifying the mechanisms of effect, it has been found that pretreatment with the cyclo-oxygenase inhibitor indomethacin and ibuprofen abolishes the ozone-induced decrements in pulmonary function. Furthermore, antioxidant supplement use appears to reduce the formation of ozonides, lipoperoxides, and oxidation products (see Figure 14.31).

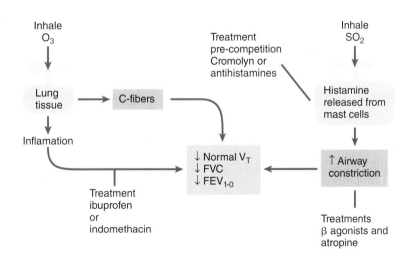

FIGURE 14.31 Flow diagram identifying the mechanisms of ozone (O_3)-induced broncho-constriction and the sulfur oxide (SO_2)– and/or exercise-induced asthma. The diagram also identifies the prophylactic uses of antioxidants, ibuprofen, and indomethacin for O_3 and cromolyn sodium and antihistamines for SO_2. Atropine and beta agonists are used by physicians only in severe asthmatic episodes. (Modified from Folins-bee, L. J., and P. B. Raven. 2001. Air pollution: Acute and chronic effects. Figure 2 in *Marathon medicine* [pp. 235–245]. edited by D. Tunstall Pedoe. London: Royal Society of Medicine Press.)

The asthmatic symptoms and lung function changes associated with the asthmatic bronchoconstriction induced by exercise and exacerbated by SO_2 exposure can be rapidly reversed using beta-2 adrenergic agonists (for example, salbutamol or terbutaline). The compound that has been shown to be more effective in preventing exercise-induced asthma is by using cromolyn sodium before starting exercise and/or being exposed to oxidants or sulfur oxides. (see Figure 14.31).

Recent anecdotal reports have implicated that the spraying of organophosphate pesticides before and during the track and field season has resulted in asthmatic bronchoconstriction-like symptoms in some athletes during their track meets. These athletes appear to have a unique sensitivity to these compounds, and the fields they play on may require a different approach to control insects and fungi.

Carbon Monoxide (CO)

CO is an odorless and colorless gas produced from combustion of fossil fuels (gasoline, oils, and coals). It has the ability to combine with the hemoglobin (Hb) in our blood 240 times stronger than oxygen. Although it is present in very small quantities (10–100 ppm) in urban areas, its strong combination with hemoglobin causes a reduction in the oxygen-carrying capacity of the blood. The combination of CO with Hb in the blood forms the compound known as carboxyhemoglobin (COHb) and is measured as a percentage of the 100 percent O_2 saturation of the total hemoglobin in the blood, or % COHb. In other words, the CO takes the place of oxygen and effectively desaturates the oxygen from the Hb. Many people die of CO poisoning (asphyxiation) when % COHb exceeds 50 percent. Emergency treatment of CO poisoning requires hyperbaric oxygen treatments to **competitively** remove the CO from the Hb.

Maximal oxygen uptake ($\dot{V}O_2$ max) of healthy individuals decreases linearly with increases in the % COHb in their blood (see Figure 14.32). The reduction in $\dot{V}O_2$ max was not statistically significant until

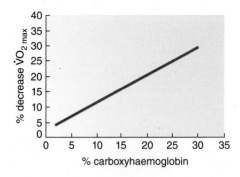

FIGURE 14.32 Graphic depiction of the percent saturation of carboxyhemoglobin and its reduction in maximal oxygen uptake ($\dot{V}O_2$ max) of healthy subjects. (From Raven, P. B., B. L. Drinkwater, R. O. Ruhling, N. Bolduan, S. Taguchi, J. Gliner, and S. M. Horvath. 1974. Effect of carbon monoxide and peroxyacetyl nitrate on man's maximal aerobic capacity. *J. Appl. Physiol.* 36:288–293.

COHb concentrations exceeded 4.3 percent; however, COHb concentrations of 2.7 percent significantly reduced maximal performance time on a treadmill. In healthy subjects, COHb concentrations less than 15 percent do not affect 35–60 percent $\dot{V}O_2$ max submaximal exercise performance, but the exercise requires a greater proportion of the cardiopulmonary reserves. However, cognitive function appears to be impaired at 5 percent COHb. The greater use of the cardiopulmonary reserves to perform 60 percent $\dot{V}O_2$ max exercise would be detrimental to an elite endurance athlete during training and competition, especially when seconds count.

When patients with angina pectoris were exposed to Los Angeles ambient air by driving in traffic for 90 minutes, their COHb was 3.9 percent and there was a significant reduction in their exercise time to angina. This reduction in exercise time to angina was confirmed in the laboratory with COHb concentrations as low as 2.7 percent after breathing 50 ppm CO in air. Other experiments have demonstrated that with COHb concentrations ranging from 4 to 9.3 percent, the healthy myocardium becomes more susceptible to fibrillation. Evidence of ischemia has been reported with COHb concentrations as low as 4 percent. Clearly, outdoor cardiac rehabilitation exercise programs require monitoring of the ambient air to ensure the patient is not being exposed to increased risk.

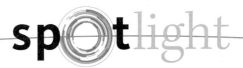

An Expert on Environmental Issues Related to Exercise: Steven M. Horvath, Ph.D.

Steven Michael Horvath was born in Cleveland, Ohio, in 1911. He earned a B.A. in chemistry and physical education in 1934 from the Miami University of Ohio and followed it up with an M.S. in physiology in 1935. After 2 years at Ohio State University, he went to Harvard University and earned a Ph.D. in physiology and biology in 1942 under the mentorship of David Bruce Dill, Director of the Harvard Fatigue Laboratory. There he met Dr. Dill's daughter, Betsy, whom he married. Through Steve Horvath's entire career, Betsy supported his work and his students. They both took great pride in his students, post-doctoral fellows, and colleagues.

When the United States entered World War II, Dr. Dill sent his graduates to work at various military institutions to support the war effort. Steve Horvath was "assigned" to the Armored Medical Research Lab at Fort Knox, where he was the major in charge of investigating adjustments of humans to varying environmental conditions. Much of his work is still classified, but it laid the groundwork for his career's work in thermal regulation and environmental stress. After the end of World War II, he went to the University of Pennsylvania, Graduate School of Medicine as an assistant professor; the next year he was promoted to associate professor. He then moved to the University of Iowa, School of Medicine and was promoted to full professor of physiology 2 years later. He

also served as Director of the Institute of Gerontology at the University of Iowa. After a year sabbatical in Denmark at the University of Copenhagen in 1958 with Dr. Erling Asmussen at the August Krogh Institute, he became the chair of the physiology department at Lankenau Hospital in Philadelphia and a visiting professor at the University of Pennsylvania in the Jefferson Medical College.

However, the portion of his career with the most scientific impact was spent at the University of California at Santa Barbara, where he founded the Institute of Environmental Stress in 1962. Horvath's research spanned many different areas using human and animal models. He was instrumental in developing physiologic and psychophysiologic investigations into temperature regulation and dietary manipulation during rest and exercise in the heat and cold, altitude, and air pollutants. In collaboration with Barbara L. Drinkwater, he encouraged investigations that identified sex differences in how the human responded to exercise and environmental challenges. His publication record included more than 500 manuscripts, books, and book chapters. The one publication he was most proud of was with his wife on the Harvard Fatigue Laboratory published in 1973. Dr. Horvath passed away in 2007 at the age of 96 after a distinguished career investigating environmental stressors related to exercise.

in*Practice*

Examples of Environmental Challenges to Exercise

The following examples are related to the environmental challenges to exercise, and the advice is based on the most current understanding of the links between the topics of environmental impact on exercise, which are continuing to evolve.

Health/Fitness: Jason is a 22-year-old college student in Texas who has a BMI of 30. He recently started walking for exercise and is interested in participating regularly in an outdoor exercise program beginning in June. What advice

can you provide him to help him prevent heat injury (for example, heat cramps, heat exhaustion, heat stroke)? How would acclimatization help him, and what benefits might he see?

It would certainly be important to educate Jason about the fact that because he is overweight, at least by BMI standards (see Chapter 13 for more information on body composition), this will cause him to overheat easily, particularly during outdoor exercise. It would also be important to help him get acclimated to the heat, which in many states and countries is often 33°C (approximately 90°F) to more than 37°C (approximately 98.6°F) with high humidity. Although encouraging Jason to exercise in a cool environment may be helpful at first to ensure his compliance to the exercise program, he will need to get acclimatized to get the maximum efforts for exercising outdoors. You should remind him that acclimatization time varies between individuals, but typically requires 8 to 14 days of participation in the heat for maximum effects. By getting acclimatized, Jason can reduce his heart rate at any intensity of exercise, cool his body more effectively, and reduce his risk for heat injuries.

Medicine: Mary is a 23-year-old college student with a BMI of 30, and her percentage of body fat has been measured at 32 percent. She was told by her physical activity instructor in her university jogging class that she should follow the "no pain, no gain" philosophy. While jogging on a warm, muggy morning in late spring, Mary started feeling nausea and a headache before approaching her instructor to complain that she did not feel well. As she started to explain her discomfort, she collapsed to the ground and started convulsing. What should this instructor have done to prevent this incident, and what should the instructor do now to help her recover?

As you have probably already thought, this instructor needs to get rid of her "no pain, no gain" philosophy and educate students to monitor their FITT (frequency, intensity, time, and type) such that they can acclimatize to the heat and minimize their risk for heat injuries. The instructor needs to also recognize that Mary's symptoms are consistent with heat exhaustion and/or heat stroke (the symptoms are often overlapping and not rigidly defined). Mary's symptoms indicate that the instructor should contact 911 and get her cooled down with whatever methods are effective (for example, place her in the shade or get her in a cool water bath) because her symptoms may be life-threatening.

Athletic Performance: Cara is a 26-year-old recreational distance runner diagnosed with asthma who likes to run local 5-kilometer races on up to marathon races. She lives in Houston, Texas (fourth largest city in the United States), and has noticed that sometimes when she runs when there is more pollution her asthma is worse than normal. She uses an inhaler that was prescribed by her general

physician but wants to know what she can do to minimize her asthma symptoms because the inhaler therapy does not seem to be that effective. What advice can you give Cara as your client?

If Cara hopes to optimize her training and performance times, she probably needs to see a pulmonary specialist who works with asthmatic athletes and be clinically evaluated. She needs to consider avoiding running in areas that have high concentrations of pollution, such as service roads next to freeways and areas with chemical plant emissions. She needs to carry her inhaler on days that she might be challenged with her asthma. A pulmonary specialist can optimize her medical regimen such that she should not have to use her inhaler more than twice in one day for effective care.

Rehabilitation: Dave is a 65-year-old man with diagnosed cardiovascular disease. He has not had a heart attack but has a 50 percent lesion of his left anterior descending coronary artery that has been treated in the last 6 months with balloon angioplasty and stent placement to treat the lesion. Dave is not taking any medications; he has been going to cardiac rehabilitation for the past 3 months and has an exercise capacity of 8 metabolic equivalents, or METS. He has been an accomplished downhill skier for several years and wants to go skiing with his family in Colorado (9,000 feet at the base and 11,000 feet at the highest peak) for 4 days. What advice can you give him to deal with the challenges of skiing at altitude?

First, it is imperative that Dave be cleared to go skiing by his physician. Once he is cleared, it is important that you educate Dave that although he has the physical working capacity required to participate in downhill skiing; he may experience the symptoms of high-altitude cerebral edema or high-altitude pulmonary edema and may need to limit his exercise. He needs to understand that his heart rate and ventilation will be increased at altitude, and he will need to stay hydrated and modify his skiing routine from years past to minimize any cardiac symptoms he might encounter. He should ski on the green slopes (easiest) the first day and build up to the blue slopes (moderately hard) by day 2 or 3, while probably avoiding any black slopes (hardest). He should also carry his cell phone and a simple one-way walkie-talkie in case he gets separated from his skiing group and encounters problems.

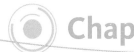

Chapter Summary

- For the naked human at rest, the thermoneutral environment ranges between 24.0°C and 26°C, or 75.2°F and 78.8°F, at a relative humidity of 50 percent and no air flow over the body.

- The body redistributes its blood flow to the skin surface when the core and skin temperatures are sensed as being hot. When the skin temperature senses that it is cold, it results in the body redistributing its blood flow to heart, lung, and brain circulation.

- The primary methods in which the body can gain or lose heat are radiation, conduction, convection, and evaporation. The primary method to dissipate heat while engaging in exercise is evaporation, which is highly dependent on the ambient temperature and humidity.

- The human's thermoregulatory control system generally involves the neural and the endocrine systems. In the human, the temperature regulatory center is located in the hypothalamus, and it attempts to maintain the body's core temperature at a set point of 37°C, or 98.6°F.

- Shivering is the main mechanism by which humans add heat to the body without exercising.

- Heat acclimatization is associated with the following physiologic adaptations: increased plasma volume, increased sweat rate, decreased heart rate, and decreased core temperature.

- A near-linear decrease in barometric pressure occurs in relation to an increase in altitude.

- At approximately 6,000 feet, the resultant reduction in PaO_2 and oxygen content of the blood precipitates an increase in the number of red blood cells, resulting in an increase in hematocrit and total hemoglobin. This adaptation is termed *polycythemia* and is the primary adaptation of low-altitude dwellers who sojourn at altitude for long periods.

- Blood doping is an illegal and unethical method of enhancing endurance performance that has been abused by endurance athletes since the 1970s.

- An important point for teachers, coaches, parents, and athletes to remember is that all airborne pollutants exhibit a dose–response relationship summarized in the following relationship: Air pollutant concentration × ventilation volume (L/min) × time of exposure.

Exercise Physiology Reality

CENGAGE brain   To reinforce the exercise physiology concepts presented above, complete the laboratory exercises for Chapter 14. To access labs and other course materials for this text, please visit www.cengagebrain.com. See the preface on page xiii for details. Once you complete the exercises, have your instructor evaluate your work. Remember to use your lab experience to help guide you toward future success in exercise physiology.

Exercise Physiology Web Links

Access the following websites for further study of topics covered in this chapter:

- Find updates and quick links to these and other exercise sites at our website. To access labs and other course materials for this text, please visit www.cengagebrain.com. See the preface on page xiii for details.

- Search for further information about environmental stress and exercise at the Centers for Disease Control and Prevention (CDC) website: http://www.cdc.gov.

- Search for information about environmental stress and exercise at the American College of Sports Medicine website: http://www.acsm.org.

- Search for more information about environmental stress and exercise at the Institute for Exercise and Environmental Medicine website: http://www.ieemphd.org.

- Search for more information about environmental stress and exercise at the U.S. government health information site: http://www.healthierUS.gov.

- Search for more information about environmental stress and exercise at the Center for College and University Sports Medicine Environmental Policies and Procedures website: http://www.csmfoundation.org.

- Search for video clips that depict examples of environmental challenges and exercise at the YouTube website: http://www.youtube.com.

Study Questions

Review the Warm-Up Pre-Test questions you were asked to answer before reading Chapter 14. Test yourself once more to determine what you know now that you have completed the chapter.

The questions that follow will help you review this chapter. You will find the answers in the discussions on the pages provided.

1. Define the term *thermoneutral environment* and how it influences exercise for your clients. *pp. 469–471*

2. Why does your body redistribute blood in hot or cold environments? *pp. 471–472*

3. What is radiation? How does your body lose or gain heat via this mechanism? *pp. 472–473*

4. What is acclimatization? How does one acclimatize to hot and cold environments? *pp. 481–487*

5. What is wind chill and how does it influence cold-related injuries? *pp. 489–490*

6. How does barometric pressure influence exercise at high altitudes? *pp. 491–492*

7. Describe and explain three physiologic adaptations that occur with altitude acclimatization. *pp. 495–496*

8. What would you expect to see happen to endurance performance at altitudes greater than 6,000 feet? *p. 498*

9. Why would athletes turn to blood doping as a method to enhance their endurance performances? *p. 499*

10. Describe and explain three ways in which exposure to air pollution might limit your client's exercise performances. *pp. 499–502*

Selected References

American College of Sports Medicine position stand on prevention of thermal injuries during distance running. *Med. Sci. Sports Exerc.* 1984;16:ix–xiv.

Benzinger, T. H. 1969. Heat regulation: Homeostasis of central temperature in man. *Physiol. Rev.* 49:671–759.

Buskirk, E. R. 1966. Variation in heat production during acute exposures of men and women to cold air or water. *Ann. N. Y. Acad. Sci.* 134:733–742.

Buskirk, E. R., and J. Kollias. 1969. Total body metabolism in the cold. *Bull. N. J. Acad. Sci.* (Spec. Symp. Issue):17–25.

Crandall, C. G, and J. Gonzalez-Alonzo. 2010. Cardiovascular function in the heat stressed human. *Acta Physiol. Scand.* 199:407–423.

Dill, D. B., E. F. Adolph, and C. G. Wilber, editors. 1964. *Adaptation to the environment, Section 4: Handbook of physiology.* Bethesda, MD: American Physiological Society.

Folinsbee, L. J., and P. B. Raven. 2001. Air pollution: Acute and chronic effects. In *Marathon medicine* (pp. 235–245), edited by D. Tunstall Pedoe. London: Royal Society of Medicine Press.

Grover, R. F., and J. T. Reeves. 1966. Exercise performance of athletes at sea level and 3,100 meters altitude. *Med. Thorac.* 23:129–143.

Pandolf, K. B., M. N. Sawka, and R. R. Gonzalez, editors. 1989. *Human performance physiology and environmental medicine at terrestrial extremes.* Dubuque, IA: Brown and Benchmark.

Rowell, L. B. 1974. Human cardiovascular adjustments to exercise and thermal stress. *Physiol. Rev.* 54:75–159.

West, J. B. 1982. Respiratory and circulatory control at high altitudes. *J. Exp. Biol.* 100:147–157.

appendix

This appendix is designed to provide examples of more detailed exercise plans and programs than found in the text, to help you develop skills to meet the goals (allowing for health limitations) of your clients related to the exercise physiology principles and applications you have learned. The cases are provided to help you assist your clients in meeting the various global challenges of avoiding sedentary lifestyles. We have specifically developed the case examples from the areas of focus in the text: health & fitness, medicine, athletics, and rehabilitation. Each case integrates exercise physiology concepts with the scientific aspects of effective exercise techniques (explained in the text), which are readily available via the hard copy or online references cited at the end of Chapters 1 to 14. In addition, the following resources were used to help design the sample exercise plans and programs:

www.acsm.org
www.ispah.org
www.cdc.gov
www.health.gov/paguidelines
www.healthierUS.gov
www.faseb.org
www.physicalactivityplan.org
www.americanheart.org
www.diabetes.org
www.nsca-lift.org
www.nata.org
www.apta.org
www.ieemphd.org
www.gssiweb.com
www.exrx.net
www.fitnessgram.net
www.brianmac.co.uk
www.topendsports.com
www.cnpp.usda.gov/DietaryGuidelines.htm

Before developing exercise programs for clients, remember to review the health and medical screening suggestions in Chapter 2. Also, use the references throughout the text and this appendix to help you understand the approaches provided for each case, and develop alternative plans and programs based on your own skills.

Health/Fitness

Case 1

Casandra is a 14-year-old girl in Pittsburgh, Pennsylvania, who is interested in improving her personal fitness because she gained 20 pounds in the past year when her parents divorced, and she moved (in May) with her mother to a different school district, so she will attend a new high school in September. She would like to try out for the school dance team (freshman squad) that she has heard about, but she's unsure that her fitness level is high enough for her to succeed, and she does not want to be embarrassed even if she does try out. Casandra knows that her dietary habits need to improve, and she has become completely sedentary since her parents divorced (6 months ago). She has been watching four hours of television per day and has spent most of her other waking hours during the spring at school or electronically staying in touch with friends. She is motivated to improve her fitness level and lose some weight over the summer for a chance at trying out for dance, but she knows she does not presently have the skills to be successful.

One option might be to have Casandra contact the dance director of her new school and discuss her goals and ask for help in developing a nutrition and exercise training plan to prepare for tryouts. An experienced dance director would probably suggest that Casandra develop a plan similar to the following:

1. Determine the specific skills and fitness levels she needs to achieve to make the high school dance team. These skills would include not only specific dance moves and basic routines, but also basic fitness items that are measured by health-related fitness assessments such as the FITNESSGRAM®: body mass index (BMI), cardiovascular fitness (mile run), muscular strength (push-ups), muscular endurance (curl-ups), and flexibility (sit and reach and

trunk lift). For instance, Casandra could initially assess herself on the following basic fitness factors that all contribute to dance success and then set goals for improvement as needed over the next 12 weeks before tryouts.

2. Work with one of the current school dancers on the team to learn the basic tryout routines as specified in the dance program tryout manual. Also, befriend one or more of the current dance team members, if possible, and make arrangements to work out/dance together two to three times per week during the summer. A primary goal would be to learn dance moves but also enjoy dance as a potential lifelong activity.

3. Locate, use, and try to achieve the goals presented for teens in the *2008 Physical Activity Guidelines for Americans* (60 minutes including aerobic, muscle-strengthening, and bone-strengthening activities for children and adolescents) and the *2010 Dietary Guidelines for Americans* (via www.choosemyplate.gov).

4. Conduct an Internet search for national and regional dance association websites such as the National Dance Association, American Dance/Drill Team, National Spirit Group, Varsity Spirit Corporation, and Dance USA to learn more about dance and personal fitness–related topics.

Case 2

Sam is a 68-year-old retired (at age 65) university professor emeritus from the University of California at Berkeley, who continues to write and publish in his discipline; he also likes to travel throughout the year with his wife of 40 years. He taught at Berkeley for 35 years and exercised 5 days/week at the university fitness center (walking, jogging, stationary cycling, and light weight lifting on machines) while teaching, but he and his wife have become sedentary since his retirement, and both have gained 15 pounds in the last 3 years. Although he is considered healthy by his physician (he is taking only one low-level medication for elevated cholesterol, without side effects), he has noticed lately that he gets short of breath quicker than he used to when he has to climb a couple of flights of stairs or when he does yard work. Although he is motivated to regain his previous levels of fitness, he is not sure what exercises he should do at his age and/or whether he would benefit much from changing his current lifestyle. Following is a recommended course of action for Sam:

1. Design and begin a home-based fitness program with his wife using the key guidelines for older adults as listed in the *2008 Physical Activity Guidelines for Americans* (p. 30):

   - All older adults should avoid inactivity. Some physical activity is better than none, and older adults who participate in any amount of physical activity gain some health benefits.

   - For substantial health benefits, older adults should do at least 150 minutes (2 hours 30 minutes) a week of moderate-intensity, or 75 minutes (1 hour 15 minutes) a week of vigorous-intensity aerobic physical activity, or an equivalent combination of moderate- and vigorous-intensity aerobic activity. Aerobic activity should be performed in episodes of at least 10 minutes, and preferably, it should be spread throughout the week.

   - For additional and more extensive health benefits, older adults should increase their aerobic physical activity to 300 minutes (5 hours) a week of moderate-intensity, 150 minutes a week of vigorous-intensity aerobic physical activity, or an equivalent combination of moderate- and vigorous-intensity activity. Additional health benefits are gained by engaging in physical activity beyond this amount.

   - Older adults should also do muscle-strengthening activities that are moderate or high intensity and involve all major muscle groups on two or more days a week, as these activities provide additional health benefits.

   - When older adults cannot do 150 minutes of moderate-intensity aerobic activity a week because of chronic conditions, they should be as physically active as their abilities and conditions allow.

   - Older adults should do exercises that maintain or improve balance if they are at risk for falling.

   - Older adults should determine their level of effort for physical activity relative to their level of fitness.

   - Older adults with chronic conditions should understand whether and how their conditions affect their ability to do regular physical activity safely.

2. Sam and his wife would also benefit from learning more about how to develop and follow a healthy eating plan and maintaining a healthy weight by using the *2010 Dietary Guidelines for Americans* (via http://www.choosemyplate .gov). (Also see American College of Sports Medicine; W. J. Chodzko-Zajko, D. N. Proctor, M. A. Fiatarone Singh, C. T. Minson, C. R. Nigg, G. J. Salem, and J. S. Skinner. 2009. American College of Sports Medicine position stand on exercise and physical activity for older adults. *Med. Sci. Sports Exerc.* 41:1510–1530.)

Medicine (Clinical)

Case 1

Gerald is a 45-year-old male executive (6 feet, 268 pounds) who works at a large petro-chemical company in downtown Houston, Texas. He is married to his high school sweetheart, has two teenage daughters, commutes from the suburbs daily (45 minutes one-way, minimum), and works 50+ hours per week. He was a high school football player (offensive lineman) and exercised regularly (walked, jogged, lifted weights) in college but became sedentary at age 25 (6 feet, 190 pounds). He is not presently physically active at work or at home. During a recent company-recommended medical checkup, his results were as follows:

BMI = 36.3; waist circumference = 42 inches; resting heart rate = 80; blood pressure = 150/90; total cholesterol = 245; low-density lipoprotein (LDL) = 160; high-density lipoprotein (HDL) = 40; triglycerides = 240; fasting glucose = 115; and fasting insulin level = 12.

The physician told Gerald that he is obese and has five factors associated with metabolic syndrome. He is also prediabetic based on his glucose and insulin levels. The physician asked him to return for further evaluation in 3 months.

The checkup results surprised Gerald because except for knowing that he was overweight, he felt healthy, although he had not challenged himself much physically in a long time. The physician actually scared Gerald when he let him know he was a "walking time bomb" for problems such as a myocardial infarction and type 2 diabetes, which has long-term complications, including the potential for blindness, amputation, and/or renal failure requiring dialysis. Gerald wants to get healthier for his family as well as himself, and he is motivated to try, but he is unsure where to begin because he has been inactive for 20 years. A problem generic to ex-athletes is that they think that starting an exercise program after 20 years of a sedentary lifestyle is easy and that they can start their exercise program at the same intensity as when they were in training. An initial simple and safe way to get Gerald started moving from being sedentary toward achieving functional health (see Chapter 1) is as follows:

Have him develop a time-management plan to begin a moderate-intensity walking program (about 4 miles/hour) by walking at work during three 10-minute breaks during the day (because he commutes and spends most waking hours at work) by himself or with a group of colleagues. He should use a pedometer initially to get a baseline of the number of steps he takes per day. After week 1, have him try to progressively increase his steps per day (shooting for 2,000/day above baseline in the next 10–12 weeks) and begin to focus on the goal of achieving 150 minutes of walking per week at work and home (minimum to achieve the *2008 Physical Activity Guidelines* for adults that can have metabolic benefits) and lifting 20-pound dumbbells at his desk (five to six exercises like overhead press, curls, etc., with eight to ten repetitions per set, working up to

three to four sets over the course of 3 to 4 weeks) two to three times per week. He could also evaluate his dietary habits via http://www.choosemyplate.gov, with a goal of improving his nutrient intake, adjusting his caloric intake, and reducing his BMI initially to less than 30. If Gerald can get started on this type of suggested program and stay with it for 12 weeks, his medical follow-up screening should be more positive; then he can seek other options for improved functional health (for example, dietitian consultation, join a fitness facility, hire a personal trainer, or develop a home gym and program for the family). (Also see Donnelly, J. E., S. N. Blair, J. M. Jakicic, M. M. Manore, J. W. Rankin, B. K. Smith; American College of Sports Medicine. 2009. American College of Sports Medicine position stand. Appropriate physical activity intervention strategies for weight loss and prevention of weight regain for adults. *Med. Sci. Sports Exerc.* 41:459–471.)

Case 2

Maria is a 50-year-old female artist living in Monterrey, Mexico, who has had type 2 diabetes for the past 5 years. She works very hard to support her family (older husband and two teenage sons). Maria was very active in her youth and as a young adult, but her husband cannot work anymore, and she has had to increase her productivity of drawing, painting, and selling her art in the downtown El Mercado and plaza to support her family. She presently is very sedentary and feels that she overeats because she is stressed and bored by sitting long hours in her art display space at the plaza.

Her physician recently changed and upgraded her medication regimen (based on DeFronzo, R. A. 2009. From the triumvirate to the ominous octet: A new paradigm for the treatment of type 2 diabetes mellitus. *Diabetes* 58:773–795.) to include thiazolidinedione, metformin, and exenatide to help reduce her HB1c to less than 6.0 percent. She presently does not have any vascular disease symptoms or peripheral neuropathies. However, to optimize Maria's medical management, her physician knows he needs to encourage her and get her to adhere to also adding lifestyle changes that will increase her physical activity levels to a minimum of 150 min/week of moderate-intensity exercise (like walking and light resistance training). The lifestyle modifications together with medications can more optimally control her insulin and blood glucose levels, as well as increase/maintain her functional health (aerobic, muscle mass, and strength). To help Maria improve her diabetes management, her physician recommended the following plan:

1. Try to walk around the plaza for up to 30 min/day in short segments or in a continuous manner. Encourage her art friends and other vendors in the plaza to join her by

walking and discussing her stress levels with others to learn coping skills that can reinforce an active lifestyle (creativity via art and physical health via achieving functional health and management control of her diabetes).

2. Recognize the signs of hypoglycemia and hyperglycemia. Because she has type 2 diabetes and is not taking insulin, she probably will not experience hypoglycemia with moderate exercise (American College of Sports Medicine; American Diabetes Association. 2010. Exercise and type 2 diabetes: American College of Sports Medicine and the American Diabetes Association: Joint position statement. Exercise and type 2 diabetes. *Med. Sci. Sports Exerc.* 42:2282–2303). However, she should conduct comprehensive foot care including the daily inspection of her feet for the detection of sores or ulcers and report them immediately. Although she may be on a family budget, she should invest in a good pair of walking shoes (cushioned and comfortable) to minimize foot problems and improve her long-term care.

3. Learn about caloric intake and monitor daily caloric intake for a week. Follow up with the nurse clinician to develop a dietary plan to be followed until the next clinical checkup in 2 months.

Athletic Performance

Case 1

Katherine is a 23-year-old female collegiate cross-country and track runner from Sydney, Australia. She has run a personal best of 17:49 for 5 kilometers (5K; on the track). She has been coaching herself for the past year because her former coach moved to another university and her interim coach is a sprints coach who knows little about the specifics of distance running. Fortunately for Katherine, an assistant distance coach has been hired to begin in the fall, and she is looking forward to optimizing her training to improve on her personal best and to win the province championship in what will be her final year of eligibility.

Katherine's new coach (who was a collegiate runner himself) has a training philosophy that has been heavily influenced by what he has learned from reading the training theories of Jack. T. Daniels, Ph.D. (for example, Daniels, J. T. 2005. *Daniels' running formula.* Champaign, IL: Human Kinetics). Katherine's new coach decided to meet with the distance runners at the end of August, 2 weeks before the beginning of the school session and cross-country season. He provided the distance runners with an overview of his coaching philosophy, and he briefly described the following types of training that

he will design into their new training regimen: easy distance (75 to 80 percent of total training volume at 5K pace plus 90 seconds to 2 minutes); a weekly long run (approximately ≥25 kilometers [15.5 miles] based on a weekly training volume of approximately 100 kilometers) to optimize central and peripheral cardiorespiratory adaptations; 12,000 kilometers (12%) of weekly training volume, run at lactate threshold pace (5K pace plus 25 to 45 seconds) to improve her lactate threshold; 8,000 kilometers (8%) of weekly training volume, run at interval pace to increase maximal oxygen uptake ($\dot{V}O_2$ max; 5K pace minus 10 to 20 seconds per 1,500 meters); 2,000 kilometers of weekly training volume, run at repetition pace (5K pace minus 40 to 80 seconds per 1,500 meters) to improve her running economy; and a periodized resistance training program with muscular endurance training focusing on the core and upper body.

To determine the specific training paces for his distance runners, Katherine's coach schedules a 3,000-meter time trial for all the distance runners and uses the final time to help him predict their individual $\dot{V}O_2$ max levels and training paces (http://www.coacheseducation.com/endur/jack-daniels-nov-00.htm). Based on Katherine's preseason 3K time of 10:27, he developed the following training data for her that will be used in an additional detailed periodization plan to help her reach her performance goals:

> Predicted relative $\dot{V}O_2$ max = 56 ml/kg/min; current predicted 5K time = 18:05; easy distance pace = 4:40 per kilometer (or 7:31 per mile); weekly long run pace of 6:37 per 1,600 kilometers; lactate threshold pace = 93 seconds per 400 meters; interval pace of 86 seconds per 400 meters; repetition pace = 39 seconds per 200 meters.

Case 2

George is a 20-year-old soccer, rugby, and cricket player from London, England, who plays for the Southwark Rugby Club and has been asked to try out for the national rugby team of England. George is 187.96 cm (6 feet, 2 inches) tall and weighs 100 kg (220 pounds) of what appears to be solid muscle. He has not really worked out formally in the past for sports because he is very much a natural athlete (good genetics as both his mom and dad were outstanding athletes when they were his age).

George is very excited about his tryout scheduled 6 weeks from now, but he feels that he needs to focus on practicing and enhancing his rugby sport-specific conditioning if he is going to be selected for the national team. He also thinks he should work with a sports-specific trainer to help him focus on optimizing his performance on the various assessments conducted during the tryout, which include BMI, skinfold measures for percentage of body fat, a 40-meter sprint, a 3 RM bench press, a 3 RM squat, a vertical jump, a standing long jump, a three-on-two passing accuracy drill, a three-cone agility test, and a Yo-Yo intermittent test.

Fortunately for George, one of the master's players (William) from his club is a former coach and scout who previously participated in judging the national tryouts, and he has volunteered to help George prepare for the rugby combine. Because George was unfamiliar with most of the rugby assessments (except the passing drill) and has limited time to prepare himself, William decided to waive pretesting George. However, he developed a 6-week microcycle program (two-a-day workouts, 45 minutes maximum each session, for 5 days each per week, saving a final week for taper) to specifically help George learn how to perform each assessment (practicing starts and techniques) and to fine-tune his skill and conditioning for each test as follows:

1. Speed, agility, and aerobic endurance training—mornings: sample workouts include a daily warm-up of two to four laps jogging around a 400-meter track; lunges and plyometric jumps, 3 days per week; 40-meter sprint practice, five times with 5-minute recovery, 2 days per week; endurance practice on the Yo-Yo intermittent test, once a week; sprint agility practice, three-cone drill five times with 5-minute recovery, 3 days per week; cooldown includes a one-lap jog and stretching major muscle groups followed by drinking a recovery sports drink (containing electrolytes, carbohydrate, and protein) within 15 to 30 minutes after practice.

2. Passing accuracy, vertical jump, standing long jump, strength, and muscular endurance conditioning—in the late afternoon: sample workouts include a daily warm-up of 5 to 10 minutes of jump rope or stationary cycling followed by three to five sets of five repetitions, 3 to 5 minutes of rest between sets, focused on six exercises (for example, bench press, squats, dead lifts) per session, 2 days per week; three to five sets of 15 repetitions, 1-minute rest between sets focused on six exercises (for example, curls, lat pulls, seated rows) per session, 2 days per week; practice passing drills with three-on-two, game speed one length of the field with walk back five times, 2 days per week; 2 to 3 days per week, practice vertical-jump and long-jump procedures; during rest, cooldown includes a 1-lap jog and stretching of major muscle groups followed by drinking a recovery sports drink (containing electrolytes, carbohydrate, and protein) within 15 to 30 minutes after practice. William also encouraged George to remember to hydrate with meals throughout each day and to use the restoration techniques (massage, contrast whirl pools, etc.) available to him, including getting 8 to 10 hours of sleep each night. (Also see American College of Sports Medicine. 2009. American College of Sports Medicine position stand. Progression models in resistance training for healthy adults. *Med. Sci. Sports Exerc.* 41:687–708.)

In the last week, 5 days before his tryout, George posted the following results following his preparation (rated based on national level team profiles): BMI = 28.3; skinfold percentage body fat = 10% (better than average); 40 meters = 4.8 seconds (above average); 3 RM bench press = 140 kg (above average); 3 RM squat = 190 kg (above average); vertical jump = 76.2 cm (30 inches; above average); standing long jump = 3.0 meters (10 feet, 6 inches; above average); the three-on-two passing accuracy drill, five of five successes (above average); three-cone agility test = 6.7 (above average); and the Yo-Yo intermittent test = stage 13 (above average).

Rehabilitation

Case 1

Dan is a 52-year-old former marathon runner (in his 20s and 30s) and an exercise science professional in Amsterdam, the Netherlands, who was running 30 to 40 min/day at 7- to 8-min/mile pace, 6 to 7 days/week; cycling about 1 day/week, 70 minutes moderately; and participating in general resistance training 3 days/week before suffering a mild inguinal hernia (likely because of aging and the average age-associated weight gain, 20 to 30 pounds). When he consulted his exercise science colleagues (athletic trainers, physical therapists, physicians, etc.) and friends (other runners and active folks) in the week after his injury, he got a mixed bag of advice about what he should do concerning continuing to exercise with the hernia, as well as whether he should get the hernia surgically repaired first and then return to exercise. Some of his colleagues said he could continue to run but not cycle, whereas others suggested he cycle but discontinue running. There was consensus from all the people he consulted that he should discontinue resistance work to minimize the risk of making the hernia worse. Most suggested he could still be physically active without getting the hernia surgically repaired but that it would probably get worse over time.

In the following 4 weeks, Dan elected to have an indirect hernioplasty surgical repair so that he could resume his normal physical activity routine without limitations. During the 4 weeks before surgery, Dan jogged for the first 2 weeks for 30 min/day at 8 to 9 min/mile and then cycled for the next 2 weeks moderately for 35 min/day. He successfully underwent surgery, where the surgeon used a mesh plug and overlay patch repair procedure, and was advised to do no vigorous activities (running or cycling) for 14 days. On day 4 after surgery, he returned to light jogging and cycling (contrary to physician's orders); he returned to normal running (about 8 min/mile) by day 10, 4 days before physician clearance to resume all physical activities.

During his postoperative follow-up visit, Dan shared his self-prescribed daily rehabilitation program and physical activity log with his physician. The physician requested permission to copy and share the program/log with some of his other middle-age patients to encourage them in their own recovery and rehabilitation programs because little is known or has been reported in the literature about acute long-term hernia repair and recovery (Murray, T., J. Ransone, W. Lockett, and R. Markus. 2006. Acute recovery from hernioplasty. *Athl. Ther. Today* 11:58–59.). *Note:* Although Dan was successful at fast-tracking his acute rehabilitation regimen (likely because of his past extensive experience with training and injury recovery), most clients will need to follow protocols closely because non-adherence usually results in another injury, delayed rehabilitation, or incomplete rehabilitation.

Dan's acute rehabilitation program/log was as follows:

Day 1

Standing several times in PM, post AM surgery, ice/rest, pain before bedtime (2 Vicodin tablets taken). No other complications.

Day 2

Standing, naps × 2, 30-minute walk, ibuprofen × 2. No complications.

Day 3

Point tenderness, some swelling at incision site, 40-minute walk, ibuprofen × 2. No complications.

Day 4

1/2 day @ work, point tenderness (incision), 45-minute walk (4 × 300-yard very slow jogs included on grass), ibuprofen × 2. No complications.

Day 5

Full/busy day @ work, pain @ site of incision (dry/itchy), worse in late afternoon, no exercise, ibuprofen × 2, Motrin × 1. No other complications.

Day 6

200-mile auto trip for academic meeting, pain @ incision site (pinching), 15-minute walk, ibuprofen × 2. No other complications.

Day 7

50-mile auto trip to visit friend, no exercise, increased incision pain. Ibuprofen × 2. No other complications.

Day 8

Less incision site pain, bandage applied at incision site, 1-hour, 15-minute brisk walk. No other complications.

Day 9

Incision site discomfort, getting better bandage, 30-minute stationary cycle @ resistance level 3 on Model #4500 Lifecycle. No other complications.

Day 10

Full day @ work, incision site discomfort, getting even better with bandage coverage, 30-minute slow (9 minute/mile) jog, No other complications.

Day 11

60-mile auto trip for academic meeting, 30-minute slow (9 minute/mile) jog, removed bandage to air out wound. No other complications.

Day 12

Minimal incision pain, 30-minute slow (9 minute/mile) jog, tired from busy/full day @ work. No other complications.

Day 13

30-mile auto trip to attend academic meeting, no exercise, very tired. No pain.

Day 14

200-mile auto trip to attend academic meeting, 30-minute faster jog (8 min/mile). No pain.

Day 15

Visited general surgeon for follow-up: cleared for all physical activity. 40 minutes around park jogging at 8-min/mile pace.

Case 2

Lee and May are a married couple (60+ years) who grew up in small towns 30 miles apart in the Dust Bowl, Great Depression era (1930s) of the panhandle of Oklahoma. They are both in their early 80s now, very independent, and have lived close to the Gulf Coast of Texas for the past 45+ years. Lee and May have faced the typical physical challenges of aging, as well as individual health challenges that have required them to participate in rehabilitation programming. The following summaries describe the unique rehabilitation plans that they developed themselves based on medical/surgical feedback, sound physical therapy concepts, and their own tenacity and modifications of their personal lifestyles to regain and maintain functional health. *Note:* Although the following cases for Lee and May are success stories, many clients will need to participate in supervised rehabilitation (limited by their financial means) to experience successful rehabilitation to regain their fitness and health.

Lee was very active as a youngster; he was involved in hunting and fishing, planting and harvesting crops, playing baseball, and hustling for food to get enough to eat during hard times. He began heavy smoking as a young teen (2+ packs/day). Later, he worked for the railroad and joined the army during the Korean War, where he became a Master Sergeant.

After his military service, Lee earned his Bachelor's of Science in math and physics while working 40 hours/week. He then worked professionally as an aerospace engineer in "high-stress" positions for large firms until age 55, when he retired with a partial disability. He had experienced development of emphysema from smoking, and his physician told him to quit smoking, take his prescribed medications, and get healthier, or else he faced a very early death.

Motivated to move on after his retirement, Lee spent most of his days participating in his favorite hobby, metal detecting. At first, he hunted for treasure (coins, jewelry) for 4 to 5 hours most days. Because he lived close to the coast, he began driving to the beach and using a new detector that allowed him to wade into the gulf and search on the beach, as well as underwater. By pursuing his hobby (later for about 6 hours most days), Lee knowingly or unknowingly increased/maintained his physical work capacity of the past 25+ years by walking (aerobic), bouncing off the rocks in the surf (balance), and doing resistance work by digging with a scoop and carrying his metal detector. He also benefited by seeing physicians regularly, using his nebulizer daily, taking his other medications regularly, and eating healthy meals prepared by May.

May grew up on a farm where she learned early to do various chores, eat healthy, and cook nutritious meals; she also adored her heroine, her grandmother, who lived to age 93. May had three sons with Lee and worked as a traditional housewife as the boys grew up, but she also worked as an expert seamstress and pursued her main hobby, gardening, with a passion. May was always healthy and rarely had the need to see a physician after her last son was born (1957). As Lee experienced health problems and retired, she took over most of the yard maintenance duties (1/2-acre lot) and continued to shop, clean, and cook (all activities she enjoyed).

Six months before her 80th birthday, May tripped and fell while walking the family's two dogs (caught up in leashes).

As a result, she broke her hip (probably a combination of the twisting force of the fall and osteoporosis) and was hospitalized. She had a partial hip replacement by an excellent surgeon with a standard Medicare hospital stay of 14 days with inpatient rehabilitation (physical therapy). May was eager to get home after a couple of days in the hospital (as all patients are) but was encouraged by Lee and one son to be a "good patient" and adhere to all physical therapy requests to facilitate her recovery.

May did an excellent job in the rehabilitation program, although she found it silly and very easy compared with others of her same age who did not progress as well, probably partly because of their histories (10 to 20 years) of physical inactivity. She was discharged with a walker and told to keep her wound clear and begin to resume household activities slowly. She had decided with Lee that she did not want home health care, and she set a course of further rehabilitation for herself based on what she had watched her grandmother do; her grandmother had broken her own hip (in her 80s), requiring her to use a cane the remainder of her life.

May's plan involved getting up and moving regularly throughout each day until she could get medically released via medical follow-up, which was scheduled 6 weeks after surgery. Her main goals were to get back to gardening and mowing the grass. Because 25 percent of 80-year-olds die within the first year after surgery and only about 25 percent of individuals return to a normal lifestyle 1 year after surgery, it did not seem possible that May would meet her goals in her time frame. But with a positive surgical outcome, her strong will to regain her fitness and health, and her experience and ability to withstand minor joint/muscle discomfort, she mowed the grass and returned to tend her plants, flowers, and trees 6 months to the day of her hospital release. She remains mobile and active 1 year after surgery.

glossary

(a − v) O$_2$ difference The amount of oxygen extracted by the tissues from one liter of blood.

1 repetition maximum (1 RM) Method of monitoring intensity based on the weight lifting concept of determining what your client can lift maximally in one lift such as a standard bench press lift.

2,3-diphosphoglycerate (DPG) Produced during metabolism within the RBC. As the DPG concentration increases, the O$_2$ − Hb shifts to the right enabling an unloading of oxygen from the RBC at a higher PO$_2$.

absolute intensity Expressed as intensity values such as kcals/min, METS, or walking 3 miles per hour or jogging at 6 miles per hour (see discussion of methods to determine intensity for more). For resistance exercise, absolute intensity is expressed as the amount of weight lifted or force exerted (e.g., pounds, kilograms).

accelerometers Usually worn on the hip at waist level, these assess the intensity, frequency, and duration of acceleration of movement associated with participation in exercise.

acid−base balance The balance between the hydrogen ion (acid) and the bicarbonate ion (base) in the blood.

activities of daily living (ADL) Physical activities one must perform daily for self-care.

acute mountain sickness (AMS) A complex of symptoms that present acutely and include severe headache, lassitude, irritability, nausea, vomiting, anorexia, indigestion, flatus, constipation, and sleep disturbances characterized by periodic breathing.

acute muscle soreness The feeling of sore muscles immediately after exercise.

adaptive thermogenesis Adjustments to thermogenesis due to factors like environmental stress (hot or cold), injury, or changes in hormone regulation.

adenosine monophosphate-activated protein kinase (AMPK) An enzyme that is under covalent and allosteric regulation. It accelerates pathways involved in energy production and decelerates pathways involved in energy consumption.

adenosine triphosphate (ATP) A molecule comprised of adenine, ribose, and three phosphate ions. It is formed by the breakdown of nutrients and serves as the common energy currency for cellular reactions.

adequate intake The average daily amount of a nutrient that is thought to be adequate to maintain a healthy criterion level if the RDA is not known.

adherence Developing the client's ability to stick to a program of exercise.

adipokines Protein hormones such as adiponectin and leptin that transmit information related to the size of adipocytes. They act in diverse tissues involved in metabolic regulation. Leptin sensitively inhibits brain feeding centers.

adrenergic stimulation The stimulation of adrenergic receptors by the catecholamines. This is increased in many cell types during exercise. Effects of adrenergic stimulation are cell type dependent.

adrenocorticotropic hormone (ACTH) A polypeptide hormone produced and secreted by the anterior pituitary gland. It acts through receptors on the adrenal cortex to promote the synthesis and secretion of gluco- and mineralo-corticoids. ACTH release is increased by exercise.

aerobic (oxidative) Activities that depend heavily on metabolic reactions in muscle cells that do require large amounts of oxygen and allow the individual to reach steady state.

aerobic capacity ($\dot{V}O_2$ max or oxygen uptake) Activities that last longer than 15–20 minutes and require large amounts of oxygen to be delivered to the working muscles.

aerobic power Activities that last 3–15 minutes and also require a large delivery of oxygen to be available to the working muscles.

afterload, or arterial pressure Generally thought of as the "load" that the heart ejects blood against. In simple terms, the afterload is closely related to the mean aortic pressure.

albumin The predominant protein in plasma. It maintains osmotic pressure gradient between plasma and the interstitial space. It plays an important role in transport of fatty acids, cations, hormones, and other molecules in the blood.

alpha- and beta-adrenergic receptors The two major types of adrenergic receptors. They bind to and are activated by the catecholamines.

alpha cells Endocrine cells located in the istet of Langerhans that secrete glucagon.

alveolar ventilation The effective tidal volume (VT).

alveolar volume The area of the lung where gas exchange between the air and blood occurs and is often referred to as the alveolar ventilation volume or the effective VT.

amenorrhea Absence or cessation of menstruation.

anabolic steroids Drugs derived from the hormone testosterone; their ingestion in combination with exercise promotes male characteristics, increases muscle mass, and decreases recovery time from vigorous exercise.

anaerobic (nonoxidative) Activities that depend heavily on metabolic reactions (or bioenergetics) in muscle cells that do not require oxygen.

anaerobic capacity (mean anaerobic power) High-intensity activities that last for longer than 10 seconds and may last up to 2–3 minutes.

anaerobic power (peak anaerobic power) Activities lasting < 10 seconds performed at high intensity with limited amounts of oxygen available to the working muscles.

anorexia nervosa (AN) Eating disorder where a person refuses to maintain a minimally normal body weight and has a distorted view of their body shape and weight.

antioxidant vitamin Another class of vitamins that helps scavenge the free radicals from many metabolic and inflammatory reactions.

aorta The large artery exiting the left ventricle.

apolipoprotein Proteins that regulate biochemical reactions by stabilizing lipoprotein particles, providing recognition sites for cell membranes, and acting as cofactors for enzymes.

arterial baroreflexes These include pressure-sensitive receptors in the carotid sinus and aortic arch, which signal the central nervous system that the blood pressure is too low or too high. (Chapter 7)

arterial baroreflexes Negative feedback neural control circuits that have sensors located in the aortic arch and the carotid sinus that monitor arterial pressure and relay afferent information regarding changes in arterial pressure to the cardiovascular center in the central nervous system. (Chapter 10)

arteriovenous difference technique This uses the amount of a molecule entering and leaving an organ or tissue bed to calculate the production or release of a molecule.

asthma A disease that produces spasmodic contractions of the bronchi, which results from direct irritation or reflex irritation of the bronchial mucosal membranes, especially in sensitized individuals.

atherosclerosis Narrowing and hardening of the arteries.

athlete's heart Describes the enlarged ventricular chambers that result from endurance training without a change in ventricular wall thickness (eccentric hypertrophy) and a decrease in resting and submaximal heart rates.

ATP synthase The enzyme that harnesses energy from the movement of proteins down the inner mitochondrial membrane electromotive gradient to the synthesis of ATP.

autonomic nervous system (ANS) Includes both the sympathetic and parasympathetic (vagal) nerves.

autoregulation An intrinsic mechanism that enables a blood vessel to automatically alter its diameter.

axons (motor neurons) The individual motor neurons.

Bainbridge reflex An increase in heart rate due to an increase in right atrial pressure caused by an increase in venous return. Sometimes called the *atrial reflex*.

bariatric Refers to the treatment of obesity or obesity-related problems.

bariatric banding surgery A procedure that makes the stomach very small and increases the level of satiety for individuals, although they are consuming much less food.

bariatric bypass surgery A procedure that alters the digestive tract so that only small amounts of food can be consumed or digested.

basal metabolic rate (BMR) A measure of baseline metabolism conducted under standardized conditions (for example, quiet room; lying still; following 5-hour fast; avoiding caffeine, nicotine, and alcohol for 4 hours; and abstaining from exercise for at least 2 hours).

basal metabolism The energy needed to maintain life when a body is at complete rest.

beta cells Endocrine cells located in the islets of Langerhans that secrete insulin.

beta-endorphin A peptide neurotransmitter in both the central and peripheral nervous systems. It also may have an endocrine function. It is formed from the same precursor gene as ACTH (pro-opiomelanocortin). Its levels may increase with exercise.

bicarbonate ion (HCO_3-) The base (salt) of carbonic acid.

bigorexia Lay term for muscle dysmorphia.

binge eating/purging Eating extreme amounts at one meal/self-induced vomiting.

bioelectrical impedance (BIA) A simplified method used to evaluate body composition; based on the concepts of TOBEC.

biological plausibility The theory that there is a causal link between preventable diseases or health outcomes and exercise.

blood doping To transfuse whole blood or synthetic blood into a competitor to increase their oxygen-carrying capacity. (Chapter 9)

blood doping Often defined as transfusion, storage, and reinfusion of RBCs or the supplemental use of the hormone EPO to increase RBCs. (Chapter 12)

blood doping The acute infusion 1.0 blood just before competition. (Chapter 14)

blood pressure (BP) The pressure exerted by the blood against the blood vessel walls.

blood vessel autoregulation The ability of the blood vessel to adjust its diameter to its initial diameter in response to stretch (vasodilatation) or contraction (vasoconstriction).

body composition Components such as the amount of water, bone, muscle, and fat in the body. (Chapter 1)

body composition The distribution of fat, lean mass (muscle and bone), and minerals in the body. (Chapter 13)

body temperature pressure saturated (BTPS) A correction factor used to standardize (equilibrate) the measured ventilation volumes to the body's temperature of 37°C to the absolute temperature of 273° K and the barometric pressure plus the 47 mm Hg water vapor pressure at 37°C.

Bohr effect Occurs when excess H^+ and or CO_2 bind with the Hb molecule and reduces the Hb molecule's affinity for oxygen.

branched-chain amino acid An amino acid having a side-chain with a branch (a carbon atom bound to more than two other carbon atoms). There are three branched-chain amino acids. They are the essential amino acids: leucine, isoleucine, and valine.

buffering capacity The capacity of a buffer to resist changes in pH by removing excess hydrogen ions and by adding hydrogen ions when they are reduced.

bulimia nervosa (BN) Eating disorder where a person has repeated episodes of binge eating, usually followed by self-induced vomiting, misuse of laxatives or diuretics, or engaging in excessive exercise.

carbohydrate loading The ingestion of a high carbohydrate diet to maximize glycogen stores.

carbon monoxide (CO) An odorless and colorless gas produced from combustion of fossil fuels (gasoline, oils, and coals). It has the ability to combine with the hemoglobin (Hb) in our blood 240 times stronger than oxygen.

carbonic acid (H_2CO_3) The combination of H^+ (ion) or acid with the bicarbonate (ion) or base.

carbonic anhydrase The enzyme catalyst for the rapid breakdown of carbonic acid to CO_2 and H_2O.

cardiac output ($\dot{Q}$) The volume of blood pumped by the heart in one minute.

cardiac tamponade patient A patient with a life-threatening situation in which there is such a large amount of blood or other fluid inside the pericardial sac around the heart that it interferes with the performance of the heart.

cardiovascular drift Occurs during prolonged (>30 minutes) submaximal exercise, resulting in reduced stroke volume (SV) and mean arterial pressure with a concomitant increase in heart rate in an attempt to maintain cardiac output constant.

cardiovascular system Consists of the heart and blood vessels that circulate blood to all major organs of the body.

case–control This type of study uses individuals with and without a disease or health problem and compares past participation in regular exercise to determine if there was any relationship to the disease or health problem.

catecholamines Released from the adrenal medulla and sympathetic nerves in response to exercise or stressful conditions. These include norepinephrine, epinephrine, and dopamine.

cell bodies The body of the nerve cell.

central (neural) fatigue A condition when an individual's Ratings of Perceived Exertion (RPE) progressively increases and his or her neuromuscular coordination decreases.

central blood volume (CBV) The volume of blood in the heart chambers, lungs and central arterial blood vessels.

central body or core temperature The temperature of the blood near the heart, brain, gut or rectum.

central chemoreceptors Located in the medulla oblongata and separate from the respiratory centers, sense changes in hydrogen ion concentration caused by changes in CO_2 within the brain's extracellular fluid (ECF).

central command A concept that requires there to be a feed-forward set of neural signals emanating from the motor cortex that, in parallel, activate cardiovascular control centers in the brainstem. This activation rapidly withdraws parasympathetic control of the heart, increasing the heart rate, and at the same time increases sympathetic outflow to the heart and vasculature, increasing heart rate and regulating the sympathetic outflow to alter the vasomotor function of the blood vessels to ultimately regulate blood pressure. (Chapter 3)

central command (CC) A feed-forward mechanism that controls the cardiovascular system. (Chapter 7)

central nervous system (CNS) A network of cell bodies, axons, nuclei, and ganglia encased within the brain and spinal cord.

cerebral autoregulation (CA) A primary means of regulating brain blood flow using blood vessel autoregulation over a wide range of blood pressures (60 mm Hg to 150 mm Hg).

cerebral circulation The network of blood vessels that circulates blood throughout the brain.

chemical energy The energy released when the covalent bonds of a molecule are broken.

cholecystokinin Hormone produced by cells of the intestinal wall that targets the gallbladder and causes the release of bile and slows GI mobility.

cholesterol A fat-like substance that is manufactured in the body and found in animal foods.

cholesteryl ester transfer protein A lipolytic enzyme that has been linked to HDL particles and is one of several transfer proteins that mediates the transfer of esterified cholesterol from HDL-C to VLDL and is involved in the formation of a subfraction of HDL-C.

chylomicron Lipoproteins assembled from dietary fat in the intestinal mucosa. (Chapter 6)

chylomicron Type of lipoprotein that transfers lipids from the intestinal cells to the rest of the body. (Chapter 11)

classical method Method of carbohydrate loading that requires a glycogen depletion bout of exercise on day 1 followed by a low carbohydrate diet for 3 days, and then a diet rich in carbohydrates for next 4 days.

client education Educating clients about goals/outcomes so they can perform more effectively and resist injuries or rehabilitate more effectively.

clinical trial This type of study uses individuals free of disease or a health problem of interest who are randomly assigned to receive an exercise intervention or no exercise intervention. The groups are followed over time to determine if they differ in terms of the percentage of people who develop the disease or health problem.

complex carbohydrate Consist of large molecules composed of chains of monosaccharides called *polysaccharides* (these include glycogen, starches, and fibers). Examples of complex carbohydrates include vegetables, breads, cereals, pasta, rice, and beans.

compliance (C) The change in volume (ΔV) over the change in pressure (ΔP).

concentric This type of contraction is when the muscle develops force by causing the length of the muscle to shorten.

conductance (C) A measurement of a blood vessel's ability to convey blood.

conduction (K) The transfer of heat from a hot surface to a colder surface while the two surfaces are in contact with each other.

confounders Variables, such as age, body composition, or baseline health status, which might influence interpretation of the data.

convection (C) A type of heat transfer that requires a disturbance of a temperature gradient by air or fluid flow.

corticospinal tracts Connect the motor cortex to the alpha motor neurons (motor nerve) via the pyramidal tracts.

cortisol A steroid hormone, or a glucocorticoid, that is released from the adrenal cortex in response to strenuous exercise. It has effects that can accelerate glucose, fat, and protein metabolism. It also suppresses the immune system.

creatine A nitrogen-containing compound that combines with phosphate to form the high-energy compound creatine phosphate.

criterion-referenced values Based on an individual score and are often expressed as pass/fail or the achievement of a health standard (that is, systolic blood pressure ≤140/90 mm Hg).

critical power The work rate at which a person can maintain a constant submaximal power output for several minutes without fatigue.

cross-sectional This type of study uses individuals with and without a disease or health problem and compares subjects at one point in time to determine if participation in regular exercise has any relationship to the disease or health problem.

cytokines Encompass a large and diverse family of protein or glycoprotein regulators produced throughout the body by cells of diverse embryological origin. Responsiveness to exercise and their actions are dependent on the individual member of this broad family of molecules.

Dallas bed-rest study A historical classic study conducted at the University of Texas Southwestern Medical Center in Dallas under the direction of Jere H. Mitchell M.D and Bengt Saltin M.D./Ph.D.

Dalton's law Dalton's law of partial pressures states that the total pressure of a mixture of gases is equal to the sum of the pressure that each gas independently exerts.

dead space Space made up of the airways and alveoli of the lung where no gas exchange occurs. In healthy lungs this usually the conducting airways only.

deep vein thrombosis Usually a blood clot in the internal veins of the legs.

delayed onset of muscular soreness (DOMS) Usually associated with more severe pain than felt with acute muscle soreness, this occurs 24 to 48 hours following high intensity exercise, especially for the beginning exerciser, or after a period of detraining.

densitometry The estimation of body composition from body density, which is determined from body mass and volume.

detraining The loss of positive physiological effects of participating in a program of exercise after a client stops participating.

diabetic complications Cardiovascular, neural, and metabolic impairments that often accompany diabetes. They are far less common and less severe in people who have well-controlled blood sugar levels.

diastolic blood pressure (DBP) The lowest pressure exerted by the pressure wave of the blood against the blood vessel walls.

dietary reference intake (DRI) A set of nutrient intake values for healthy people in the United States and Canada.

dietary supplements Defined by the U.S. Dietary Supplement Health and Education Act as something added to the diet, mainly vitamins, minerals, amino acids, herbs or botanicals, metabolites/constituents/extracts, or a combination of any of these ingredients.

diffusion The net movement of solutes and gases across a semi-permeable membrane from a high concentration/pressure to a low concentration/pressure. The high to low difference in concentrations/pressure is known as the diffusion gradient.

direct observation A common measure of epidemiological and physical activity research; an example is charting minutes of participation during a middle-school physical education class.

disordered eating Includes a variety of eating patterns that are irregular, excessive, or too sparse.

distress Excess negative stress, caused by fear, anger, confusion, or other similar mood states in one's life.

dose–response relationship The amount of exercise needed to get the desired health or performance outcomes for a client.

double product (HR × SBP) The mathematical product of heart rate times the systolic blood pressure; an index of the workload of the heart.

doubly labeled water A biochemical marker that estimates energy expenditure through the use of isotopes of water ingested by study subjects.

dual-energy X-ray absorptiometry (DEXA) Uses two low doses of X-rays that differentiate between total body bone mineral, lean soft tissue, and fat in a 3-C model.

dynamic exercise Activities that depend mostly on oxidative energy pathways involving concentric (shortening) and eccentric (lengthening) muscle contractions that produce work.

dynamic or aerobic exercise Involves rhythmic muscle contractions that primarily uses aerobic energy production.

dyspnea index The ratio of the ventilation volume at maximal workload (Ve max in L/min) to their clinically measured maximal voluntary ventilation in 15 seconds (MVV.15; expressed as L/min).

eating disorder Abnormal eating behaviors that compromise a person's physical and/or psychological health.

eccentric This type of contraction is when the muscle develops force and the external force causes the muscle to lengthen.

ectomorph Body type associated with low body fat, small bone mass, and a small amount of muscle mass and size.

efficiency A description of the percentage of energy expended that goes to performing mechanical work (force × distance). When we perform work (exercise), the energy expended is usually much higher than the energy required because of the aforementioned loss of heat energy, friction, and other mechanically inefficient movements. $E_{Required}/E_{expended} \times 100 =$ efficiency, where E = energy. The measurements of mechanical efficiency of a human performing cycling exercise range from 23 to 27 percent.

ejection fraction The amount of blood pumped each beat (stroke volume) divided by the end-diastolic volume, expressed as a percentage.

electromyographic (EMG) This type of recording is obtained by using electrodes on the surface of or needle electrodes placed in the belly of the skeletal muscle. It measures and integrates the electrical activity of the active action potentials of the muscle. During its contraction, a linear relation between the force of the contraction and the amount of electromyographic (EMG) activity has been demonstrated. The amount of EMG activity is greater during shortening (concentric or positive) contractions than during lengthening (eccentric or negative) contractions.

electron transport chain This couples electron transfer between an electron donor (such as NADH) and an electron acceptor (such as O_2) with the transfer of protons across the inner mitochondrial membrane. The resulting proton gradient is used to generate chemical energy in the form of ATP.

emphysema An obstructive disease of the lung where the alveolar membrane is destroyed.

end-diastolic volume (EDV) The volume of blood in the heart when the end of the heart muscle's relaxation is complete or when filling is complete.

endomorph Body type characterized by large quantities of body fat and large bone size, and is muscular but not as well proportioned as the mesomorphs.

end-systolic volume (ESV) The volume of blood in the heart when the heart muscle's contraction is maximal and emptying is complete.

energy (caloric) balance The balance of caloric intake (kcals) and caloric expenditure (kcals) associated with the maintenance of homeostasis and a healthy body weight.

energy balance equation The relationship between energy intake and energy expenditure.

energy cost Calculated in calories from the amount of oxygen used to perform the work.

energy substrates In a biological system, these are nutrients that yield ATP.

ephedrine Substance that simulates the sympathetic nervous system to cause physiologic effects like increased heart rate and blood pressure.

epidemiology The study of how a disease or health outcome is distributed in populations and what risk factors influence or determine this distribution. Epidemiologists study infectious or communicable diseases such as influenza or tuberculosis, as well as chronic diseases such as heart disease and cancer. They also study behaviors that may positively impact those chronic diseases.

epigenetic markers These sit on top of the genes and help regulate gene function (or gene expression), at least in part, by up-regulating or down-regulating their cellular actions.

EPO Erythropoietin is the hormone released from the kidney in response to low PO_2 in the blood that stimulates RBC production in the bone marrow. (Chapter 9)

ergogenic aids Substances, devices, or strategies to improve an individual's energy use, production, or recovery.

erythropoietin (EPO) Hormone that stimulates the formation of red blood cells (RBCs). (Chapter 12)

erythropoietin (EPO) An endogenous hormone produced by the kidney in response to low PaO_2 and stimulates the production of red blood cells in the bone marrow. (Chapter 14)

esophageal temperature (Tes) The temperature measured in the esophagus by a thermistor or thermocouple.

essential amino acid Amino acid that the body cannot synthesize in sufficient quantity to meet its needs.

essential fat The amount of fat necessary for normal bodily functions. Essential fat includes fat in and around the nervous system, heart, lungs, kidneys, spleen, intestines, and muscles.

esterification The formation of an ester bond between glycerol and a fatty acid. Three ester bonds link fatty acids to the glycerol backbone in triglyceride molecules.

euhydrated The normal hydrated state.

eustress Positive stress that is healthy.

evaporation (E) The cooling effect associated with the changing of water into vapor, or, in this case, sweat into vapor. The specific heat of sweat evaporation is a measure of the heat energy required to vaporize the sweat. About 600 calories of energy are needed for every gram of water at room temperature.

excess postexercise oxygen consumption (EPOC) The amount of $\dot{V}O_2$ that is above the resting $\dot{V}O_2$ values during the time of recovery. The end of recovery is at the time that the $\dot{V}O_2$ returns to the resting $\dot{V}O_2$ value measured before the beginning of exercise.

exercise Physical activity that is planned, structured, and repetitive and that results in a desired outcome.

exercise economy Energy required to perform the work divided by the actual energy cost measured performing the work; see efficiency.

exercise-induced arterial hypoxemia (EIAH) When the hemoglobin is not completely saturated with oxygen after passing through the lung during exercise.

exercise physiology The study of both the functional changes that occur in response to a single session of exercise and the adaptations that occur as a result of regular, repeated exercise sessions.

exercise physiology integration The understanding and the development of exercise physiology strategies to promote exercise to achieve functional fitness and higher levels of human performance.

exercise prescriptions Individual or group exercise guides that provide the type, intensity, frequency, and duration of physical activities to achieve personal fitness goals.

exercise pressor reflex (EPR) A feedback mechanism from the skeletal muscle to the brain to maintain oxygen delivery.

exercise questionnaires and surveys Tools that can be simple or detailed that use a time frame of recall (e.g. days, weeks, months, years, or a lifetime), and types of activities assessed (e.g. leisure, occupational, household/self-care, and/or transportation) to provide the researcher with exercise data.

experimental A study where the researcher can assign individuals to groups of exercise or control (inactivity) and various confounders can be statistically controlled.

FADH$_2$ The reduced form of flavin adenine dinucleotide. It is important in the transport of electrons used for oxidative phosphorylation.

fatigue index The ability to maintain a high percentage of peak anaerobic power for several seconds.

fat-soluble vitamin Vitamins carried by fat in your food and can be stored in large quantities. The fat-soluble vitamins are A, D, E, and K.

fatty acid binding protein A family of carrier proteins for fatty acids and other lipophilic substances. These proteins facilitate the transfer of fatty acids between extracellular space to and within intracellular compartments.

fatty acids Comprised of unbranched carbon chains, they contain a terminal carboxylic acid. They can be consumed from the diet or synthesized in the body and are an abundant source of energy.

female athlete triad A combination of interrelated conditions like disordered eating, amenorrhea, and increased risk of osteoporosis.

ferritin A protein that helps receive iron from food and helps in its storage.

Fick's law Fick's law of diffusion of gases states that the rate (velocity) at which a gas (V gas) is transferred across a tissue membrane is proportional to the tissue membrane's surface area (A), the diffusion coefficient (D) of the gas, and the difference between the partial pressures of the gas on each side of the tissue membrane ($P_1 - P_2$), and is inversely proportional to the thickness (T) of the tissue membrane.

field tests Exercise physiology-related tests that are conducted in more practical settings, where multiple clients can often be tested at one time and performance times or distances are measured and related to estimated physiologic measures.

FITT Frequency, intensity, time, and type of exercise.

fluid balance Consuming the appropriate amounts and types of fluids to maintain normal hydration and homeostasis.

forearm blood flow (FBF) The blood flow measured in the forearm by invasive or non-invasive measurement techniques.

Frank–Starling mechanism As the length of the ventricular fibers are stretched, the contraction force of the fiber becomes greater.

free fatty acids Blood fatty acids that are associated with albumin via non-polar interactions.

frequency How often you work.

functional abilities Activities such as physical movement used for transportation (walking, preventing avoidable falls, etc.).

functional health The ability to maintain high levels of health and wellness by reducing or controlling your health risks for developing health problems and maintaining your physical movement independence.

gastrointestinal hormones Constitute a group of hormones secreted by enteroendocrine cells in the stomach, pancreas, and small intestine. These control digestive function, but they have also been implicated in systemic metabolic regulation and in control of feeding centers in the brain.

gene transcription The formation of mRNA from the gene that encodes it in the nucleus, and to a lesser extent in the mitochondria, of a cell. This is an enzymatic process that is regulated by complex activators and activation sites on the gene.

genetic predisposition Increased health risk for various disease processes.

ghrelin A protein by the stomach cells that enhances appetite and decreases energy expenditure.

global positional systems (GPS) Geographical location devices that use satellite technology to document participation in exercise.

glucagon A hormone released from pancreatic islet alpha cells that stimulates glucose release, fat oxidation, and ureagenesis by the liver. It counters the glucose lowering effect of insulin.

gluconeogenesis The pathway, primarily in the liver, that converts lactate, pyruvate, glycerol, and amino acids into glucose. It is important in sustaining blood glucose in a fast or during prolonged exercise.

glucose A simple sugar that can be derived from diet or formed in the body. Cells use it as a primary source of energy.

glucose flux The rate at which glucose enters and leaves the blood. It is accelerated by exercise.

GLUT4 A protein that transports glucose into muscle and other specialized cell types (heart and adipose tissue) GLUT4 is regulated by stimuli that result in its incorporation into the cell membrane.

GLUT4 translocation The movement of the GLUT4 transport protein from intracellular vesicles to the plasma membrane where it facilitates glucose entry into cells. It is increased in response to exercise.

glycemic index A way of classifying foods according to their potential to increase blood glucose (generally the lower the index, the better the glucose control).

glycerol The three-carbon backbone that binds fatty acids to form triglycerides.

glycogen A molecule that serves as the storage form of glucose. It consists of long polymer chains of glucose and is synthesized and stored mainly in the liver and the muscles.

glycogen depletion Results from prolonged fasting or long distance exercise. Low levels of glycogen correspond to exercise fatigue.

glycogen loading Another term for carbohydrate loading.

glycogenolysis The enzyme-catalyzed conversion of glycogen polymers to glucose monomers.

glycolysis The metabolic pathway that results in the conversion of glucose pyruvate. It results in a small energy yield.

goal setting/reality A needs analysis based on specific individual characteristics.

Golgi tendon organs Respond to tension within the muscle by inhibiting the agonist muscles and facilitating the antagonist muscles during contraction.

gonadal hormones Steroid hormones made in the ovaries or testes. These hormones have diverse actions. In addition to those involved with development, they have synthetic and metabolic actions.

growth hormone (GH) A peptide hormone secreted from the anterior pituitary. It is regulated by a number of stimuli, including exercise. It is postulated to be involved with adaptations to regular physical activity.

Harvard step test A simple cardiorespiratory fitness test developed by the Harvard Fatigue Laboratory prior to World War II.

health-related fitness The ability to stay healthy and fit; includes obtainable optimal levels of cardiovascular fitness, body composition, muscular strength, muscular endurance, and flexibility.

heart rate (HR) The number of times the heart beats (contracts) in one minute.

heart rate monitor Heart rate transmitters worn by study participants used to estimate energy expenditure.

heart rate variability A physiological phenomenon where the time interval between consecutive heart beats or R-R intervals varies.

heat acclimatization The adaptation of the physiological responses to heat stress that occurs after repeated daily exposures to a given hot environment for a period of 8 days.

hemodynamics The study of the forces that move the blood within the cardiovascular system.

hemoglobin (Hb) The large iron-bearing protein molecule contained in the red blood cells, which primarily combines with oxygen in the lungs to carry it to body's tissues via circulation.

Henry's law Henry's law of solubility of gases states that at equilibrium, the amount of a gas dissolved in a fluid is directly proportional to the partial pressure of the gas in the air.

hepatic lipase A lipolytic enzyme that interacts with lipoproteins in the liver and may play a role in the reconversion of HDL-C.

Heritage Study Funded by the National Heart, Lung, and Blood Institute of NIH since 1992. Its main goal is to study the role of the genotype in the cardiovascular.

hexokinase This enzyme catalyzes the conversion of glucose to glucose 6-phosphate inside the cytosolic compartment of the cell.

high-altitude cerebral edema (HACE) A severe form of AMS and its symptoms with the presence of edema in the brain and is potentially fatal if left untreated.

high-altitude pulmonary edema (HAPE) A non-cardiogenic pulmonary edema that usually results 12 to 96 hours from rapid ascent to high altitude (10,000 ft). Active adults appear to be more susceptible than middle-aged and older adults. Symptoms include those of AMS, rapid and shallow breathing, rapid heart rate, and rale lung sounds.

high-density lipoprotein (HDL) A fat transporter called *good cholesterol* because it has a higher proportion protein and lower proportion of triglyceride and cholesterol.

high-density lipoprotein cholesterol (HDL-C) Type of lipoprotein that transports cholesterol back to the liver from the cells; composed primarily of protein.

histochemistry The chemistry of identifying living tissues by using different stains that can be identified by light microscopy, electron microscopy. It is used to identify different fiber types.

homeostasis The maintenance of a relatively stable internal environment at rest.

hormone-sensitive lipase (HSL) An intracellular neutral lipase that is capable of hydrolyzing a variety of esters.

hormones Chemicals released by a cell or a gland in one part of the body that sends out messages that are transmitted through the blood to target cells in other parts of the organism. Hormones act through specific receptors.

human genome The nucleic acid sequences that comprise genes that make up chromosomes. Genes encode the proteins that lead to human development and physiological function. Errors or mutations can result in abnormalities or disease.

human growth hormone (HGH) Hormone produced by the pituitary gland and initially used in the 1950s to help children with growth problems. HGH has been synthetically produced and used/abused by those interested in enhancing speed, strength, and power performances.

hydrometry The measurement of TBW, which can be determined from stable isotope dilution techniques.

hypercapnia An arterial carbon dioxide partial pressure of greater than 40 mm Hg.

hyperglycemia High blood glucose characteristic of diabetes. Can occur transiently with stress or in response to a glucose-rich meal.

hyperplasia An increase in the number of fibers.

hypertrophy An increase in muscle fiber size.

hyperventilation An excess ventilation, which causes a reduction in the arterial carbon dioxide tension, or $PaCO_2$.

hypocapnia An arterial carbon dioxide partial pressure of less than 40 mm Hg.

hypoglycemia A fall in blood glucose that is most prevalent in people treated with insulin. Exercise can increase the risk of insulin-induced hypoglycemia. Hypoglycemia may lead to seizure and death in extreme cases.

hypoxia A reduction in ambient PO_2 or a low oxygen pressure environment.

hypoxic hypoxia The reduction in arterial oxygen tension (PaO_2) associated with hypoxia.

ideal body fat Term often used to describe the hypothetical optimal percentage of body fat a person should have.

ideal body weight Term often used to describe the hypothetical optimal body weight a person should have.

immunocytochemistry A technique using the chemical reaction that occurs between proteins and its antibodies within a cell and can be identified by imaging techniques, such as confocal or fluorescence microscopy.

incidence Rate or range of occurrence.

indirect calorimetry Measuring oxygen consumption and energy expenditure in an exercise laboratory. (Chapter 1)

indirect calorimetry A method by which the oxidation of carbohydrates and fats are calculated from the rate of uptake of O_2 and the rate of production of CO_2. Accurate application of this method requires an estimate of protein oxidation. (Chapter 5)

inherent ability Analyzing the genetic or heredity traits of the individual as related to exercise.

insulin A hormone released from pancreatic islet beta cells that lowers blood glucose by stimulating its uptake from the blood into muscle, liver, and fat and suppressing the release of glucose from the liver into the blood.

insulin-dependent diabetes Diabetes that requires insulin therapy. All people with type 1 diabetes require insulin therapy and many people with type 2 diabetes.

insulin sensitivity A variable that defines insulin action. It is increased during and after exercise. It can increase as an adaptive response to long term exercise.

intensity How hard you work.

interval training Participation in a high-intensity (anaerobic) bout of activity followed by participation in a lower intensity (aerobic) bout of activity, or vice versa. (Chapter 2)

interval training Based on the idea of using timed speed runs over distances; for example, 100 m in 12 seconds, 200 m in 30 seconds, 300 in 45 seconds, and 400 m in 60–70 seconds. At completion of the speed run, the athlete walks or jogs back to the beginning of the speed run while measuring his or her heart rate. When the heart rate recovers to less than 120 beats/min, the athlete repeats the speed run and recovery walk/jog/rest paradigm. (Chapter 3)

intrinsic heart rate (IHR) The heart rate that is measured when the sympathetic and parasympathetic neural influence is fully blocked by metoprolol (ß-1 selective receptor) and atropine (muscarinic receptor), respectively.

intrinsic motivation Encouraging motivation from the client to reinforce positive feedback.

iron deficiency anemia Refers to the severe depletion of iron stores that reduces hemoglobin concentration.

isokinetics A dynamic muscle contraction (concentric or eccentric) that is accomplished at the same speed of contraction throughout the complete contraction.

isometric (static) This type of contraction is when the muscle develops force but its length does not change.

isometric exercise Involves a static muscle contraction that primarily uses anaerobic energy production.

isotopic approaches These have many applications. Isotopes are used in exercise physiology research to calculate the flux of energy substrates in and out of the bloodstream.

ketogenesis The process by which ketone bodies are produced as a result of fatty acid breakdown in the liver.

ketone body A water soluble byproduct of fat oxidation in the liver. There are three ketone bodies: acetone, acetoacetate, and beta-hydroxybutyrate. They achieve their highest concentrations when liver fatty acid oxidation is high, as it is during a fast or prolonged exercise. Ketone bodies can be oxidized in the heart and brain.

ketosis High concentration of ketone bodies associated with incomplete fat metabolism that can lower pH and produce acid–base imbalances.

kilocalories (kcal) The amount of energy required to raise the temperature of 1 kilogram of water 1 degree centigrade. The term kilocalorie or Calorie is also used to describe the energy value of food or for energy expenditure during exercise.

kilocalories/minute (kcal/min) Method that requires you be able to accurately measure or estimate your client's $\dot{V}O_2$ max (or peak $\dot{V}O_2$) and then use the following conversion factor: 1 liter of oxygen consumed is approximately equal to 5 kcal/min.

Kosraeans Natives of the island of Kosrae that is part of the Federated States of Miconesia in the South Pacific. Their isolation for many centuries resulted in a limited genetic diversity, making them a unique population for studying the genetics of obesity. Obesity and diabetes became highly prevalent among the inhabitants of Kosrae during World War II as military installations imported processed foods rich in fat and sucrose.

laboratory tests Exercise physiology-related tests that are very controlled and focused on one client at a time. Physiologic variables are measured using invasive and non-invasive techniques, whereas exercise performances are directly measured.

lactate paradox The apparent lack of an increase in anaerobic glycolysis during exercise in chronic hypoxia (altitude acclimatization).

lactate threshold (LT) Method that requires that you be able to accurately measure or estimate your client's lactate threshold (LT)—the point at which the body recruits greater percentages of intermediate and fast twitch muscle fibers via anaerobic metabolic pathways, and the accumulation of lactic acid occurs when the lactate clearance becomes less than the lactate production.

Laplace's law States that there is an inverse relationship between the inside surface tension of a sphere and its radius. In the cardiovascular system a small heart chamber or blood vessel exhibits a greater inward force than a large heart chamber or blood vessel. Also called the *Law of Laplace.*

lecithin A phospholipid important for cell membrane function.

lecithin cholesterol acetyltransferase A lipolytic enzyme that catalyzes esterified cholesterol while binding to HDL.

leptin A protein produced by fat cells that decreases appetite and increases energy expenditure.

lipolysis The means by which triglycerides are mobilized to fatty acids and glycerol.

lipoprotein lipase A water soluble enzyme that hydrolyzes triglycerides in lipoproteins, such as those found in chylomicrons and very low-density lipoproteins (VLDL), into two free fatty acids and one monoacylglycerol molecule. (Chapter 6)

lipoprotein lipase A lipolytic enzyme that controls triglyceride hydrolysis and is the rate-limiting step in the uptake of lipoprotein, triglyceride, and free fatty acids into adipose tissue and muscle. (Chapter 11)

lipoproteins These are diverse in the body. Important species are assembled from proteins and fat in the liver and used to transport lipids, such as triglycerides and cholesterol, in the blood. Low-density lipoproteins, intermediate density lipoproteins, and high-density lipoproteins are important lipoproteins in the blood.

long-chain fatty acids (LCFA) Free fatty acids greater than 12 carbons in length.

low-density lipoprotein (LDL) A fat transporter called *bad cholesterol* because it has a moderate proportion of protein, a low proportion of triglyceride, and a high proportion of cholesterol.

low-density lipoprotein cholesterol (LDL-C) Type of lipoprotein that is derived from VLDLs as VLDL triglycerides are removed and broken down; composed primarily of cholesterol.

Master's step test A clinical version of the Harvard step test—see Rosenfeld, I. The Master Two-Step Test, 1959. *Canadian Medical Association Journal*, March 15; 80(6):480–481 for more.

maximal expired (e) ventilation (Ve max) The maximal volume of air moved for 1 minute (L/min) when maximal exercise is being performed.

maximal oxygen uptake ($\dot{V}O_2$ max) The maximal rate of oxygen uptake ($\dot{V}O_2$) achieved during a progressive increase in work load exercise test. (Chapter 7)

maximal oxygen uptake ($\dot{V}O_2$ max) Measured using the general principle of progressively increasing workloads and measuring the increase in $\dot{V}O_2$ until a plateau of $\dot{V}O_2$ is achieved (that is, $\dot{V}O_2$ max) that increases no further despite a continued increase in workload. (Chapter 10)

maximal voluntary contraction (MVC) The force generated by an individual's voluntary muscle contraction.

mean anaerobic power The ability to maintain a high percentage of peak anaerobic power for several seconds.

mean blood pressure or mean arterial pressure (MAP) The average pressure exerted by the pressure wave of the blood against the blood vessel walls.

mean skin temperature (or Tsk) A calculated summation of different body segments (arm, legs thorax, etc.) weighed to the ratio of the segment's surface area of the total body surface area.

mechanical efficiency (ME) ME of a muscle can be calculated as a ratio of the external work (W) performed divided by the extra Energy (E) required to perform the work above the resting energy (e). This ratio is expressed as a percentage and is summarized in the following equation: ME = W/E − e × 100.

mesomorph Body type characterized by a low-to-medium body fat and medium-to-large bone size, and is muscular and well proportioned.

metabolic acids The most abundant metabolic acid is CO_2 and although not a true acid, it is the end result of the breakdown of carbonic acid; by reason of its exchange at the lung, CO_2 is a primary regulator of the acid-base status during exercise.

metabolic efficiency Primarily refers to the ability of the body to use fat and carbohydrates as fuel for energy expenditure.

metabolic equivalents (METs) Method that is based on the concept of identifying the work intensity as the metabolic equivalents, expressed in METS, where the resting metabolic rate defined as 1 MET. In healthy adults, 1 MET = 3.5 ml kg^{-1} min^{-1}.

metabolic syndrome The state characterized by the coexistence of multiple pathologies associated with obesity.

mineral balance Consuming the appropriate amounts of minerals to maintain energy balance based on the U.S. Dietary Guidelines.

moderate-to-vigorous physical activity (MVPA) Threshold for physical activity or exercise where intensities between 3 to 5.9 METs are considered moderate intensity and those above 6 METs are considered to be vigorous intensity.

modified method Effective alternative to classic method that requires an exercise taper followed by mixed diet of carbohydrates (50%) for 3 days, and then a diet rich in carbohydrates for next 4 days.

monounsaturated fat A fat containing only one double bond between carbons. Olive oil is an example.

morbidity The rate of incidence of a disease.

mortality Death.

motor cortex The outer layer of the brain that contains the cell bodies and axons of the motor nerves.

motor neurons (nerves) The axons that possess a motor function that enclose the nucleus.

motor unit The body's fundamental structural unit that functionally integrates the neural activity with that of the skeletal muscle contraction.

muscle biopsy A muscle sample obtained to measure the composition of muscle.

muscle dysmorphia Body image disorder where individuals think that their muscles are too small and they workout excessively to obtain a "perfect" physique.

muscle fibers (or cells) Fibers composed of myofibrils.

muscle pump The contracting skeletal muscles work in conjunction with competent venous valves to effectively drive blood back to heart.

muscle spindles Receptors in connective tissue capsules located between muscle fibers.

myocardial oxygen consumption The amount of oxygen consumed by the heart in a given unit of time (1 minute); directly related to the double product.

myogenic tone The intrinsic muscle tone of the blood vessels.

myoglobin (Mb) The large iron-bearing protein molecule contained in the muscle.

myokines Molecules released from the muscle that serve an endocrine or paracrine function. It is thought that they transmit a signal related to the metabolic, structural, or inflammatory state of the muscle.

myoplasticity The adaptation that a muscle fiber and its metabolic capacity undergoes as a result of a period of exercise training.

myotendinous junction The junction between bones and tendons.

NADH A reducing agent that donates electrons for various reactions, including those that drive the formation of ATP.

neural reflexes Involve four components: a receptor located in the muscle, the gamma afferent neurons arising from the receptor and synapse in the gray matter of the spinal cord, the alpha motor neurons exiting from the cell bodies within the spinal cord, and the muscle fibers of the motor unit.

neuroendocrine regulators Molecules that are secreted by nerves or glands to control the functions of an organism.

neuromuscular integration The communication between nerves and muscles.

neuromuscular junction The junction between a nerve and a muscle.

neuropeptide Y A chemical produced in the brain that stimulates appetite, diminishes energy expenditure, and increases fat storage.

nomogram A two-dimensional graphical device that helps predict a third variable.

nonessential amino acid Amino acids that the body can synthesize itself from foods consumed or from metabolic action.

norepinephrine A catecholamine with multiple roles including as a hormone and a neurotransmitter. It is also called noradrenalin.

normative values Based on the performance of a group of people and are often expressed as percentages (that is, within the 10th to 90th percentile).

normocapnia An arterial carbon dioxide partial pressure of 40 mm Hg.

nutrient (carbohydrates, fats, proteins) balance Consuming the appropriate amounts of carbohydrates, fats, and proteins to maintain energy balance based on the U.S. Dietary Guidelines.

nutrition The science of foods and the nutrients and other substances they contain. In addition, the study of nutrition involves understanding the actions within the body that enable us to make use of our food.

obesity Excessive accumulation of body fat.

obesity syndrome The condition of being overweight due to excess fat mass. It is defined as having a BMI >30%.

objectivity Tests that have a defined scoring system, are administered by trained personnel, and where at least two trained testers score the same test and get similar scores.

observational A study that evaluates self-selected intensities of exercise by study subjects and often does not control for confounders that might influence the conclusions made by the researcher.

Ohm's law The relationship between the voltage (V), current (I) and resistance (R), and is usually written V = IR.

omega-3 fat A polyunsaturated fatty aid in which the first double bond is three carbons away from the methyl (CH3) end of carbon chain.

omega-6 fat A polyunsaturated fatty aid in which the first double bond is six carbons away from the methyl (CH3) end of carbon chain.

overcompensation The overload principle where improvements occur by imposing new and higher training demands on your client to ensure that they are successfully adapting to training.

overload A progressive increase in the work of a muscle or group of muscles (by increases in frequency duration or load) within one period of exercise or over a multiple number of exercise periods.

overload/progression Changing the FITT to improve physiological adaptations.

overreaching Planned acute overtraining that lasts no more than 2–3 weeks.

overtraining Engaging in intensities, durations, and frequencies of an exercise program that results in negative physiological effects, which, if continued, have been found to cause clinical depression and overuse injuries such as stress fractures.

overuse Participating in too much exercise, where an individual cannot adapt to the workload, often leading injuries and addictive behaviors.

overweight Excess weight for a given height.

oxidants A substance that oxidizes another substance. In air pollution, a mixture of oxidative substances and usually consists of ozone and nitrogen oxides.

oxidative phosphorylation A process that uses energy released by the oxidation of nutrients to produce ATP in the electron transport chain.

oxygen deficit The difference between the $\dot{V}O_2$ measured in the initial minutes of the exercise and the calculated $\dot{V}O_2$ required to perform the exercise.

oxygen delivery The organization of the circulatory system related to providing blood flow and oxygen to skeletal muscles.

oxygen uptake ($\dot{V}O_2$) The rate of oxygen uptake usually measured in liters/min.

oxyhemoglobin (O_2–Hb) dissociation curve Describes the relationship between the pressure of O_2 and the percentage of the Hb that is saturated with O.

oxyhemoglobin desaturation When the hemoglobin is not 100% saturated with oxygen.

particulates Can be a mixture of one or more pieces of soot, sand, smoke, etc., that is in the air we breathe. During inspiration, settles on lung tissue depending on the size of the particles.

peak anaerobic power The maximum anaerobic power, whereas the predominant energy source is ATP/CP and the anaerobic breakdown of carbohydrate.

pedometers Monitors worn on the hip that use stride length and steps taken throughout the day to estimate exercise and energy expenditure. Pedometers can help measure distances but do not measure intensity, an important component in assessing exercise.

percent of maximal speed Method of monitoring intensity often used by coaches who have their athletes run at a percentage of their maximal speed (like 90%).

percentage of maximal oxygen uptake (% $\dot{V}O_2$ max) Method that utilizes a simple percentage calculation from an individual's measured, or estimated, $\dot{V}O_2$ max.

percentage of maximum heart rate (% MHR) Method that uses the simple prediction of max heart rate (MHR) as 220 − age multiplied by the percentage of intensity desired.

percentage of maximum heart rate reserve (% HHR) Method that uses the simple prediction of max heart rate MHR) as 220 − age, but then requires that resting heart rate (RHR) be considered in the following equation: MHR Reserve = MHR − RHR; then, THR = (MHR − RHR) × (desired percentage) + RHR.

periodization A systematic approach altering program variables (like FITT), which improves training efficiency and specificity, allowing for general adaptations and a decrease in the likelihood of overtraining.

peripheral chemoreceptors The aortic and carotid bodies located in the aortic arch and the bifurcation of the carotid artery and respond to increases in $PaCO_2$, arterial H^+, and potassium ion concentrations by increasing ventilation. A reduction in PaO_2 to less than 75 to 80 mm Hg (identified as a hypoxic threshold) also stimulates the peripheral chemoreceptors and increase ventilation.

personal fitness Individual attainment and maintenance of both functional health and physical fitness.

phosphofructokinase-1 (PFK-1) This enzyme catalyzes an important regulatory step of glycolysis, the conversion of fructose 6-phosphate and ATP to fructose 1,6-bisphosphate and ADP. It is sensitively controlled by allosteric regulation.

phospholipid A fat that is similar to a triglyceride but contains phosphate.

phosphorylase kinase A serine-/threonine-specific protein kinase that activates glycogen phosphorylase to degrades glycogen.

physical activity Any movement that works larger muscles of the body, such as the arm, leg, and back muscles.

physical fitness The outcome of participating in physical activity exercise that improves the body's ability to carry out daily tasks and still have enough reserve energy to respond to unexpected demands.

physical inactivity An independent risk factor for coronary heart disease.

plasma lipoprotein Clusters of lipids associated with proteins that serve as transport vehicles for lipids in the lymph and blood.

plyometric Movements (quick, powerful muscular movements where the muscle is pre stretched prior to contractions like jumping, resistance ball drills, etc.) or resistance training such as weight training.

plyometric exercise training This involves repeated, rapid stretching and contracting of muscles that, when the activated muscles are stretched, the kinetic energy is stored as potential energy in the series of elastic elements of the muscles.

polycythemia An excess number of red blood cells above normal sea level values.

polyunsaturated fat A fatty acid with two or more double bonds between carbons.

postexercise hypotension A decrease in mean arterial pressure ranging from 5 to 10 mm Hg below resting baseline measures obtained before exercise in healthy individuals and up to −20 mm Hg in hypertensive patients.

potassium ATP (KATP) A cell membrane channel that allows passage of potassium ions into and out of the cell.

potential energy The energy stored in a molecule due to its composition and configuration.

power spectral density Describes how the power of a signal or time series is distributed with respect to frequency is used to analyze heart rate variability and breathing variability by transforming (using a mathematical process termed **Fast Fourier Transform analysis**) the time domain to the frequency domain.

preload The right atrial pressure for the right ventricle and the pulmonary wedge pressure for the left ventricle.

preload, or cardiac filling pressure (end-diastolic fiber length) The initial stretching of the cardiac myocytes prior to contraction. Preload, therefore, is related to the sarcomere length. Because sarcomere length cannot be determined in the intact heart, other indices of preload are used such as ventricular end-diastolic volume or pressure.

prevalence The total number of cases of a disease in a given population at a specific point in time.

prevention of weight regain Consistent with a change in weight of 3 percent to less than 5 percent.

prospective This type of study uses individuals who are free of the disease or health problem of interest and monitors baseline exercise. Subjects are evaluated over time for the development of disease or the outcome with regards to their exercise.

protein content The abundance and type of proteins that are contained in or surrounding a cell or tissue.

pulmonary capillary wedge pressure (PCWP) An indirect measurement of the left atrial pressure obtained by wedging a catheter into a small pulmonary artery tightly enough to block flow from behind and in order to sample the pressure beyond. This measurement is used as a measure of the filling pressure of the left ventricle.

pulmonary gas exchange The movement of O_2 from the environment to the pulmonary circulation and the movement of CO_2 from the pulmonary circulation to the environment. The process requires bulk flow of air into the lungs and diffusion of gases between air and blood.

pulmonary ventilation The movement of air into and out of the lungs during the act of breathing.

pyruvate dehydrogenase (PDH) A protein complex that catalyzes the conversion of pyruvate to acetyl CoA. CO_2 The end product of complete fat, carbohydrate, and protein oxidation.

radiation (R) The transfer of heat from a hot surface to a cool surface without physical contact between the two surfaces.

randomly Individuals or groups are assigned by chance.

rating of perceived exertion (RPE) Method that requires your clients to rate "how hard" they are working during exercise.

recommended daily allowances (RDA) A goal for dietary intake of various nutrients based on the U.S. Dietary Guidelines.

recruitment As the required force and speed of contraction increases, the number of slow motor units increases, as does the frequency of their use, until the force requirement increases to a level that causes a further recruitment of the motor units with larger cell bodies (soma) until maximal force output is achieved.

regular exercise Working most days of the week at the MVPA threshold for several minutes (30 minutes total, per session, or accumulated in multiple sessions each day).

rehydration The replacement of body fluids, orally intravenously, following heat stress dehydration, vomiting, or diarrhea.

relapse Discontinuing a regular program of exercise.

relative intensity Expressed as an intensity value or percentage of a client's aerobic capacity ($\dot{V}O_2$ max) or $\dot{V}O_2$ reserve ($\dot{V}O_2$ max – resting $\dot{V}O_2$), as a percentage of a person's measured heart rate or heart rate reserve (max heart rate – resting heart rate), as a perceived exertion rating (how hard a client feels they are working from light to very hard), or as a percentage of 1 repetition maximum (maximum one can lift in one trial).

reliability The ability to obtain repeatable results during different testing sessions. (Chapter 1)

reliability The ability of a test to repeatedly measure performance abilities or physiologic variables and provide the same result. (Chapter 10)

renin A peptide hormone released by the kidney that acts as an enzyme to cleave angiotensinogen to angiotensin I, which is then converted to angiotensin II. Angiotensin II constricts blood vessels and stimulates the release of antidiuretic hormone and aldosterone.

resistance (R) Calculated from the pressure difference from one end of a blood vessel to the other end divided by the blood flow in the blood vessel.

resistance exercise When the isometric exercise involves some rhythmic dynamic contractions (for example, weight training).

respiratory exchange ratio (RER) The ratio of the amount of CO_2 expired to the amount of O_2 used in the metabolic processes, that is, $VCO_2/\dot{V}O_2$. (Chapter 9)

respiratory exchange ratio (RER – $\dot{V}O_2/VCO_2$) The ratio of expired carbon dioxide to the amount of oxygen uptake. Values over 1.00 indicate hyperventilation. (Chapter 10)

respiratory pump Inspiration increases venous return, and expiration decreases venous return.

respiratory sinus arrhythmia (RSA) A naturally occurring variation in heart rate that occurs during respiration.

respiratory system Designed to obtain oxygen from the ambient air for use by the body's cells and to utilize and eliminate the carbon dioxide produced.

resting metabolism rate (RMR) Estimated energy expenditure while sitting at rest, which is slightly higher than BMR.

restoration Enhancing recovery from program of exercise.

risk factors Conditions and behaviors that represent a potential threat to an individual's well-being.

risk stratification Strategies to categorize clients as apparently healthy (low risk), possibly at risk (moderate risk), or at higher risk.

RNA translation The synthesis of peptide chains from the nucleic acids that comprise mRNA. An enzyme-catalyzed process that has diverse and stringently controlled regulatory sites.

sarcomeres The smallest contractile units in the muscle fibers.

satiation The feeling of satisfaction and fullness that occurs during a meal and halts eating.

satiety The feeling of satisfaction that occurs after a meal and inhibits eating until the next meal.

saturated fat A fat that contains no double bonds between carbons.

scientific method A systematic process for testing hypotheses.

screen time The compilation of time spent in using computers, video games, and television. This may contribute to decreased physical activity if it is excessive in duration.

secondary amenorrhea The absence of three to six consecutive menstrual cycles in previously menstruating women.

sedentary Inactive lifestyle with regard to participating regularly in physical activity or exercise. Expending few calories above resting levels and associated with lots of sitting.

sensitivity The ability of the method or assessment tool to measure and detect change in exercise patterns.

set point The central nervous system's temperature (similar to setting the thermostat temperature of a heating and cooling system) that is the reference temperature the core, mean body, and mean skin temperatures are compared with to activate the regulatory physiological responses if a difference between the two temperatures exists.

set-point theory The control or maintenance of a specific body weight by an individual's internal controls (primarily the hypothalamus).

simple carbohydrate Include the monosaccharides (that is, simple sugars such as glucose, fructose, and galactose) and disaccharides (such as maltose, sucrose, and lactose).

skeletal muscle The largest tissue type in healthy people. Shortening of muscle by energy-driven contraction of muscle fibers causes physical movement.

skill-related fitness (Sometimes called motor-skill, athletic, or performance fitness.) The ability to perform successfully in various games and sports. The components of skill-related fitness include the ability to demonstrate high levels of agility, balance, speed, power, coordination, and reaction time.

sliding filament (cross-bridging) theory of contraction A common psychological theory explaining how skeletal muscles contract.

somatic nerves (axons) Peripheral nerves that control skeletal muscles.

special situations Adjusting the exercise program or exercise prescription based on illness, disability, medications, and so on.

specificity Understanding the specific physiological adaptations that occur because of the specific demands applied.

spectrum of energy demands Continuum that contains a variety of common physical activities and exercises that require varying amounts of anaerobic and aerobic energy pathway contributions (percentages) based on estimated metabolic requirements.

spinal cord The cord-like structure contained within the spinal canal.

standard temperature pressure dry (STPD) A correction factor used to standardize (equilibrate) the measured ventilation volumes to the absolute temperature of 273° K and the barometric pressure without 47 mm Hg water vapor pressure at 37°C.

static exercise (isometric) A static exercise contraction includes an increase in force generated over a very limited range of motion (ROM).

steady state exercise The body's ability to maintain homeostatic-like conditions during movement.

sterol A fat whose core structure contains four rings.

stress The physical and psychological responses of your body as you try to adapt to a new situation that can be threatening, frightening, or exciting.

stressor Anything that requires one to adapt and cope with either positive or negative situations.

stroke volume (SV) The volume of blood pumped during one heart beat.

structural hierarchy The structure and branches of skeletal muscles.

sucrose A disaccharide comprised of glucose and fructose.

sulfur oxides Result from fossil fuel combustion and include sulfur dioxide (SO_2), sulfuric acid, and sulfate. SO_2 is a soluble gas that irritates the upper respiratory tract and causes reflex bronchoconstriction.

sucrose A disaccharide comprised of glucose and fructose.

sympathetic activity The rate of release of sympathetic neurotransmitter (usually norepinephrine) from sympathetic nerves of the autonomic nervous system.

syncope Fainting.

systolic blood pressure (SBP) The peak pressure exerted by the pressure wave of the blood against the blood vessel walls.

talk test Method for monitoring intensity that evaluates the ability of your client to carry on a conversation during exercise.

taper A planned segment of time in a periodization plan where an individual in training reduces the frequency and/or volume of training while maintaining high intensities to achieve a peaking of performance, usually for competition.

temperature regulation The neural process by which the body senses whether it is hot or cold and reflexively activates physiologic responses to cool or heat the body, respectively.

thermal sensors or receptors Temperature-sensitive endings of neurons that increase the neurons firing rate in response to heating or cooling.

thermic effect of food An estimate of the energy required to process food.

thermogenesis The amount of heat generated by the body; used as an index of how much energy the body is expending.

thermoneutral environment The state in which the ambient environment surrounding the naked human does not activate the physiological mechanism to gain or lose body heat.

thrifty genes The name given to those genes that encode the proteins that are used for nutrient storage. These genes were necessary for survival in hunter and gatherer societies. They are now hypothesized to be a cause of obesity in societies where food is always available.

thyroid hormone Releases hormones tridothyronine and thyroxine that participate in the control of how the body uses energy and makes proteins and controls how sensitive the body is to other hormones.

tidal volume The volume of air that is moved into or out of the lung in each breath (ml/breath).

time or duration How long you work.

total body electrical conductivity (TOBEC) A method used to determine body composition based on the concept that water and lean body tissue (like muscle) conducts electricty better than fat tissue.

total energy expenditure Resting metabolism plus the thermic effect of food, and the amount of energy expended in physical activity daily.

total peripheral resistance (TPR) The total resistance to blood flow within the cardiovascular system.

trainability Evaluating the rate at which an individual improves for a specific FITT.

training plateau Normal period of time during training when little, if any, improvement occurs.

trans fat Fatty acids with hydrogens on opposite sides of the double bonds.

transcranial magnetic stimulation A non-invasive technology that can provide a focused magnetic stimulation of specific areas of the motor cortex.

transferrin Important protein for iron transport in the body.

transtheoretical model The transtheoretical model of behavioral change (or Stages of Change Model) is one of most popular models currently used by researchers and includes levels labeled pre-contemplation, contemplation, preparation, action, maintenance, and relapse.

tricarboxylic acid (TCA) cycle A series of enzyme catalyzed reactions in the mitochondria of living cells that result the chemical conversion of carbohydrates, fats, and protein into carbon dioxide and water. NADH formed in these reactions contributes electrons to the electron transport chain, leading to the formation of ATP.

triglyceride A fat made up of three fatty acids attached to a glycerol molecule; major storage form of fat in humans. (Chapter 1)

triglyceride A molecule that serves as the storage form of fat. It consists of glycerol and three fatty acids. It is concentrated in adipose tissue. (Chapter 4)

triglyceride Lipid-containing glycerol bonded to three fatty acids; the chief form of fat in the diet and the major storage form of fat in the body. (Chapter 11)

type 1 diabetes This was initially thought to be a genetic disease. However, type 1 diabetes has been diagnosed in people of all ages and causes an individual's immune system to attack and destroy the insulin producing beta cells of the islets of Langerhans in the pancreas (treatable with insulin). (Chapter 1)

type 1 diabetes A form of diabetes mellitus that results from autoimmune destruction of insulin-producing beta cells of the pancreas. Hyperglycemia occurs if insulin treatment is inadequate. (Chapter 6B)

type 2 diabetes Also known as adult onset diabetes, type 2 diabetes was initially linked to excessive weight gain and causes insulin resistance at the tissues, thereby slowing down or inhibiting the glucose uptake. Type 2 diabetes is linked to lack of physical activity, being overweight (increased waist circumference), and genetic factors predisposing the individual to obesity. (Chapter 1)

type 2 diabetes Usually develops from resistance to the actions of insulin due to excess body fat. Ultimately both type 1 and type 2 are characterized by inadequate pancreatic beta cell insulin response. (Chapter 6B)

type I A muscle fiber that is classified by histochemistry or immunocytochemistry as a slow oxidative red fiber. With light microscopy the type I fiber appears pinky-red.

type IIa A fast-twitch fiber with a higher oxidative capacity that also appears pinky red with light microscopy.

type IIb A fast-twitch fiber that has low oxidative capacity and appears pale white in color with light microscopy.

type IIx A muscle fiber that is only in the rat and appears to have high oxidative capacity and resists fatigue.

type The specific type or mode of physical activity or exercise you choose.

U.S. Dietary Guidelines The *Dietary Guidelines for Americans, 2010* provides evidence-based nutrition information and advice for people age 2 and older. They serve as the basis for federal food and nutrition education programs.

underweight Low weight for a given height.

validity The degree to which an instrument measures what it is supposed to measure. (Chapter 1)

validity The ability of a selected test to evaluate what you want it to test. (Chapter 10)

velocity at $\dot{V}O_2$ max (v$\dot{V}O_2$ max) The performance speed of an athletic, such as running at the running speed (v$\dot{V}O_2$ max) of $\dot{V}O_2$ max occurs.

venous return The amount of venous blood measured in liters returning to the heart in one minute.

ventilation equivalent for carbon dioxide (VECO$_2$ = V_E/$\dot{V}CO_2$) The volume of ventilation required to exhale 1 liter of carbon dioxide.

ventilation equivalent for oxygen (VEO$_2$ = Ve/$\dot{V}O_2$) The volume of ventilation required to enable the uptake of 1 liter of oxygen.

ventilation threshold The exponential increases in ventilation above a threshold workload, or $\dot{V}O_2$, during a progressive increase in workload exercise test. (Chapter 9)

ventilation threshold The workload, or $\dot{V}O_2$, at which lactate appears in the venous blood, indicating a greater production of lactate than the clearance of lactate and at which time the ventilations increase exponentially. (Chapter 10)

ventilation volume The volume (ml) of air that is moved into or out of the lung per unit time, usually recorded in 1 minute (L/min).

ventilatory threshold (Tvent) When the minute ventilation increases exponentially above a threshold workload, or $\dot{V}O_2$, at which point there is an extra stimulus from the central and peripheral chemoreceptors that are sensitive to arterial carbon dioxide (CO_2) and hydrogen ion concentration (pH) to increase ventilation.

ventral (front) The anatomical front of a structure.

very-low-density lipoprotein cholesterol (VLDL-C) Type of lipoprotein made primarily by liver cells to transport lipids to various tissues in the body; composed primarily of triglycerides.

very low-density lipoprotein (VLDL) A fat transporter also called *bad cholesterol* because it has a higher proportion of triglyceride and serves as a precursor to the formation of low-density lipoproteins.

viscosity A measure of how sticky a fluid (blood) is.

vitamin balance Consuming the appropriate amounts of vitamins to maintain energy balance based on the U.S. Dietary Guidelines.

volume of workload Another method often used by coaches when their athletes perform plyometric exercises that include a sport-specific FITT.

water-soluble vitamin Those that include the B complex vitamins and vitamin C. They need to be replaced regularly by consuming nutritious foods.

weight cycling Losing weight and then regaining the lost weight and even more over time.

weight loss At least a 5 percent loss of body weight (clinically significant).

weight maintenance A weight change of less than 3 percent. Also known as *weight stability.*

weight management Understanding the physiologic influences, environmental challenges, and behavioral strategies that all impact the ability to maintain a healthy weight for functional health and wellness.

wet bulb globe temperature (WBGT) index An index that integrates the primary extrinsic risk factors of dry and wet bulb temperatures (humidity) and solar radiant energy into a practical indication of the relative risk for heat injury.

wind chill The cooling power of the environment as a function of wind velocity and ambient temperature and relates the time of cooling a given volume of water to the point of freezing.

index